Stedman's
MEDICAL EPONYMS

SECOND EDITION

Sue Bartolucci, CMT
Pat Forbis, CMT

To my husband, Bob,
our sons, Robert, Tim, Rick, and Michael, and
their beautiful families, and

to the memory of Kristen Noelle.

Pat Forbis, CMT

My thanks to my husband Gene and to my family and friends who all
understood when I was incommunicado while working to bring our
second edition to fruition. To all of you who are engaged in the
never-ending quest to "get it right," this book is dedicated to you as
we travel that road together.

Sue Bartolucci, CMT

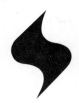

Stedman's
MEDICAL EPONYMS

SECOND EDITION

Sue Bartolucci, CMT
Pat Forbis, CMT

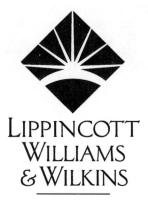

LIPPINCOTT
WILLIAMS
& WILKINS

Publisher: Julie K. Stegman
Managing Editor: Heather A. Rybacki
Production Coordinator: Jason Delaney
Typesetter: Peirce Graphic Services, LLC., and Publication Services
Printer & Binder: Malloy Litho, Inc.

R 121
F 67
2005
(0781)5443)

Printed in the United States of America

Second Edition, 2005

Library of Congress Cataloging-in-Publication Data

Bartolucci, Susan L.
Stedman's medical eponyms / Sue Bartolucci, Pat Forbis.— 2nd ed.
    p. ; cm.
Forbis's name appears first on earlier ed.
Includes bibliographical references and index.
  ISBN 0-7817-5443-7
  1. Medicine—Dictionaries. 2. Eponyms—Dictionaries. I. Title.
II. Title: Medical eponyms. III. Stedman, Thomas Lathrop, 1853–1938.
IV. Forbis, Pat, 1940–
  [DNLM: 1. Eponyms—Dictionary—English. 2. Biography—Dictionary—English.
3. Disease—Dictionary—English. WB 15
B292s 2005]
R121.F67 2005
610'.1'48—dc22

2004016660
01
1 2 3 4 5 6 7 8 9 10

Contents

Acknowledgments

It is always a pleasure to work with the editors at Lippincott Williams & Wilkins, and it is especially enjoyable to work with Heather Rybacki. Under her benevolent guidance and with her assistance, this revision took place, and we happily offer this second edition to you.

We offer out sincerest thanks to Ellen Atwood for her many skills and talents, and her willingness to share these abilities with us in our endeavor. We want to thank her for the countless hours she has spent reviewing format, editing copy, and helping this book along.

As with all *Stedman's* references, this resource incorporates the suggestions and expertise of many members of the medical community. Thanks to all who took the time to submit their ideas for ways in which this reference could be improved and for sending along new eponymous terms.

And, finally, to family, friends, and colleagues — without your support we couldn't have done it.

Pat Forbis, CMT
Sue Bartolucci, CMT

Editors' Preface

Medical language is a living thing. As such, it's no wonder that new terms are added and old terms sometimes fall into disuse. When the time came for us to update our first edition, we approached the project with some trepidation, knowing there would be a substantial amount of time committed to researching new terms and adding information to existing terms. Yet there was excitement at the thought of finding new and useful eponyms from a broad range of fields to include in the second edition. There was also a great deal of frustration when we came to dead ends in our research, unable to add a term because it could not be verified accurately. This book is the result of our best efforts to provide you with the most correct information about an eponymic term and its "parent" word.

Individuals whose daily work requires the appropriate use of words never cease to be amazed at the continual need to increase their vocabularies. Medical eponyms are no different than other areas of language, in that new terms are constantly being introduced while the existing terms gradually evolve. One must pause to wonder how many names are left to affiliate with new procedures, instruments, and the like. We suggest that it is impossible to capture all of them, but within these pages are the names of important persons whose contributions to medicine are duly recognized and defined.

Some eponyms continue to be challenging, such as names with von, van, de, and la, which are commonly used with and without their prefix. The appropriate placement of full names, such as Marcus Gunn, is debatable. Variant spellings have been captured as best we understand them.

No company recognizes the value of recommendations from medical language specialists more than Lippincott Williams & Wilkins. Therefore, there is a postpaid card in the back of the book for your convenience, and you are encouraged to use it.

Pat Forbis, CMT
Sue Bartolucci, CMT

Publisher's Preface

Medical language is teeming with procedures, syndromes, instruments, signs, phenomena, and techniques that have been named after the person (or persons) who first discovered, invented, or, in the case of some diseases, acquired it. Additional medical conditions are described by the geographical location in which a particular illness occurs. Due to the potential variances in the spelling and pronunciation of names from nationality to nationality and place to place, eponyms are often among the most difficult medical terminology for healthcare professionals to absorb and recall. Unlike most medical terms, eponyms cannot be broken down into word parts to determine which medical condition it describes, making eponyms a truly challenging area of medical teminology.

Stedman's Medical Eponyms, Second Edition, provides members of the healthcare community, including practitioners, educators, and students, along with the wordsmiths of the healthcare profession—medical transcriptionists, medical editors and copyeditors, health information management personnel, and court reporters—with an authoritative resource for these often problematic eponyms.

In an effort to provide a clear understanding of the eponyms used in medical language today, this reference includes not only names and related terms, but also full biographical information, when available, on each individual, such as nationality, specialty, and birth/death dates. Related terms appear underneath each main entry, and include clear, concise definitions. Every term is fully cross-referenced so users can quickly locate the information they need.

New to this edition is a Keyword Index, allowing readers to find eponymic terms by their key words. For example, by looking up the word "test" in the index, one will encounter a comprehensive list of all of the eponymously named tests contained in this reference, along with the corresponding page number for each entry.

The pages that follow encompass thousands of equipment names, diagnostic and therapeutic procedures, operations, techniques and maneuvers, incisions, methods and approaches, syndromes and diseases, anatomic terms, and more, from all the major specialties and subspecialties of medicine.

This compilation contains nearly 18,000 eponyms and their associated terms. The extensive A–Z list was initially developed from entries found in *Stedman's Medical Dictionary* and supplemented by the authors with terminology found in current medical literature (please see the list of References on page xvii).

We at Lippincott Williams & Wilkins strive to provide you with the most up-to-date and accurate word references available. Your use of this reference will prompt new editions, which we will publish as often as updates and revisions justify. We welcome your suggestions for improvements, changes, corrections, and additions—whatever will make this Stedman's product more useful to you. Please complete the postage-paid card in this book for future suggestions and recommendations, or visit us online at www.stedmans.com.

Explanatory Notes

While the use of eponyms in medical language has been widely debated throughout the years, they continue to be found extensively in both medical documentation and conversation. New eponyms creep into the medical lexicon daily, and because of the nature of these terms, it is often difficult to determine the correct spelling and usage. *Stedman's Medical Eponyms, Second Edition,* seeks to clarify some of the ambiguity surrounding eponyms, and provides variant spellings and phrasings for thousands of eponymic terms. This reference is an invaluable resource for determining the validity of terms as they are encountered.

Organization and Order

Terms in this reference are listed in a main entry-subentry format. Main entries are listed in alphabetical order by the individual's last name or the name of a geographical location. Subentries consist of any eponymic terms associated with that individual or place, and appear, indented, under the main entry. The alphabetization of both names and their associated terms is letter by letter as spelled, ignoring punctuation, spaces, prefixes, accented letters, or other characters. For example:

Debré, Robert, French pediatrician and bacteriologist, *1882.
    Debré-De Toni-Fanconi syndrome
    Debré-Marie syndrome
    Debré phenomenon

de Clérambault, G., French psychiatrist, 1872–1934.

Deetjen, Hermann, German physician, 1867–1915.

Format and Style

All main entries and subentries are in **boldface** to expedite locating a sought-after entry, to enhance distinction between the entries and their associated explanatory information, and to relieve the textual density of the pages.

As often as possible, the style of the book follows the style recommendations put forth by the American Medical Association (AMA) in the *AMA Manual of Style, 9th edition,* and the American Association for Medical Transcription (AAMT) in *The AAMT Book of Style for Medical Transcription, 2nd edition.*

Biographical/Geographical Information

Every attempt has been made to provide comprehensive biographical and geographical information about the individuals listed in this text. In some cases, when information could not be located or verified, only partial information has been provided. When a birth date or death date is not known, or if the death date is not yet applicable, the following conventions are used:

Date of birth is represented by an asterisk (*) followed by a date. For example, *1896 indicates that the person was born in 1896 and he or she is either still living or the date of death is unknown.

Date of death is represented by "d." followed by a date. For example, d. 1896 indicates that the person died in 1896 and his or her birth date is unknown.

Variant Forms

Variant spellings of eponyms are listed alphabetically, and refer the user to the preferred spelling. For example:

Lewandowsky, var. of Lewandowski
Lewandowski, (Lewandowsky), Felix, German dermatologist, 1879–1921.

American spellings are used for words with variant spellings, such as orthopedic/orthopaedic and curet/curette, with the understanding that popular variant spellings remain a matter of preference.

Diacritical Marks

Diacritical marks, or accents, are used to show pronunciation and syllabic emphasis, and occur quite frequently in proper names. Every effort has been made to preserve the appropriate diacritical marks within this reference. The *AMA Book of Style, 9th edition,* asserts that accent marks should be retained in proper names. However, per *The AAMT Book of Style, 2nd edition*, it is acceptable to omit these accents when word processing software does not accommodate special characters or if an employer permits their omission.

Possessives

Possessive forms have been dropped in this reference for the sake of consistency and conformance with the guidelines of the American Medical Association (AMA), the American Association for Medical Transcription (AAMT), and other groups. Please note, however, that in many cases, retaining the possessive is a question of style, not of accuracy, and thus is a matter of choice. To form the possessive of a word, simply add an apostrophe or apostrophe "s" to the end of the word.

Cross-Indexing

Multiple eponymic terms are cross-referenced under all names listed in the term. For example, Dollinger-Bielschowsky syndrome is listed both under Max Bielschowsky and Albert Dollinger. This format provides the user with more than one way to locate and identify a multiple eponymic term. It also allows the user to see together all terms that contain a certain name.

In some cases, the order of the names within a term can vary. Based on the medical literature, a preferred order for that term has been identified. Any explanatory information about the term will only appear under the *first* name of the *preferred* term.

See under

Consider the above example of Bielschowsky and Dollinger. Bielschowsky-Dollinger syndrome is the nonpreferred term, so its entry reads, "Syn: Dollinger-Bielschowsky syndrome." A little further down the list is "Dollinger-Bielschowsky syndrome," the preferred term. Since it is not under Dollinger, but under Bielschowsky, no explanatory material appears here. Instead, a "see under Dollinger" reference points the user to Dollinger for any necessary explanatory material. Where more than one entry shares the same surname, the first name also appears at "see under."

Synonyms

Explanatory information about a term can be of several types. When the eponymic term is the preferred term in *Stedman's Medical Dictionary*, a brief definition and any applicable synonyms follow it. These synonyms can be other eponyms, or they can be noneponymic terms. For example:

Marjolin, Jean N., French physician, 1780–1850.
    Marjolin syndrome—*SYN*: Marjolin ulcer
    Marjolin ulcer—well-differentiated but aggressive squamous cell carcinoma occurring in cicatricial tissue at the epidermal edge of a sinus draining underlying osteomyelitis. *SYN*: Marjolin syndrome; epidermoid ulcer

In other cases, a noneponymic term is the preferred term in *Stedman's Medical Dictionary*. Where the noneponymic synonym is sufficient for the user to determine that the appropriate condition, anatomical structure, or procedure is being discussed, the noneponymic synonym will stand for all eponymic entries. For example:

Keith, Sir Arthur, Scottish anatomist, 1866–1955.
    Keith and Flack node—*SYN*: sinuatrial node
    Keith bundle—*SYN*: atrioventricular bundle
    Keith node—*SYN*: sinuatrial node

Flack, Martin, English physiologist, 1882–1931.
    Flack node—*SYN*: sinuatrial node
    Keith and Flack node—*SYN*: sinuatrial node

Using synonyms alone saves the user time flipping back and forth to find explanatory material.

On the other hand, at times the preferred noneponymic synonym in *Stedman's Medical Dictionary* is ambiguous anatomically or contains uncommon medical vocabulary. In those cases, explanatory material appears at an eponymic term and all eponymic synonyms refer back to that term.

References

Books

American Medical Association Manual of Style. 9th ed. Baltimore: Lippincott Williams & Wilkins; 1998.

Barankin B, Lin AN, Metelitsa AI. *Stedman's Illustrated Dictionary of Dermatology Eponyms.* Baltimore: Lippincott Williams & Wilkins; 2005.

Dorland's Illustrated Medical Dictionary. 30th ed. Philadelphia: Saunders; 2003.

Firkin BG, Whitworth JA. *Dictionary of Medical Eponyms.* 2nd ed. New York: The Parthenon Publishing Group Inc.; 2002.

Hughs P, ed. *The AAMT Book of Style for Medical Transcription.* 2nd ed. Modesto, CA: American Association for Medical Transcription; 2002.

Jablonski S. *Jablonski's Dictionary of Syndromes & Eponymic Diseases.* 2nd ed. Malabar, FL: Krieger Publishing Company; 1991.

Lourie JA. *Medical Eponyms: Who Was Coudé?* London: Pitman Publishing Limited; 1982.

Marcucci L. *Marcucci's Handbook of Medical Eponyms.* Baltimore: Lippincott Williams & Wilkins; 2002.

Stedman's Alternative Medicine Words. Baltimore: Lippincott Williams & Wilkins; 2000.

Stedman's Cardiovascular & Pulmonary Words. 4th ed. Baltimore: Lippincott Williams & Wilkins; 2004.

Stedman's Dermatology & Immunology Words. 2nd ed. Baltimore: Lippincott Williams & Wilkins; 2002.

Stedman's GI & GU Words. 3rd ed. Baltimore: Lippincott Williams & Wilkins; 2002.

Stedman's Medical Dictionary. 27th ed. Baltimore: Lippincott Williams & Wilkins; 2000.

Stedman's Neurology & Neurosurgery Words. 3rd ed. Baltimore: Lippincott Williams & Wilkins; 2003.

Stedman's OB-GYN & Genetic Words. 3rd ed. Baltimore: Lippincott Williams & Wilkins; 2001.

Stedman's Oncology Words. 4th ed. Baltimore: Lippincott Williams & Wilkins; 2004.

Stedman's Organisms & Infectious Disease Words. Baltimore: Lippincott Williams & Wilkins; 2002.

Stedman's Orthopaedic & Rehab Words. 4th ed. Baltimore: Lippincott Williams & Wilkins; 2003.

Stedman's Pediatric Words. Baltimore: Lippincott Williams & Wilkins; 2001.

Stedman's Plastic Surgery/ENT/Dentistry Words. 3rd ed. Baltimore: Lippincott Williams & Wilkins; 2003.

Stedman's Psychiatry Words. 3rd ed. Baltimore: Lippincott Williams & Wilkins; 2003.

Taber's Cyclopedic Medical Dictionary. 19th ed. Philadelphia, PA: F.A. Davis Company; 2001.

Web Sites

http://bmj.bmjjournals.com/cgi/content/full/325/7362/497

http://members.lycos.co.uk/Magill_Department/hp.html

http://merck.praxis.md/

http://wotug.ukc.ac.uk/parallel/www/occam/occam-bio.html

http://www.02.dokmed.de/2031.htm

http://www.almaz.com/nobel/

http://www.amershamhealth.com/medcyclopaedia/medical/index.asp

http://www.baillement.chez.tiscali.fr/lettres/babinski.html

http://www.bartleby.com/65/ba/Babcock.html

http://www.barttersite.com/westnile.htm

http://www.bdid.com/defectaa.com

http://www.behavenet.com/capsules/people/binil.htm

http://www.biomet.com

http://www.blc.arizona.edu/marty/411/Modules/okazaki.html

http://www.bmjjournals.com

http://www.books.md/W/dic/Wrightssyndrome.php

http://www.brookes.ac.uk/schools/bms/medical/synopses/burkitt1.html

http://www.cincypost.com/news/1998/obits081598.html

http://www.clinicalcardiology.org

http://www.dictionarybarn.com

http://www.emedicine.com

http://www.ich.ucl.ac.uk/cmgs/wolfram.htm

http://www.lankalibrary.com/

http://www.loggia.com/myth/olympians.html

http://www.mblab.gla.ac.uk/~julian/dict2.cgi?300-1K

http://www.mcbrideclinic.com

http://www.medterms.com/script/main/art.asp?articlekey=24172

http://www.members.aol.com/savilon/nmantel.html

http://www.mercksource.com

http://www.mhhe.com/mayfieldpub/psychtesting/pdf/vol1no2.pdf

http://www.mrcophth.com/ophthalmologyhalloffame/mainpage.html

http://www.mythweb.com

http://www.nap.edu

http://www.naspe.org/ep-history/

http://www.orthoteers.co.uk

http://www.pantheon.org/articles/c/caenis.html

http://www.pbs.org/wnet/redgold/innovators/bio_diamond.html

http://www.press.uchicago.edu

http://www.st-andrews.ac.uk/~sshm/history.htm

http://www.texasheartinstitute.org/starr.html

http://www.umdnj.edu

http://www.upstate.edu

http://www.webelements.com

http://www.whonamedit.com

http://www.wiem.onet.pl/wiem/009d41.html

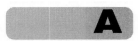

Aagenaes, Oystein, Norwegian pediatrician, *1925.
Aagenaes syndrome – inherited condition of lymphedema and arrested bile flow.

Aaron, in the Old Testament of the Bible, Moses' brother.
Aaron rod – walking stick (rod) with one serpent twined around it, used as a symbol for medicine.

Aaron, Charles Dettie, U.S. physician, 1866-1951.
Aaron sign – in acute appendicitis, a referred pain or feeling of distress in the epigastrium or precordial region on continuous firm pressure over McBurney point.

Aarskog, Dagfinn, Norwegian pediatrician, *1928.
Aarskog-Scott syndrome – *SYN:* faciodigitogenital dysplasia

Aase, Jon Morton, U.S. pediatrician, *1936.
Aase syndrome – affiliated with multiple birth defects; may be inherited recessive.

Abadie, Charles A., French ophthalmologist, 1842-1932.
Abadie sign of exophthalmic goiter – spasm of the musculus levator palpebrae superioris in Graves disease.

Abadie, Joseph Louis Irénée Jean, French neurosurgeon, 1873-1946.
Abadie sign of tabes dorsalis – insensibility to pressure over the Achilles tendon.

Abaza, Alphonse, French physician, *1909.
Hoet-Abaza syndrome – see under Hoet, Joseph Jules

Abbé, Ernst Karl, German physicist, 1840-1905.
Abbé condenser – a system of two or three wide-angle, achromatic, convex, and planoconvex lenses.

NOTES

Abbé-Zeiss apparatus – instrument for counting red blood cells in blood sample. *SYN:* Thoma-Zeiss apparatus

Abbe, Robert, U.S. surgeon, 1851-1928.
Abbe-Estlander cheiloplasty
Abbe flap – a full-thickness flap of the middle portion of the lower lip that is transferred into the upper lip, or vice versa.
Abbe intestinal anastomosis
Abbe neurectomy
Abbe operation – use of an Abbe flap in plastic surgery of the lips.
Abbe refractometer
Abbe repair
Abbe ring
Abbe small-bowel operation
Abbe stage I cheiloplasty
Abbe stage II cheiloplasty

Abbott, Alexander C., U.S. bacteriologist, 1860-1935.
Abbott stain for spores

Abbott, Edville Gerhardt, U.S. orthopedic surgeon, 1871-1938.
Abbott approach
Abbott arthrodesis
Abbott elevator
Abbott method – a method of treatment for scoliosis.

Abbott, William Osler, U.S. physician, 1902-1943.
Abbott tube – *SYN:* Miller-Abbott tube
Miller-Abbott catheter – *SYN:* Miller-Abbott tube
Miller-Abbott tube – see under Miller, Thomas Grier

Abegg, Richard, Danish chemist, 1869-1910.
Abegg rule – the tendency of the sum of the maximum positive and negative valence of an element to equal 8.

Abel, Rudolf, German bacteriologist, 1868-1942.
Abel bacillus – *Klebsiella pneumoniae* subspecies ozaenae.

Abelin, Isaak, Swiss physiologist, 1883-1965.
Abelin reaction – qualitative reaction that determines the presence of arsphenamine (Salvarsan) and neoarsphenamine (Neosalvarsan) in urine and/or blood.

Abels, Dietrich, 20th century German psychologist.
Abels test – number-sorting test for evaluating concentration and diagnosing disturbances thereof.

A

Abelson, Herbert T., U.S. pediatrician, *1941.
  Abelson murine leukemia virus – a retrovirus belonging to the type C retrovirus group subfamily (family Oncovirinae), which is associated with leukemia.

Abercrombie, John, English physician, 1780-1844.
  Abercrombie degeneration – pathological condition in which amyloid deposits occur between cells of organs and tissues. *SYN:* Abercrombie syndrome; amyloidosis
  Abercrombie syndrome – *SYN:* Abercrombie degeneration

Aberfeld, D.C., 20th century English physician.
  Schwartz-Jampel-Aberfeld syndrome – see under Schwartz, Oscar

Aberhalden, Emil, Swiss physiologist and biochemist, 1877-1950.
  Aberhalden-Kauffman-Lignac syndrome – renal rickets with widespread deposits of cystine crystals throughout the body.

Abernethy, John, English surgeon and anatomist, 1764-1831.
  Abernethy fascia – a layer of subperitoneal areolar tissue in front of the external iliac artery.
  Abernethy operation

Abrahams, Robert, U.S. physician, 1861-1935.
  Abrahams sign – rales and other adventitious sounds indicating progress from incipient to advanced tuberculosis.

Abrami, Pierre, French physician, 1879-1943.
  Widal and Abrami test – see under Widal

Abrams, Albert, U.S. physician, 1863-1924.
  Abrams heart reflex – a contraction of the myocardium when the skin of the precordial region is irritated.

Abrikosov, (Abrikossoff), Aleksei Ivanovich, Russian physician, 1875-1955.
  Abrikosov myoblastoma – generally benign skin tumor. *SYN:* Abrikosov tumor
  Abrikosov tumor – *SYN:* Abrikosov myoblastoma

NOTES

Abrikossoff, var. of Abrikosov

Abt, Arthur Frederic, U.S. physician, 1867-1955.
Abt-Letterer-Siwe syndrome – *SYN:* Letterer-Siwe disease

Achalme, Pierre Jean, French physician, *1866.
Achalme bacillus – bacillus discovered by Achalme in 1891.

Achard, Émile Charles, French physician, 1860-1941.
Achard syndrome – arachnodactyly with small, receding mandible, broad skull, and joint laxity limited to the hands and feet.
Achard-Thiers syndrome – one form of a virilizing disorder of adrenocortical origin in women.

Achenbach, Walter, German internist, *1921.
Achenbach syndrome – hematoma of the finger pad with accompanying edema.

Achilles, mythical Greek warrior who was vulnerable only in the heel.
Achilles bursa – bursa between the tendo calcaneus and the upper part of the posterior surface of the calcaneum. *SYN:* bursa of tendo calcaneus
Achilles reflex – a contraction of the calf muscles when the tendo calcaneus is sharply struck. *SYN:* ankle jerk; ankle reflex; tendo Achillis reflex; triceps surae reflex
Achilles tendon – the tendon of insertion of the triceps surae (gastrocnemius and soleus) into the tuberosity of the calcaneus. *SYN:* tendo calcaneus

Achor, Richard William Paul, U.S. physician, *1922.
Achor-Smith syndrome – potassium deficiency leading to pernicious anemia, severe diarrhea, muscle wasting, renal insufficiency. *SYN:* nutritional deficiency syndrome with hypopotassemia

Achúcarro, Nicolás, Spanish histologist, 1881-1918.
Achúcarro stain – stain for impregnating connective tissue.

Ackerman, James L., U.S. orthodontist.
Ackerman syndrome – familial syndrome characterized by pyramidal molars, abnormal upper lip, glaucoma, hyperpigmentation and hardening of interphalangeal skin of the hand.

Ackerman, Lauren Vedder, U.S. histopathologist, *1905.
Ackerman tumor – rare verrucous carcinoma of the larynx.

Acland, Robert D., U.S. physician.
Acland-Banis arteriotomy clamp – instrument that allows surgeon to create a hole in a vessel for end-to-side anastomosis.

A

Acosta, Joseph (José) de, Spanish Jesuit missionary, 1539-1600.
   Acosta disease – *SYN:* altitude sickness

Acree, Salomon Farley, U.S. chemist, *1875.
   Acree color test – used to detect preservatives in milk.

Acrel, Olof, Swedish surgeon, 1717-1806.
   Acrel ganglion – a cyst on a tendon of an extensor muscle at the level of the wrist.

Adair, G.S.
   Adair-Koshland-Némethy-Filmer model – *SYN:* Koshland-Némethy-Filmer model

Adam, first man, according to the Bible.
   Adam's apple – *SYN:* laryngeal prominence

Adamantiades, Benediktos, Greek ophthalmologist, 1875-1962.
   Adamantiades-Behçet syndrome – *SYN:* Behçet syndrome

Adamkiewicz, Albert, Polish pathologist, 1850-1921.
   artery of Adamkiewicz – largest of the medullary arteries which supply the spinal cord by anastomosing with the anterior (longitudinal) spinal artery. *SYN:* arteria radicularis magna

Adams, Forrest H., 20th century U.S. pediatrician.
   Adams-Oliver syndrome – autosomal dominant condition characterized by aplasia cutis congenita of the scalp with underlying skull defects and distal limb abnormalities.

Adams, James Alexander, Scottish gynecologist, 1857-1930.
   Alexander-Adams operation – *SYN:* Alexander operation

Adams, R.D., U.S. physician.
   Bickers-Adams syndrome – see under Bickers
   Hakim-Adams syndrome – *SYN:* Hakim syndrome

Adams, Robert, Irish physician, 1791-1875.
   Adams-Stokes disease – *SYN:* Adams-Stokes syndrome

NOTES

Adams-Stokes syncope – syncope due to complete atrioventricular block.

Adams-Stokes syndrome – characterized by slow or absent pulse, vertigo, syncope, convulsions, and sometimes Cheyne-Stokes respiration. *SYN:* Adams-Stokes disease; Morgagni-Adams-Stokes syndrome; Morgagni disease; Spens syndrome; Stokes-Adams disease; Stokes-Adams syndrome

Morgagni-Adams-Stokes syndrome – *SYN:* Adams-Stokes syndrome

Stokes-Adams disease – *SYN:* Adams-Stokes syndrome

Stokes-Adams syndrome – *SYN:* Adams-Stokes syndrome

Adams, Sir William, English surgeon, 1760-1829.

Adams operation

Adams saw

Adamson, Horatio George, English dermatologist and mycologist, 1866-1955.

Adamson fringe – zone of the hair follicle that separates the stem and the bulb.

Adanson, Michel, French naturalist, 1727-1806.

adansonian classification – the classification of organisms based on giving equal weight to every characteristic of the organism.

Addis, Thomas, U.S. internist, 1881-1949.

Addis count – a quantitative enumeration of the red and white blood counts, and casts in a 12-hour urine specimen, used to follow the progress of renal disease.

Addison, Christopher, English anatomist, 1869-1951.

Addison clinical planes – a series of planes used as landmarks in thoracoabdominal topography.

Addison, Thomas, English physician, 1793-1860.

Addison anemia – a chronic, progressive anemia of older adults due to failure of absorption of vitamin B_{12}. *SYN:* Addison-Biermer disease; addisonian anemia; Biermer anemia; Biermer disease; pernicious anemia

Addison-Biermer disease – *SYN:* Addison anemia

Addison disease – *SYN:* chronic adrenocortical insufficiency

addisonian anemia – *SYN:* Addison anemia

addisonian crisis – *SYN:* acute adrenocortical insufficiency

Addison-Schilder disease – *SYN:* Schilder disease

Adie, William John, Australian physician, 1886-1935.

Adie pupil – *SYN:* Adie syndrome

Adie syndrome – an idiopathic postganglionic denervation of the parasympathetically innervated intraocular muscles. *SYN:* Adie pupil; Holmes-Adie pupil; Holmes-Adie syndrome; pupillotonic pseudotabes; Weill syndrome

Holmes-Adie pupil – *SYN:* Adie syndrome

Holmes-Adie syndrome – *SYN:* Adie syndrome

Adler, Alfred, Austrian psychiatrist, 1870-1937.

adlerian psychoanalysis – a theory of human behavior emphasizing humans' social nature, strivings for mastery, and drive to overcome, by compensation, feelings of inferiority. *SYN:* individual psychology; adlerian psychology

adlerian psychology – *SYN:* adlerian psychoanalysis

Adler, Oscar, German physician, 1879-1932.

Adler test – a test to detect the presence of blood. *SYN:* benzidine test

Adrian, Lord Edgar Douglas, English physiologist, 1889-1977, joint winner of the 1932 Nobel Prize for discovery of neuron functions.

Adrian of Cambridge, var. of Adrian, Lord Edgar Douglas

Adson, Alfred Washington, U.S. neurosurgeon, 1887-1951.

Adson aneurysm needle
Adson angular hook
Adson brain clip
Adson brain-exploring cannula
Adson brain forceps
Adson brain hook
Adson brain retractor
Adson brain suction tip
Adson brain suction tube
Adson cerebellar retractor
Adson cranial rongeur
Adson drainage cannula
Adson dural hook

NOTES

Adson dural knife
Adson dural protector
Adson forceps
Adson Gigli saw
Adson Gigli-saw guide
Adson head rest
Adson maneuver – *SYN:* Adson test
Adson microbipolar forceps
Adson microdressing forceps
Adson microtissue forceps
Adson procedure – *SYN:* Adson test
Adson scalp clip
Adson scalp clip-applying forceps
Adson syndrome – (1) thoracic outlet syndrome. *SYN:* Naffziger syndrome; (2) cerebral sphingolipidosis.
Adson test – a test for thoracic outlet syndrome. *SYN:* Adson maneuver; Adson procedure
Brown-Adson forceps – see under Brown, James

Aeby, Christopher Theodore, Swiss anatomist, 1835-1885.
   Aeby muscle – a labial muscle formed by sagittal fibers running from the skin to the mucous membrane. *SYN:* cutaneomucous muscle
   Aeby plane – in craniometry, a plane perpendicular to the median plane of the cranium.

Afzelius, Arvid, Swedish physician, 1857-1923.
   Afzelius erythema – single lesions of erythema annulare centrifugum which erupt and spread. *SYN:* erythema chronicum migrans; Lipschütz erythema

Agatston, Arthur, U.S. cardiologist.
   Agatston method – protocol used for screening of coronary calcium.
   Agatston score – in CT scanning, the measure of coronary calcium present.

Aguecheek, Sir Andrew, Shakespearean character known for his consumption of beef.
   Aguecheek disease – chronic dementia in cases of liver disease due to intolerance of nitrogen produced after ingestion of large amounts of protein.

Ahumada, Juan Carlos, 20th century Argentinian physician.
   Ahumada-del Castillo syndrome – unphysiological lactation and amenorrhea not following pregnancy characterized by

hyperprolactinemia and a pituitary adenoma. *SYN:* Argonz-del Castillo syndrome

Aicardi, Jean Dennis, French neurologist, *1924.
  Aicardi syndrome – agenesis of the corpus callosum with infantile spasms in female babies.

Aird, Robert B., U.S. neurologist, *1903.
  Flynn-Aird syndrome – see under Flynn

Åkerlund, A. Olof, Swedish radiologist, 1885-1958.
  Åkerlund deformity – indentation (incisura) with niche of duodenal cap as demonstrated radiographically.
  Åkerlund diaphragm

Åkesson, Hand Olof, Swedish psychiatrist.
  Åkesson syndrome – X-linked recessive condition featuring cutis verticis gyrata, shagreen patch, hypoplastic thyroid disease, mental retardation, skull abnormality, and short stature.

Akureyri, a town in Iceland where approximately 1,000 cases were reported in 1948.
  Akureyri disease – epidemic neuromyasthenia.

Alagille, Daniel B., French pediatrician, *1925.
  Alagille syndrome – *SYN:* syndromatic paucity of interlobular bile ducts

Alajouanine, Théophile, French neurologist, 1890-1980.
  Foix-Alajouanine myelitis – see under Foix
  Foix-Alajouanine syndrome – see under Foix

Alanson, Edward, English surgeon, 1747-1823.
  Alanson amputation – a circular amputation, the stump shaped like a cone.

Albarran y Dominguez, Joaquin Maria, Cuban urologist, 1860-1912.
  Albarran bridge

NOTES

Albarran cystoscope

Albarran glands – minute submucosal glands or branching tubules in the subcervical region of the prostate gland. *SYN:* Albarran y Dominguez tubules

Albarran test – a test for renal insufficiency. *SYN:* polyuria test

Albarran urethroscope

Albarran y Dominguez tubules – *SYN:* Albarran glands

Albatross, large sea bird that figures prominently in Coleridge's poem, "The Rime of the Ancient Mariner."

Albatross syndrome – *SYN:* Münchausen syndrome

Albee, Fred Houdlet, U.S. orthopedic surgeon, 1876-1945.

Albee acetabuloplasty

Albee arthrodesis

Albee bone graft

Albee bone graft calipers

Albee bone saw

Albee drill

Albee fracture table

Albee fusion

Albee graft

Albee hip reconstruction

Albee operation – orthopedic hip procedure.

Albee orthopedic table

Albee osteotome

Albee osteotomy

Albee shelf procedure

Albee spinal fusion

Albers-Schönberg, Heinrich Ernst, German radiologist, 1865-1921.

Albers-Schönberg disease – excessive formation of dense trabecular bone and calcified cartilage. *SYN:* osteopetrosis

Albert, Eduard, Austrian surgeon, 1841-1900.

Albert disease – inflammation of the bursa between the Achilles tendon and the os calcis. *SYN:* Swediauer disease

Albert suture – a modified Czerny suture, the first row of stitches passing through the entire thickness of the wall of the gut.

Albert, Henry, U.S. physician, 1878-1930.

Albert stain – a stain for diphtheria bacilli.

Albertini, Ambrosius von, Swiss physician, 1894-1971.

Fanconi-Albertini-Zellweger syndrome – see under Fanconi, Guido

Albini, Giuseppe, Italian physiologist, 1827-1911.
Albini nodules – minute fibrous nodules on the margins of the mitral and tricuspid valves of the heart, representing fetal tissue rests.

Albinus, Bernhard Siegfried, German anatomist and surgeon, 1697-1770.
Albinus muscle – a facial muscle that draws angle of mouth laterally. *SYN:* risorius muscle; scalenus minimus muscle

Albrecht, Karl Martin Paul, German anatomist, 1851-1894.
Albrecht bone – a small bone between the basioccipital and basisphenoid.
Albrecht syndrome

Albright, Fuller, U.S. physician, 1900-1969.
Albright disease – *SYN:* McCune-Albright syndrome
Albright-Hadorn syndrome – softening and bending of bones associated with abnormally small concentration of potassium in blood.
Albright hereditary osteodystrophy – an inherited form of hyperparathyroidism associated with ectopic calcification and ossification and skeletal defects. *SYN:* Albright syndrome (1)
Albright syndrome (1) *SYN:* Albright hereditary osteodystrophy; (2) *SYN:* McCune-Albright syndrome
Albright IV syndrome – *SYN:* Martin-Albright syndrome
Albright synovectomy
Forbes-Albright syndrome – see under Forbes, Anne P.
Martin-Albright syndrome – see under Martin, August E.
McCune-Albright syndrome – see under McCune

Alcock, Benjamin, Irish anatomist, *1801.
Alcock bag
Alcock bladder syringe
Alcock canal – the space within the obturator internus fascia lining the lateral wall of the ischiorectal fossa that transmits the pudendal vessels and nerves. *SYN:* pudendal canal
Alcock catheter

NOTES

Alcock catheter adapter
Alcock catheter plug
Alcock hemostatic bag
Alcock hemostatic catheter
Alcock lithotrite
Alcock obturator

Alder, Albert von, *1888.
Alder anomaly – coarse azurophilic granulation of leukocytes, especially granulocytes, which may be associated with gargoylism and Morquio disease.
Alder bodies – granular inclusions in polymorphonuclear leukocytes.
Alder-Reilly anomaly – *SYN:* Reilly bodies

Aldrete, Antonio, U.S. physician and pain specialist.
Aldrete needle

Aldrich, Robert Anderson, U.S. pediatrician, *1917.
Aldrich syndrome – *SYN:* Wiskott-Aldrich syndrome
Wiskott-Aldrich syndrome – see under Wiskott

Alè, G., Italian radiologist.
Alè-Calò syndrome – *SYN:* Langer-Giedion syndrome

Aleutian Islands, chain of islands in the North Pacific Ocean.
Aleutian disease – plasma cell disorder of minks with characteristics similar to multiple myeloma.

Alexander, Benjamin, U.S. physician, *1909.
Alexander syndrome – congenital disorder resulting in hemophilia-like hemorrhagic diathesis, epistaxis, hematomas, and internal hemorrhaging.

Alexander, Frederick Matthias, Australian elocutionist, 1869-1955.
Alexander technique – used to develop kinesthetic sense of normal movements and posture.

Alexander, Gustav, Austrian otolaryngologist, *1873.
Alexander antrostomy punch
Alexander deafness – high-frequency deafness due to membranous cochlear dysplasia.
Alexander mastoid bone gouge
Alexander mastoid chisel
Alexander otoplasty
Alexander tonsil needle

Alexander, William Stuart, 20th century New Zealand pathologist.
  Alexander disease – a rare, fatal, central nervous system degenerative disease of infants.

Alexander, William, English surgeon, 1844-1919.
  Alexander-Adams operation – *SYN:* Alexander operation
  Alexander operation – repair of uterine displacement. *SYN:* Alexander-Adams operation

Alezzandrini, Arturo Alberto, Argentinian ophthalmologist, *1932.
  Alezzandrini syndrome – a rare syndrome appearing in adolescents and young adults, characterized by unilateral degenerative retinitis, followed by ipsilateral poliosis and facial vitiligo, and occasionally bilateral perceptive deafness.

Alfidi, Ralph J., U.S. physician.
  Alfidi syndrome – occlusion of the celiac axis leading to hypertension. *SYN:* renal-splanchnic steal

Alfvén, Hannes Olof Gosta, Swedish plasma physicist and astronomer, 1908-1995, winner of the 1970 Nobel Prize for Physics.
  Alfvén wave – transverse electromagnetic wave propagated along lines of magnetic force in plasma.

Alibert, Jean Louis Marc, French dermatologist, 1768-1837.
  Alibert-Bazin syndrome – heterogenous group of malignant lymphomas characterized by the expansion of a clone of CD4+ (or helper) memory cells, primarily affecting the skin. *SYN:* Alibert disease III; Auspitz dermatosis; cutaneous T-cell lymphoma; granuloma fungoides; mycosis fungoides
  Alibert disease I – firm, thickened, irregularly shaped, pink or red growth that arises on and extends beyond an area of the skin that has been injured. *SYN:* Alibert keloid; cicatricial keloid
  Alibert disease II – infection caused by *Leishmania tropica*. *SYN:* Baghdad boil; chiclero ulcer; cutaneous leishmaniasis; oriental sore
  Alibert disease III – *SYN:* Alibert-Bazin syndrome

NOTES

Alibert keloid – *SYN:* Alibert disease I

Alice in Wonderland, character created by author Lewis Carroll.
    Alice in Wonderland syndrome – syndrome characterized by distortion of time perception, distortion of body perception, and visual hallucinations; migraine is often involved.

Allemann, Richard, Swiss physician, 1893-1958.
    Allemann syndrome – hereditary double kidney, clubbing of fingers; may be associated with facial asymmetry and motor nerve degeneration.

Allen, Alfred Henry, U.S. chemist, 1846-1904.
    Allen test – a test for phenol.

Allen, Arthur W., U.S. surgeon, 1887-1958.
    Buerger-Allen exercises – see under Buerger

Allen, Edgar, U.S. endocrinologist, 1892-1943.
    Allen-Doisy test – a test for estrogenic activity.
    Allen-Doisy unit – the quantity of estrogen capable of producing in a spayed mouse a characteristic change in the vaginal epithelium. *SYN:* mouse unit

Allen, Edgar Van Nuys, U.S. physician, 1900-1961.
    Allen test – a test for radial or ulnar patency.

Allen, Frederick Madison, U.S. physician, 1879-1964.
    Allen paradoxic law – that more sugar is utilized by nondiabetics as more is given; the opposite in those with diabetes.

Allen, Willard Myron, U.S. gynecologist, *1904.
    Allen fetal stethoscope
    Allen-Masters syndrome – pelvic pain resulting from old lacerations of the broad ligament during delivery.
    Allen uterine forceps
    Corner-Allen test – see under Corner, George W.
    Corner-Allen unit – see under Corner, George W.

Allingham, William, English physician, 1829-1908.
    Allingham colotomy
    Allingham rectal speculum
    Allingham rectum excision
    Allingham ulcer – anal ulcer. *SYN:* fissure in ano

Allis, Oscar Huntington, U.S. surgeon, 1836-1921.
    Allis forceps – a straight grasping forceps.
    Allis hemostat

Allis intestinal forceps
Allis Micro-Line pediatric forceps
Allis sign – in fracture of the neck of the femur, the trochanter rides up, relaxing the fascia lata, so that the finger can be sunk deeply between the great trochanter and the iliac crest.

Allison, Nathaniel, U.S. physician, 1876-1932.
Allison atrophy – non-use of bones resulting in atrophy and demineralization.

Allport, Gordon Willard, U.S. psychologist, 1897-1967.
Allport A-S Reaction Study – a personality test designed to determine whether a subject is dominant or submissive in dealing with situations.
Allport personality-trait theory – theory that personality traits are the key to individuality and consistency of behavior.

Almeida, Floriano Paulo de, Brazilian physician, *1898.
Almeida disease – a chronic mycosis caused by *Paracoccidioides brasiliensis*. *SYN:* paracoccidioidomycosis
Lutz-Splendore-Almeida disease – see under Lutz

Almén, August Teodor, Swedish physiologist, 1833-1903.
Almén test for blood – a test for occult blood. *SYN:* guaiac test; Schönbein test; van Deen test

Alpers, Bernard J., U.S. neurologist, 1900-1981.
Alpers disease – familial progressive spastic paresis of extremities with destruction and disorganization of nerve cells of the cerebral cortex. *SYN:* poliodystrophia cerebri progressiva infantalis

Alport, Arthur Cecil, South African physician, 1880-1959.
Alport syndrome – progressive microscopic hematuria.

Alsever, John Bellows, U.S. hematologist, *1908.
Alsever solution – solution used to preserve red blood cells.

NOTES

Alström, Carl-Henry, Swedish geneticist, *1907.
Alström syndrome – retinal degeneration with nystagmus and loss of central vision.

Altherr, Franz.
Meyenburg-Altherr-Uehlinger syndrome – *SYN:* Meyenburg disease

Altmann, Richard, German histologist, 1852-1900.
Altmann anilin-acid fuchsin stain – a mixture of picric acid, anilin, and acid fuchsin which stains mitochondria crimson against a yellow background.
Altmann fixative – a bichromate-osmic acid fixative.
Altmann-Gersh method – the method of rapidly freezing a tissue and dehydrating it in a vacuum.
Altmann granule – a granule that has an affinity for fuchsin. *SYN:* fuchsinophil granule; mitochondrion
Altmann theory – a theory that protoplasm consists of granular particles that are clustered and enclosed in indifferent matter.

Alvarez, Walter C., U.S. physician.
Alvarez syndrome – neurotic or hysterical bloating of the abdomen without clinical cause. *SYN:* accordion abdomen; hysterical nongaseous abdominal bloating; pseudoileus

Alzheimer, Alois, German neurologist, 1864-1915.
Alzheimer dementia – *SYN:* Alzheimer disease
Alzheimer disease – progressive mental deterioration. *SYN:* Alzheimer dementia; presenile dementia; primary neuronal degeneration; primary senile dementia
Alzheimer sclerosis – hyaline degeneration of the medium and smaller blood vessels of the brain.

Amann, Josef Albert, German physician, d. 1919.
Amann operation – surgery for creation of an artificial vagina in cases of congenital absence.

Ambard, Léon, French pharmacologist, 1876-1962.
Ambard constant
Ambard laws – laws for output of urea.

Amberg, Emil, U.S. otologist, 1868-1948.
Amberg lateral sinus line – a line dividing the angle formed by the anterior edge of the mastoid process and the temporal line.

Amendola, F., Brazilian physician.
    Amendola syndrome – a form of pemphigus foliaceus that is endemic to Brazil. *SYN:* Brazilian pemphigus; fogo selvagem; wildfire pemphigus

Ames, Adelbert, Jr., U.S. educator, 1880-1955.
    Ames demonstrations – series of illusions designed to test depth perception.

Ames, Bruce N., U.S. molecular geneticist, *1928.
    Ames assay – a screening test for possible carcinogens. *SYN:* Ames test
    Ames test – *SYN:* Ames assay

Amici, Giovanni Battista, Italian physicist, 1786-1863.
    Amici disk – thin membrane seen as a line which serves as delimiter of sarcomeres in striated muscle. *SYN:* Amici striae; Z band
    Amici line
    Amici striae – *SYN:* Amici disk

Amish, religious group found in 22 states and Canada; stresses community life and separation from the modern world.
    Amish brittle hair syndrome – syndrome noted in the Amish, characterized by short stature, brittle hair, decreased fertility, mild intellectual impairment; hair noted to be without scales. *SYN:* hair-brain syndrome

Ammon, Greek name of the Egyptian god Amun.
    Ammon horn – one of the two interlocking gyri composing the hippocampus, the other being the dentate gyrus. *SYN:* cornu ammonis

Ammon, Friedrich von, German ophthalmologist and pathologist, 1799-1861.
    Ammon blepharoplasty
    Ammon blue dye
    Ammon canthoplasty
    Ammon dacryocystotomy
    Ammon eyelid repair

NOTES

Ammon fissure – a pear-shaped opening in the sclera during early embryogenesis.

Ammon prominence – an external prominence in the posterior pole of the eyeball during early embryogenesis.

Ammons, Henry R., U.S. physician, 1857-1923.
Ammons Full Range Picture Vocabulary Test

Amoss, Harold Lindsay, U.S. physician, 1886-1956.
Amoss sign – in painful flexion of the spine, it is necessary to support a sitting position by extending the arms behind the torso with the weight placed on the hands.

Ampère, André-Marie, French physicist, 1775-1836.
ampere – the practical unit of electrical current.
Ampère postulate – *SYN:* Avogadro law
statampere – the electrostatic unit of current, equal to 3.335641×10^{-10} ampere.

Amplatz, Kurt, 20th century U.S. cardiologist.
Amplatz angiography needle
Amplatz aortography catheter
Amplatz cardiac catheter
Amplatz coronary catheter
Amplatz II curve
AMPLATZER septal occluder
Amplatz fascial dilator
Amplatz femoral catheter
Amplatz guide
Amplatz injector
Amplatz Super Stiff guide wire
Amplatz torque wire

Amreich, Isidor Alfred, German gynecologist, 1885-1972.
Schauta-Amreich operation – *SYN:* Schauta operation

Amsler, Marc, Swiss ophthalmologist, 1891-1968.
Amsler chart – a 10-cm square divided into 5-mm squares upon which an individual may project a defect in the central visual field.
Amsler chart marker
Amsler corneal graft operation
Amsler needle
Amsler operation
Amsler scleral marker
Amsler test – projection of a visual field defect onto an Amsler chart.

A

Amussat, Jean Z., French surgeon, 1796-1856.
Amussat incision
Amussat operation
Amussat probe
Amussat valve – a series of crescentic folds of mucous membrane in the upper part of the cystic duct. *SYN:* spiral fold of cystic duct
Amussat valvula – anomalous folds occurring at the level of the seminal colliculus. *SYN:* posterior urethral valves

Amyand, Claudius, English surgeon.
Amyand hernia – inguinal hernia with involvement of appendix.

Anagnostakis, Andrei, Cretan ophthalmologist, 1826-1897.
Anagnostakis operation – (1) a procedure for entropion; (2) a procedure for trichiasis.

Ancell, Henry A., English physician, 1802-1863.
Ancell-Spiegler cylindroma – *SYN:* Brooke disease (1)
Ancell-Spiegler syndrome – *SYN:* Brooke disease (1)
Ancell syndrome – *SYN:* Brooke disease (1)

Andermann, Frederick, Canadian physician.
Andermann syndrome – recessive gene causing agenesis of the corpus callosum. *SYN:* Charlevoix disease

Andernach, Johann Winther von (Guenther von), German physician, 1505-1574.
Andernach ossicles – small irregular bones found along the sutures of the cranium. *SYN:* sutural bones

Anders, James Meschter, U.S. physician, 1854-1936.
Anders disease – a condition characterized by a deposit of symmetrical nodular or pendulous masses of fat in various regions of the body, with discomfort or pain. *SYN:* adiposis dolorosa; adiposis tuberosa simplex

NOTES

Andersch, Carolus Samuel, German anatomist, 1732-1777.
  Andersch ganglion – the lower of two sensory ganglions on the
    glossopharyngeal nerve as it traverses the jugular foramen. *SYN:* inferior
    ganglion of glossopharyngeal nerve
  Andersch nerve – *SYN:* tympanic nerve

Andersen, Dorothy Hansine, U.S. pediatrician, 1901-1963.
  Andersen disease – familial cirrhosis of the liver with storage of abnormal
    glycogen. *SYN:* type 4 glycogenosis
  Andersen syndrome – cystic fibrosis of the pancreas, vitamin A
    deficiency, and disease of the abdominal cavity. *SYN:* Andersen triad
  Andersen triad – *SYN:* Andersen syndrome

Anderson, Evelyn, U.S. physician, *1899.
  Anderson-Collip test – a procedure for evaluating the thyrotropic activity
    of an extract of the anterior lobe of the pituitary gland.

Anderson, James C., English urologist, *1899.
  Anderson-Hynes pyeloplasty – disjoined or dismembered pyeloplasty.

Anderson, L.G., U.S. physician.
  Anderson syndrome – syndrome characterized by multiple osseous
    abnormalities with associated hyperuricemia and elevated diastolic
    pressure.

Anderson, Roger, U.S. orthopedic surgeon, 1891-1971.
  Anderson splint – a skeletal traction splint.
  Anderson tibial lengthening
  Anderson traction bow

Anderson, Rose G., U.S. psychologist, *1893.
  Kuhlmann-Anderson tests – see under Kuhlmann

Anderson, W., English surgeon and dermatologist, 1842-1900.
  Anderson-Fabry disease – *SYN:* Fabry disease

Andes, mountains in Peru.
  Andes disease – chronic altitude sickness.

Andogskii, var. of Andogsky

Andogsky, (Andogskii), N., Russian physician.
  Andogsky syndrome – development of total soft cataracts in adults who
    have a history of chronic dermatologic eczema. *SYN:* cataracta
    dermatogenes; cataracta syndermatotica; dermatogenic cataract

Andrade, Corino M. de, 20th century Portuguese physician.
Andrade syndrome – accumulation of amyloid in organs and tissues of the body.

Andrade, Eduardo Penny, U.S. bacteriologist, 1872-1906.
Andrade indicator – solution used to culture acid-producing organisms.

Andral, Gabriel, French physician, 1797-1876.
Andral decubitus – position assumed by a patient who lies on the sound side in cases of beginning pleurisy.

Andre, M., French physician.
Andre syndrome – syndrome characterized by osseous defects and orofacial anomalies in infants; usual fatal within weeks.

André Thomas, see under Thomas, André Antoine Henri

Andresen, Viggo, Norwegian orthodontist, 1870-1950.
Andresen activator
Andresen monoblock appliance
Andresen removable orthodontic appliance

Andrews, C.J., U.S. surgeon.
Andrews gouge
Andrews iliotibial band reconstruction
Andrews iliotibial band tenodesis
Andrews knee reconstruction
Andrews lateral tenodesis
Andrews spinal surgery table
Andrews technique
Brandt-Andrews maneuver – see under Brandt, Thure

Andrews, George Clinton, U.S. dermatologist, 1891-1978.
Andrews bacterid – eruption of pustules on palms of hands and soles of feet, usually following an infection of the teeth, sinuses, or tonsils. *SYN:* Andrews disease; pustular bacterid of Andrews
Andrews disease – *SYN:* Andrews bacterid

NOTES

pustular bacterid of Andrews – *SYN:* Andrews bacterid

Andry, Nicholas, French physician who first used term "orthopedics" (derived from the Greek words for "straight" and "child"), 1658-1759.
tree of Andry – illustration of postural defects.

Anel, Dominique, French surgeon, 1679-1725.
Anel lacrimal duct dilation
Anel method – ligation of an artery immediately above (on the proximal side of) an aneurysm.
Anel probe
Anel syringe

Angelman, Harry, 20th century English physician.
Angelman syndrome – recessive gene causing motor dysfunction, mental retardation, and hypotonia. *SYN:* happy puppet syndrome

Angelucci, Arnaldo, Italian ophthalmologist, 1854-1934.
Angelucci syndrome – extreme excitability, vasomotor disturbances, and palpitation associated with vernal conjunctivitis.

Anger, Hal, U.S. electrical engineer, *1920.
Anger camera – a scintigraphic imaging system or type of gamma camera.

Anghelescu, Constantin, Romanian surgeon, 1869-1948.
Anghelescu sign – in vertebral tuberculosis, painful or impossible flexion of the spine when the patient attempts to rest weight on the heels and occiput.

Angle, Edward Hartley, U.S. orthodontist, 1855-1930.
Angle classification of malocclusion

Anglesey, an island off the north-west coast of Wales.
Anglesey leg – first prosthetic wooden leg, designed for Henry William Paget, first marquis of Anglesey, 1768-1854.

Ångström, Anders J., Swedish physicist, 1814-1874.
ångström – a unit of wavelength, 10^{-10} m, roughly the diameter of an atom; equivalent to 0.1 nm. *SYN:* Ångström unit
Ångström law – a substance absorbs light of the same wavelength as it emits when luminous.
Ångström scale – a table of wavelengths of a large number of light rays corresponding to as many Fraunhofer lines in the spectrum.
Ångström unit – *SYN:* ångström

Anichkov, var. of Anitschkow

Anitschkow, (Anichkov), Nikolai, Russian pathologist, 1885-1964.
　Anitschkow cell – a large mononuclear cell found in connective tissue of the heart wall in inflammatory conditions. *SYN:* Anitschkow myocyte; cardiac histiocyte
　Anitschkow myocyte – *SYN:* Anitschkow cell

Annandale, Thomas, English surgeon, 1838-1907.
　Annandale operation – use of preperitoneal approach to repair groin hernia.

Anrep, G.V., 20th century Lebanese physiologist in Britain.
　Anrep phenomenon – homeometric autoregulation of the heart whereby cardiac performance improves as the aortic pressure is increased.

Ansbacher, Stefan, German-born U.S. biologist, *1905.
　Ansbacher unit – vitamin K unit.

Antley, Ray M., U.S. physician.
　Antley-Bixler syndrome – syndrome characterized by craniofacial defects and extremity anomalies.

Anton, Gabriel, German neuropsychiatrist, 1858-1933.
　Anton syndrome – in cortical blindness, lack of awareness of being blind.

Antoni, Nils, Swedish neurologist, 1887-1968.
　Antoni type A neurilemoma – relatively solid or compact arrangement of neoplastic tissue that consists of Schwann cells arranged in twisting bundles associated with delicate reticulin fibers.
　Antoni type B neurilemoma – relatively soft or loose arrangement of neoplastic tissue that consists of Schwann cells in a nondescript arrangement among reticulin fibers and tiny cystlike foci.

Antopol, William, U.S. physician.
　Antopol disease – cardiomegaly caused by glycogen deposits in the heart, thought to be caused by recessive transmission.

NOTES

Antyllus, Greek physician, ca. 150 A.D.
Antyllus method – ligation of the artery above and below an aneurysm, followed by incision into and emptying of the sac.

Apert, Eugène, French pediatrician, 1868-1940.
Apert hirsutism – excessive body or facial hair caused by a virilizing disorder of adrenocortical origin.
Apert syndrome – type I acrocephalosyndactyly. *SYN:* Crouzon-Apert disease
Crouzon-Apert disease – *SYN:* Apert syndrome

Apgar, Virginia, U.S. anesthesiologist, 1909-1974.
Apgar score – evaluation of a newborn infant's physical status by assigning numerical values to each of 5 criteria.
Apgar timer

Apley, Alan Graham, English orthopedic surgeon, 1917-1996.
Apley grinding test – orthopedic test related to a meniscal tear.
Apley knee test
Apley maneuver
Apley sign
Apley traction

Apollo, Greek god of the arts, archery, and divination.
Apollo disease – *SYN:* acute hemorrhagic conjunctivitis

Appian of Alexandria, Greek historian, 2nd century A.D.
Appian-Plutarch syndrome – condition caused by atropine intoxication; characterized by various neurological reactions. Appian and Plutarch wrote about symptoms exhibited by hungry soldiers who ate strange plants during war.

Applebaum, L., 20th century German physician.
Recklinghausen-Applebaum disease – see under Recklinghausen

Arakawa, Tsuneo, Japanese physician.
Arakawa syndrome – (1) formiminotransferase deficiency; (2) tetrahydrofolate methyltransferase deficiency.

Aran, François, French physician, 1817-1861.
Aran-Duchenne disease – *SYN:* Lou Gehrig disease
Aran-Duchenne dystrophy – *SYN:* Lou Gehrig disease
Duchenne-Aran disease – *SYN:* Lou Gehrig disease

Arantius, (Aranzio), Giulio C., Italian anatomist and physician, 1530-1589.
    Arantius ligament – a thin fibrous cord, lying in the fissure of the ligamentum venosum; the remains of the ductus venosus of the fetus. *SYN:* ligamentum venosum
    Arantius nodule – a nodule at the center of the free border of each semilunar valve at the beginning of the pulmonary artery and aorta. *SYN:* corpus arantii; nodule of semilunar valve
    Arantius ventricle – inferior part of the rhomboid fossa. *SYN:* calamus scriptorius
    corpus arantii – *SYN:* Arantius nodule
    ductus venosus arantii – rarely used term for ductus venosus.

Aranzio, var. of Arantius

Arber, Werner, Swiss microbiologist, *1929, joint winner of the 1978 Nobel Prize for medicine and physiology for his work on restriction enzymes.

Archambault, LaSalle, U.S. neurologist, 1879-1940.
    Meyer-Archambault loop – see under Meyer, Adolf

Arey, Leslie B., U.S. anatomist, 1891-1988.
    Arey rule – rule related to size of embryo or fetus.

Argand, Aimé, Swiss physicist, 1755-1803.
    Argand burner – oil or gas burner with air supplied to flame by an inner tube.

Argonz, J., Argentinian physician.
    Argonz-del Castillo syndrome – *SYN:* Ahumada-del Castillo syndrome

Argyll Robertson, see under Robertson, Douglas M.C.L.

Arias, Irwin Monroe, U.S. physician, *1926.
    Arias syndrome – *SYN:* Crigler-Najjar syndrome

NOTES

Arias-Stella, Javier, Peruvian pathologist, *1924.
  Arias-Stella effect – focal, unusual, decidual changes in endometrial epithelium that may be associated with ectopic or uterine pregnancy. *SYN:* Arias-Stella phenomenon; Arias-Stella reaction
  Arias-Stella phenomenon – *SYN:* Arias-Stella effect
  Arias-Stella reaction – *SYN:* Arias-Stella effect

Aristotle, Greek philosopher and scientist, 384-322 B.C.
  Aristotelian method – a method of study that stresses the relation between a general category and a particular object.
  Aristotle anomaly

Arlt, Carl Ferdinand von, Austrian ophthalmologist, 1812-1887.
  Arlt epicanthus repair
  Arlt eyelid repair
  Arlt fenestrated lens scoop
  Arlt lens loupe
  Arlt operation – transplantation of the eyelashes back from the edge of the lid in trichiasis.
  Arlt pterygium excision
  Arlt recess
  Arlt sinus – an inconstant depression on the lower portion of the internal surface of the lacrimal sac.
  Arlt sutures
  Arlt trachoma

Armanni, Luciano, Italian pathologist, 1839-1903.
  Armanni-Ebstein change – glycogen vacuolization of the loops of Henle, seen in diabetics before the introduction of insulin. *SYN:* Armanni-Ebstein kidney
  Armanni-Ebstein kidney – *SYN:* Armanni-Ebstein change
  Armanni-Ebstein nephropathy – diabetic glycogen vacuolization of renal convoluted tubules; related to glycosuria.

Armendares, S.
  Armendares syndrome – syndrome characterized by growth retardation, craniofacial defects, and other congenital malformations.

Armstrong, Arthur Riley, Canadian physician, *1904.
  King-Armstrong unit – *SYN:* King unit

Arndt, Georg, German dermatologist, 1874-1929.
  Arndt-Gottron syndrome – generalized lichen myxedematosus with diffuse thickening of the skin underlying the papules. *SYN:* scleromyxedema

Arndt, Rudolph, German psychiatrist, 1835-1900.

Arndt law – obsolete law stating that weak stimuli excite physiologic activity, moderately strong ones favor it, strong ones retard it, and very strong ones arrest it.

Arneth, Joseph, German physician, 1873-1955.

Arneth classification – a classification of the polymorphonuclear neutrophils according to the number of their nuclear lobes.

Arneth count – the percentage distribution of polymorphonuclear neutrophils, based on the number of lobes in the nuclei (from 1 to 5).

Arneth formula – the normal, approximate ratio of polymorphonuclear neutrophils, based on the number of lobes in the nuclei.

Arneth index – an expression based on adding percentages of polymorphonuclear neutrophils.

Arneth stages – a differential grouping of polymorphonuclear neutrophils in accordance with the number of lobes in their nuclei.

Arning, Eduard, German physician, *1855.

Arning carcinoid – multiple flat skin tumors that heal spontaneously over time, found on face and trunk.

Arnold, Friedrich, German anatomist, 1803-1890.

Arnold bundle – a fiber group originating in the cerebral cortex of the temporal lobe and terminating in the pontine nuclei or the ventral part of the pons. *SYN:* Arnold tract; temporopontine tract

Arnold canal – the small opening in the petrous bone lateral to the hiatus of facial canal that gives passage to the lesser petrosal nerve. *SYN:* hiatus of canal of lesser petrosal nerve

Arnold ganglion – an autonomic ganglion situated below the foramen ovale medial to the mandibular nerve. *SYN:* otic ganglion

Arnold nerve – a branch of the superior ganglion of the vagus, supplying the back of the pinna and the external acoustic meatus. *SYN:* auricular branch of vagus nerve

Arnold tract – *SYN:* Arnold bundle

NOTES

foramen of Arnold – an occasional opening in the greater wing of the sphenoid bone, between the foramen spinosum and foramen ovale, which transmits the lesser petrosal nerve. *SYN:* petrosal foramen

Arnold, Julius, German pathologist, 1835-1915.
Arnold bodies – small portions or minute fragments of erythrocytes.
Arnold-Chiari deformity – *SYN:* Arnold-Chiari malformation
Arnold-Chiari malformation – malformed posterior fossa structures. *SYN:* Arnold-Chiari deformity; Arnold-Chiari syndrome; cerebellomedullary malformation syndrome
Arnold-Chiari syndrome – *SYN:* Arnold-Chiari malformation

Arnold Pick, see under Pick, Arnold

Arnott, Neil, Scottish physician, 1788-1874.
Arnott bed – a type of waterbed used to treat bed sores.

Arrhenius, Svante, Swedish chemist and Nobel laureate, 1859-1927.
Arrhenius doctrine – the theory of electrolytic dissociation that became the basis of modern understanding of electrolytes. *SYN:* Arrhenius law
Arrhenius equation – an equation relating chemical reaction rate to the absolute temperature.
Arrhenius law – *SYN:* Arrhenius doctrine
Arrhenius-Madsen theory – that the reaction of an antigen with its antibody is a reversible reaction.

Arrillaga, student of Abel Ayerza who wrote the thesis correlating clinical findings of Ayerza syndrome with pulmonary artery sclerosis.
Ayerza-Arrillaga disease – *SYN:* Ayerza syndrome

Arroyo, Carlos F., U.S. physician, 1892-1928.
Arroyo expressor
Arroyo implant
Arroyo protector
Arroyo sign – sluggish pupillary reaction to light. *SYN:* asthenocoria

Arruga, Count Hermenegildo, Spanish ophthalmologist, 1886-1972.
Arruga capsular forceps
Arruga cataract extraction
Arruga eye expressor
Arruga eye implant
Arruga eye retractor
Arruga eye speculum
Arruga eye trephine
Arruga forceps – for the intracapsular extraction of a cataract.

Arruga globe retractor
Arruga keratoplasty
Arruga lacrimal trephine
Arruga needle holder
Arruga protector
Arruga retinal detachment operation

Arslan, Michele, Italian otorhinolaryngologist, 1904-1988.
Arslan ultrasonic operation

Arthur, Mary Grace, U.S. psychologist, 1883-1967.
Arthur Point Scale of Performance – nonverbal test of intellectual performance.

Arthus, Nicolas Maurice, French bacteriologist, 1862-1945.
Arthus phenomenon – a form of immediate hypersensitivity observed in rabbits after injection of antigen to which the animal has already been sensitized and has specific IgG antibodies. *SYN:* Arthus reaction
Arthus reaction – *SYN:* Arthus phenomenon

Asboe-Hansen, Gustav, Danish physician, 1917-1989.
Asboe-Hansen disease – congenital disturbance occurring predominantly in female newborns; charcterized by irregularly shaped pigmented macules as well as defects of the integumentary system.
Asboe-Hansen sign – vertical pressure on a blister causes the blister to extend laterally.

Asch, Solomon E., U.S. psychologist, *1907.
Asch situation – a test designed to determine the degree to which subject conforms to group opinion.

Ascher, Karl Wolfgang, U.S. ophthalmologist, 1887-1971.
Ascher aqueous influx phenomenon – the filling of the aqueous vein, which normally carries blood and aqueous, with aqueous, when the junction of the aqueous vein and the recipient vein is partially occluded. *SYN:* aqueous influx phenomenon

NOTES

Ascher syndrome – a condition in which a congenital double lip is associated with blepharochalasis and nontoxic thyroid gland enlargement.
Laffer-Ascher syndrome

Ascherson, Ferdinand Moritz, German physician, 1798-1879.
Ascherson membrane – casein covering enclosing milk globules.

Aschheim, Selmar, German obstetrician and gynecologist, 1878-1965.
Aschheim-Zondek test – an obsolete test for pregnancy. *SYN:* A-Z test; Zondek-Aschheim test
Zondek-Aschheim test – *SYN:* Aschheim-Zondek test

Aschner, Bernhard, Austrian gynecologist, 1883-1960.
Aschner-Dagnini reflex – *SYN:* Aschner phenomenon
Aschner phenomenon – decrease in pulse rate associated with traction on extraocular muscles or compression of the eyeball; may produce asystolic cardiac arrest. *SYN:* Aschner-Dagnini reflex; Aschner reflex; oculocardiac reflex
Aschner reflex – *SYN:* Aschner phenomenon

Aschoff, Karl Ludwig, German pathologist, 1866-1942.
Aschoff bodies – a form of granulomatous inflammation characteristically observed in acute rheumatic carditis. *SYN:* Aschoff nodules
Aschoff cell – a large-cell component of rheumatic nodules in the myocardium.
Aschoff nodules – *SYN:* Aschoff bodies
node of Aschoff and Tawara – a small node of modified cardiac muscle that gives rise to the atrioventricular bundle of the conduction system of the heart. *SYN:* atrioventricular node; Tawara node
Rokitansky-Aschoff sinuses – see under Rokitansky

Ascoli, Alberto, Italian serologist, 1877-1957.
Ascoli reaction – a method for confirming the diagnosis of anthrax.
Ascoli test – a precipitin test for anthrax using a tissue extract and anthrax antiserum.

Aselli, (Asellio, Asellius), Gasparo, Italian anatomist, 1581-1626.
Aselli gland – a single large lymph node ventral to the abdominal aorta that receives all the lymph from the intestines in many smaller mammals. *SYN:* Aselli pancreas
Aselli pancreas – *SYN:* Aselli gland

Asellio, var. of Aselli

Asellius, var. of Aselli

Ashby, Winifred, 20th century hematologist.
   Ashby method – a differential agglutination method for estimating erythrocyte life span.

Asherman, Joseph G., Czech gynecologist, *1889.
   Asherman syndrome – synechiae within the endometrial cavity, often causing amenorrhea and infertility.

Asherson, Nehemiah, English physician, *1897.
   Asherson syndrome – dysphagia caused by neuromuscular incoordination, resulting in liquids entering air passages during swallowing.

Ashley, R.K., U.S. physician.
   Ashley syndrome – syndrome characterized by multiple musculoskeletal anomalies and abnormalities.

Ashman, R., 20th century U.S. physiologist.
   Ashman phenomenon – aberrant ventricular conduction of a beat ending a short cycle that is preceded by a longer cycle most commonly during atrial fibrillation.

Askanazy, Max, German pathologist, 1865-1940.
   Askanazy cell – *SYN:* Hürthle cell

Ask-Upmark, Erik, Swedish pathologist, 1901-1985.
   Ask-Upmark kidney – true renal hypoplasia with decreased lobules and deep transverse grooving of the cortical surfaces of the kidney.

Asperger, Hans, Austrian physician, 1844-1954.
   Asperger syndrome – personality disorder characterized by insensitivity to others and speaking in a manner which is one-sided. *SYN:* autistic psychopathy

Assézat, Jules, French anthropologist, 1832-1876.
   Assézat triangle – a triangle formed by lines connecting the nasion with the alveolar and nasal point; used to indicate prognathism in comparative craniology.

NOTES

Assmann, Herbert, German internist, 1882-1950.
　Assmann focus – *SYN:* Assmann tuberculous infiltrate
　Assmann tuberculous infiltrate – an incipient lesion of tuberculous infection. *SYN:* Assman focus; infraclavicular infiltrate

Astrup, Poul, Danish clinical chemist, *1915.
　micro-Astrup method – an interpolation technique for acid-base measurement.

Astwood, Edwin B., U.S. endocrinologist, 1909-1976.
　Astwood test – a test for the assay of estrogenic substances. *SYN:* metrotrophic test

Atkins, Robert C., U.S. physician, 1930-2003.
　Atkins diet – eating plan that stresses high intake of protein and low intake of carbohydrates.

Aub, Joseph C., U.S. physician, 1890-1973.
　Aub-DuBois table – table of basal metabolic rates in calories per square meter of body surface per hour or day for different ages.

Auberger, name of a French woman in whom this blood group was detected.
　Auberger blood group – blood group found in 82% of Caucasians.

Aubert, Hermann, German physiologist, 1826-1892.
　Aubert phenomenon – a bright perpendicular line appearing to incline to one side when the observer turns the head to the opposite side in a dark room.

Audouin, Jean-Victor, French physician, 1797-1841.
　Audouin microsporon – ringworm fungus causing tinea capitis.

Audry, Charles, French physician, 1865-1934.
　Audry syndrome – digital clubbing, coarsening of facial features, hyperostosis of hands and feet; genetic disorder. *SYN:* pachydermoperiostosis syndrome

Auenbrugger, Leopold, Austrian physician, 1722-1809.
　Auenbrugger sign – an epigastric prominence seen in cases of marked pericardial effusion.

Auer, John, U.S. physician, 1875-1948.
　Auer bodies – rod-shaped structures of uncertain nature in the cytoplasm of immature myeloid cells in acute myelocytic leukemia. *SYN:* Auer rods
　Auer rods – *SYN:* Auer bodies

Auerbach, Leopold, German anatomist, 1828-1897.
　Auerbach ganglia – collections of parasympathetic nerve cells in the myenteric plexus.
　Auerbach plexus – a plexus of unmyelinated fibers and postganglionic autonomic cell bodies lying in the muscular coat of the esophagus, stomach, and intestines. *SYN:* myenteric plexus

Aufrecht, Emanuel, German physician, 1844-1933.
　Aufrecht sign – diminished breath sounds in the trachea just above the jugular notch, in cases of stenosis.

Aujeszky, Aládar, Hungarian pathologist, 1869-1933.
　Aujeszky disease – a highly contagious disease caused by porcine herpesvirus. *SYN:* pseudorabies
　Aujeszky disease virus – a herpesvirus causing pseudorabies in swine. *SYN:* pseudorabies virus

Auspitz, Heinrich, Austrian dermatologist, 1835-1886.
　Auspitz dermatosis – *SYN:* Alibert-Bazin syndrome
　Auspitz sign – scratching or lifting of the scale over a psoriatic papule or plaque reveals pin-point bleeding; also may be observed in actinic keratosis and seborrheic keratosis.

Austin, James H., U.S. physician.
　Austin syndrome – autosomal recessive disorder whose clinical features include developmental delay during infancy, and mild ichthyosis and progressive neurological degeneration in the second or third year of life. *SYN:* juvenile sulfatidosis of Austin type
　juvenile sulfatidosis of Austin type – *SYN:* Austin syndrome

Austin Flint, see under Flint, Austin

Austin Moore, see under Moore, Austin Talley

Australia, a continent commonly referred to as "the land down under."
　Australian antigen – hepatitis B antigen first identified in serum of Australian aborigines.

NOTES

Australian Q fever – acute rickettsial infection transmitted by ticks and caused by Coxiella burnetii, most often found in Australian bandicoots.
Australian X disease – *SYN:* Murray Valley encephalitis
Australian X disease virus *–SYN:* Murray Valley virus
Australian X encephalitis – *SYN:* Murray Valley encephalitis

Austrian, Charles Robert, U.S. physician, 1885-1956.
Austrian reaction – intracutaneous test once used to diagnose typhus abdominalis.

Avellis, Georg, German laryngologist, 1864-1916.
Avellis syndrome – unilateral paralysis of the larynx and velum palati, with contralateral loss of pain and temperature sensibility in the parts below. *SYN:* jugular foramen syndrome

Avogadro, Amadeo, Italian physicist, 1776-1856.
Avogadro constant – *SYN:* Avogadro number
Avogadro hypothesis – *SYN:* Avogadro law
Avogadro law – equal volumes of gases contain equal numbers of molecules, the conditions of pressure and temperature being the same. *SYN:* Ampère postulate; Avogadro hypothesis; Avogadro postulate
Avogadro number – the number of molecules in one gram-molecular weight (1 mol) of any compound. *SYN:* Avogadro constant
Avogadro postulate – *SYN:* Avogadro law

Axelrod, Julius, joint winner of 1970 Nobel Prize for work related to neural transmitters.

Axenfeld, Karl Theodor Paul Polykarpus, German ophthalmologist, 1867-1930.
Morax-Axenfeld conjunctivitis – see under Morax
Morax-Axenfeld diplobacillus – *SYN: Moraxella lacunata*; see under Morax

Ayala, G., Italian neurologist, 1878-1943.
Ayala index – the cerebrospinal index when 10 ml of cerebrospinal fluid has been removed. *SYN:* Ayala quotient; spinal quotient
Ayala quotient – *SYN:* Ayala index

Ayer, James Bourne, U.S. neurologist, 1882-1963.
Ayer test – used with spinal block to test pressure in lumbar puncture.
Ayer-Tobey test
Tobey-Ayer test

Ayerza, Abel, Argentinian physician, 1861-1918.
Ayerza-Arrillaga disease – *SYN:* Ayerza syndrome

A

Ayerza disease – *SYN:* Ayerza syndrome

Ayerza syndrome – sclerosis of the pulmonary arteries in chronic cor pulmonale. *SYN:* Ayerza-Arrillaga disease; Ayerza disease; cardiopathia nigra; plexogenic pulmonary arteriopathy

Ayre, J. Ernest, U.S. gynecologist, *1910.

Ayre brush – a device for collecting gastric mucosal cells in cancer detection studies.

Ayurveda, "science of life" from ancient Vedic tradition of India.

Ayurvedic medicine – ancient science of natural medicine which promotes health of mind and body.

Azua, see under De Azua y Suarez, Juan

Azzopardi, John G., pathologist.

Azzopardi effect – deposition of DNA within vessel wall of oat cell carcinoma of the lung.

NOTES

Baader, Ernst, German physician.
　Baader dermatostomatitis – *SYN:* Stevens-Johnson syndrome

Baastrup, Christian Ingerslev, Danish physician, 1885-1950.
　Baastrup syndrome – compression of spinous processes related to various degenerative diseases. *SYN:* kissing osteophytes; kissing spine; Michotte syndrome

Babbitt, Isaac, U.S. inventor, 1799-1862.
　Babbitt metal – an alloy used occasionally in dentistry.

Babcock, Stephen Moulton, U.S. chemist, 1843-1931.
　Babcock tube – a tube in which milk, after treatment with sulfuric acid, is centrifuged and its fat content then determined in a graduated neck.

Babès, Victor, Romanian bacteriologist, 1854-1926.
　Babès-Ernst bodies – intracellular granules present in many species of bacteria, which possess a strong affinity for nuclear stains. *SYN:* Babès-Ernst granules; Ernst-Babès granules
　Babès-Ernst granules – *SYN:* Babès-Ernst bodies
　Babesia – a protozoan parasite.
　Babès nodes – collections of lymphocytes in the central nervous system found in rabies.
　Babès nodules – *SYN:* Babès tubercles
　Babès tubercles – cellular aggregations found around medulla oblongata and spinal ganglia in the presence of rabies or encephalitis. *SYN:* Babès nodules
　Ernst-Babès granules – *SYN:* Babès-Ernst bodies

Babington, B.G., English physician, 1794-1866.
　Babington disease – hereditary telangiectasia.

Babinski, Joseph François Félix, French neurologist, 1857-1932.
    Babinski-Nageotte syndrome – brain lesions resulting in Horner syndrome.
    Babinski phenomenon – *SYN:* Babinski sign (1)
    Babinski reflex – *SYN:* Babinski sign (1)
    Babinski sign – (1) extension of the great toe and abduction of the other toes instead of normal flexion reflex to plantar stimulation. *SYN:* Babinski phenomenon; Babinski reflex; Babinski test; (2) in hemiplegia, weakness of platysma muscle on affected side; (3) when patient is in supine position with hands crossed on chest and attempts to sit up, the thigh on the side of an organic paralysis is flexed and heel raised, whereas unaffected side remains flat; (4) in hemiplegia, the forearm on the affected side turns to a pronated position when placed in a position of supination.
    Babinski syndrome – the combination of cardiac, arterial, and central nervous system manifestations of tertiary syphilis.
    Babinski test – *SYN:* Babinski sign (1)

Babkin, Boris Petrovich, Russian neurologist, 1877-1950.
    Babkin reflex – congenital reflex of the newborn.

Baccelli, Guido, Italian physician, 1832-1916.
    Baccelli sign – an obsolete sign; good conduction of whisper in nonpurulent pleural effusions. *SYN:* aphonic pectoriloquy

Bachman, George W., U.S. parasitologist, *1890.
    Bachman-Pettit test – modification of the Kober test for the detection of estrogenic hormones in the urine.

Bachmann, Jean George, U.S. physiologist, 1877-1959.
    Bachmann bundle – division of the anterior internodal tract that continues into the left atrium, providing a specialized path for interatrial conduction.

Bacon, Harry E., U.S. proctologist, *1900.
    Bacon anoscope – an instrument resembling a rectal speculum, with a long slit on one side and an electric light opposite.
    Bacon proctoscope

Bacon, Sir Francis, English author and philosopher, 1561-1626.
    Bacon syndrome – syndrome based on Baconian principles that man exists to control nature, man and nature are enemies, and man intervenes and regulates nature through repetition and predictability. Physicians adhering to these principles destroy diseases without regard for danger to nature/environment.

Baddeley, Alan D., professor and memory specialist.
    Baddeley model – central processor in brain coordinates activity of two subsystems; also posits existence of phonological and visual/spatial memory.

Baehr, George, U.S. physician, 1887-1978.
    Baehr-Lohlein lesion – focal embolic glomerulonephritis occurring in bacterial endocarditis. *SYN:* Lohlein-Baehr lesion
    Baehr-Schiffrin disease – *SYN:* Moschcowitz syndrome
    Lohlein-Baehr lesion – *SYN:* Baehr-Lohlein lesion

Baelz, Erwin, German physician in Tokyo, 1849-1913.
    Baelz disease – an acquired disorder of unknown etiology of the lower lip characterized by swelling, ulceration, crusting, mucous gland hyperplasia, abscesses, and sinus tracts. *SYN:* cheilitis glandularis

Baer, Benjamin Franklin, U.S. obstetrician and surgeon, 1846-1920.
    Baer operation – simplified method for performing abdominal hysterectomy.

Baer, Karl Ernest von, German-Russian embryologist, 1792-1876.
    Baer law – concept of embryonic recapitulation.
    Baer vesicle – obsolete term for vesicular ovarian follicle.

Baeyer, Johann F.W.A. von, German chemist and Nobel laureate, 1835-1917.
    Baeyer theory – that carbon bonds are set at fixed angles and that those carbon rings are most stable that least distort those angles.

Bäfverstedt, Bo Erik, Swedish dermatologist, 1905-1990.
    Bäfverstedt ichthyosis – a form of ichthyosis hystrix.

Baggenstoss, Archie H., U.S. pathologist, *1908.
    Baggenstoss change – distention of pancreatic acini by proteinaceous secretion, seen in dehydration.

Baghdad, capital of Iraq.
    Baghdad boil – *SYN:* Alibert disease II

NOTES

Bagolini, B., 20th century Italian ophthalmologist.
Bagolini lens
Bagolini test – a test for retinal correspondence.

Bahima, "Hamitic" Bahima people of Uganda.
Bahima disease – disease seen in Africa; may be due to iron deficiency when cow's milk is the exclusive diet.

Bahnson, Henry T., U.S. cardiologist.
Bahnson aortic clamp

Bail, Oskar, German bacteriologist, hygienist, and immunologist, 1869-1927.
Bail phenomenon – rapid death within 6-18 hours due to hemorrhagic peritonitis with hypothermia.

Bailey, Charles, U.S. cardiac surgeon.
Bailey aortic clamp
Bailey aortic valve-cutting forceps
Bailey aortic valve rongeur
Bailey catheter

Baillarger, Jules Gabriel François, French neurologist, 1809-1890.
Baillarger bands – *SYN:* Baillarger lines
Baillarger lines – two laminae of white fibers that course parallel to the surface of the cerebral cortex. *SYN:* Baillarger bands
Baillarger sign – in cases of partial or incomplete paralysis, inequality of the pupils may occur.
Baillarger striae
Baillarger stripes
Baillarger syndrome

Bailliart, Paul, French ophthalmologist, 1877-1969.
Bailliart goniometer
Bailliart ophthalmodynamometer – an instrument used to measure the blood pressure of the central retinal artery.
Bailliart tonometer

Bainbridge, Francis A., English physiologist, 1874-1921.
Bainbridge clamp
Bainbridge hemostatic forceps
Bainbridge reflex – rise in right atrial pressure causing increased heart rate.
Bainbridge vessel clamp

Bairnsdale, Australian town.
Bairnsdale ulcer – infection due to *Mycobacterium*.

B

Baker, Henry A., U.S. surgeon, 1848-1934.
   Baker velum – cleft palate obturator.

Baker, James Porter, U.S. physician, *1902.
   Charcot-Weiss-Baker syndrome – see under Charcot

Baker, John Randal, English zoologist, *1900.
   Baker acid hematein – an acidic solution of oxidized hematoxylin used on frozen sections for staining phospholipids.
   Baker pyridine extraction – hot pyridine treatment of tissues fixed in dilute Bouin fixative.

Baker, Thomas J., U.S. dermatologist, *1925.
   Baker-Gordon formula – solution used for deep chemical peel.

Baker, William Marrent, English surgeon, 1839-1896.
   Baker cyst – a collection of synovial fluid seen in degenerative or other joint diseases.

Balbiani, Edouard G., French embryologist, 1823-1899.
   Balbiani rings – *SYN:* chromosome puffs

Baldwin, Ruth Workman, U.S. pediatrician, *1915.
   Bessman-Baldwin syndrome – see under Bessman

Baldy, John M., U.S. gynecologist, 1860-1934.
   Baldy operation – an obsolete operation for retrodisplacement of the uterus. *SYN:* Webster operation

Balestra, G., Italian physician.
   De Martini-Balestra syndrome – *SYN:* Burke syndrome

Balfour, Donald Church, Canadian-born surgeon, 1882-1963.
   Balfour retractor

Balint, Rudolph, Hungarian neurologist and psychiatrist, 1874-1929.
   Balint syndrome – an entity characterized by optic ataxia and simultanagnosia.

NOTES

Balkans, the countries of the Balkan Peninsula, which include Romania, Bulgaria, and Yugoslavia.

> **Balkan frame** – metal frame above a bed which provides for limb suspension, named for the Balkan wars, 1908-1913.
>
> **Balkan nephrectomy**
>
> **Balkan nephritis** – chronic progressive nephritis seen predominantly in Balkan countries.
>
> **Balkan nephropathy** – interstitial nephritis occurring in the Balkan countries.

Ball, Sir Charles, Irish surgeon, 1851-1916.

> **Ball operation** – division of the sensory nerve trunks supplying the anus, for relief of pruritus ani.

Ballance, Sir Charles Alfred, English surgeon, 1856-1936.

> **Ballance sign** – the presence of a dull percussion note in both flanks, constant on the left side but shifting with change of position on the right, said to indicate ruptured spleen; the dullness is due to the presence of blood, fluid on the right side but coagulated on the left.
>
> **Koerte-Ballance operation** – see under Koerte

Ballantyne, John William, English gynecologist, 1861-1923.

> **Ballantyne syndrome** – triad consisting of edema in the mother, fetal hydrops, and large placenta.

Baller, Friedrich, 20th century German physician.

> **Baller-Gerold syndrome** – autosomal recessive syndrome resulting in premature closing of skull sutures. *SYN:* Gerold-Baller syndrome
>
> **Gerold-Baller syndrome** – *SYN:* Baller-Gerold syndrome

Ballet, Gilbert, French neurologist, 1853-1916.

> **Ballet sign** – the appearance of partial or complete external ophthalmoplegia in Graves disease.

Ballingall, Sir George, English physician, 1780-1855.

> **Ballingall disease** – *SYN:* Madura foot

Balme, Paul Jean, French physician, *1857.

> **Balme cough** – nasopharyngeal obstruction causing coughing when patient lies down.

Balmoral, castle in Scotland.

> **Balmoral shoe** – a type of laced shoe.

Baló, Jozsef Matthias, Hungarian neurologist, *1896.

> **Baló disease** – encephalitis that is clinically similar to adrenoleukodystrophy, but pathologically characterized by concentric

globes or circles of demyelination of cerebral white matter separated by normal tissue. *SYN:* encephalitis periaxialis concentrica

Balser, Wilhelm August, German physician, d. 1892.
  Balser fatty necrosis – fat necrosis accompanying pancreatitis.

Baltic Sea, a sea in northern Europe.
  Baltic myeloma – autosomal recessive condition with onset between 8 and 13 years of age, characterized by myoclonic and generalized seizures, relatively frequent in the Baltic region, particularly Finland.

Baltimore, David, joint winner of 1975 Nobel Prize for work related to tumor viruses and cell material.

Bamatter, Frédéric, Swiss physician, 1899-1988.
  Bamatter syndrome – genetic trait causing birdlike facies, alopecia, premature dryness, and wrinkling of the skin in children after the first year of normal development. *SYN:* premature senility syndrome

Bamberger, Eugen von, Austrian physician, 1858-1921.
  Bamberger disease – chronic inflammation with effusions in several serous cavities resulting in fibrous thickening of serosa and constrictive pericarditis.
  Bamberger-Marie disease – *SYN:* Bamberger-Marie syndrome
  Bamberger-Marie syndrome – expansion of the distal ends, or the entire shafts, of the long bones that occurs in chronic pulmonary disease, heart disease, and other acute and chronic disorders. *SYN:* Bamberger-Marie disease; hypertrophic pulmonary osteoarthropathy
  Bamberger sign – jugular pulse in tricuspid insufficiency. *SYN:* allochiria

Bamberger, Heinrich von, Austrian physician, 1822-1888.
  Bamberger albuminuria – obsolete term for hematogenous albuminuria that is sometimes observed during the later phases of advanced anemia.
  Bamberger disease – a spasmodic affection of the muscles of the lower extremities.

NOTES

Bancroft, Sir Joseph, English physician in Australia, 1836-1894.
  Bancroft filariasis – nematode which lives in body tissues and cavities; upon death of adult worm, granulomatous inflammation and permanent fibrosis develop.

Bandl, Ludwig, German obstetrician, 1842-1892.
  Bandl obstetric ring – *SYN:* Bandl ring
  Bandl ring – a constriction of the uterus resulting from obstructed labor. *SYN:* Bandl obstetric ring; pathologic retraction ring

Banff, city in Alberta in the Canadian Rockies.
  Banff Classification – internationally accepted standard for assessment of renal allograft biopsies; first agreed upon at meeting in this city in 1991.

Bang, Bernhard L.F., Danish veterinarian and physician, 1848-1932.
  Bang bacillus – *SYN: Brucella abortus*
  Bang disease – a disease in cattle caused by *Brucella abortus. SYN:* bovine brucellosis

Banis, Joseph, U.S. physician.
  Acland-Banis arteriotomy clamp – see under Acland
  Banis forceps

Bankart, Arthur S.B., English surgeon, 1876-1951.
  Bankart dislocation
  Bankart lesion – related to shoulder dislocation.
  Bankart procedure – surgical repair of Bankart lesion.
  Bankart reconstruction
  Bankart repair
  Bankart retractor
  Bankart shoulder repair set

Bannister, Henry M., U.S. physician, 1844-1920.
  Bannister disease – recurrent large circumscribed areas of subcutaneous edema, frequently an allergic reaction to foods or drugs. *SYN:* angioedema

Bannwarth, Alfred, German neurologist, 1903-1970.
  Bannwarth syndrome – neurologic manifestations of Lyme disease.

Banti, Guido, Italian physician, 1852-1925.
  Banti disease – *SYN:* Banti syndrome
  Banti syndrome – chronic congestive splenomegaly occurring primarily in children as a sequel to hypertension in the portal or splenic veins. *SYN:* Banti disease; splenic anemia

Banting, Sir Frederick G., Canadian physician, 1891-1941, co-winner of the 1923 Nobel Prize for isolating insulin from the pancreas.

Banting, William, English carpenter, 1796-1878.
   Banting diet – diet high in fats and protein and low in refined carbohydrates, successfully used by Banting in 1862.

Bar, Paul, French obstetrician, 1853-1945.
   Bar incision

Baraitser, M., 20th century English pediatrician.
   Baraitser syndrome I – rare autosomal recessive disorder presenting with total scalp alopecia, absent eyelash and eyebrows, and mental retardation.
   Baraitser syndrome II – rare disorder presenting with low birth weight, short stature, mental retardation, multiple pigmented nevi, and birdlike facies. Lack of facial subcutaneous fat gives appearance of premature aging.

Bárány, Robert, Austrian-Hungarian otologist and Nobel laureate, 1876-1936.
   Bárány alarm apparatus
   Bárány apparatus
   Bárány box
   Bárány caloric test – a test for vestibular function. *SYN:* caloric test; nystagmus test
   Bárány chair
   Bárány noise apparatus
   Bárány noise apparatus whistle
   Bárány sign – nystagmus induced by injecting either hot or cold water into the external ear canal in the caloric test.
   Bárány syndrome – the direction of a fall is influenced by changing head position in the presence of equilibrium disturbance.
   Bárány test
   positional vertigo of Bárány – brief attacks of paroxysmal vertigo and nystagmus due to labyrinthine dysfunction. *SYN:* benign positional vertigo

NOTES

Barbeau, Andre, Canadian physician.
　Giroux-Barbeau syndrome – see under Giroux

Barber, Glenn, 20th century U.S. orthopedic surgeon.
　Blount-Barber disease – *SYN:* Blount disease

Barber, Harold W., English dermatologist, 1886-1955.
　Barber psoriasis

Barclay, Alfred E., English physician, 1877-1949.
　Barclay-Baron disease – dysphagia caused by food becoming lodged
　above the epiglottis. *SYN:* vallecular dysphagia

Barcroft, Sir Joseph F., English physiologist, 1872-1947.
　Barcroft-Warburg apparatus – *SYN:* Warburg apparatus
　Barcroft-Warburg technique – *SYN:* Warburg apparatus

Bard, Louis, French physician, 1857-1930.
　Bard sign – eye oscillations related to nystagmus.

Bard, Philip, U.S. physiologist, 1898-1945.
　Cannon-Bard theory – see under Cannon, Walter B.

Bardet, Georges, French physician, *1885.
　Bardet-Biedl syndrome – mental retardation, pigmentary retinopathy,
　polydactyly, obesity, and hypogenitalism.

Bardinet, Barthélemy A., French physician, 1809-1874.
　Bardinet ligament – the posterior band of the ulnar collateral ligament of
　the elbow.

Barkan, Otto, U.S. ophthalmologist, 1887-1958.
　Barkan cyclodialysis
　Barkan forceps
　Barkan goniolens
　Barkan gonioscope
　Barkan illuminator
　Barkan implant
　Barkan iris forceps
　Barkan knife
　Barkan lens
　Barkan operation – goniotomy for congenital glaucoma under direct
　observation of the anterior chamber angle.
　Barkan scissors

Barkman, Åke, 20th century Swedish internist.
　Barkman reflex – contraction of the ipsilateral rectus muscle in response to a stimulus applied to the skin below a nipple.

Barkow, Hans K.L., German anatomist, 1798-1873.
　Barkow ligaments – the anterior and posterior portions of the fibrous capsule of the elbow joint.

Barlow, John, 20th century South African cardiologist.
　Barlow syndrome – late apical systolic murmur or (so-called "mid-late") systolic click, or both, due to massive billowing of the anterior and/or posterior (mural) mitral valvular leaflet into the left atrial cavity.

Barlow, Sir Thomas, English physician, 1845-1945.
　Barlow disease – a cachectic condition in infants, resulting from malnutrition. *SYN:* infantile scurvy

Barnard, Christiaan, South African surgeon who performed first successful heart transplant in 1967.

Barnard, William George, English physician, *1892.
　Barnard carcinoma – metastatic tumor of the mediastinum, pericardium, lung hilum, and bronchus. *SYN:* oat cell carcinoma

Barnes, Robert, English obstetrician, 1817-1907.
　Barnes curve – a curve corresponding in general with Carus curve, being the segment of a circle whose center is the promontory of the sacrum.
　Barnes zone – the lower fourth of the pregnant uterus, attachment of the placenta to any part of which may cause dangerous hemorrhage. *SYN:* cervical zone

Barr, Murray Liewellyn, Canadian microanatomist, *1908.
　Barr body – *SYN:* Barr chromatin body
　Barr chromatin body – a small condensed mass of the inactivated X-chromosome usually located just inside the nuclear membrane of the interphase nucleus. *SYN:* Barr body; sex chromatin

NOTES

Barr, Yvonne M., English virologist, *1932.
Epstein-Barr virus – see under Epstein, Michael Anthony

Barraquer, Hignacio, Spanish ophthalmologist, 1884-1965.
Barraquer ciliary forceps
Barraquer corneal forceps
Barraquer hemostatic mosquito forceps
Barraquer irrigator spatula
Barraquer keratoplasty knife
Barraquer method – dissolution of the zonula ciliaris by enzymes
(α-chymotrypsin) to facilitate surgical removal of a cataract. *SYN:* zonulolysis
Barraquer microkeratome
Barraquer needle carrier
Barraquer shield

Barraquer Roviralta, Luis, Spanish physician, 1855-1928.
Barraquer disease – a condition characterized by a complete loss of the
subcutaneous fat of the upper part of the torso, the arms, neck, and
face. *SYN:* Barraquer-Simons disease; progressive lipodystrophy; Simons
disease
Barraquer-Simons disease – *SYN:* Barraquer disease

Barré, Jean A., French neurologist, 1880-1971.
Barré sign – a hemiplegic placed in the prone position with the limbs
flexed at the knees is unable to maintain the flexed position on the side
of the lesion but extends the leg.
Barré-Liéou syndrome – irritation of a nerve plexus around a vertebral
artery produces symptoms of dizziness, headache, tinnitus.
SYN: Liéou-Barré syndrome
Guillain-Barré reflex – see under Guillain
Guillain-Barré syndrome – see under Guillain
Landry-Guillain-Barré syndrome – *SYN:* Landry syndrome
Liéou-Barré syndrome – *SYN:* Barré-Liéou syndrome

Barrett, Norman Rupert, English surgeon, 1903-1979.
adenocarcinoma in Barrett esophagus – an adenocarcinoma arising in
the lower third of the esophagus that has become columnar cell lined
(Barrett mucosa) due to gastroesophageal reflux.
Barrett epithelium – columnar esophageal epithelium seen in Barrett
syndrome.
Barrett esophagus – chronic peptic ulceration of the lower esophagus
acquired as a result of long-standing chronic esophagitis. *SYN:* Barrett
syndrome; Barrett ulcer

Barrett syndrome – *SYN:* Barrett esophagus
Barrett ulcer – *SYN:* Barrett esophagus
Eagle-Barrett syndrome – *SYN:* prune belly syndrome

Barrière, Henri, French physician.
Bureau-Barrière syndrome – see under Bureau
Bureau-Barrière-Thomas syndrome – see under Bureau

Bart, nickname of St. Bartholomew's Hospital in London, England.
Bart hemoglobin – abnormal hemoglobin with affinity for oxygen; named for hospital where this hemoglobin was first isolated in a patient.

Bart, Bruce Joseph, U.S. dermatologist, *1936.
Bart syndrome – autosomal dominant trait resulting in extremity blistering, mouth erosions, and deformed nails, often with spontaneous improvement and no residual scarring.

Bart, Robert S., U.S. dermatologist, *1933.
Bart-Pumphrey syndrome – an autosomal dominant syndrome consisting of knuckle pads, leukonychia, and mixed sensorineural and conductive deafness. *SYN:* knuckle pads, leukonychia, and sensorineural deafness

Bartenwerfer, Kurt, German physician, 1892-1942.
Bartenwerfer syndrome – a form of dwarfism.

Barth, Jean, French physician, 1806-1877.
Barth hernia – a loop of intestine between a persistent vitelline duct and the abdominal wall.

Barthel, D.W., 20th century U.S. physiatrist.
Barthel ADL score – *SYN:* Barthel index
Barthel index – assessment tool which uses standardized classifications to determine level of function for skills such as mobility and activities of daily living. *SYN:* Barthel ADL score

NOTES

Barthélemy, P. Toussaint, French dermatologist, 1850-1906.

Barthélemy disease – a tuberculid reaction characterized by symmetrical eruption of papulonecrotic lesions on the face, hands, and trunk. *SYN:* acne agminata; acne scrofulosorum; nodular tuberculid

Bartholin, Casper, Danish anatomist, 1655-1738.

Bartholin abscess – an abscess of the vulvovaginal gland.

Bartholin cyst – a cyst arising from the major vestibular gland or its ducts.

Bartholin cystectomy – removal of a cyst of a major vestibular gland. *SYN:* vulvovaginal cystectomy

Bartholin duct – the duct that drains the anterior portion of the sublingual gland. *SYN:* major sublingual duct

Bartholin gland – one of two mucoid-secreting tubuloalveolar glands on either side of the lower part of the vagina. *SYN:* greater vestibular gland

Bartholin, Thomas, Danish anatomist, 1616-1680.

Bartholin anus – entrance to the cerebral aqueduct (of Sylvius) from the caudal part of the third ventricle. *SYN:* anus cerebri

Bartholin-Patau syndrome – *SYN:* Patau syndrome

Bartley, Samuel H., U.S. psychologist, *1901.

Brücke-Bartley phenomenon – see under Brücke

Barton, Alberto Leopaldo, Peruvian physician, 1871-1950.

Bartonella – bacterium transmitted by Andean sandflies, causing bartonellosis.

bartonellosis – infection with *Bartonella bacilliformis* causing acute febrile illness followed by benign skin eruptions.

Barton, John Rhea, U.S. surgeon, 1794-1871.

Barton bandage – a figure-of-eight bandage supporting the mandible below and anteriorly.

Barton blade

Barton dressing

Barton forceps – obstetrical forceps with one fixed curved blade and a hinged anterior blade for application to a high transverse head.

Barton fracture – fracture of the distal radius with dislocation of the radiocarpal joint.

Barton hook

Barton operation

Barton sling

Barton tongs

Barton traction handle

Bärtschi-Rochaix, Werner, Swiss physician, *1911.

    Bärtschi-Rochaix syndrome – a complex of symptoms resulting from traumatic compression of the cerebral artery. *SYN:* cervical vertigo syndrome; vertebral artery compression syndrome

Bartsocas, Christos S., Greek physician.

    Bartsocas-Papas syndrome – severe autosomal recessive trait causing bone abnormalities, microcephaly, facial abnormalities.

Bartter, Frederic Crosby, U.S. physician, 1914-1983.

    Bartter syndrome – primary juxtaglomerular cell hyperplasia with secondary hyperaldosteronism, reported in children with hypokalemic alkalosis and elevated renin or angiotensin levels.

    Schwartz-Bartter syndrome – see under Schwartz, William

Baruch, Simon, U.S. physician, 1840-1921.

    Baruch law – the effect of any hydriatric procedure is in direct proportion to the difference between the temperature of the water and that of the skin.

Basan, Marianne, 20th century German dermatologist.

    Basan syndrome – autosomal dominant ectodermal dysplasia with hypohidrosis and dryness of the skin and mucosa, dental caries, sparse body hair, and thick, short nails.

Basedow, Karl Adolph von, German physician, 1799-1854.

    Basedow disease – *SYN:* Graves disease; thyrotoxicosis

    Basedow goiter – colloid goiter which becomes hyperfunctional after the ingestion of excess iodine, causing Jod-Basedow phenomenon.

    Basedow pseudoparaplegia – weakness of the thigh muscles in thyrotoxicosis.

    Basedow syndrome – myeloneuropathy seen in the presence of thyrotoxicosis.

    Jod-Basedow phenomenon – induction of thyrotoxicosis in a previously euthyroid individual as a result of exposure to large quantities of iodine. *SYN:* iodine-induced hyperthyroidism

NOTES

Bass, Harold N.
  Bass syndrome – autosomal dominant disorder featuring abnormalities of fingers and toes.

Bassen, Frank A., U.S. physician, *1903.
  Bassen-Kornzweig disease – *SYN:* Bassen-Kornzweig syndrome
  Bassen-Kornzweig syndrome – autosomal recessive trait causing retinal pigmentary degeneration, malabsorption, engorgement of upper intestinal absorptive cells with dietary triglycerides, and neuromuscular abnormalities. *SYN:* abetalipoproteinemia; Bassen-Kornzweig disease

Basset, Antoine, French surgeon, 1882-1951.
  Basset operation – dissection of inguinal glands during surgery for vulvar cancer.

Bassini, Edoardo, Italian surgeon, 1844-1924.
  Bassini herniorrhaphy
  Bassini operation – an operation for an inguinal hernia repair.

Bassler, Anthony, U.S. physician, 1874-1959.
  Bassler sign – in chronic appendicitis, pinching the appendix between the thumb and the iliacus muscle causes sharp pain.

Bastedo, Walter A., U.S. physician, 1873-1952.
  Bastedo sign – an obsolete sign; in chronic appendicitis, pain and tenderness in the right iliac fossa on inflation of the colon with air.

Bastian, Henry Charlton, English neurologist, 1837-1915.
  Bastian aphasia – *SYN:* Wernicke aphasia
  Bastian-Bruns law – deep-reflex loss in lower limbs due to disruption of spinal cord above lumbar enlargement. *SYN:* Bastian-Bruns sign
  Bastian-Bruns sign – *SYN:* Bastian-Bruns law

Bateman, Thomas, English dermatologist, 1778-1821.
  Bateman disease – infectious disease of the skin caused by a member of the pox virus.
  Bateman purpura – purpura caused by lack of support of blood vessels secondary to old age. Can also be caused by corticosteroid therapy.

Batson, Oscar V., U.S. otolaryngologist, 1894-1979.
  Batson plexus – any of four interconnected venous networks surrounding the vertebral column. *SYN:* vertebral venous system
  Carmody-Batson operation – see under Carmody

Batten, Frederick Eustace, English ophthalmologist, 1865-1918.
    Batten disease – cerebral sphingolipidosis, late infantile and juvenile types. *SYN:* Batten-Mayou disease; Spielmeyer-Stock disease; Spielmeyer-Vogt disease; Vogt-Spielmeyer disease
    Batten-Mayou disease – *SYN:* Batten disease
    Curschmann-Batten-Steinert syndrome – see under Curschmann

Battey, a state hospital in Georgia, USA.
    Battey bacillus – mycobacterium causing lung disease similar to tuberculosis; first isolated at Battey State Hospital in Georgia.
    Battey-type mycobacteriosis

Battle, William H., English surgeon, 1855-1936.
    Battle incision
    Battle operation
    Battle sign – postauricular ecchymosis in cases of fracture of the base of the skull.

Baudelocque, Jean L., French obstetrician, 1746-1810.
    Baudelocque diameter – the distance in a straight line between the depression under the last spinous process of the lumbar vertebrae and the upper edge of the pubic symphysis. *SYN:* external conjugate
    Baudelocque uterine circle – a constriction of the uterus resulting from obstructed labor, one of the classic signs of threatened rupture of the uterus. *SYN:* pathologic retraction ring

Baudelocque, Louis A., French obstetrician, 1800-1864.
    Baudelocque operation – an incision through the posterior cul-de-sac of the vagina for the removal of the ovum, in extrauterine pregnancy.

Bauer, Hans, 20th century German anatomist.
    Bauer chromic acid leucofuchsin stain – a stain for glycogen and fungi.

Bauer, Walter, U.S. internist, *1898.
    Bauer reaction

NOTES

Bauer syndrome – aortitis and aortic endocarditis as a little recognized manifestation of rheumatoid arthritis.

Baughman, Fred A., U.S. neurologist.
> **Baughman syndrome** – an autosomal recessive syndrome characterized by curly hair and hypoplastic nails with congenital ankyloblepharon (fusion of eyelids). *SYN:* curly hair, ankyloblepharon, nail dysplasia syndrome (CHANDS)

Bauhin, Gaspard, Swiss anatomist, 1560-1624.
> **Bauhin gland** – one of the small mixed glands deeply placed near the apex of the tongue on each side of the frenulum. *SYN:* anterior lingual gland
> **Bauhin valve** – *SYN:* ileocecal valve

Baumé, Antoine, French chemist and pharmacist, 1728-1805.
> **Baumé scale** – a hydrometer scale for determining the specific gravity of liquids.

Baumgarten, Paul Clemens von, German pathologist, 1848-1928.
> **Baumgarten glands** – *SYN:* Henle glands
> **Baumgarten veins** – nonobliterated remnants of the vena umbilicalis.
> **Cruveilhier-Baumgarten disease** – *SYN:* Cruveilhier-Baumgarten syndrome
> **Cruveilhier-Baumgarten murmur** – see under Cruveilhier
> **Cruveilhier-Baumgarten sign** – see under Cruveilhier
> **Cruveilhier-Baumgarten syndrome** – see under Cruveilhier

Bayer, Joseph F., U.S. physician.
> **Braun-Bayer syndrome** – see under Braun, Frederick C., Jr.

Bayes, Thomas, English mathematician, 1702-1761.
> **Bayes theorem** – to determine the impact of new data on the evidential merits of competing scientific hypotheses.

Bayle, Antoine L.J., French physician, 1799-1858.
> **Bayle disease** – a disease of the brain, syphilitic in origin.

Bayle, Gaspard Laurent, French physician, 1774-1816.
> **Bayle granulations** – tubercular lung nodules.

Bayley, Nancy, U.S. psychologist, *1899.
> **Bayley Scales of Infant Development** – a psychological test used to measure the developmental progress of infants.

Bayliss, William M., English physiologist, 1860-1924.
  Bayliss theory – distention of a vessel results in vasomotor constriction
    which results in hypertrophy of muscle if constriction is sustained.

bayou, swampy, sluggishly moving inlet found predominantly in Louisiana and
Mississippi.
  Bayou virus – a form of hantavirus carried by the rice rat, found in
    Louisiana and Texas, causing human hantavirus pulmonary syndrome.

B

Bazett, Henry, English cardiologist, *1885.
  Bazett formula – used for correcting the observed Q-T interval in the
    electrocardiogram for cardiac rate.

Bazex, A., 20th century French physician.
  Bazex syndrome – lesions of an eczematous or psoriatic nature seen in
    patients with upper respiratory tract or digestive tract carcinomas. *SYN:*
    paraneoplastic acrokeratosis

Bazex, J., 20th century French dermatologist.
  Bazex syndrome I – congenital disorder with generalized telangiectasia,
    alopecia and multiple abnormalities.

Bazin, Antoine Pierre Ernest, French dermatologist, 1807-1878.
  Bazin disease – recurrent, hard, subcutaneous nodules that frequently
    break down and form necrotic ulcers, usually on the calves; lesions are
    sterile and probably a form of nodular vasculitis. *SYN:* erythema
    induratum; nodular tuberculid

Beadle, George Wells, joint winner of 1958 Nobel Prize for work related to
genetics.

Beale, Lionel S., English physician, 1828-1906.
  Beale cell – a bipolar ganglion cell of the heart with one spiral and one
    straight prolongation.

Beals, Rodney Kenneth, U.S. orthopedic surgeon, *1931.
  Beals syndrome – congenital condition resulting in abnormally long hands
    and fingers and often feet and toes. *SYN:* arachnodactyly

NOTES

Bean, William Bennett, U.S. physician born in Philippines, 1909-1989.
Bean syndrome – multiple cutaneous venous malformations that present as soft, compressible, blue nodules, which may be painful. *SYN:* blue rubber bleb nevus syndrome

Beard, George Miller, U.S. physician, 1839-1883.
Beard disease – *SYN:* Beard syndrome
Beard syndrome – may be associated with chronic fatigue syndrome. *SYN:* Beard disease; nervous exhaustion
Beard test

Beare, John Martin, English dermatologist, 1920-1998.
Beare syndrome – an autosomal dominant syndrome characterized by mental retardation, twisted hair, sparse body hair, and fragile nails.

Bearn, Alexander Gordon, English-U.S. physician, 1923-1983.
Bearn-Kunkel-Slater syndrome – *SYN:* Bearn-Kunkel syndrome
Bearn-Kunkel syndrome – lupoid hepatitis. *SYN:* Bearn-Kunkel-Slater syndrome; Kunkel syndrome

Beau, Joseph H.S., French physician, 1806-1865.
Beau lines – transverse depressions on the fingernails following severe febrile disease, malnutrition, trauma, myocardial infarction, etc.
Beau syndrome – cardiac insufficiency.

Bechterew, var. of Bekhterev

Beck, var. of Bek

Beck, Carl, U.S. surgeon, 1856-1911.
Beck gastrostomy
Beck gastrostomy scoop

Beck, Claude Schaeffer, U.S. surgeon, 1894-1971.
Beck triad – the rising venous pressure, falling arterial pressure, and decreased heart sounds of pericardial tamponade. *SYN:* acute compression triad

Beck, Emil G., U.S. surgeon, 1866-1932.
Beck method – a permanent opening into the stomach made from its greater curvature.

Beck, Soma Cornelius, German physician, 1872-1930.
Beck disease – *SYN:* Beck-Ibrahim syndrome
Beck-Ibrahim syndrome – an erythematous eruption of the perineal and perigenital regions of newborns, with multiple pustules filled with

Candida albicans. *SYN:* Beck disease; candidiasis; cutaneous anergy; Ibrahim disease; moniliasis

Becker, J.P.
   Becker disease – an obscure South African cardiomyopathy leading to rapidly fatal congestive heart failure and idiopathic mural endomyocardial disease.

Becker, Peter Emil, German geneticist, *1908.
   Becker muscular dystrophy – a muscular dystrophy that has many of the clinical features of Duchenne muscular dystrophy. *SYN:* adult pseudohypertrophic muscular dystrophy; Becker-type tardive muscular dystrophy
   Becker-type tardive muscular dystrophy – *SYN:* Becker muscular dystrophy

Becker, Samuel W., U.S. dermatologist, 1894-1964.
   Becker nevus – a nevus first seen as an irregular pigmentation of the shoulders, upper chest, or scapular area, gradually enlarging irregularly and becoming thickened and hairy. *SYN:* pigmented hair epidermal nevus

Beckmann, Ernst O., German chemist, 1853-1923.
   Beckmann apparatus – apparatus for the accurate measurement of melting points and boiling points in connection with molecular weight determinations.
   Beckmann thermometer

Beckwith, John Bruce, U.S. pediatric pathologist, *1933.
   Beckwith syndrome – *SYN:* Beckwith-Wiedemann syndrome
   Beckwith-Wiedemann syndrome – exomphalos, macroglossia, and gigantism, often with neonatal hypoglycemia; autosomal recessive inheritance. *SYN:* Beckwith syndrome; EMG syndrome

Béclard, Pierre A., French anatomist, 1785-1825.
   Béclard anastomosis – an anastomosis between the right and the left end-branch of the deep lingual artery. *SYN:* arcus raninus

NOTES

Béclard hernia – a hernia through the opening for the saphenous vein.

Béclard triangle – area bounded by the posterior border of the hyoglossus muscle, the posterior belly of the digastric and the greater horn of the hyoid bone.

Becquerel, Antoine H., French physicist and Nobel laureate, 1852-1908.
becquerel – the SI unit of measurement of radioactivity.
Becquerel rays – obsolete term for radiation given off by uranium and other radioactive substances.

Bednar, Alois, Austrian physician, 1816-1888.
Bednar aphthae – traumatic ulcers located bilaterally on either side of the midpalatal raphe in infants.
Bednar-Parrot syndrome – *SYN:* Parrot I syndrome

Bednar, Blahoslav, 20th century Czech pathologist.
Bednar tumor – an uncommon variant of dermatofibrosarcoma protuberans containing heavily pigmented dendritic melanocytes scattered between spindle cells of the tumor. *SYN:* pigmented dermatofibrosarcoma protuberans

Beemer, Frits A., Dutch physician.
Beemer syndrome – syndrome characterized by ascites and hydrops, dwarfing abnormalities, malrotation of intestine. *SYN:* short rib syndrome, Beemer type
short rib syndrome, Beemer type – *SYN:* Beemer syndrome

Beer, August, German physicist, 1825-1863.
Beer-Lambert law – the absorbance of light is directly proportional to the thickness of the ligand through which the light is being transmitted multiplied by the concentration of absorbing chromophore.
Beer law – the intensity of a color or of a light ray is inversely proportional to the depth of liquid through which it is transmitted.

Beer, Georg Joseph, Austrian ophthalmologist, 1763-1821.
Beer canaliculus knife
Beer cataract flap operation
Beer cataract knife
Beer cilia forceps
Beer knife – a triangular knife with a sharp point and one sharp edge, formerly used for incision for cataract.

Beevor, Charles E., English neurologist, 1854-1908.
Beevor phenomenon

Beevor sign – with paralysis of the lower portions of the recti abdominis muscles, the umbilicus moves upward.

Begbie, James, Scottish physician, 1798-1869.
Begbie disease – localized chorea.

Begg, P. Raymond, Australian orthodontist, *1898.
Begg appliance
Begg light wire differential force technique
Begg paralleling
Begg slots
Begg straight-wire combination bracket
Begg technique
Begg theory
Begg torquing

Béguez César, Antonio, 20th century Cuban pediatrician.
Béguez César disease – *SYN:* Chédiak-Steinbrinck-Higashi syndrome

Behçet, Hulusi, Turkish dermatologist, 1889-1948.
Adamantiades-Behçet syndrome – *SYN:* Behçet syndrome
Behçet disease – *SYN:* Behçet syndrome
Behçet syndrome – severe uveitis with ulceration of mouth and genitalia. *SYN:* Adamantiades-Behçet syndrome; Behçet disease; cutaneomucouveal syndrome; iridocyclitis septica; recurrent hypopyon; triple symptom complex

Behn-Eschenburg, H., German psychologist.
Behn-Rorschach Test – alternative to standard Rorschach test.

Behr, Carl, German ophthalmologist, 1874-1943.
Behr disease – adult or presenile form of heredomacular degeneration. *SYN:* Behr syndrome
Behr syndrome – *SYN:* Behr disease

Behring, Emil A. von, German bacteriologist and Nobel laureate, 1854-1917.
   Behring law – parenteral administration of serum from an immunized
   person provides a relative, passive immunity to that disease.

Beigel, Hermann, German physician, 1830-1879.
   Beigel disease – fungal disease which affects hair shafts. *SYN:* tinea
   nodosa

Bek, (Beck), E.V.V., Russian physician.
   Kashin-Bek disease – see under Kashin

Békésy, Georg von, Hungarian biophysicist in U.S. and Nobel laureate,
1899-1972.
   Békésy audiometer – an automatic audiometer.
   Békésy audiometry – automatic audiometry.

Bekhterev, (Bechterew), Vladimir M., Russian neurologist, 1857-1927.
   band of Kaes-Bekhterev – see under Kaes
   Bekhterev band – *SYN:* band of Kaes-Bekhterev
   Bekhterev disease – arthritis and osteitis deformans involving the spinal
   column. *SYN:* spondylitis deformans
   Bekhterev-Mendel reflex – percussion of the dorsum of the foot causes
   flexion of the toes in a pyramidal lesion. *SYN:* dorsum pedis reflex;
   Mendel-Bekhterev reflex
   Bekhterev nucleus – one of the nuclei raphes. *SYN:* nucleus centralis
   tegmenti superior
   Bekhterev sign – paralysis of automatic facial movements, the power of
   voluntary movement being retained.
   layer of Bekhterev – *SYN:* band of Kaes-Bekhterev
   line of Bekhterev – *SYN:* band of Kaes-Bekhterev
   Mendel-Bekhterev reflex – *SYN:* Bekhterev-Mendel reflex

Bell, John, Scottish surgeon and anatomist, 1763-1820.
   Bell muscle – a band of muscular fibers forming a slight fold in the wall of
   the bladder.

Bell, Julia, English scientist, *1879.
   Bell brachydactyly – abnormal shortness of digits on hands and feet.

Bell, Luther Vose, U.S. physician, 1806-1862.
   Bell delirium – *SYN:* Bell mania
   Bell disease – *SYN:* Bell mania
   Bell mania – syndrome characterized by delusions, hallucinations,
   hyperactivity, and frequent fevers, similar to symptoms of schizophrenia,
   but now attributed to encephalopathy. *SYN:* Bell delirium; Bell disease

Bell, Sir Charles, Scottish surgeon, anatomist, and physiologist, 1774-1842.
  Bell law – the ventral spinal roots are motor, the dorsal are sensory. *SYN:* Bell-Magendie law; Magendie law
  Bell-Magendie law – *SYN:* Bell law
  Bell palsy – paresis or paralysis, usually unilateral, of the facial muscles, caused by dysfunction of the 7th cranial nerve. *SYN:* peripheral facial paralysis
  Bell phenomenon – upward movement of the eye on attempted eyelid closure in a patient with peripheral facial paralysis.
  Bell respiratory nerve – *SYN:* long thoracic nerve
  Bell spasm – involuntary twitching of the facial muscles. *SYN:* facial tic
  external respiratory nerve of Bell – *SYN:* long thoracic nerve

Bellini, Lorenzo, Italian physician and anatomist, 1643-1704.
  Bellini ducts – the largest straight excretory ducts in the kidney medulla and papillae whose openings form the area cribrosa. *SYN:* papillary ducts
  Bellini ligament – a fasciculus from the ischiofemoral portion of the articular fibrous capsule of the hip which extends to the greater trochanter.
  Bellini tubules

Belsey, Ronald, 20th century English surgeon.
  Belsey antireflux operation
  Belsey esophagoplasty
  Belsey herniorrhaphy
  Belsey hiatal hernia repair
  Belsey Mark II fundoplication
  Belsey Mark IV operation – a transthoracic antireflux procedure.
  Belsey Mark IV procedure – a transthoracic hiatal hernia repair that restores the lower esophageal sphincter zone to the high pressure region below the diaphragm.
  Belsey Mark V procedure – a modified Belsey Mark IV procedure.
  Belsey perfusor

NOTES

Benacerraf, Baruj, joint winner of 1980 Nobel Prize for work related to cell structures and regulation of immunological reactions.

Bence Jones, Henry, English physician, 1814-1873.

Bence Jones albumin

Bence Jones cylinders – slightly irregular, relatively smooth, rod-shaped or cylindroid bodies of fairly tenacious, viscid proteinaceous material in the fluid of the seminal vesicles.

Bence Jones myeloma – multiple myeloma in which the malignant plasma cells excrete only light chains of one type (either kappa or lambda). *SYN:* L-chain disease; L-chain myeloma

Bence Jones proteins – proteins with unusual thermosolubility found in the urine of patients with multiple myeloma, consisting of monoclonal immunoglobulin light chains.

Bence Jones reaction – the classic means of identifying Bence Jones protein.

Bence Jones test

Bencze, J., Hungarian physician.

Bencze syndrome – syndrome characterized by cleft palate, amblyopia, esotropia, hemifacial hyperplasia. *SYN:* hemifacial hyperplasia with strabismus

Bender, Lauretta, U.S. psychiatrist, 1897-1987.

Bender gestalt test – a psychological test used for measuring visuospatial and visuomotor coordination to detect brain damage. *SYN:* Bender Visual Motor Gestalt test

Bender Visual Motor Gestalt test – *SYN:* Bender gestalt test

Benedek, Ladislaus (László), Austrian neurologist, 1887-1945.

Benedek reflex – plantar flexion of the foot by tapping the anterior margin of the lower part of the fibula, while the foot is slightly dorsiflexed.

Benedict, Francis Gano, U.S. chemist, 1870-1957.

Benedict-Roth apparatus – a device to measure the amount of oxygen utilized in quiet breathing for the estimation of the basal metabolic rate.

Benedict-Roth calorimeter

Benedict, Stanley R., U.S. chemist, 1884-1936.

Benedict-Hopkins-Cole reagent – magnesium glyoxalate, made from a mixture of oxalic acid and magnesium, used for testing proteins for the presence of tryptophan.

Benedict solution – used to demonstrate a reducing sugar such as glucose in the urine.

Benedict test for glucose – a copper reduction test for glucose in the urine.

Benedikt, Moritz, Austrian physician, 1835-1920.
Benedikt syndrome – hemiplegia with clonic spasm or tremor and oculomotor paralysis on the opposite side.

Benjamin, E., German pediatrician.
Benjamin pediatric operating laryngoscope
Benjamin syndrome – genetic trait resulting in hypochromic anemia and other abnormalities: megalocephaly, carious lesions, cardiac murmur, splenic tumors.

Bennett, Edward H., Irish surgeon, 1837-1907.
Bennett fracture – fracture dislocation of the first metacarpal bone at the carpometacarpal joint.
Bennett lesion
Bennett nail biopsy
Bennett posterior shoulder approach
Bennett retractor

Bennett, George Kettner, U.S. psychologist, *1904.
Bennett Differential Aptitude Test – aptitude test administered to children in grades 8 through 12.

Bennett, John Hughes, English physician, 1812-1875.
Bennett disease – disease characterized by progressive proliferation of abnormal leukocytes found in hemopoietic tissues, other organs, and usually in the blood in increased numbers; often fatal. *SYN:* leukemia

Bennett, Norman G., English dentist, 1870-1947.
Bennett angle – the angle formed by the sagittal plane and the path of the advancing condyle during lateral mandibular movement as viewed in the horizontal plane.
Bennett movement – the bodily lateral movement or lateral shift of the mandible during a laterotrusive movement.

NOTES

Bennhold, H., German physician, *1893.
   Bennhold Congo red stain – a stain for amyloid detection in pathologic tissue.

Bensaude, Raoul, French physician.
   Launois-Bensaude syndrome – see under Launois

Bensley, Robert R., U.S.-Canadian anatomist, 1867-1956.
   Bensley osmic dichromate fluid
   Bensley specific granules – granules in the cells of the islets of Langerhans in the pancreas.

Benson, Alfred Hugh, Irish ophthalmologist, 1852-1912.
   Benson disease – small spherical bodies in corpus vitreum, a unilateral age change which does not affect vision. *SYN:* asteroid hyalosis

Benton, Arthur Lester, U.S. psychologist, *1909.
   Benton Visual Retention Test – test of ability to reproduce geometric designs from memory.

Bérard, Auguste, French surgeon, 1802-1846.
   Bérard aneurysm – an arteriovenous aneurysm in the tissues outside the injured vein.

Berardinelli, Waldemar, Argentinian physician, 1903-1956.
   Berardinelli syndrome – accelerated growth, lipodystrophy with muscular hypertrophy, hepatomegaly, and lipemia.

Béraud, Bruno J., French surgeon, 1825-1865.
   Béraud valve – a small fold in the interior of the lacrimal sac at its junction with the lacrimal duct. *SYN:* Krause valve

Berenberg, William, U.S. physician, *1915.
   Neuhauser-Berenberg syndrome – see under Neuhauser

Berger, Emil, Austrian ophthalmologist, 1855-1926.
   Berger space – the space between the patellar fossa of the vitreous and the lens.

Berger, Hans, German neurologist, 1873-1941.
   Berger rhythm – a wave pattern in the encephalogram in the frequency band of 8 to 13 Hz. *SYN:* alpha rhythm; Berger wave
   Berger wave – *SYN:* Berger rhythm

Berger, Jean, 20th century French nephrologist.
   Berger disease – *SYN:* focal glomerulonephritis
   Berger focal glomerulonephritis – *SYN:* focal glomerulonephritis

Berger, Oskar, German physician, 1845-1908.
    Berger paresthesia – lower extremity paresthesia and accompanying weakness with no objective symptoms.

Bergeron, E.J., French physician, 1817-1900.
    Bergeron chorea – involuntary and usually self-limiting muscle spasm occurring at long intervals; may follow Sydenham chorea. *SYN:* Bergeron disease
    Bergeron disease – *SYN:* Bergeron chorea

Bergmann, Gottlieb H., German neurologist and anatomist, 1781-1861.
    Bergmann cords – *SYN:* medullary striae of fourth ventricle
    Bergmann fibers – filamentous glia fibers traversing the cerebellar cortex perpendicular to the surface.

Bergmann, Gustav von, German physician, 1878-1955.
    Bergmann syndrome – condition which simulates angina pectoris due to protrusion of stomach above diaphragm, accompanied by dysphagia, tachycardia, hiccups. *SYN:* hiatus hernia syndrome; von Bergmann syndrome
    von Bergmann syndrome – *SYN:* Bergmann syndrome

Bergmeister, O., Austrian ophthalmologist, 1845-1918.
    Bergmeister papilla – a small mass of glial tissue that forms in the hyaloid artery during fetal life.

Bergstrand, Hilding, Swedish physician, 1886-1967.
    Bergstrand disease – benign tumor usually found in long bones of young or adolescent males. *SYN:* osteoid osteoma

Bergstrom, Lavonne, U.S. physician.
    Rosenberg-Bergstrom syndrome – see under Rosenberg, Alan L.

Bergström, Sune K., joint winner of 1982 Nobel Prize for work related to prostaglandins.

Berke, Raynold N., U.S. ophthalmologist, *1901.
    Berke cilia forceps

NOTES

Berke clamp
Berke forceps
Berke operation – correction of eyelid ptosis.
Berke ptosis clamp
Berke ptosis correction
Berke ptosis forceps

Berkefeld, name of a mine owner from which material to make filter was taken.
Berkefeld filter – filter for bacteria.

Berlin, Chaim, 20th century Israeli dermatologist.
Berlin syndrome – ectodermal dysplasia described in two brothers and two sisters, featuring stunted growth, mental retardation, birdlike legs, fine dry skin with mottled pigmentation, flat nose, thick lips, and wrinkling around mouth and eyes.

Berlin, Rudolf, German ophthalmologist, 1833-1897.
Berlin disease
Berlin edema – retinal edema after blunt trauma to the globe.

Bernard, Claude, French physiologist, 1813-1878.
Bernard canal – the excretory duct of the head of the pancreas. *SYN:* accessory pancreatic duct; Bernard duct
Bernard duct – *SYN:* Bernard canal
Bernard puncture – a puncture at a point in the floor of the fourth ventricle of the brain which causes glycosuria. *SYN:* diabetic puncture
Bernard syndrome – *SYN:* Horner syndrome
Bernard-Cannon homeostasis – the set of mechanisms responsible for the cybernetic adjustment of physiological and biochemical states in postnatal life. *SYN:* physiological homeostasis
Bernard-Horner syndrome – *SYN:* Horner syndrome
Bernard-Sergent syndrome – *SYN:* acute adrenocortical insufficiency

Bernard, Jean, 20th century French physician.
Bernard-Soulier syndrome – a coagulation disorder characterized by thrombocytopenia, giant platelets, and a bleeding tendency.

Bernays, Augustus C., U.S. surgeon, 1854-1907.
Bernays sponge – a compressed disk of aseptic cotton used in packing cavities.

Berndorfer, Alfred, Hungarian physician.
Berndorfer syndrome – syndrome of unknown etiology that causes cleft palate, harelip, and cleft hands and feet.

Bernhardt, Martin, German neurologist, 1844-1915.

Bernhardt disease – tingling, formication, itching, and other forms of paresthesia in the outer side of the lower thigh in the area of distribution of the lateral femoral cutaneous nerve. *SYN:* Bernhardt-Roth syndrome; meralgia paraesthetica; Roth-Bernhardt disease; Roth disease

Bernhardt-Roth syndrome – *SYN:* Bernhardt disease

Roth-Bernhardt disease – *SYN:* Bernhardt disease

Bernheim, Hippolyte-Marie, French psychologist, 1840-1919.

Bernheim therapy – obsolete term for hypnotic psychotherapy.

Bernheim, P., early 20th century French physician.

Bernheim syndrome – systemic congestion resembling consequences of right heart failure without pulmonary congestion in subjects with left ventricular enlargement from any cause.

Bernoulli, Daniel, Swiss mathematician, 1700-1782.

Bernoulli effect – the decrease in fluid pressure that occurs in converting potential to kinetic energy when motion of the fluid is accelerated in accordance with Bernoulli law.

Bernoulli law – when friction is negligible, the velocity of flow of a gas or fluid through a tube is inversely related to its pressure against the side of the tube. *SYN:* Bernoulli principle; Bernoulli theorem

Bernoulli principle – *SYN:* Bernoulli law

Bernoulli theorem – *SYN:* Bernoulli law

Bernreuter, Robert G., U.S. psychologist, *1901.

Bernreuter Personal Adjustment Inventory – test designed to measure personality and behavior.

Bernstein, Lionel M., U.S. internist, *1923.

Bernstein test – a test to establish that substernal pain is due to reflux esophagitis. *SYN:* acid perfusion test

Bernuth, Fritz Von, German physician.

Bernuth syndrome – sporadic hemophilia.

NOTES

Berry, George Andreas, English physician, 1853-1929.
Berry syndrome – mandibulofacial dysostosis.

Berry, Sir James, Canadian surgeon, 1860-1946.
Berry ligaments – thickened elastic bundle connecting the superior horn of thyroid cartilage to the tip of the greater horn of hyoid cartilage. *SYN:* lateral thyrohyoid ligament

Berson, Solomon A., U.S. internist, 1918-1972.
Berson test – a test of thyroid clearance of ^{131}I from the plasma by the thyroid gland.

Berthelot, Pierre Eugene Marcellin, French chemist, 1827-1907.
Berthelot reaction – the reaction of ammonia with phenol-hypochlorite, used to analyze ammonia concentration in body fluids.

Berthollet, Claude L., French chemist, 1748-1822.
Berthollet law – salts in solution will always react with each other so as to form a less soluble salt, if possible.

Bertillon, Alphonse, chief of criminal investigation for Paris police, 1853-1914.
Bertillon system – identification system. *SYN:* anthropometry
Bertillon cephalometer

Bertin, Exupère Joseph, French anatomist, 1712-1781.
Bertin bones – paired ossicles of pyramidal shape, the bases forming the roof of the nasal cavity. *SYN:* Bertin ossicles; sphenoidal conchae
Bertin columns – the prolongations of cortical substance separating the pyramids of the kidney. *SYN:* renal columns
Bertin ligament – among the strongest of the body's ligaments, it limits extension at the hip joint. *SYN:* iliofemoral ligament
Bertin ossicles – *SYN:* Bertin bones

Bertolotti, Mario, Italian physician, *1876.
Bertolotti syndrome – fifth lumbar vertebra sacralization with concomitant scoliosis and sciatica.

Bertrand, Ivan Georges, 20th century French neurologist.
Canavan-van Bogaert-Bertrand disease – *SYN:* Canavan disease

Besnier, Ernest, French dermatologist, 1831-1909.
Besnier-Boeck disease – systemic granulomatous disease of unknown cause which involves lungs with resulting fibrosis; also involving lymph nodes, skin, liver, spleen, eyes, phalangeal bones, and parotid glands. *SYN:* Besnier-Boeck-Schaumann disease; Besnier-Boeck-Schaumann

syndrome; Boeck disease; Boeck sarcoid; sarcoidosis; Schaumann syndrome

Besnier-Boeck-Schaumann disease – *SYN:* Besnier-Boeck disease

Besnier-Boeck-Schaumann syndrome – *SYN:* Besnier-Boeck disease

Besnier prurigo – an atopic form which may be associated with asthma, hay fever, or other allergic conditions.

Besredka, Alexandre Mikhailovich, Russian-born French serologist and immunologist, 1870-1940.

Besredka antivirus – bacterial broth cultures used to produce local immunity.

Besredka desensitization – method for avoiding anaphylactic shock.

Besredka egg substrate – liquid substrate for cultivation of bacteria related to tuberculosis.

Besredka reaction – complement deviation reaction for tuberculosis.

Besredka vaccine

Bessman, Samuel Paul, U.S. physician, *1921.

Bessman-Baldwin syndrome – autosomal recessive trait in individuals with cerebromacular degeneration and blindness, causing excretion of large amounts of carnosine, anserine and histidine.

Best, Franz, German pathologist, 1878-1920.

Best carmine stain – a method for the demonstration of glycogen in tissues.

Best disease – autosomal dominant retinal degeneration beginning during the first years of life.

Bethea, Oscar Walter, U.S. physician, 1878-1963.

Bethea sign – unilateral impairment of chest expansion seen when examiner places fingers on upper surfaces of ribs in patient's axillae; there is less respiratory movement on affected side. *SYN:* Bethea method

Bethea method – *SYN:* Bethea sign

NOTES

Bethesda, city in Maryland.
   Bethesda system – classification system for cervical Papanicolaou smears; originated in Bethesda, Maryland.
   Bethesda unit – measure of inhibitor activity; originated in Bethesda, Maryland.

Bettendorff, Anton J., German chemist, 1839-1902.
   Bettendorff test – a test for arsenic.

Betz, Vladimir A., Russian anatomist, 1834-1894.
   Betz cells – large pyramidal cells in the motor area of the precentral gyrus of the cerebral cortex. *SYN:* Bevan-Lewis cells

Beuermann, Charles Lucien, French physician, 1851-1923.
   Beuermann disease – *SYN:* Schenck disease
   Beuermann-Gougerot disease – *SYN:* Schenck disease

Beuren, Alois J.
   Beuren syndrome – supravalvular aortic stenosis with multiple areas of peripheral pulmonary arterial stenosis, mental retardation, and dental anomalies.

Bevan-Lewis, William, English physician and physiologist, 1847-1929.
   Bevan-Lewis cells – *SYN:* Betz cells

Bezold, Albert von, German physiologist, 1836-1868.
   Bezold ganglion – an aggregation of nerve cells in the interatrial septum.
   Bezold-Jarisch reflex – a reflex with afferent and efferent pathways in the vagus, originating in unidentified chemoreceptors in the heart and resulting in sinus bradycardia, hypotension, and probable peripheral vasodilation.

Bezold, Friedrich, German otologist, 1842-1908.
   Bezold abscess – an abscess deep in the neck's parapharyngeal space associated with suppuration in the mastoid tip cells.
   Bezold mastoiditis – mastoiditis with perforation medially into the digastric groove, forming a deep neck abscess.
   Bezold sign – inflammatory edema at the tip of the mastoid process in mastoiditis. *SYN:* Bezold symptom
   Bezold symptom – *SYN:* Bezold sign
   Bezold triad – diminished perception of the deeper tones, retarded bone conduction, and negative Rinne test, pointing, in the absence of objective signs, to otosclerosis.

Bial, Manfred, German physician, 1869-1908.
   Bial reagent

Bial test – a test for pentoses with orcinol. *SYN:* orcinol test

Bianchi, Giovanni, Italian anatomist, 1681-1761.
Bianchi nodule – a nodule at the center of the free border of each semilunar valve at the beginning of the pulmonary artery and aorta. *SYN:* nodule of semilunar valve
Bianchi valve – a fold of mucous membrane guarding the lower opening of the nasolacrimal duct. *SYN:* lacrimal fold

Bianchi, Leonardo, Italian psychiatrist, 1848-1927.
Bianchi syndrome – lesions in right parietal lobe causing alexia, aphasia, apraxia, and hemianesthesia of right hand and foot.

Bichat, Marie F.X., French anatomist, physician, and biologist, 1771-1802.
Bichat canal – *SYN:* cistern of great cerebral vein.
Bichat fat pad – an encapsuled mass of fat in the cheek on the outer side of the buccinator muscle. *SYN:* buccal fat pad
Bichat fissure – the nearly circular fissure corresponding to the medial margin of the cerebral (pallial) mantle, marking the hilus of the cerebral hemisphere.
Bichat foramen – *SYN:* cistern of great cerebral vein
Bichat fossa – sphenomaxillary fossa, a small pyramidal space, housing the pterygopalatine ganglion, between the pterygoid process, the maxilla, and the palatine bone. *SYN:* pterygopalatine fossa
Bichat ligament – the lower fasciculus of the posterior sacroiliac ligament.
Bichat membrane – the inner elastic membrane of arteries.
Bichat protuberance – *SYN:* buccal fat pad
Bichat tunic – the tunica intima of the blood vessels.

Bickel, Gustav, 19th century German physician.
Bickel ring – the broken ring of lymphoid tissue, formed of the lingual, faucial, and pharyngeal tonsils. *SYN:* lymphoid ring

Bickers, D.S., U.S. physician.
Bickers-Adams syndrome – congenital hydrocephalus caused by recessive gene. *SYN:* X-linked hydrocephalus

NOTES

Bickerstaff, Edward R., English physician, *1920.
   Bickerstaff encephalitis – *SYN:* brainstem encephalitis
   Bickerstaff migraine

Bidder, Heinrich Friedrich, Estonian anatomist, 1810-1894.
   Bidder ganglia – cardiac nerve ganglia found at the atrial septum. *SYN:*
     Bidder organ
   Bidder organ – *SYN:* Bidder ganglia

Bidwell, Shelford, English physicist, 1848-1909.
   Bidwell ghost – visual afterimage in response to stimulus. *SYN:* Purkinje
     afterimage

Biebl, M.
   Biebl loop – a continuous loop of small intestine brought through the
     abdominal wall to a subcutaneous location, for observation of motility.

Biederman, Joseph, U.S. physician, *1907.
   Biederman sign – a dusky redness of the lower portion of the anterior
     pillars of the fauces in certain cases of syphilis.

Biedl, Artur, Austrian physician, 1869-1933.
   Bardet-Biedl syndrome – see under Bardet
   Biedl disease
   Laurence-Moon-Biedl syndrome – see under Laurence

Bielschowsky, Alfred, German ophthalmologist, 1871-1940.
   Bielschowsky disease – early childhood type of lipofuscinosis.
   Bielschowsky sign – in paralysis of a superior oblique muscle, tilting the
     head to the side of the involved eye causes that eye to rotate upward.
   Roth-Bielschowsky syndrome – see under Roth, W.

Bielschowsky, Max, German neuropathologist, 1869-1940.
   Bielschowsky-Dollinger syndrome – *SYN:* Dollinger-Bielschowsky
     syndrome
   Bielschowsky head tilt test
   Bielschowsky-Jansky disease – *SYN:* Jansky-Bielschowsky disease
   Bielschowsky method
   Bielschowsky stain – a method of treating tissues with silver nitrate to
     demonstrate reticular fibers, neurofibrils, axons, and dendrites.
   Bielschowsky syndrome – *SYN:* Dollinger-Bielschowsky syndrome
   Dollinger-Bielschowsky syndrome – see under Dollinger
   Jansky-Bielschowsky disease – see under Jansky

Biemond, A., French neurologist, *1902.
   Biemond ataxia – *SYN:* Friedreich ataxia

Biemond syndrome – iris coloboma, mental retardation, obesity, hypogenitalism, and postaxial polydactyly.

Bier, August K.G., German surgeon, 1861-1949.
Bier amputation – osteoplastic amputation of the tibia and fibula.
Bier amputation saw
Bier block anesthesia
Bier combined treatment
Bier hyperemia
Bier method – (1) *SYN:* intravenous regional anesthesia; (2) treatment of various surgical conditions by reactive hyperemia.
Bier spots – *SYN:* Marshall-White syndrome
Bier syndrome – *SYN:* Marshall-White syndrome

Biermer, Anton, German physician, 1827-1892.
Addison-Biermer disease – *SYN:* Addison anemia
Biermer anemia – *SYN:* Addison anemia
Biermer disease – *SYN:* Addison anemia
Biermer sign – *SYN:* Gerhardt sign

Biernacki, Edmund A., Polish pathologist, 1866-1912.
Biernacki sign – analgesia to percussion of the ulnar nerve in tabes dorsalis and dementia paralytica.

Biesiadecki, Alfred von, Polish physician, 1839-1888.
Biesiadecki fossa – a peritoneal recess between the psoas muscle and the crest of the ilium. *SYN:* iliacosubfascial fossa

Biett, Laurent, Swiss-born French dermatologist, 1781-1840.
Biett collarette – collarette of scales around a papule of secondary syphilis.
Biett disease – a chronic form of cutaneous lupus erythematosus.

NOTES

Bietti, Giambattista, Italian ophthalmologist, *1907.
    Bietti dystrophy – autosomal recessive trait characterized by Bowman membrane opacification, common in climates with bright sunlight. *SYN:* Bietti keratopathy; Bietti tapetoretinal degeneration
    Bietti keratopathy – *SYN:* Bietti dystrophy
    Bietti tapetoretinal degeneration – *SYN:* Bietti dystrophy
    Bietti syndrome – pathologic dryness of skin, conjunctivae, and/or mucous membranes accompanied by anomalies of iris and pupil.

Bigelow, Henry J., U.S. surgeon, 1818-1890.
    Bigelow clamp
    Bigelow evacuator – instrument used to remove fragments of bladder calculi.
    Bigelow forceps
    Bigelow ligament – among the strongest of the body's ligaments, it limits extension at the hip joint. *SYN:* iliofemoral ligament
    Bigelow litholapaxy – process of crushing a bladder stone and using a catheter to wash out fragments.
    Bigelow lithotrite
    Bigelow septum – a bony spur springing from the underside of the neck of the femur above and anterior to the lesser trochanter. *SYN:* calcar femorale
    Bigelow sutures

Bignami, Amico, Italian physician, 1862-1929.
    Marchiafava-Bignami disease – see under Marchiafava

Bilharz, T.M., German parasitologist, 1825-1862.
    Bilharzia – schistosomiasis; tumorlike swelling of the skin due to infection by *Schistosoma* organism. *SYN: Schistosoma*

Bill, Arthur H., U.S. obstetrician, 1877-1961.
    Bill maneuver – forceps rotation of the fetal head at midpelvis before extraction of the head.

Billig, Harvey E., Jr., U.S. orthopedic surgeon.
    Billig exercise – an exercise for dysmenorrhea; used to counteract tendency toward lordosis and to stretch tight fascia around the pelvis.

Billroth, Christian Albert Theodor, Austrian surgeon, 1829-1894.
    Billroth I anastomosis – *SYN:* Billroth operation I
    Billroth II anastomosis – *SYN:* Billroth operation II
    Billroth cords – the tissue occurring between the venous sinuses in the spleen. *SYN:* splenic cords
    Billroth disease

Billroth forceps
Billroth gastrectomy – *SYN:* Billroth operation I and II
Billroth gastroduodenoscopy
Billroth gastroenterostomy
Billroth gastrojejunostomy
Billroth hypertrophy
Billroth operation I – excision of the pylorus with end-to-end anastomosis of stomach and duodenum. *SYN:* Billroth I anastomosis; Billroth gasterectomy
Billroth operation II – resection of the pylorus with the greater part of the lesser curvature of the stomach, closure of the cut ends of the duodenum and stomach, followed by a gastrojejunostomy. *SYN:* Billroth II anastomosis; Billroth gasterectomy
Billroth ovarian retractor
Billroth venae cavernosae – small tributaries of the splenic vein in the pulp of the spleen. *SYN:* venae cavernosae of spleen

Binder, K.H., German dentist.
Binder syndrome – *SYN:* maxillonasal dysplasia; nasomaxillary hypoplasia

Binet, Alfred, French psychologist, 1857-1911.
Binet age – the age of the normal child with whose intelligence (as measured by the Stanford-Binet scale) the intelligence of the abnormal child corresponds.
Binet scale – *SYN:* Binet-Simon scale
Binet-Simon scale – forerunner of individual intelligence tests desinged for children and adults, sometimes referred to as the Binet scale. *SYN:* Binet scale
Binet test – *SYN:* Stanford-Binet intelligence scale
Stanford-Binet intelligence scale – see under Stanford

NOTES

Bing, J., Scandinavian physician.
   Bing-Neel syndrome – central nervous system response to macroglobulinemia.

Bing, Paul Robert, German neurologist, 1878-1956.
   Bing reflex – when the foot is passively dorsiflexed, plantar flexion occurs if any point on the ankle between the two malleoli is tapped. *SYN:* Bing sign
   Bing sign – *SYN:* Bing reflex

Bing, Richard J., U.S. physician, *1909.
   Taussig-Bing disease – *SYN:* Taussig-Bing syndrome
   Taussig-Bing syndrome – see under Taussig

Bingham, E.C., U.S. chemist, 1878-1945.
   Bingham flow – the flow characteristics exhibited by a Bingham plastic.
   Bingham model – a model representing the flow behavior of a Bingham plastic, in the idealized case.
   Bingham plastic – a material that, in the idealized case, does not flow until a critical stress (yield stress) is exceeded, and then flows at a rate proportional to the excess of stress over the yield stress.

Binswanger, Otto Ludwig, German neurologist, 1852-1929.
   Binswanger dementia – *SYN:* Binswanger disease
   Binswanger disease – one of the causes of multiinfarct dementia, in which there are many infarcts and lacunes in the white matter, with relative sparing of the cortex and basal ganglia. *SYN:* Binswanger dementia; Binswanger encephalopathy; encephalitis subcorticalis chronica; subcortical arteriosclerotic encephalopathy
   Binswanger encephalopathy – *SYN:* Binswanger disease

Binz, Carl, German pharmacologist, 1832-1913.
   Binz test – a qualitative test for the presence of quinine in the urine.

Biondi, Aldolpho, Italian pathologist, 1846-1917.
   Biondi-Heidenhain stain – an obsolete stain for spirochetes, using acid fuchsin and orange G.

Biot, Camille, French physician, *1878.
   Biot breathing – *SYN:* Biot respiration
   Biot breathing sign – irregular periods of apnea alternating with four or five deep breaths, seen with increased intracranial pressure.
   Biot respiration – abrupt, irregular alternating periods of apnea with constant rate and depth of breathing, as that resulting from lesions due

to increased intracranial pressure. *SYN:* ataxic breathing; Biot breathing; respiratory ataxia

Birbeck, Michael S., English cancer researcher.
Birbeck granule – *SYN:* Langerhans granule

Birch-Hirschfeld, Felix V., German pathologist, 1842-1899.
Birch-Hirschfeld stain – an obsolete stain for demonstrating amyloid.

Bird, Golding, English physician, 1814-1854.
Bird formula – formula related to specific gravity of urine.

Bird, Samuel D., Australian physician, 1833-1904.
Bird sign – the presence of a zone of dullness on percussion with absence of respiratory signs in hydatid cyst of the lung.

Birkett, John, English physician, 1815-1904.
Birkett forceps
Birkett hemostatic forceps
Birkett hernia – inguinal hernia with sac extending into the anterior or inferior wall. *SYN:* ascending hernia; intermuscular hernia

Bischof, W., 20th century German neurosurgeon.
Bischof corona
Bischof myelotomy – longitudinal incision of the spinal cord through the lateral column for treatment of spasticity of the lower extremities.
Bischof operation

Bishop, J. Michael, joint winner of 1989 Nobel Prize for work related to oncogenes.

Bishop, Louis F., U.S. physician, 1864-1941.
Bishop sphygmoscope – an instrument for measuring the blood pressure.

Bissell, G.W.
Bissell lines – longitudinal brown lines on the nail plate caused by melanin deposition, associated with adrenal insufficiency.

NOTES

Bitot, Pierre A., French physician, 1822-1888.
Bitot patches – *SYN:* Bitot spots
Bitot spots – small, circumscribed, lusterless, grayish-white, foamy, greasy, triangular deposits on the bulbar conjunctiva adjacent to the cornea; occurs in vitamin A deficiency. *SYN:* Bitot patches

Bittner, John J., U.S. oncologist, 1904-1961.
Bittner agent – member of the retrovirus subfamily Oncornavirinae. *SYN:* Bittner factor; Bittner milk factor; mammary tumor virus of mice
Bittner factor – *SYN:* Bittner agent
Bittner milk factor – *SYN:* Bittner agent

Bittorf, Alexander, German physician, 1876-1949.
Bittorf reaction – in cases of renal colic, pain radiating to the kidney upon squeezing the testicle or pressing the ovary.

Bixler, David, U.S. dentist and geneticist, *1929.
Antley-Bixler syndrome – see under Antley

Bizzozero, Giulio, Italian physician, 1846-1901.
Bizzozero corpuscle – an irregularly shaped disklike cytoplasmic fragment of a megakaryocyte found in the peripheral blood; functions in clotting. *SYN:* platelet

Bjerrum, Jannik P., Danish ophthalmologist, 1851-1926.
Bjerrum scotoma – a comet-shaped scotoma, occurring in glaucoma. *SYN:* Bjerrum sign; sickle scotoma
Bjerrum scotometer
Bjerrum screen – a flat, usually black surface used to measure the central 30 degrees of the field of vision. *SYN:* tangent screen
Bjerrum sign – *SYN:* Bjerrum scotoma

Björk, V.O., 20th century Swedish cardiothoracic surgeon.
Björk-Shiley valve – prosthetic aortic/mitral valve.

Björnstad, R., Swedish dermatologist.
Björnstad syndrome – autosomal dominant trait causing sensorineural hearing loss.

Black, Douglas A.K., Scottish physician, *1909.
Black formula – a translation of Pignet formula into British measurements.

Black, Greene V., U.S. dentist, 1836-1915.
Black classification – a classification of cavities of the teeth based upon the tooth surface(s) involved.

Black, Sir James W., joint winner of 1988 Nobel Prize for work related to drug treatment.

Blackfan, Kenneth Daniel, U.S. physician, 1883-1941.
  Diamond-Blackfan anemia – see under Diamond
  Diamond-Blackfan syndrome – *SYN:* Diamond-Blackfan anemia

Blagden, Sir Charles, English physician, 1748-1820.
  Blagden law – the depression of the freezing point of dilute solutions is proportional to the amount of the dissolved substance.

Blainville, Henri Marie Ducrotay de, French zoologist and anthropologist, 1777-1850.
  Blainville ears – asymmetry in size or shape of the auricles.

Blair, Vilray P., U.S. surgeon, 1871-1955.
  Blair ankle arthrodesis
  Blair-Brown graft – a split-thickness graft of intermediate thickness.
  Blair chisel
  Blair elevator
  Blair fusion
  Blair knife
  Blair saw guide
  Blair technique

Blaivas, Jerry D., U.S. urologist.
  Blaivas urinary incontinence classification

Blakemore, Arthur H., U.S. surgeon, 1897-1970.
  Blakemore esophageal tube
  Sengstaken-Blakemore tube – see under Sengstaken

Blalock, Alfred, U.S. surgeon, 1899-1965.
  Blalock anastomosis
  Blalock clamp
  Blalock-Hanlon operation – the creation of a large atrial septal defect as a palliative procedure for complete transposition of the great arteries.

NOTES

Blalock pulmonary clamp

Blalock shunt – subclavian artery to pulmonary artery shunt to increase pulmonary circulation in cyanotic heart disease with decreased pulmonary flow.

Blalock sutures

Blalock-Taussig operation – an operation for congenital malformations of the heart.

Blalock-Taussig shunt – a palliative subclavian artery to pulmonary artery anastomosis.

Blanc, Emile, French physician, 1901-1952.

Bonnett-Dechaume-Blanc syndrome – see under Bonnet, Paul

Bland, Edward Franklin, U.S. physician, *1901.

Bland-White-Garland syndrome – juvenile angina pectoris and myocardial infarction.

Blandin, Philipe Frédéric, French anatomist and surgeon, 1798-1849.

Blandin gland – one of the small mixed glands deeply placed near the apex of the tongue on each side of the frenulum. *SYN:* anterior lingual gland

Blaschko, Alfred, German venereologist, leprologist, and scientist, 1858-1922.

Blaschko lines – system of lines on the surface of the human body, representing developmental growth pattern of the skin. Certain nevi are distributed along these lines.

Blasius, Gerardus, 17th century Dutch anatomist.

Blasius duct – the duct of the parotid gland opening from the cheek into the vestibule of the mouth opposite the neck of the superior second molar tooth. *SYN:* parotid duct

Blaskovics, Laszlo de, Hungarian ophthalmologist, 1869-1938.

Blaskovics operation – operation for correction of eyelid ptosis.

Blatin, Marc, French physician, 1878-1943.

Blatin syndrome – the peculiar trembling or vibratory sensation felt on palpation of a hydatid cyst. *SYN:* hydatid thrill

Blau, E., 20th century U.S. pediatrician.

Blau syndrome – autosomal dominant syndrome featuring camptodactyly (flexion contracture of fingers and toes), granulomatous arthritis, uveitis, and granulomatous lesions of the skin. *SYN:* Blau type arthrocutaneouveal granulomatosis

Blau type arthrocutaneouveal granulomatosis – *SYN:* Blau syndrome

Blaud, P., French physician, 1774-1858.
    Blaud pill – ferrous sulfate used in treatment of chlorosis. *SYN:* iron pill

Blegvad, Olaf, Danish physician, 1888-1961.
    Blegvad-Haxthausen syndrome – osteogenesis imperfecta, blue sclera, and anetoderma.

Blencke, August, German orthopedic surgeon, 1868-1937.
    Blencke syndrome – ischemic necrosis of epiphyses resulting in calcaneal metaphyseal osteodystrophy.

Blesovsky, A., English physician.
    Blesovsky syndrome – folding of lung which can occur with large pleural plaques or thickened pleural membrane. *SYN:* folded lung

Bleuler, Paul Eugen, Swiss psychiatrist, 1857-1939.
    Bleuler's four A's – disturbances in affect, association, ambivalence, autism; related to schizophrenia.

Bliss, Karl (Charles), Austrian semanticist, 1897-1985.
    Blissymbolics – visual sign system, artificially constructed by Bliss in 1965, and used as communication aid for rehabilitation in persons with severely impaired speech function. *SYN:* semantography

Blobel, Günter, German-born U.S. scientist, *1936, winner of 1999 Nobel Prize for work related to protein signals governing transport and localization within cells.

Bloch, Bruno, Swiss dermatologist, 1878-1933.
    Bloch-Sulzberger disease – genodermatosis that may also involve other structures. *SYN:* Asboe-Hansen disease; Bloch-Sulzberger syndrome; incontinentia pigmenti
    Bloch-Sulzberger syndrome – *SYN:* Bloch-Sulzberger disease

Bloch, Konrad, joint winner of 1964 Nobel Prize for work related to cholesterol and metabolism of fatty acids.

B

NOTES

Bloch, Marcel, French physician, 1885-1925.
　Bloch reaction – a dark staining observed in fresh tissue sections to which a solution of dopa has been applied. *SYN:* dopa reaction

Blocq, Paul O., French physician, 1860-1896.
　Blocq disease – the inability to either stand or walk in the normal manner. *SYN:* astasia-abasia

Blondeel, Phillip, Belgian physician.
　Blondeel scissors – scissors used in breast reconstruction surgery when a perforator flap is involved.

Bloodgood, Joseph Colt, U.S. surgeon, 1867-1935.
　Bloodgood disease
　Bloodgood operation – inguinal canal reconstruction procedure.
　blue-domed cyst of Bloodgood – breast cyst.

Bloom, David, U.S. dermatologist, *1892.
　Bloom syndrome – congenital telangiectatic erythema and dwarfism with normal body proportions except for a narrow face and dolichocephalic skull.

Blount, Walter Putnam, U.S. orthopedist, *1900.
　Blount-Barber disease – *SYN:* Blount disease
　Blount bent blade
　Blount blade plate
　Blount bone retractor
　Blount bone spreader
　Blount brace
　Blount disease – nonrachitic bowlegs in children. *SYN:* Blount-Barber disease
　Blount displacement osteotomy
　Blount epiphysiodesis
　Blount hip retractor
　Blount knee retractor
　Blount knife
　Blount mallet
　Blount osteotome
　Blount osteotomy
　Blount scoliosis osteotome
　Blount splint
　Blount spreader
　Blount staple
　Blount technique for osteoclasis

Blount tibia vara
Blount tracing technique
Blount V-blade

Blücher, Gebhard von, Prussian field marshal, 1742-1819.
Blücher shoe – a type of laced shoe. *SYN:* Gibson shoe

Blum, Paul, French physician, 1878-1933.
Gougerot and Blum disease – see under Gougerot, Henri

Blumberg, Baruch S., joint winner of 1976 Nobel Prize for work related to infectious diseases.

Blumberg, Jacob Moritz, German surgeon and gynecologist, 1873-1955.
Blumberg sign – pain felt upon sudden release of steadily applied pressure on a suspected area of the abdomen, indicative of peritonitis.

Blumenau, Leonid W., Russian neurologist, 1862-1932.
Blumenau nucleus – the lateral cuneate nucleus of the medulla oblongata.

Blumenbach, Johann Friedrich, German physiologist, 1752-1840.
Blumenbach clivus – the sloping surface from the dorsum sellae to the foramen magnum. *SYN:* clivus

Blumer, George, U.S. physician, 1858-1940.
Blumer shelf – a shelf palpable by rectal examination, due to metastatic tumor cells gravitating from an abdominal cancer and growing in the rectovesical or rectouterine pouch. *SYN:* rectal shelf

Blythedale, a children's hospital in Valhalla, NY.
Blythemobile – stretcher-wheelchair combination that can be self-propelled.

Boas, Ismar I., German gastroenterologist, 1858-1938.
Boas-Oppler bacillus
Boas sign – hyperesthesia related to acute cholecystitis.
Boas test

NOTES

Bobath, Berta, English physical therapist, and Karel, English neurologist.
> **Bobath facilitation technique** – *SYN:* Bobath method
> **Bobath method** – therapeutic exercise method for individuals with central nervous system lesions. *SYN:* Bobath facilitation technique; Bobath method of exercise; Bobath proprioceptive neuromuscular facilitation
> **Bobath method of exercise** – *SYN:* Bobath method
> **Bobath proprioceptive neuromuscular facilitation** – *SYN:* Bobath method
> **Bobath test chart of motor ability**

Bochdalek, Vincent A., Czech anatomist, 1801-1883.
> **Bochdalek duct** – thyroglossal duct. *SYN:* duct of His; duct of Vater; thyrolingual duct
> **Bochdalek foramen** – a congenital defective opening through the diaphragm, connecting pleural and peritoneal cavities. *SYN:* pleuroperitoneal hiatus
> **Bochdalek ganglion** – a ganglion of the plexus of the dental nerve lying in the maxilla just above the root of the canine tooth.
> **Bochdalek gap** – a triangular area in the diaphragm devoid of muscle fibers. *SYN:* vertebrocostal trigone
> **Bochdalek hernia** – absence of the pleuroperitoneal membrane (usually on the left) or an enlarged Morgagni foramen which allows protrusion of abdominal viscera into the chest. *SYN:* congenital diaphragmatic hernia
> **Bochdalek muscle** – an occasional thin band of muscular fibers passing between the root of the tongue and the triticeal cartilage. *SYN:* musculus triticeoglossus
> **Bochdalek valve** – a fold of mucous membrane in the lacrimal canaliculus at the lacrimal punctum. *SYN:* Foltz valvule
> **flower basket of Bochdalek** – part of the choroid plexus of the fourth ventricle protruding through Luschka foramen and resting on the dorsal surface of the glossopharyngeal nerve.

Bock, August C., German anatomist, 1782-1833.
> **Bock ganglion** – a small ganglionic swelling on filaments from the internal carotid plexus, lying on the undersurface of the carotid artery in the cavernous sinus. *SYN:* carotid ganglion

Bockhart, Max, German physician, 1883-1921.
> **Bockhart impetigo** – a superficial follicular pustular eruption involving the scalp or other hairy area. *SYN:* follicular impetigo

Bodansky, Aaron, U.S. biochemist, 1887-1961.
>**Bodansky unit** – that amount of phosphatase that liberates 1 mg of phosphorus as inorganic phosphate during the first hour of incubation with a buffered substrate containing sodium β-glycerophosphate.

Bödecker, Charles F., U.S. oral histologist, embryologist, and pathologist, *1880.
>**Bödecker index** – a modification of the decayed, missing, and filled surfaces (DMFS) caries index.

Bodian, David, U.S. anatomist, *1910.
>**Bodian copper-PROTARGOL stain** – a stain employing a silver proteinate complex (PROTARGOL) to demonstrate axis cylinders and neurofibrils.
>**Bodian method**

Boeck, Caesar P.M., Norwegian dermatologist, 1845-1917.
>**Besnier-Boeck disease** – see under Besnier
>**Besnier-Boeck-Schaumann disease** – *SYN:* Besnier-Boeck disease
>**Besnier-Boeck-Schaumann syndrome** – *SYN:* Besnier-Boeck disease
>**Boeck disease** – *SYN:* Besnier-Boeck disease
>**Boeck sarcoid** – *SYN:* Besnier-Boeck disease

Boeck, Carl Wilhelm, Norwegian physician, 1808-1875.
>**Danielssen-Boeck disease** – *SYN:* anesthetic leprosy

Boehmer, F.
>**Boehmer hematoxylin** – an alum type of hematoxylin in which natural ripening occurs in about 8 to 10 days.

Boerhaave, Hermann, Dutch physician, 1668-1738.
>**Boerhaave glands** – *SYN:* sweat glands
>**Boerhaave syndrome** – spontaneous rupture of the lower esophagus, a variant of Mallory-Weiss syndrome.

Bogaert, Ludo van, see under van Bogaert

B

NOTES

Bogalusa, a city in Louisiana.
    Bogalusa Heart Study – study of children in semirural area of Louisiana, focusing on natural history of coronary artery disease and essential hypertension; largest and longest study of its kind.

Bogomolets, Alexander Alexandrovich, biologist and pathophysiologist, 1881-1946.
    Bogomolets serum – antiaging serum.

Bogorad, F.A., 20th century Russian physician.
    Bogorad syndrome – in cases of facial nerve palsy, tearing occurs from one eye after eating or drinking; facial tic and taste loss may occur concurrently.

Bogros, Antoine, 19th century French anatomist.
    Bogros serous membrane – a membrane of the episcleral space (of Tenon).

Bogros, Jean-Annet, French anatomist, 1786-1823.
    Bogros space – a triangular space between the peritoneum and the transversalis fascia. *SYN:* retroinguinal space

Böhler, Lorenz, Austrian orthopedic surgeon, 1885-1973.
    Böhler exerciser – a device used to exercise knee extensors.
    Böhler frame – orthopedic device.
    Böhler iron – orthopedic device.
    Böhler splint – orthopedic device.

Bohn, Heinrich, German physician, 1832-1888.
    Bohn nodules – tiny multiple cysts in newborns.

Bohr, Christian, Danish physiologist, 1855-1911.
    Bohr effect – the influence exerted by carbon dioxide on the oxygen dissociation curve of blood.
    Bohr equation – an equation to calculate respiratory dead space.

Bohr, Niels H.D., Danish physicist and Nobel laureate, 1885-1962.
    Bohr atom – a concept or model of the atom in which the negatively charged electrons move in circular or elliptical orbits around the positively charged nucleus, energy being emitted or absorbed when electrons change from one orbit to another.
    Bohr magneton – the net magnetic moment of one unpaired electron; used in electron spin resonance spectrometry for detection and estimation of free radicals. *SYN:* electron magneton
    Bohr theory – that spectrum lines are produced by the quantized emission of radiant energy when electrons drop from an orbit of a higher to one of

a lower energy level, or by absorption of radiation when an electron rises from a lower to a higher energy level.

Boll, Franz C., German histologist and physiologist, 1849-1879.
 Boll cells – basal cells in the lacrimal gland.

Bollinger, Otto, German pathologist, 1843-1909.
 Bollinger bodies – intracytoplasmic inclusion bodies observed in the infected tissues of birds with fowlpox.
 Bollinger granules – irregular aggregates or colonizations of gram-positive cocci, usually staphylococci, observed in lesions of botryomycosis.

Bollman, Jesse L., U.S. physiologist, *1896.
 Mann-Bollman fistula – see under Mann, Frank C.

Bolton, Joseph S., English neurologist, 1867-1946.
 Bolton-Broadbent plane – *SYN:* Bolton plane
 Bolton-nasion line – *SYN:* Bolton plane
 Bolton-nasion plane – *SYN:* Bolton plane
 Bolton plane – a roentgenographic cephalometric plane extending from the Bolton point to nasion. *SYN:* Bolton-nasion plane; Bolton-nasion line; Bolton-Broadbent plane

Boltzmann, Ludwig, Austrian physicist who founded branch of physics known as statistical mechanics, 1844-1906.
 Boltzmann constant
 Boltzmann distribution
 Boltzmann equation

Bombay, city in India.
 Bombay blood group – red cells resembling Group O, first seen in Bombay, India.

NOTES

Bongiovanni, Alfred M., U.S. physician.
Bongiovanni-Eisenmenger syndrome – chronic liver disease of unknown etiology and characterized by hyperadrenalism and elevated glycogen levels.

Bonhoeffer, Karl, German psychiatrist, 1868-1948.
Bonhoeffer sign – loss of normal muscle tone in chorea.

Bonnet, Amédée, French surgeon, 1809-1858.
Bonnet capsule – the anterior part of the vagina bulbi.

Bonnet, Charles, Swiss naturalist, 1720-1795.
Charles Bonnet syndrome – geriatric disorder marked by hallucinations.

Bonnet, Paul, French ophthalmologist, 1884-1959.
Bonnet-Dechaume-Blanc syndrome – rare syndrome featuring unilateral retinal arteriovenous malformation, ipsilateral aneurysmal arteriovenous malformation of the brain, and ipsilateral cutaneous vascular abnormalities. *SYN:* Bonnet syndrome
Bonnet syndrome – *SYN:* Bonnet-Dechaume-Blanc syndrome

Bonnevie, Kristine, German physician, 1872-1950.
Bonnevie-Ullrich syndrome – characteristics include hand and foot lymphedema, short stature, skin laxity.

Bonney, William F.V., English gynecologist, 1872-1953.
Bonney blue – ink for marking skin.
Bonney cervical amputation
Bonney cervical dilator
Bonney clamp
Bonney clip
Bonney forceps
Bonney hysterectomy
Bonney inflator
Bonney test – bladder test.

Bonnier, Pierre, French clinician, 1861-1918.
Bonnier syndrome – ocular disturbances, deafness, nausea, thirst, and anorexia due to a lesion of the Deiters nucleus.

Bonwill, William G.A., U.S. dentist, 1833-1899.
Bonwill triangle – an equilateral triangle formed by lines from the contact points of the lower central incisors, or the medial line of the residual ridge of the mandible, to the condyle on either side and from one condyle to the other.

Böök, Jan A., Swedish geneticist, *1915.
  Böök syndrome – premolar aplasia, hyperhidrosis, and premature graying of hair.

Borda, J.M., Argentinian physician.
  Borda syndrome – syndrome characterized by genetic skin condition associated with hydrocystoma, xanthelasma, dental dysplasia.

Bordeau, Théophile de, French physician, 1722-1776.
  de Bordeau theory – that each organ of the body manufactured a specific humor which it secreted into the bloodstream.

Bordet, Jules, Belgian bacteriologist and Nobel laureate, 1870-1961.
  Bordet amboceptor
  Bordetella – a genus of strictly aerobic bacteria that are pathogens of the mammalian respiratory tract.
  Bordet-Gengou bacillus – a species that causes whooping cough. SYN: *Bordetella pertussis*
  Bordet-Gengou phenomenon – the phenomenon of complement fixation.
  Bordet-Gengou potato blood agar – glycerin-potato agar with 25% of blood, used for the isolation of *Bordetella pertussis*.
  Bordet-Gengou reaction – SYN: complement fixation

Börjeson, Mats, Swedish physician, *1922.
  Börjeson-Forssman-Lehmann syndrome – a condition characterized by mental deficiency, epilepsy, hypogonadism, hypometabolism, obesity, and narrow palpebral fissures.

Born, Gustav Jacob, German embryologist, 1851-1900.
  Born method of wax plate reconstruction – the making of three-dimensional models of structures from serial sections.

Bornholm, island in the Baltic Sea.
  Bornholm disease – infection with coxsackievirus, causing severe abdominal and/or pleural pain.

NOTES

Borrel, Amédée, French bacteriologist, 1867-1936.
Borrel blue stain – a stain for demonstrating spirochetes, treponemes, and Borrelia organisms.
Borrel bodies – particles of fowlpox virus.

Borries, T., Danish physician.
Borries syndrome – encephalitis with changes in cerebrospinal fluid suggestive of brain abscess.

Borsieri, Giovanni Battista, Italian physician, 1725-1785.
Borsieri line – *SYN:* Borsieri sign
Borsieri sign – in patients with scarlet fever, drawing the fingernail across the skin creates a white line that turns red. *SYN:* Borsieri line

Borst, Maximilian, German pathologist, 1869-1946.
Borst-Jadassohn type intraepidermal epithelioma – precancerous lesions clinically suggestive of actinic or seborrheic keratosis, with nest of immature or abnormal keratinocytes within the epidermis.

Bostock, John, English physician, 1773-1846.
Bostock catarrh – *SYN:* allergic rhinitis; hay fever
Bostock disease

Boston, Leonard N., U.S. physician, 1871-1931.
Boston exanthem
Boston sign – jerky downward movement of the upper eyelid on downward rotation of the eye, characteristic of Graves disease.

Bosviel, J., French physician.
Bosviel syndrome – hemorrhage from ruptured hematoma of the uvula.

Botallo, Leonardo, Italian physician in Paris, 1530-1600.
Botallo duct – a fetal vessel connecting the left pulmonary artery with the descending aorta. *SYN:* ductus arteriosus
Botallo foramen – the orifice of communication between the two atria of the fetal heart.
Botallo ligament – the remains of the ductus arteriosus. *SYN:* ligamentum arteriosum

Botkin, Sergei Petrovich, Russian physician, 1832-1889.
Botkin disease – viral disease caused by poor hygienic conditions and ingestion of contaminated foods or liquids. *SYN:* hepatitis A; hepatitis epidemica; infectious hepatitis

Böttcher, Arthur, Estonian anatomist, 1831-1889.

Böttcher canal – a duct that connects the inner aspect of the utricle with the endolymphatic duct a short distance from its origin from the saccule. *SYN:* utriculosaccular duct

Böttcher cells – cells of the basilar membrane of the cochlea.

Böttcher crystals – small crystals observed microscopically in prostatic fluid.

Böttcher ganglion – ganglion on the cochlear nerve in the internal acoustic meatus.

Böttcher space – the dilated blind extremity of the endolymphatic duct. *SYN:* endolymphatic sac

Charcot-Böttcher crystalloids – see under Charcot

Bouchard, Charles Jacques, French physician, 1837-1915.

Bouchard disease – myopathic dilation of the stomach.

Bouchard nodes – interphalangeal joint nodes, related to osteoarthritis or gout.

Bouchut, Jean A.E., French physician, 1818-1891.

Bouchut tube – a short cylindrical tube used in intubation of the larynx.

Bouillaud, Jean, French physician, 1796-1881.

Bouillaud disease – obsolete term for acute rheumatic fever with carditis.

Bouillaud sign

Bouin, Paul, French histologist, 1870-1962.

Bouin fixative – a solution of glacial acetic acid, formalin, and picric acid.

Bourdon, Eugène, French engineer and inventor, 1808-1884.

Bourdon tube – a curved tube used as a transducer to move the pointer of an aneroid manometer.

Bourgery, Marc-Jean, French anatomist and surgeon, 1797-1849.

Bourgery ligament – a fibrous band that extends across the back of the knee from its separation from the direct tendon of insertion on the

NOTES

medial condyle of the tibia to the lateral condyle of the femur. *SYN:* oblique popliteal ligament

Bourneville, Désiré-Magloire, French physician, 1840-1909.
  Bourneville disease – phacomatosis characterized by the formation of multisystem hamartomas. *SYN:* Bourneville syndrome; tuberous sclerosis
  Bourneville-Pringle disease – facial lesions with tuberous sclerosis.
  Bourneville syndrome – *SYN:* Bourneville disease

Bourquin, Anne, U.S. chemist, *1897.
  Sherman-Bourquin unit of vitamin B$_2$ – see under Sherman, Henry C.

Bouveret, Leon, French physician, 1850-1926.
  Bouveret disease
  Bouveret syndrome – (1) paroxysmal supraventricular tachycardia; (2) gastric outlet obstruction due to gallstone passing into the duodenal bulb through a choledochoduodenal or cholecystoduodenal fistula.

Bouvrain, Y., French physician.
  Sézary-Bouvrain syndrome – *SYN:* Sézary syndrome

Bovero, Renaldo, 20th century Italian dermatologist.
  Bovero muscle – "the sucking muscle," compressor muscle of the lips. *SYN:* cutaneomucous muscle

Bovet, Daniel, Swiss-Italian pharmacologist, *1907, winner of the 1957 Nobel Prize for developing muscle relaxants and antihistamines.

Bowditch, Henry P., U.S. physiologist, 1840-1911.
  Bowditch effect – homeometric autoregulation of cardiac function induced by changing heart rate.
  Bowditch law – consistently total response to any effective stimulus. *SYN:* all or none law

Bowen, John T., U.S. dermatologist, 1857-1941.
  Bowen disease – a form of intraepidermal carcinoma. *SYN:* Bowen precancerous dermatosis
  bowenoid cells – cells characteristic of Bowen disease.
  bowenoid papulosis – a clinically benign form of intraepithelial neoplasia that microscopically resembles Bowen disease or carcinoma in situ, occurring in young individuals of both sexes on the genital or perianal skin usually as multiple well-demarcated pigmented warty papules.
  Bowen precancerous dermatosis – *SYN:* Bowen disease

Bowman, Sir William, English ophthalmologist, anatomist, and physiologist, 1816-1892.

   Bowman capsule – the expanded beginning of a nephron. *SYN:* glomerular capsule

   Bowman disk – disk resulting from transverse segmentation of striated muscular fiber treated with weak acids, certain alkaline solutions, or freezing.

   Bowman eye knife

   Bowman gland

   Bowman iris needle

   Bowman iris scissors

   Bowman lacrimal dilator

   Bowman lacrimal probe

   Bowman membrane – *SYN:* anterior limiting layer of cornea

   Bowman muscle – *SYN:* ciliary muscle

   Bowman probe – a double-ended probe for the lacrimal duct.

   Bowman space – the slitlike space between the visceral and parietal layers of the capsule of the renal corpuscle. *SYN:* capsular space

   Bowman strabismus scissors

   Bowman theory – that urine is formed by passive filtration through the glomeruli and secretion by the epithelium of the tubules.

Boyce, Frederick F., U.S. physician, *1903.

   Boyce sign – hand pressure on side of neck causes gurgling sound when esophageal diverticulum is present.

Boyce, William H., U.S. urologist, *1918.

   Smith-Boyce operation – an incision into the posterolateral renal parenchyma used for removal of renal calculi. *SYN:* anatrophic nephrotomy

B

NOTES

Boyd, Julian Deigh, U.S. physician, *1894.
  Boyd-Stearns syndrome – syndrome characterized by rickets during infancy, dwarfism, osteoporosis, and malnutrition, and associated with metabolic disorders.

Boyden, Edward A., U.S. anatomist, 1886-1977.
  Boyden meal – a meal used to test the evacuation time of the gallbladder.
  Boyden sphincter – smooth muscle sphincter that controls the flow of bile in the duodenum. *SYN:* sphincter of the common bile duct

Boyer, Baron Alexis, French surgeon, 1757-1833.
  Boyer bursa – a bursa between the posterior surface of the body of the hyoid bone and the thyrohyoid membrane. *SYN:* retrohyoid bursa
  Boyer cyst – a subhyoid cyst.

Boyle, Hon. Robert, English physicist and chemist, 1627-1691.
  Boyle law – at constant temperature, the volume of a given quantity of gas varies inversely with its absolute pressure. *SYN:* Mariotte law

Bozeman, Nathan, U.S. surgeon, 1825-1905.
  Bozeman clamp
  Bozeman curette
  Bozeman dilator
  Bozeman dressing forceps
  Bozeman forceps
  Bozeman-Fritsch catheter – a slightly curved double-channel uterine catheter with several openings at the tip.
  Bozeman hook
  Bozeman needle holder
  Bozeman operation – an operation for uterovaginal fistula, the cervix uteri being attached to the bladder and opening into its cavity.
  Bozeman position – knee-elbow position, the patient being strapped to supports.
  Bozeman speculum
  Bozeman sutures
  Bozeman uterine forceps

Bozzolo, Camillo, Italian physician, 1845-1920.
  Bozzolo sign – pulsating vessels in the nasal mucous membrane, noted occasionally in thoracic aneurysm.

Braasch, William F., U.S. urologist, 1878-1975.
  Braasch bladder specimen forceps
  Braasch bulb
  Braasch catheter – a bulb-tipped catheter used for dilation and calibration.

Braasch cystoscope
Braasch forceps
Braasch ureteral catheter
Braasch ureteral dilator

Bracht, E., 20th century German pathologist.
Bracht-Wächter bodies – myocardial microabscesses observed in the presence of bacterial endocarditis.
Bracht-Wächter lesion – a focal collection of lymphocytes and mononuclear cells within the myocardium in bacterial endocarditis.

Bracht, Erich Franz, German obstetrician and gynecologist, *1882.
Bracht maneuver – delivery of a fetus in the breech position by extension of the legs and trunk of the fetus over the symphysis pubis and abdomen of the mother.

Bradbury, Samuel, U.S. physician, 1883-1947.
Bradbury-Eggleston syndrome – impaired peripheral vasoconstriction causing visual disturbances, dizziness, syncope, and other symptoms. *SYN:* Eggleston-Bradbury syndrome
Eggleston-Bradbury syndrome – *SYN:* Bradbury-Eggleston syndrome

Bradford, Edward H., U.S. orthopedist, 1848-1926.
Bradford frame – an oblong rectangular frame that permits trunk and lower extremities to move as a unit.

Bradley, W.H., 20th century English physician.
Bradley disease – nausea and vomiting which are epidemic.

Braham, R.L., Canadian dentist.
Braham syndrome – rare syndrome characterized by multiple congenital abnormalities and mental retardation. *SYN:* hyperostotic dwarfism

Brahmachari, Upendra Nath, 20th century Indian physician.
Brahmachari leishmanoid – A type of cutaneous leishmaniasis caused by *Leishmania donovani*, occurring in patients who had recovered from kala-azar. *SYN:* dermal leishmanoid

NOTES

Braille, Louis, French educator, 1809-1852.
Braille – system of raised dots placed in patterns to allow the blind to read.
Braillophone – a combination telephone and braille system.

Brailsford, James Frederick, English radiologist, 1888-1961.
Brailsford-Morquio disease – *SYN:* Morquio syndrome

Brain, Lord W. Russell, English physician, 1895-1966.
Brain reflex – extension of the arm of a hemiplegic patient when turned prone as if on all fours. *SYN:* quadripedal extensor reflex

Brainerd, city in Minnesota.
Brainerd diarrhea – multiple watery, explosive episodes of diarrhea accompanied by urgency and fecal incontinence; first outbreak occurred in this city in 1983.

Brandt, M.L., U.S. obstetrician, *1894.
Brandt brassiere
Brandt treatment

Brandt, Thore Edvard, Finnish dermatologist, *1901.
Brandt syndrome – symptoms include fat in feces, baldness, paronychia, and pustular eruptions around the mouth and anus. *SYN:* Danbolt-Closs syndrome; Danbolt syndrome

Brandt, Thure, Swedish obstetrician and gynecologist, 1819-1895.
Brandt-Andrews maneuver – method of delivering the placenta.
Brandt massage – a gynecologic massage used to correct the faulty position of the uterus. *SYN:* Thure Brandt massage
Thure Brandt massage – *SYN:* Brandt massage

Branham, H.H., 19th century U.S. surgeon.
Branham bradycardia – *SYN:* Branham sign
Branham sign – bradycardia following compression or excision of an arteriovenous fistula. *SYN:* Branham bradycardia

Branham, Sara Elizabeth, U.S. bacteriologist, 1888-1962.
Branhamella – a subgenus of the genus *Moraxella*, occurring in mucous membranes of the upper respiratory tract.

Brasdor, Pierre, French surgeon, 1721-1798.
Brasdor method – treatment of aneurysm by ligation of the artery immediately below the tumor.

Brauer, August, German dermatologist, 1883-1945.

Brauer syndrome – autosomal dominant disorder featuring sweat gland aplasia, pigmented nevi of chin and forehead, absent eyelashes, or double row of eyelashes. *SYN:* focal facial dermal dysplasia

Buschke-Fischer-Brauer syndrome – see under Buschke

Braun, Christopher Heinrich, German surgeon, 1847-1911.

Braun anastomosis – after gastroenterostomy, anastomosis between afferent and efferent loops of jejunum.

Braun, Frederick C., Jr., U.S. physician.

Braun-Bayer syndrome – syndrome characterized by nephrosis, deafness, urinary tract anomalies, bifid uvula, and digital defects.

Braune, Christian W., German anatomist, 1831-1892.

Braune canal – the birth canal formed by the uterine cavity, dilated cervix, vagina, and vulva.

Braune muscle – *SYN:* puborectalis muscle

Braune valve – a fold of mucous membrane at the junction of the esophagus with the stomach.

Braun-Falco, Otto, German physician.

Marghescu and Braun-Falco syndrome – see under Marghescu

Braunwald, Eugene, U.S. cardiologist, *1929.

Braunwald sign – weak pulse occurring immediately after a premature ventricular contraction.

Braxton Hicks, John, English gynecologist, 1825-1897.

Braxton Hicks contraction – rhythmic myometrial activity, occurring during the course of a pregnancy, which causes no pain for the patient.

Braxton Hicks sign – irregular uterine contractions occurring after the third month of pregnancy.

Braxton Hicks version – obsolete term for internal version of the fetus, substituting the breech for the head as the leading pole.

NOTES

Bray, Charles William, U.S. otologist, *1904.
  Wever-Bray effect – *SYN:* Wever-Bray phenomenon
  Wever-Bray phenomenon – see under Wever

Brazelton, T. Terry, U.S. pediatrician.
  Brazelton Neonatal Behavioral Assessment Scale – a scale to assess the development of the neonate.

Breda, Achille, Italian dermatologist, 1850-1933.
  Breda disease – a type of American leishmaniasis. *SYN:* espundia

Breen, William, U.S. physician, *1930.
  Cross-McKusick-Breen syndrome – *SYN:* Cross syndrome

Bregeat, P.
  Bregeat syndrome – angiomatosis of the eye and orbit, ipsilateral thalamencephalic angiomatosis that involves the choroids plexus, and cutaneous vascular nevus (port wine stain type) on contralateral forehead and adjacent scalp.

Brehmer, Hermann, German physician, 1826-1889.
  Brehmer method – *SYN:* Brehmer treatment
  Brehmer treatment – treatment used for pulmonary tuberculosis. *SYN:* Brehmer method

Breisky, August, Czech gynecologist, 1832-1889.
  Breisky disease – eruption of papules with vulvar involvement. *SYN:* lichen sclerosus

Brenn, Lena, 20th century U.S. researcher.
  Brown-Brenn stain – see under Brown, James H.
  Brown-Brenn technique

Brennemann, Joseph, U.S. pediatrician, 1872-1944.
  Brennemann syndrome – lymphadenitis of the retroperitoneal and mesenteric regions as a result of throat infection.

Brenner, Fritz, German pathologist, *1877.
  Brenner tumor – a relatively infrequent benign neoplasm of the ovary.

Brenner, Sydney, South African-born English scientist, *1927, joint winner of 2002 Nobel Prize for work related to genetic regulation of organ development and cell death.

Breschet, Gilbert, French anatomist, 1784-1845.
  Breschet bones – one of the small ossicles occasionally found in the ligaments of the sternoclavicular articulation. *SYN:* os suprasternale

Breschet canals – channels in the diploë that accommodate the diploic veins. *SYN:* diploic canals

Breschet hiatus – a semilunar opening at the apex of the cochlea through which the scala vestibuli and the scala tympani of the cochlea communicate with one another. *SYN:* helicotrema

Breschet sinus – a paired dural venous sinus beginning on the parietal bone, running along the sphenoidal ridges, and emptying into the cavernous sinus. *SYN:* sphenoparietal sinus

Breschet vein – one of the veins in the diploë of the cranial bones. *SYN:* diploic vein

Brescia, Michael J., U.S. nephrologist, *1933.

Brescia-Cimino fistula – a direct, surgically created arteriovenous fistula used to facilitate chronic hemodialysis.

Breslow, Alexander, U.S. pathologist, 1928-1980.

Breslow thickness – maximal thickness of a primary cutaneous melanoma.

Bretonneau, Pierre F., French physician, 1778-1862.

Bretonneau angina – diphtheria. *SYN:* Bretonneau disease

Bretonneau disease – *SYN:* Bretonneau angina

Breuer, Josef, Austrian internist, 1842-1925.

Hering-Breuer reflex – see under Hering, Heinrich Ewald

Breus, Carl, Austrian obstetrician, 1852-1914.

Breus mole – an aborted ovum in which the fetal surface of the placenta presents numerous hematomata with an absence of blood vessels in the chorion.

Brewer, George E., U.S. surgeon, 1861-1939.

Brewer infarcts – dark red, wedge-shaped areas resembling infarcts, seen on section of a kidney in pyelonephritis.

Brewer operation

Brewer speculum

NOTES

Brewer vaginal speculum

Bricker, Eugene M., U.S. urologist, *1908.
   Bricker operation – an operation utilizing an isolated segment of ileum to collect urine from the ureters and conduct it to the skin surface.

Bright, Richard, English internist and pathologist, 1789-1858.
   Bright disease – nonsuppurative nephritis with albuminuria and edema.

Brill, Nathan Edwin, U.S. physician, 1860-1925.
   Brill disease – *SYN:* Brill-Zinsser disease
   Brill-Symmers disease – obsolete term for nodular lymphoma.
   Brill-Zinsser disease – an endogenous reinfection associated with the "carrier state" in persons who previously had epidemic typhus fever. *SYN:* Brill disease; recrudescent typhus fever; recrudescent typhus

Brinell, Johan August, Swedish metallurgist, 1849-1925.
   Brinell hardness number – a number related to the size of the permanent impression made by a ball indenter of specified size pressed into the surface of the material under a specified load.
   Brinell scale

Brinton, William, English physician, 1823-1867.
   Brinton disease – infiltrating scirrhous carcinoma causing extensive thickening of stomach wall. *SYN:* leather-bottle stomach; linitis plastica

Briquet, Paul, French physician, 1796-1881.
   Briquet ataxia – weakening of the muscle sense and increased sensibility of the skin, in hysteria. *SYN:* hysterical ataxia
   Briquet syndrome – a chronic but fluctuating mental disorder, usually of young women, characterized by frequent complaints of physical illness involving multiple organ systems simultaneously.

Brissaud, Edouard, French physician, 1852-1909.
   Brissaud disease – habitual, repeated contraction of certain muscles, resulting in actions that can be voluntarily suppressed for only brief periods. *SYN:* tic
   Brissaud infantilism – *SYN:* infantile hypothyroidism
   Brissaud-Marie syndrome – unilateral spasm of the tongue and lips, of hysterical nature.
   Brissaud reflex – tickling the sole causes a contraction of the tensor fasciae latae muscle, even when there is no responsive movement of the toes.

Bristol, city in England.
> **Bristol diet therapy** – diet developed at the Cancer Help Centre in Bristol, emphasizing whole foods and the use of organic produce while avoiding caffeine and dairy products.

Bristowe, John S., English physician, 1827-1895.
> **Bristowe syndrome** – symptoms caused by corpus callosum tumor.

B

Broadbent, Sir William H., English physician, 1835-1907.
> **Bolton-Broadbent plane** – *SYN:* Bolton plane
> **Broadbent apoplexy** – intracerebral bleeding which penetrates the lateral ventricle of the brain.
> **Broadbent inverted sign** – retraction of thoracic wall, synchronous with cardiac systole, visible particularly in the left posterior axillary line; sign of adherent pericardium. *SYN:* Broadbent sign
> **Broadbent law** – lesions of the upper segment of the motor tract cause less marked paralysis of muscles that habitually produce bilateral movements than of those that commonly act independently of the opposite side.
> **Broadbent sign** – *SYN:* Broadbent inverted sign

Broca, Paul, French surgeon, neurologist, and anthropologist, 1824-1880.
> **Broca angle** – the angle formed at the basion of lines drawn from the nasion and the alveolar point; the angle formed by the intersection at the biauricular axis of lines drawn from the supraorbital point and the alveolar point; the posterior superior angle of the parietal bone. *SYN:* Broca basilar angle; Broca facial angle; occipital angle of parietal bone
> **Broca aphasia** – any of the varieties of aphasia in which the power of expression by writing, speaking, or signs is lost. *SYN:* motor aphasia
> **Broca area** – *SYN:* Broca center
> **Broca basilar angle** – *SYN:* Broca angle
> **Broca center** – the posterior part of the inferior frontal gyrus of the left or dominant hemisphere, essential component of the motor mechanisms

NOTES

governing articulated speech. *SYN:* Broca area; Broca field; Brodmann area 44; motor speech center

Broca diagonal band – a white fiber bundle descending in the precommissural septum toward the base of the forebrain.

Broca facial angle – *SYN:* Broca angle

Broca field – *SYN:* Broca center

Broca fissure – the fissure surrounding Broca convolution.

Broca formula – a fully developed man should weigh as many kilograms as he is centimeters in height over and above 1 meter.

Broca parolfactory area – a small region of cerebral cortex on the medical surface of the frontal lobe demarcated from the subcallosal gyrus by the posterior parolfactory sulcus. *SYN:* parolfactory area

Broca pouch – a pear-shaped encapsulated collection of connective tissue and fat in each labium majus. *SYN:* pudendal sac

Broca visual plane – a plane drawn through the visual axes of each eye.

Brock, Sir Russell C., English surgeon, 1903-1980.

Brock operation – transventricular valvotomy for relief of pulmonic valvar stenosis; obsolete procedure.

Brock syndrome – atelectasis with chronic pneumonitis of the middle lobe of the right lung, due to compression of the middle lobe bronchus, usually by enlarged lymph nodes, which may be tuberculous. *SYN:* middle lobe syndrome

Brockenbrough, E.C., U.S. surgeon, *1930.

Brockenbrough sign – a sign of idiopathic hypertrophic subaortic stenosis.

Brocq, Anne-Jean Louis, French dermatologist, 1856-1928.

Brocq disease – a variety of parapsoriasis.

Brödel, Max, German medical artist in the U.S., 1870-1941.

Brödel bloodless line – line demarcating the areas of distribution of the anterior and posterior branches of the renal artery.

Brodie, Charles Gordon, Scottish anatomist and surgeon, 1860-1933.

Brodie ligament – a fibrous band running more or less obliquely from the greater to the lesser tuberosity of the humerus, bridging over the bicipital groove. *SYN:* transverse humeral ligament

Brodie, Sir Benjamin C., English surgeon, 1783-1862.

Brodie abscess – a chronic abscess of bone surrounded by dense fibrous tissue and sclerotic bone.

Brodie bursa – medial subtendinous bursa of gastrocnemius muscle. *SYN:* bursa of semimembranosus muscle

Brodie disease – (1) *SYN:* Brodie knee; (2) hysterical spinal neuralgia, simulating Pott disease.

Brodie knee – chronic hypertrophic synovitis of the knee. *SYN:* Brodie disease (1)

Brodie serocystic disease – usually benign and fast-growing postpubescent breast tumor.

Brodie-Trendelenburg test – test for varicosities in leg veins.

Brodie, Thomas Gregor, English physiologist, 1866-1916.

Brodie fluid – an aqueous salt solution used in manometers designed for testing gas evolution or uptake, as in cell respiration.

Brodin, M., French physician.

Brodin syndrome – stenosis of duodenum caused by lymphadenitis related to appendicitis.

Brodmann, Korbinian, German neurologist, 1868-1918.

Brodmann area 41 – *SYN:* primary auditory cortex

Brodmann area 44 – *SYN:* Broca center

Brodmann areas – areas of cerebral cortex mapped out on the basis of cortical cytoarchitectural patterns.

Brody, Irwin A., U.S. physician.

Brody syndrome – a disorder of muscle function with exercise-induced painless contractures.

Broesike, Gustav, German anatomist, *1853.

Broesike fossa – a peritoneal fossa. *SYN:* parajejunal fossa

Brompton, name of a hospital in London.

Brompton cocktail – analgesic drink given to terminal cancer patients.

Brønsted, Johannes N., Danish physical chemist, 1879-1947.

Brønsted acid – an acid that is a proton donor.

Brønsted base – any molecule or ion that combines with a proton.

NOTES

Brønsted theory – that an acid is a substance, charged or uncharged, liberating hydrogen ions in solution, and that a base is a substance that removes them from solution.

Brooke, Bryan N., English surgeon, *1915.

Brooke ileostomy – ileostomy in which the divided proximal ileum, brought through the abdominal wall, is evaginated and its edge is sutured to the dermis.

Brooke, Henry Ambrose Grundy, English dermatologist, 1854-1919.

Brooke disease – (1) multiple small benign nodules, occurring mostly on the skin of the face, derived from basal cells of hair follicles enclosing small keratin cysts. *SYN:* Ancell-Spiegler cylindroma; Ancell-Spiegler syndrome; Ancell syndrome; Brooke epithelioma; Brooke-Fordyce disease; Brooke-Fordyce trichoepithelioma; Brooke-Spiegler phatomatosis; Brooke tumor; trichoepithelioma; (2) a rare condition simulating keratosis follicularis. *SYN:* Morrow-Brooke syndrome

Brooke epithelioma – *SYN:* Brooke disease (1)

Brooke-Fordyce disease – *SYN:* Brooke disease (1)

Brooke-Fordyce trichoepithelioma – *SYN:* Brooke disease (1)

Brooke tumor – *SYN:* Brooke disease (1)

Morrow-Brooke syndrome – *SYN:* Brooke disease (2)

Brophy, Truman William, U.S. oral surgeon, 1848-1928.

Brophy bistoury

Brophy bistoury knife

Brophy cleft palate knife

Brophy dressing forceps

Brophy elevator

Brophy forceps

Brophy gag

Brophy knife

Brophy needle

Brophy operation – surgery to correct cleft palate.

Brophy periosteal elevator

Brophy periosteotome

Brophy plate

Brophy scissors

Brophy tenaculum

Brophy tenaculum retractor

Brophy tissue forceps

Brophy tooth elevator

Brown, George Elgie, U.S. physician, 1885-1935.
　Hines and Brown test – see under Hines
　Nygaard-Brown syndrome– *SYN:* Trousseau syndrome

Brown, Harold Whaley, U.S. ophthalmologist, *1898.
　Brown syndrome – limited elevation of the eye in adduction due to fascia
　　contracting the superior oblique muscle on the same side. *SYN:* tendon
　　sheath syndrome
　Paterson-Brown-Kelly syndrome – see under Paterson

Brown, James, U.S. plastic surgeon, 1899-1971.
　Blair-Brown graft – see under Blair
　Brown-Adson forceps – an Adson forceps with about 16 delicate teeth on
　　each tip.

Brown, James H., U.S. microbiologist, *1884.
　Brown-Brenn stain – a method for differential staining of gram-positive
　　and gram-negative bacteria in tissue sections.
　Brown-Brenn technique

Brown, Jason W., U.S. physician.
　Brown syndrome – syndrome occurring in individuals with light
　　complexion, blond hair, light eyes and characterized by loss of pain
　　sensitivity, pupillary abnormalities, neurogenic anhidrosis, vasomotor
　　instability. *SYN:* neural crest syndrome

Brown, Michael S., joint winner of 1985 Nobel Prize for work related to
cholesterol.

Brown, Robert, English botanist, 1773-1858.
　brownian motion – *SYN:* brownian movement
　brownian movement – rapid random motion of small particles in
　　suspension. *SYN:* brownian motion; brownian-Zsigmondy movement;
　　molecular movement; pedesis
　brownian-Zsigmondy movement – *SYN:* brownian movement

B

NOTES

Brown, Sanger, U.S. neuropsychiatrist, 1852-1928.
Sanger Brown syndrome – *SYN:* Menzel syndrome

Browne, Sir Denis John, English surgeon, 1892-1967.
Denis Browne bucket
Denis Browne forceps
Denis Browne pouch – a common lodging site for undescended testes.
SYN: superficial inguinal pouch
Denis Browne splint – a light aluminum splint used for clubfoot.
Denis Browne talipes hobble splint
Denis Browne tray

Browning, William, U.S. anatomist and neurologist, 1855-1941.
Browning vein – an inconstant vein that passes from the superficial
middle cerebral vein posteriorly over the lateral aspect of the temporal
lobe to enter the transverse sinus. *SYN:* inferior anastomotic vein

Brown-Séquard, Charles E., French physiologist and neurologist, 1817-
1894.
Brown-Séquard paralysis – *SYN:* Brown-Séquard syndrome
Brown-Séquard syndrome – syndrome with unilateral spinal cord lesions,
proprioception loss and weakness ipsilateral to the lesion, while pain
and temperature loss occur contralateral. *SYN:* Brown-Séquard paralysis

Bruce, Robert A., U.S. cardiologist.
Bruce test – exercise test for individuals with coronary disease.

Bruce, Sir David, English surgeon, 1855-1931.
Brucella – a genus of encapsulated, nonmotile bacteria (family
Brucellaceae) causing infection of the genital organs, the mammary
gland, and the respiratory and intestinal tracts.
Brucella abortus – infectious bacteria causing abortions in cattle, sheep,
mares; causes undulant fever in man and a wasting disease in chickens.
SYN: abortus bacillus; Bang bacillus
brucellosis – an infectious disease caused by *Brucella*, and transmitted by
direct contact with diseased animals or through ingestion of infected
meat, milk, or cheese. *SYN:* febris undulans; Malta fever; Mediterranean
fever; undulant fever

Bruch, Carl W.L., German anatomist, 1819-1884.
Bruch glands – lymph nodes in the palpebral conjunctiva. *SYN:* trachoma
glands
Bruch membrane – the transparent, nearly structureless inner layer of the
choroid in contact with the pigmented layer of the retina. *SYN:* lamina
basalis choroideae

Bruck, Alfred, German physician, *1865.
  Bruck disease – a disease marked by osteogenesis imperfecta, ankylosis of the joints, and muscular atrophy.

Brücke, Ernst W. von, Austrian physiologist, 1819-1892.
  Brücke-Bartley phenomenon – the sensation of glare in response to successive stimuli at frequencies just below the fusion point.
  Brücke muscle – the part of the ciliary muscle formed by the meridional fibers. *SYN:* Crampton muscle
  Brücke tunic – a term formerly used to designate the retina exclusive of the layer of rods and cones. *SYN:* tunica nervea

Brudzinski, Josef von, Polish physician, 1874-1917.
  Brudzinski sign – neck or leg flexion tests for meningitis.

Brugsch, Theodor, German internist, 1878-1963.
  Brugsch syndrome – acromegaly, acropachyderma, and hypertrophy of the long bones.

Brumpt, Emile, French parasitologist, 1877-1951.
  Brumpt white mycetoma – mycetoma caused by *Pseudallescheria boydii.*

Brunati, M., 20th century Italian physician.
  Brunati sign – corneal opacities caused by pneumonia or typhoid fever.

Brünauer, Stefan Robert, German physician, *1887.
  Brünauer syndrome – *SYN:* Unna-Thost syndrome

Brunhes, S., French physician.
  Brunhes-Chavany syndrome – *SYN:* Chavany-Brunhes syndrome
  Chavany-Brunhes syndrome – see under Chavany

Brunn, Albert von, German anatomist, 1849-1895.
  Brunn epithelial nests
  Brunn membrane – the epithelium of the olfactory region of the nose.
  Brunn nests – glandlike invaginations of surface transitional epithelium in the mucosa of the lower urinary tract.

NOTES

Brunn, Fritz, 20th century Czech physician.

Brunn reaction – the increased absorption of water through the skin of a frog when the animal is injected with pituitrin and immersed in water.

Brunner, Johann C., Swiss anatomist, 1653-1727.

Brunner gland hamartoma

Brunner glands – small glands that secrete a substance that neutralizes gastric juice. *SYN:* duodenal glands

Brunnstrom, Signe, Swedish physical therapist.

Brunnstrom facilitation technique – *SYN:* Brunnstrom method

Brunnstrom method – exercises for individuals with central nervous system lesions. *SYN:* Brunnstrom facilitation technique; Brunnstrom proprioceptive neuromuscular facilitation

Brunnstrom proprioceptive neuromuscular facilitation – *SYN:* Brunnstrom method

Bruns, Ludwig von, German neurologist, 1858-1916.

Bastian-Bruns law – see under Bastian

Bastian-Bruns sign – *SYN:* Bastian-Bruns law

Bruns ataxia – difficulty in moving the feet when they are in contact with the ground; a condition related to a frontal lobe lesion.

Bruns nystagmus – due to lateral brainstem compression, usually by a cerebellopontine angle mass such as an acoustic neuroma.

Bruns syndrome – lesions of cerebral fourth ventricle cause symptoms of headache, vertigo, and vomiting; if head position is altered, the patient may fall.

Brunschwig, Alexander, U.S. surgeon, 1901-1969.

Brunschwig operation – *SYN:* total pelvic exenteration

Brunsting, Louis Albert, U.S. dermatologist, 1900-1980.

Brunsting disease – locally recurrent and scarring subepidermal blisters of the hand and neck; believed to be a form of cicatricial pemphigoid.

Brushfield, Thomas, English physician, 1858-1937.

Brushfield spots – light-colored condensations of the surface of the mid-iris; seen in Down syndrome.

Brushfield-Wyatt disease – a familial disorder characterized by unilateral nevus, contralateral hemiplegia, hemianopia, cerebral angioma, and mental retardation. *SYN:* nevoid amentia

Bruton, Ogden Carr, U.S. pediatrician, *1908.

    Bruton agammaglobulinemia – genetic trait causing decreased quantity of gamma fraction of serum globulin; associated with increased susceptibility to pyogenic infections and observed in type III isolated growth hormone deficiency.

Bryant, Sir Thomas, English surgeon, 1828-1914.

    Bryant ampulla – that portion of an artery on the proximal side of a ligature containing the clot, its upper boundary being marked by a slight constriction.

    Bryant sign – in dislocation of the shoulder, an abnormal position of axillary folds occurs.

    Bryant traction – traction upon the lower limb placed vertically, employed especially in fractures of the femur in children.

    Bryant triangle – lines drawn on the body in fracture of the neck of the femur to determine upward displacement of the trochanter. *SYN:* iliofemoral triangle

Buchem, Francis Steven Peter van, see under van Buchem

Büchner, Eduard, German chemist and Nobel laureate, 1860-1917.

    Büchner extract – a cell-free extract of yeast.

    Büchner funnel – a porcelain funnel that contains a perforated porcelain plate on which filter paper can be laid.

Büchner, Hans E.A., German bacteriologist, 1850-1902.

    Büchner extract – see under Büchner, Eduard

Buchwald, Hermann Edmund, German physician, *1903.

    Buchwald atrophy – a progressive form of cutaneous atrophy.

Buck, Gurdon, U.S. surgeon, 1807-1877.

    Buck extension – apparatus for applying longitudinal skin traction on the leg. *SYN:* Buck traction

    Buck extension bar

    Buck extension frame

NOTES

Buck extension splint
Buck fascia – a deep layer which surrounds the three erectile bodies of the penis. *SYN:* fascia penis profunda
Buck femoral cement restrictor inserter
Buck fracture appliance
Buck hook
Buck knee brace
Buck method
Buck osteotome
Buck plug
Buck traction – *SYN:* Buck extension
Buck tractor

Bücklers, Max, German ophthalmologist, 1895-1969.
Reis-Bücklers corneal dystrophy – see under Reis

Buckley, Rebecca H., U.S. pediatrician and allergist, *1933.
Buckley syndrome – recurrent furunculosis, recurrent pneumonias, and pruritic dermatitis. Patients have a markedly elevated serum IgE. *SYN:* Job syndrome

Bucky, Gustav, U.S. radiologist, 1880-1963.
Bucky diaphragm – in radiography, a diaphragm with a moving grid that avoids grid shadows. *SYN:* Potter-Bucky diaphragm
Bucky film
Bucky grid
Bucky rays
Bucky studies
Bucky technique

Bucy, Paul C., U.S. neurosurgeon, 1904-1992.
Bucy cordotomy knife
Bucy knife
Bucy laminectomy rongeur
Bucy retractor
Bucy tube
Klüver-Bucy syndrome – see under Klüver

Budd, George, English physician, 1808-1882.
Budd-Chiari syndrome – *SYN:* Chiari syndrome
Budd cirrhosis – chronic enlargement of the liver without jaundice.
Budd disease
Budd syndrome – *SYN:* Chiari syndrome
Chiari-Budd syndrome – *SYN:* Chiari syndrome

Budde, E., Danish sanitary engineer, *1871.
  Budde process – a method of milk sterilization.

Budge, Julius L., German physiologist, 1811-1888.
  Budge center – the preganglionic motor neurons in the first thoracic
    segment of the spinal cord that give rise to the sympathetic innervation
    of the dilator muscle of the eye's pupil. *SYN:* ciliospinal center

Budin, Pierre C., French gynecologist, 1846-1907.
  Budin obstetrical joint – cartilaginous union between the squamous and
    lateral parts of the occipital bone in the newborn. *SYN:* posterior
    intraoccipital synchondrosis

Buerger, Leo, Austrian-U.S. physician, 1879-1943.
  Buerger-Allen exercises – *SYN:* Buerger exercises
  Buerger disease – inflammation of the entire wall and connective tissue
    surrounding medium-sized arteries and veins, associated with
    thrombotic occlusion and commonly resulting in gangrene. *SYN:*
    thromboangiitis obliterans; Winiwarter-Buerger disease
  Buerger exercises – exercises specifically for patients with arterial
    insufficiency of their lower limbs. *SYN:* Buerger-Allen exercises
  Winiwarter-Buerger disease – *SYN:* Buerger disease

Buhl, Ludwig Von, German physician, 1816-1880.
  Buhl disease – acute sepsis occurring in newborn infants.

Bull, Sir Graham MacGregor, South African physician.
  Bull regime – diet used in cases of acute renal failure.

Buller, Frank, Canadian ophthalmologic surgeon, 1844-1905.
  Buller bandage – *SYN:* Buller shield
  Buller shield – in eye infection, a shield used to protect the healthy eye.
    SYN: Buller bandage

Bumke, Oswald C.E., German neurologist, 1877-1950.
  Bumke pupil – dilation of the pupil in response to anxiety or other psychic
    stimuli. *SYN:* Bumke syndrome

NOTES

Bumke syndrome – *SYN:* Bumke pupil

Bunnell, Sterling, U.S. physician and surgeon, 1882-1957.
Bunnell atraumatic technique
Bunnell block – a block of wood used to exercise stiffened joints.
Bunnell dressing
Bunnell gutter splint
Bunnell hand drill
Bunnell knuckle-bender splint
Bunnell modification of Steindler flexorplasty
Bunnell needle
Bunnell outrigger splint
Bunnell probe
Bunnell pull-out wire
Bunnell solution
Bunnell suture – a method of tenorrhaphy using a pull-out wire affixed to buttons.
Bunnell tendon passer
Bunnell tendon transfer technique
Paul-Bunnell test – see under Paul, John Rodman

Bunsen, Robert W., German chemist and physicist, 1811-1899.
Bunsen burner – a gas lamp giving a very hot but only slightly luminous flame.
Bunsen-Roscoe law – in two photochemical reactions, if the product of the intensity of illumination and the time of exposure are equal, the quantities of chemical material undergoing change will be equal. *SYN:* reciprocity law; Roscoe-Bunsen law
Bunsen solubility coefficient – the milliliters of gas STPD dissolved per milliliter of liquid and per atmosphere (760 mmHg) partial pressure of the gas at any given temperature.
Roscoe-Bunsen law – *SYN:* Bunsen-Roscoe law

Burchard, H., 19th century German chemist.
Burchard-Liebermann reaction – a blue-green color produced by acetic anhydride with cholesterol (and other sterols) dissolved in chloroform, when a few drops of concentrated sulfuric acid are added.
Liebermann-Burchard test – see under Liebermann

Burdach, Karl F., German anatomist and physiologist, 1776-1847.
Burdach column – the larger lateral subdivision of the posterior funiculus. *SYN:* Burdach fasciculus; Burdach tract; cuneate fasciculus
Burdach fasciculus – *SYN:* Burdach column

Burdach nucleus – *SYN:* cuneate nucleus
Burdach tract – *SYN:* Burdach column

Bureau, Yves, French dermatologist, 1900-1993.
Bureau-Barrière syndrome – severe diffuse keratoderma and osteolysis of the forefoot, associated with painless foot ulcer and polyneuropathy of lower legs.
Bureau-Barrière-Thomas syndrome – an autosomal recessive form of keratosis palmaris and plantaris and Hippocratic fingers and toes. *SYN:* Bureau syndrome
Bureau syndrome – *SYN:* Bureau-Barrière-Thomas syndrome

Buren, William H. van, see under van Buren

Burgdorfer, Willy, Swiss-born U.S. zoologist and entomologist.
Borrelia burgdorferi – the spirochete that causes Lyme disease.

Bürger, Max, German physician, *1885.
Bürger-Grütz disease – obsolete term for idiopathic hyperlipemia.
Bürger-Grütz syndrome – an inherited disorder of lipoprotein metabolism. *SYN:* type I familial hyperlipoproteinemia

Burghart, Hans G., German physician, 1862-1932.
Burghart sign – *SYN:* Burghart symptom
Burghart symptom – fine lung rales seen in early stages of pulmonary tuberculosis. *SYN:* Burghart sign

Burk, Dean, U.S. scientist, *1904.
Lineweaver-Burk equation – see under Lineweaver
Lineweaver-Burk plot – see under Lineweaver

Burke, Richard M., U.S. physician, *1903.
Burke syndrome – advanced pulmonary emphysema leading to loss of pulmonary markings on x-ray. *SYN:* vanishing lung; solitary lobar atrophy; cotton candy lung; idiopathic pulmonary atrophy; De Martini-Balestra syndrome

B

NOTES

Burkitt, Denis P., English physician in Uganda, 1911-1993.

Burkitt lymphoma – a form of malignant lymphoma reported in African children, caused by Epstein-Barr virus; a member of the family Herpesviridae.

Burkitt tumor

Burn, J.H.

Burn and Rand theory – that stimulation of sympathetic fibers results first in the production of acetylcholine in the postganglionic nerve endings, which then release norepinephrine to act on the active site of the effector cell.

Burnet, Sir Frank MacFarlane, joint winner of 1960 Nobel Prize for work related to immunology.

Burnett, Charles H., U.S. physician, 1901-1967.

Burnett syndrome – a chronic disorder of the kidneys, induced by ingestion of large amounts of calcium and alkali in the therapy of peptic ulcer. *SYN:* milk-alkali syndrome

Burns, Allan, Scottish anatomist, 1781-1813.

Burns falciform process – *SYN:* superior horn of falciform margin of saphenous opening

Burns ligament – *SYN:* superior horn of falciform margin of saphenous opening

Burns space – a narrow interval between the deep and superficial layers of the cervical fascia above the manubrium of the sternum through which pass the anterior jugular veins. *SYN:* suprasternal space

Burns, F.S.

Burns syndrome – syndrome featuring keratitis, hearing loss, and ichthyosis.

Burow, Karl August von, German military surgeon and anatomist, 1809-1874.

Burow operation – an operation in which triangles of skin adjacent to a sliding flap are excised to facilitate movement of the flap.

Burow solution – a preparation of aluminium subacetate and glacial acetic acid, used for its antiseptic and astringent action on the skin.

Burow triangle – a triangle of skin and subcutaneous fat excised so that a pedicle flap can be advanced without buckling the adjacent tissue.

Burow vein – one of the renal veins.

Burton, Henry, English physician, 1799-1849.

Burton line – a bluish line on the free border of the gingiva, occurring in lead poisoning. *SYN:* lead line

Buruli, district in Uganda.
> **Buruli lesion** – infection with *Mycobacterium ulcerans*, causing painless nodule which ulcerates on leg or forearm; common in children and first noted in Buruli.

Bury, Judson Sykes, English dermatologist, 1852-1944.
> **Bury disease** – a chronic symmetrical eruption of flattened pinkish nodules. *SYN:* erythema elevatum diutinum

Busacca, Archimede, Italian physician, *1893.
> **Busacca floccule** – *SYN:* Busacca nodule
> **Busacca nodule** – nodule that appears on the iris in the anterior mesodermal layers. *SYN:* Busacca floccule

Buschke, Abraham, Polish-born German dermatologist, 1868-1943.
> **Buschke disease** – obsolete eponym for cryptococcosis. *SYN:* scleredema adultorum
> **Buschke-Löwenstein tumor** – a large type of condyloma acuminatum found in the genitals. *SYN:* giant condyloma
> **Buschke-Ollendorf syndrome** – *SYN:* osteopoikilosis
> **Busse-Buschke disease** – see under Busse

Buselmeier, T.J., 20th century U.S. nephrologist.
> **Buselmeier shunt**

Busquet, G. Paul, French physician, 1866-1930.
> **Busquet disease** – an osteoperiostitis of the metatarsal bones, leading to exostoses on the dorsum of the foot.

Busse, Otto, German pathologist, 1867-1922.
> **Busse-Buschke disease** – an acute, subacute, or chronic infection by *Cryptococcus neoformans*, causing a pulmonary, disseminated, or meningeal mycosis. *SYN:* cryptococcosis
> **Busse saccaromyces**

Butcher, Richard George H., Irish surgeon, 1819-1891.
> **Butcher saw** – amputating saw.

NOTES

Buzzard, Thomas, English physician, 1831-1919.
> **Buzzard maneuver** – testing the patellar reflex while the sitting patient makes firm pressure on the floor with the toes.

Buzzi, Fausto, late 19th century German dermatologist.
> **Schweninger-Buzzi anetoderma** – see under Schweninger

Bwamba, forest in Uganda.
> **Bwamba virus** – genus *Bunyavirus,* family Bunyaviridae; causes mild infection and unidentified fevers; often mistaken for malaria.

Byler, Amish kindred in the U.S.
> **Byler disease** – genetic trait in Amish children that causes fatal intrahepatic arrest of bile flow.

Bywaters, Eric George Lapthorne, English rheumatologist, *1910.
> **Bywaters syndrome** – lower nephron nephrosis. *SYN:* crush syndrome

Cabot, Richard Clarke, U.S. physician, 1868-1939.

> **Cabot-Locke murmur** – an early diastolic murmur, like that of aortic insufficiency, heard best at the left lower sternal border in severe anemia.
>
> **Cabot ring bodies** – ring-shaped or figure-of-eight structures found in red blood cells in severe anemias. *SYN:* Cabot rings
>
> **Cabot rings** – *SYN:* Cabot ring bodies

Cacchi, Roberto, Italian physician.

> **Cacchi-Ricci syndrome** – *SYN:* cystic disease of the renal pyramids; medullary polycystic kidney; Ricci-Cacchi syndrome; sponge kidney
>
> **Ricci-Cacchi syndrome** – *SYN:* Cacchi-Ricci syndrome

Cacchione, Aldo, 20th century Italian psychiatrist.

> **De Sanctis-Cacchione syndrome** – see under De Sanctis

Caenis, Greek mythological character raped by Poseidon, transformed into a fearsome male warrior in order to exact revenge.

> **Caenis syndrome** – syndrome characterized by diminished or perverted appetite, hysterical personality, and female genital self-mutilation.

Caffey, John Patrick, U.S. physician, radiologist, and pediatrician, the father of pediatric radiology, 1895-1978.

> **Caffey disease** – *SYN:* Caffey syndrome
>
> **Caffey-Silverman syndrome** – *SYN:* Caffey syndrome
>
> **Caffey syndrome** – neonatal subperiosteal bone formation over many bones, especially the mandible and clavicles and the shafts of long bones. *SYN:* Caffey disease; Caffey-Silverman syndrome; infantile cortical hyperostosis

Cain, character in Old Testament of the Bible who killed his brother Abel out of jealousy.

Cain complex – hatred of a brother due to envy or jealousy. *SYN:* brother complex

Cajal, Santiago, Spanish histologist and Nobel laureate, 1852-1934.

Cajal astrocyte stain – a method for demonstrating astrocytes by impregnation in a solution containing gold chloride and mercuric chloride.

Cajal cell – *SYN:* horizontal cell of Cajal

Cajal formol ammonium bromide solution

Cajal gold-sublimate method

Cajal uranium silver method

horizontal cell of Cajal – a small fusiform cell found in the superficial layer of the cerebral cortex with its long axis placed horizontally. *SYN:* astrocyte; Cajal cell

interstitial nucleus of Cajal – a group of neurons believed to be involved in the integration of head and eye movements. *SYN:* interstitial nucleus

Calcutta, city in India.

Calcutta technique – a technique used in therapeutic irradiation by infrared rays; first observed in Calcutta, India.

Caldani, Leopoldo M.A., Italian anatomist, 1725-1813.

Caldani ligament – the strong ligament that unites the clavicle to the coracoid process. *SYN:* coracoclavicular ligament

Caldwell, George W., U.S. physician, 1834-1918.

Caldwell-Luc operation – an intraoral procedure for opening into the maxillary antrum through the supradental (canine) fossa above the maxillary premolar teeth. *SYN:* intraoral antrostomy; Luc operation

Caldwell, William E., U.S. obstetrician, 1880-1943.

Caldwell-Moloy classification – a classification of the variations in the female pelvis.

California, 31st state, admitted to the United States in 1850.

California encephalitis – encephalitis caused by genus *Bunyavirus*; may be seen in domestic animals and rodents.

California Psychological Inventory Test – personality inventory with emphasis on social interaction.

californium – man-made radioactive actinide, chemical symbol Cf, used in radiotherapy.

Calkins, Leroy Adelbert, U.S. obstetrician-gynecologist, 1894-1960.
   Calkins sign – the change of shape of the uterus from discoid to ovoid, indicating placental separation from the uterine wall.

Call, Friedrich von, Austrian physician, 1844-1917.
   Call-Exner bodies – small fluid-filled spaces between granulosa cells in ovarian follicles and in ovarian tumors of granulosal origin.

Callahan, John R., U.S. endodontist, 1853-1918.
   Callahan method – a method of filling the root canals of teeth by dissolving gutta-percha cones in a chloroform-rosin medium within the root canal. *SYN:* chloropercha method

Callander, Latimer, U.S. surgeon, 1892-1947.
   Callander amputation – tenontoplastic amputation through the femur at the knee.
   Callander derotational brace
   Callander technique hip prosthesis

Calleja, Camilo, Spanish anatomist, d. 1913.
   islands of Calleja – dense clusters of very small nerve cells (granule cells) characteristic of the olfactory tubercle at the base of the forebrain.

Callison, James S., U.S. physician, *1873.
   Callison fluid – a diluting fluid for counting red blood cells.

Calmette, Leon Charles Albert, French bacteriologist, 1863-1933.
   Bacille bilié de Calmette-Guérin – an attenuated strain of *Mycobacterium bovis* used for immunization against tuberculosis and in cancer chemotherapy. *SYN:* Bacille Calmette-Guérin; Calmette-Guérin bacillus
   Bacille Calmette-Guérin – *SYN:* Bacille bilié de Calmette-Guérin
   bacillus Calmette-Guérin vaccine – a vaccine for tuberculosis prophylaxis. *SYN:* BCG vaccine
   Calmette-Guérin bacillus – *SYN:* Bacille bilié de Calmette-Guérin
   Calmette-Guérin vaccine – *SYN:* bacillus Calmette-Guérin vaccine
   Calmette test – conjunctival reaction to tuberculin.

NOTES

Calò, S.
  Alè-Calò syndrome – *SYN:* Langer-Giedion syndrome

Calori, Luigi, Italian anatomist, 1807-1896.
  Calori bursa – a bursa between the arch of the aorta and the trachea.

Calot, Jean-François, French surgeon, 1861-1944.
  Calot node
  Calot operation
  Calot triangle – a triangle bounded by the cystic artery, cystic duct, and hepatic duct.

Calvé, Jacques, French orthopedic surgeon, 1875-1954.
  Calvé disease – vertebral osteochondrosis.
  Calvé-Perthes disease – *SYN:* Legg-Calvé-Perthes disease
  Legg-Calvé-Perthes disease – see under Legg

Calvert, A.H., English oncologist.
  Calvert formula – calculation of carboplatin dose from glomerular filtration rate (GFR) and target area under the curve (AUC) of carboplatin.

Camera, Ugo, Italian physician.
  Camera syndrome – *SYN:* neuralgic lumbosciatic osteopathy syndrome

Camerer, Johann F.W., German pediatrician, 1842-1910.
  Camerer law – child's weight rather than age determines food requirement.

Cammann, George P., U.S. physician, 1804-1863.
  Cammann stethoscope

Campanacci, Mario, Italian physician, 1932-1999.
  Campanacci syndrome – syndrome characterized by pain, swelling, café-au-lait spots, and at times hypogonadism and developmental delay. *SYN:* Jaffe-Campanacci syndrome
  Jaffe-Campanacci syndrome – *SYN:* Campanacci syndrome

Campbell, Meredith F., 20th century U.S. pediatric urologist.
  Campbell sound – a miniature sound with a short round-tipped beak, especially curved for the deep urethra of the young male.

Campbell, William F., U.S. surgeon, 1867-1926.
  Campbell ligament – maintains the characteristic hollow of the armpit. *SYN:* suspensory ligament of axilla

Camper, Pieter, Dutch physician and anatomist, 1722-1789.
  Camper chiasm – *SYN:* tendinous chiasm of the digital tendons
  Camper fascia – *SYN:* fatty layer of superficial fascia

Camper ligament – the layer of fascia extending between the ischiopubic rami inferior to the sphincter urethrae and the deep transverse perineal muscles. *SYN:* inferior fascia of urogenital diaphragm

Camper line – the line running from the inferior border of the ala of the nose to the superior border of the tragus of the ear.

Camper plane – a plane running from the tip of the anterior nasal spine (acanthion) to the center of the bony external auditory meatus on the right and left sides.

Camurati, Mario, Italian physician, 1896-1948.
Camurati-Engelmann syndrome – *SYN:* Engelmann disease

Canada, Wilma Jeanne, 20th century U.S. radiologist.
Cronkhite-Canada syndrome – see under Cronkhite

Canavan, Myrtelle M., U.S. pathologist, 1879-1953.
Canavan disease – autosomal recessive degenerative disease of infancy. *SYN:* Canavan sclerosis; Canavan-van Bogaert-Bertrand disease; spongy degeneration of infancy
Canavan sclerosis – *SYN:* Canavan disease
Canavan-van Bogaert-Bertrand disease – *SYN:* Canavan disease

Cannizzaro, Stanislao, Italian chemist, 1826-1910.
Cannizzaro reaction – formation of an acid and an alcohol by the simultaneous oxidation of one aldehyde molecule and reduction of another.

Cannon, A. Benson, U.S. dermatologist, 1888-1950.
Cannon nevus – familial disorder characterized by painless, shaggy, and folded lesions on the buccal mucosa. *SYN:* Cannon syndrome; familial white folded dysplasia; oral epithelial nevus; white sponge nevus
Cannon syndrome – *SYN:* Cannon nevus

Cannon, Walter B., U.S. physiologist, 1871-1945.
Bernard-Cannon homeostasis – see under Bernard, Claude

Cannon-Bard theory – the view that the feeling aspect of emotion and the pattern of emotional behavior are controlled by the hypothalamus.

Cannon law – reaction of excessive sensitivity to chemical neurotransmitters in tissue with deficiency of autonomic supply.

Cannon point – the location in the midtransverse colon at which innervation by superior and inferior mesenteric plexuses overlap at the junction of the primitive midgut and hindgut. *SYN:* Cannon ring

Cannon ring – *SYN:* Cannon point

Cannon syndrome – perspiration and palpitations due to increased secretion of adrenalin.

Cannon theory – a theory of the emotions that animal and human organisms respond to emergency situations by increased sympathetic nervous system activity. *SYN:* emergency theory

Cantor, Meyer O., U.S. physician, *1907.

Cantor tube – a long, single-lumen intestinal tube.

Cantú, Jose-Maria, 20th century Mexican human geneticist.

Cantú syndrome – an X-linked syndrome of dwarfism, microcephaly, keratosis follicularis, delayed psychomotor development, and absence of hair, eyebrows, and eyelashes. *SYN:* dwarfism, cerebral atrophy, and keratosis follicularis

Cantú syndrome I – an autosomal recessive disorder that may be associated with congenital generalized hypertrichosis. *SYN:* osteochondrodysplasia with hypertrichosis

Capdepont, Charles, French dentist, 1867-1917.

Capdepont-Hodge syndrome – *SYN:* Capdepont syndrome

Capdepont syndrome – dentinogenesis imperfecta. *SYN:* Capdepont-Hodge syndrome; Capdepont teeth; Stainton-Capdepont syndrome

Capdepont teeth – *SYN:* Capdepont syndrome

Stainton-Capdepont syndrome – *SYN:* Capdepont syndrome

Capgras, Jean Marie Joseph, French psychiatrist, 1873-1950.

Capgras phenomenon – *SYN:* Capgras syndrome

Capgras syndrome – the delusional belief that a person close to the schizophrenic patient has been replaced by an impostor. *SYN:* Capgras phenomenon; illusion of doubles

Caplan, Anthony, English physician, 1907-1976.

Caplan nodules – *SYN:* Caplan syndrome

Caplan syndrome – intrapulmonary nodules, histologically similar to subcutaneous rheumatoid nodules, associated with rheumatoid arthritis and pneumoconiosis in coal workers. *SYN:* Caplan nodules

Capps, Joseph A., U.S. physician, 1872-1964.
Capps reflex – obsolete eponym for vasomotor collapse at the time of crisis in pneumonia.

Capuron, Joseph, French physician, 1767-1850.
Capuron points – the iliopubic eminences and the sacroiliac joints, constituting four fixed points in the pelvic inlet.

Carabelli, George (Edler von Lunkaszprie), Austrian dentist, 1787-1842.
Carabelli tubercle – a small tubercle, resembling a supernumerary cusp, found occasionally on the lingual surface of the mesiolingual cusp of a permanent maxillary first molar. *SYN:* cusp of Carabelli
cusp of Carabelli – *SYN:* Carabelli tubercle

Carcassonne, Bernard Gauderic, 18th century French surgeon.
Carcassonne perineal ligament – thickened anterior border of perineal membrane; runs across subpubic angle posterior to deep dorsal vein of the penis.

Cardarelli, Antonio, Italian physician, 1831-1927.
Cardarelli sign – laryngotracheal tube pulsation related to aortic arch dilatation and aneurysms.

Carden, Henry D., English surgeon, d. 1872.
Carden amputation – transcondylar amputation of the leg in which the femur is sawed through the condyles just above the articular surface.

Carey Coombs, see under Coombs, Carey

Carini, Antonino, Italian physician, 1872-1950.
Carini syndrome – skin disease of the newborn characterized by fissures and shedding of membrane encasing the body to reveal red skin underneath. *SYN:* alligator baby; congenital ichthyosiform erythroderma; lamellar desquamation of the newborn; lamellar ichthyosis

NOTES

Carlen, Eric, 20th century Swedish otolaryngologist.
Carlen mediastinoscope

Carlsson, Arvid, Swedish physician, *1923, joint winner of 2000 Nobel Prize for work related to nervous system signal transduction.

Carman, Russell D., U.S. radiologist, 1875-1926.
Carman sign – on a gastric radiograph, the appearance of a contrast-filled malignant ulcer.

Carmi, Rivka, Israeli geneticist, *1948.
Carmi syndrome – autosomal recessive disorder, featuring junctional epidermolysis bullosa with pyloric atresia.

Carmody, Thomas Edward, U.S. oral surgeon, *1875.
Carmody-Batson operation – reduction of fractures of the zygoma and zygomatic arch through an intraoral incision above the maxillary molar teeth.

Carnett, J.B., 20th century U.S. physician.
Carnett sign – pain of intraabdominal origin with likely source in abdominal wall.

Carney, John A., Irish-born U.S. pathologist, *1934.
Carney complex – autosomal dominant disorder characterized by multiple lentigines, cardiac and cutaneous myxomas, and endocrine overactivity.

Carnoy, Jean Baptiste, French biologist, 1836-1899.
Carnoy fixative – an extremely rapid fixative used for glycogen preservation and as a nuclear fixative.

Caroli, Jacques, French gastroenterologist, 1902-1979.
Caroli disease – congenital cystic dilation of the intrahepatic bile ducts.

Carpenter, Charles J., U.S. immunologist, *1931.
Carpenter syndrome – acrocephalopolysyndactyly.

Carpenter, George Alfred, English physician, 1859-1910.
Carpenter syndrome – the association of primary hypothyroidism, primary adrenocortical insufficiency, and diabetes mellitus.

Carpentier, Alain, 20th century French cardiothoracic surgeon.
Carpentier annuloplasty
Carpentier annuloplasty ring prosthesis
Carpentier-Edwards aortic valve prosthesis
Carpentier-Edwards bioprosthesis
Carpentier-Edwards bioprosthetic valve
Carpentier-Edwards mitral annuloplasty valve

Carpentier-Edwards pericardial valve
Carpentier-Edwards porcine prosthetic valve
Carpentier-Edwards valve
Carpentier ring
Carpentier stent
Carpentier tricuspid valvuloplasty
Carpentier valve

Carpue, Joseph, English surgeon, 1764-1846.
   Carpue method – rhinoplasty utilizing a flap from the forehead. *SYN:* Indian rhinoplasty

Carr, Francis H., English chemist, 1874-1969.
   Carr-Price reaction – the basis of several quantitative techniques for the determination of vitamin A.

Carraro, Arturo, Italian physician.
   Cararro syndrome – recessive trait causing orthopedic deformities and deaf-mutism.

Carrel, Alexis, French-U.S. surgeon and Nobel laureate, 1873-1944.
   Carrel clamp
   Carrel-Lindbergh pump – a perfusion device designed for use in culture of whole organs.
   Carrel method
   Carrel mosquito forceps
   Carrel operation
   Carrel patch
   Carrel sutures
   Carrel treatment – treatment of wound surfaces by intermittent flushing with Dakin solution. *SYN:* Dakin-Carrel treatment
   Carrel tube
   Dakin-Carrel treatment – *SYN:* Carrel treatment

NOTES

Carrión, Daniel Alcides, Peruvian medical student, 1859-1885, who inoculated himself with a disease later designated as Carrión disease, and died thereof.

    Carrión disease – a generalized, acute, febrile, endemic, and systemic form of bartonellosis.

Carteaud, Alexandre, French dermatologist, *1897.

    Gougerot-Carteaud syndrome – see under Gougerot, Henri

Carter, Henry V., Anglo-Indian physician, 1831-1897.

    Carter black mycetoma – mycetoma caused by *Madurella mycetomatis*.

    Carter fever – an Asiatic relapsing fever caused by *Borrelia carteri*.

Carus, Karl G., German anatomist and zoologist, 1789-1869.

    Carus circle – *SYN:* Carus curve

    Carus curve – an imaginary curved line obtained from a mathematical formula, supposed to indicate the outlet of the pelvic canal. *SYN:* Carus circle

Carvallo, José Manuel Rivero-, see under Rivero-Carvallo, José Manuel

Casal, Gasper, Spanish physician, 1691-1759.

    Casal collar – *SYN:* Casal necklace

    Casal necklace – a dermatitis partly or completely encircling the lower part of the neck in pellagra. *SYN:* Casal collar

Caslick, Edward, 20th century U.S. veterinarian.

    Caslick operation – an operation for the correction of faulty conformation of the vulva of a mare.

Casoni, Tommaro, Italian physician, 1880-1933.

    Casoni intradermal test – a test for hydatid disease. *SYN:* Casoni skin test

    Casoni skin test – *SYN:* Casoni intradermal test

Cass, John W., U.S. physician.

    Meigs-Cass syndrome – *SYN:* Meigs syndrome

Casselberry, William E., U.S. laryngologist, 1858-1916.

    Casselberry position – a prone position assumed when drinking, after intubation, in order to prevent the entrance of fluid into the tube.

Casser, Giulio, Italian anatomist, 1556-1616.

    Casser fontanel – the membranous interval on either side between the mastoid angle of the parietal bone, the petrous portion of the temporal bone, and the occipital bone. *SYN:* mastoid fontanel

    Casser perforated muscle – *SYN:* coracobrachialis muscle

Cassirer, Richard, German physician, 1868-1925.
Cassirer syndrome

Castellani, Sir Aldo, Italian physician, 1877-1971.
Castellani bronchitis – chronic bronchitis due to infection with spirochetes and characterized by cough and bloody sputum. *SYN:* hemorrhagic bronchitis
Castellani disease
Castellani-Low sign – a fine tremor of the tongue observed in sleeping sickness.
Castellani paint – a paint used in the treatment of superficial mycotic infections. *SYN:* carbol-fuchsin paint
Castellani test

Castle, William B., U.S. physician, 1897-1990.
Castle intrinsic factor – a relatively small mucoprotein required for adequate absorption of vitamin B_{12}. *SYN:* intrinsic factor

Castleman, Benjamin, U.S. pathologist, 1906-1982.
Castleman disease – solitary masses of lymphoid tissue containing concentric perivascular aggregates of lymphocytes. *SYN:* benign giant lymph node hyperplasia; Castleman tumor
Castleman tumor – *SYN:* Castleman disease

Castroviejo, Ramon, Spanish physician, *1904.
Castroviejo clip-applying forceps
Castroviejo corneal transplant marker
Castroviejo corneal transplant scissors
Castroviejo discission knife
Castroviejo electrokeratotome
Castroviejo iridocapsulotomy scissors
Castroviejo lacrimal sac probe
Castroviejo lens clamp
Castroviejo lens spoon
Castroviejo lid forceps

NOTES

Castroviejo lid retractor
Castroviejo orbital aspirator
Castroviejo razor blade
Castroviejo refractor
Castroviejo scleral fold forceps
Castroviejo scleral shortening clip
Castroviejo snare enucleator
Castroviejo speculum
Castroviejo suturing forceps
Castroviejo synechia scissors
Castroviejo trephine

Cavallazzi, C., Italian physician.
Cavallazzi syndrome – a syndrome of mandibular hypoplasia, acroosteolysis, stiff joints, and skin atrophy of the hands and feet. *SYN:* mandibuloacral dysplasia

Cawthorne, Terence, English physician.
Cawthorne exercises – exercises for patients with vertigo and Ménière disease.

Cayler, Glen G., U.S. physician.
Cayler syndrome – unilateral facial weakness associated with cardiac defects. *SYN:* cardiofacial syndrome

Cazenave, Pierre L. Alphée, French dermatologist, 1795-1877.
Cazenave disease
Cazenave vitiligo – obsolete term for alopecia areata.

Cecil, Arthur Bond, U.S. urologist, 1885-1967.
Cecil operation – hypospadias repair.

Ceelen, Wilhelm, 1884-1964.
Ceelen-Gellerstedt syndrome – repeated sudden attacks of dyspnea and hemoptysis leading to diffuse pulmonary hemosiderosis. *SYN:* idiopathic pulmonary hemosiderosis

Cegka, Josephus J., Czech physician, 1812-1862.
Cegka sign – cardiac dullness related to adherent pericardium.

Celestin, Felix, French physician, *1900.
Celestin tube – a plastic tube introduced through a tumor in the esophagus.

Celsius, Anders, Swedish astronomer, 1701-1744.
Celsius scale – a temperature scale that is based on the triple point of water (defined to be 273.16 K) and assigned the value of 0.01°C.

Celsius thermometer

Celsus, Aulus (Aurelius) Cornelius, Roman physician and medical writer, ca. 30 B.C.-45 A.D.

Celsus alopecia – *SYN:* Celsus vitiligo

Celsus area – *SYN:* Celsus vitiligo

Celsus 4 cardinal signs of inflammation – heat, redness, tenderness, and swelling.

Celsus kerion – an inflammatory fungus infection of the scalp and beard. *SYN:* tinea kerion

Celsus papules – acute papular eczema of severe type. *SYN:* lichen agrius

Celsus vitiligo – obsolete term for alopecia areata. *SYN:* Celsus alopecia; Celsus area

Cerenkov, (Cherenkov), Pavel A., Russian physicist and Nobel laureate, 1904-1990.

Cerenkov radiation – light given off by a transparent medium when a high-energy particle speeds through it at a velocity greater than that of light in that medium.

Cervenka, Jaroslav.

Cervenka syndrome – autosomal dominant trait causing facial abnormalities, joint deformity, and myopia.

Cestan, Raymond, French neurologist, 1872-1934.

Cestan-Chenais syndrome – contralateral hemiplegia, hemianesthesia, with ipsilateral hemiasynergia and lateropulsion, paralysis of the larynx and soft palate, enophthalmia, miosis, and ptosis, due to lesions of the brainstem.

Ceylon, island situated in Indian Ocean, now known as Sri Lanka.

Ceylon cinnamon – dried inner bark of evergreen tree in laurel family, used for medicinal purposes or as a spice.

Ceylon moss – red seaweed which is a source of agar (culture medium).

NOTES

Chaddock, Charles G., U.S. neurologist, 1861-1936.
    Chaddock reflex – *SYN:* Chaddock sign
    Chaddock sign – when the external malleolar skin area is irritated, extension of the great toe occurs in cases of organic disease of the corticospinal reflex paths. *SYN:* Chaddock reflex; external malleolar sign

Chadwick, James R., U.S. gynecologist, 1844-1905.
    Chadwick sign – a bluish discoloration of the cervix and vagina, a sign of pregnancy.

Chagas, Carlos J.R., Brazilian physician and parasitologist, 1879-1934.
    Chagas-Cruz disease – *SYN:* Chagas disease
    Chagas disease – parasitic infection transmitted by certain species of reduviid (triatomine) bugs. *SYN:* Chagas-Cruz disease; Chagas-Mazza disease; Cruz trypanosomiasis; South American trypanosomiasis
    Chagas-Mazza disease – *SYN:* Chagas disease

Chailey, Chailey Heritage Craft School & Hospital, Sussex, England.
    Chailey go-cart – vehicle for children who cannot walk.

Chain, Sir Ernst Boris, 1906-1979, co-winner of 1945 Nobel Prize for work related to penicillin.

Chamberlain, W.E., U.S. radiologist, 1891-1947.
    Chamberlain line – a line drawn from the posterior margin of the hard palate to the dorsum of the foramen magnum.

Chamberlen, Peter, English obstetrician, 1560-1631.
    Chamberlen forceps – the original obstetrical forceps, without a curvature.

Champy, Christian, French physician, *1885.
    Champy fixative – cytologic fixative.

Chanarin, I., 20th century English hematologist.
    Dorfman-Chanarin syndrome – see under Dorfman, Maurice L.

Chance, G.Q., 20th century English radiologist.
    Chance fracture – a transverse fracture, usually in the thoracic or lumbar spine, through the body of the vertebra extending posteriorly through the pedicles and the spinous process.

Chandler, Fremont A., U.S. orthopedic surgeon, 1893-1954.
    Chandler arthrodesis
    Chandler bone elevator
    Chandler felt collar splint
    Chandler forceps

Chandler hip fusion
Chandler laminectomy retractor
Chandler patellar advancement
Chandler spinal perforating forceps
Chandler splint
Chandler table – a table used for upper limb exercises.
Chandler unreamed interlocking tibial nail

Chandler, Paul A., U.S. ophthalmologist, *1896.
Chandler iridectomy
Chandler iris forceps
Chandler syndrome – iris atrophy with corneal edema. *SYN:* iridocorneal syndrome

Changeux, Jean-Pierre, 20th century French biochemist.
Monod-Wyman-Changeux model – see under Monod

Chantemesse, André, French bacteriologist, 1851-1919.
Chantemesse reaction – a conjunctival reaction, especially as applied to typhoid.

Chaoul, Henri, Lebanese radiologist, 1887-1964.
Chaoul therapy – x-ray therapy using low voltage.
Chaoul tube – x-ray tube designed to allow intense but superficial irradiation of an area.

Chapple, Charles Culloden, U.S. pediatrician, *1903.
Chapple syndrome – (1) unilateral facial weakness in newborn caused by lateral flexion of the head in utero; (2) congenital syndrome believed to be caused by abnormal position of the fetus in utero. *SYN:* duosyndrome of laryngeal nerve; genu recurvatum-uterine retroversion-dysmenorrhea syndrome

Chaput, Henri, French surgeon, 1857-1919.
Chaput tubercle – tibial tubercle.

NOTES

Charcot, Jean Martin, French neurologist, 1825-1893.

Charcot arteries – any one of a variety of small cerebral arteries. *SYN:* lenticulostriate arteries

Charcot arthritis

Charcot arthropathy

Charcot bath – for patients with arterial disorders.

Charcot-Böttcher crystalloids – spindle-shaped crystalloids found in human Sertoli cells.

Charcot change

Charcot disease – *SYN:* Lou Gehrig disease

Charcot fever – *SYN:* Charcot intermittent fever

Charcot gait – the gait of hereditary ataxia.

Charcot intermittent fever – fever, chills, right upper quadrant pain, and jaundice associated with intermittently obstructing common duct stones. *SYN:* Charcot fever

Charcot joint – a neuropathic arthropathy that occurs with tabes dorsalis (tabetic neurosyphilis). *SYN:* tabetic arthropathy

Charcot laryngeal vertigo – fainting as a result of a coughing spell, most often occurring in heavy-set male smokers with chronic bronchitis. *SYN:* Charcot vertigo; tussive syncope

Charcot-Leyden crystals – crystals found in the sputum in bronchial asthma. *SYN:* asthma crystals; Charcot-Neumann crystals; Charcot-Robin crystals; Leyden crystals

Charcot-Marie-Tooth disease – a group of three familial peripheral neuromuscular disorders, sharing the common feature of marked wasting of the more distal extremities. *SYN:* peroneal muscular atrophy; Tooth disease

Charcot-Neumann crystals – *SYN:* Charcot-Leyden crystals

Charcot-Robin crystals – *SYN:* Charcot-Leyden crystals

Charcot spine

Charcot syndrome – a condition caused by ischemia of the muscles. *SYN:* intermittent claudication

Charcot triad (1) in multiple (disseminated) sclerosis, the three symptoms: nystagmus, tremor, and scanning speech; (2) combination of jaundice, fever, and upper abdominal pain that occurs as a result of cholangitis.

Charcot vertigo – *SYN:* Charcot laryngeal vertigo

Charcot-Weiss-Baker syndrome – stimulation of a hyperactive carotid sinus, causing a marked fall in blood pressure. *SYN:* carotid sinus syndrome

Charcot-Wilbrand syndrome – inability to recognize objects by sight, usually caused by bilateral parieto-occipital lesions.
Erb-Charcot disease – see under Erb

Chargaff, Erwin, Austrian-U.S. biochemist, *1905.
Chargaff rule – in double-stranded DNA the content of adenine residues equals the number of thymine and the number of cytosine equals the number of guanine.

Charles, Jacques, French physicist, 1746-1823.
Charles law – all gases expand equally on heating. *SYN:* Gay-Lussac law

Charles Bonnet, see under Bonnet, Charles

Charlevoix, county in Quebec, Canada, where the disease occurred.
Charlevoix disease – *SYN:* Andermann syndrome

Charlin, C. Carlos, Chilean ophthalmologist, 1886-1945.
Charlin syndrome – multiple symptoms of the nose resulting from neuralgia of the nasociliary nerve. *SYN:* nasociliary neuralgia

Charlouis, M., 19th century Dutch army surgeon in Java.
Charlouis disease – an infectious tropical disease caused by *Treponema pertenue* and characterized by the development of crusted granulomatous ulcers on the extremities. *SYN:* yaws

Charlton, Willy, German physician, *1889.
Schultz-Charlton phenomenon – *SYN:* Schultz-Charlton reaction
Schultz-Charlton reaction – see under Schultz, Werner

Charmot, Guy Denis, French physician, *1914.
Charmot syndrome – macroglobulinemia with splenomegaly, abdominal pain, emaciation, anemia, erythroblastosis, asthenia; thought to be caused by a parasite and first observed in the Congo. *SYN:* African macroglobulinemia

Charnley, Sir John, English surgeon, 1911-1988.
Charnley acetabular cup prosthesis

NOTES

Charnley arthrodesis
Charnley arthrodesis clamp
Charnley bone clamp
Charnley bone clasp
Charnley brace handle
Charnley cemented hip prosthesis
Charnley centering drill
Charnley compression arthrodesis
Charnley compression fusion
Charnley device
Charnley femoral broach
Charnley femoral condyle drill
Charnley femoral prosthesis pusher
Charnley hip arthroplasty – a form of total hip replacement consisting of the application of an acetabular cup and a femoral head prosthesis.
Charnley hip prosthesis
Charnley implant
Charnley incision
Charnley knee prosthesis
Charnley narrow stem component
Charnley pilot drill
Charnley pin
Charnley pin clamp
Charnley pin retractor
Charnley rasp
Charnley reamer
Charnley self-retaining retractor
Charnley standard stem retractor
Charnley towel

Charrière, Joseph F.B., French instrument maker, 1803-1876.
Charrière scale – a scale for grading sizes of sounds, tubules, and catheters. *SYN:* French scale

Charters, W.J., U.S. dentist.
Charters method – a method of tooth brushing utilizing a restricted circular motion with the bristles inclined coronally at a 45-degree angle.

Chaslin, Philippe, French physician, *1857.
Chaslin gliosis – sclerosis of glial fibers in brain tissue of epileptics causing pathological changes.

Chassaignac, Edouard P.M., French surgeon, 1804-1879.
  Chassaignac space – potential space between the pectoralis major and the mammary gland.
  Chassaignac tubercle – the anterior tubercle of the transverse process of the sixth cervical vertebra, against which the carotid artery may be compressed by the finger. *SYN:* carotid tubercle

Chastek, S.J., U.S. breeder of foxes.
  Chastek paralysis – disease of foxes and mink caused by eating certain types of raw fish which contain a thiamin-destroying enzyme with resultant loss of appetite, emaciation, paralysis, and death.

Chaudhry, Anand P., U.S. maxillofacial surgeon, *1922.
  Gorlin-Chaudhry-Moss syndrome – see under Gorlin, Robert James

Chauffard, Anatole Marie Émile, French physician, 1855-1932.
  Chauffard syndrome – the symptoms of Still disease in one suffering from bovine or other nonhuman form of tuberculosis. *SYN:* Still-Chauffard syndrome
  Minkowski-Chauffard syndrome – see under Minkowski
  Still-Chauffard syndrome – *SYN:* Chauffard syndrome

Chaussier, François, French physician, 1746-1828.
  Chaussier areola – a ring of indurated tissue surrounding the lesion of cutaneous anthrax.
  Chaussier line – the anteroposterior line of the corpus callosum as appearing on median section of the brain.
  Chaussier sign – severe pain in the epigastrium, a prodrome of eclampsia.

Chauveau, J.-B. Auguste, French veterinarian, physiologist, and microbiologist, 1827-1917.
  Chauveau bacterium – former name for *Clostridium chauvoei*.

Chavany, Jean A.E., French physician, 1892-1959.
  Brunhes-Chavany syndrome – *SYN:* Chavany-Brunhes syndrome

C

NOTES

Chavany-Brunhes syndrome – persistent headaches and various mental disorders caused by calcification of the falx cerebri. *SYN:* Brunhes-Chavany syndrome

Chayes, Herman E.S., U.S. prosthodontist, 1880-1933.
Chayes method – a method of replacing lost teeth.

Cheadle, Walter Butler, English pediatrician, 1835-1910.
Cheadle disease – a cachectic condition in infants, resulting from malnutrition. *SYN:* infantile scurvy

Cheatle, Sir George L., English surgeon, 1865-1951.
Cheatle slit – a longitudinal incision into the antimesenteric border of the small intestine.

Chédiak, Moisés, Cuban physician, *1903.
Chédiak-Higashi anomaly – *SYN:* Chédiak-Steinbrinck-Higashi syndrome
Chédiak-Higashi disease – *SYN:* Chédiak-Steinbrinck-Higashi syndrome
Chédiak-Steinbrinck-Higashi anomaly – *SYN:* Chédiak-Steinbrinck-Higashi syndrome
Chédiak-Steinbrinck-Higashi syndrome – hereditary, fatal disorder of granulation and nuclear structure of all types of leukocytes. *SYN:* Béguez César disease; Chédiak-Higashi anomaly; Chédiak-Higashi disease; Chédiak-Steinbrinck-Higashi anomaly
Chédiak test

Chenais, Louis J., French physician, 1872-1950.
Cestan-Chenais syndrome – see under Cestan

Chenantais, J., Jr., French physician.
Malherbe-Chenantais epithelioma – *SYN:* Malherbe calcifying epithelioma

Cheney, William D., U.S. radiologist, *1918.
Cheney-Hajdu syndrome – *SYN:* Hajdu-Cheney syndrome
Cheney syndrome – acroosteolysis with osteoporosis and changes in the skull and mandible.
Hajdu-Cheney syndrome – see under Hajdu

Cherenkov, var. of Cerenkov

Chevassu, Maurice, French physician, *1877.
Chevassu tumor – testicular germ-cell tumor affecting men over 30 years of age. *SYN:* seminoma

Cheyne, John, Scottish physician, 1777-1836.
Cheyne nystagmus
Cheyne-Stokes breathing – *SYN:* Cheyne-Stokes respiration

Cheyne-Stokes psychosis – a mental state characterized by anxiety and restlessness, accompanying Cheyne-Stokes respiration.

Cheyne-Stokes respiration – the pattern of breathing characteristically seen in coma. *SYN:* Cheyne-Stokes breathing

Chiari, Hans, German pathologist, 1851-1916.

Arnold-Chiari deformity – *SYN:* Arnold-Chiari malformation

Arnold-Chiari malformation – see under Arnold, Julius

Arnold-Chiari syndrome – *SYN:* Arnold-Chiari malformation

Budd-Chiari syndrome – *SYN:* Chiari syndrome

Chiari-Budd syndrome – *SYN:* Chiari syndrome

Chiari disease – *SYN:* Chiari syndrome

Chiari net – abnormal fibrous or lacelike strands in the right atrium.

Chiari syndrome – thrombosis of the hepatic vein with great enlargement of the liver and extensive development of collateral vessels, intractable ascites, and severe portal hypertension. *SYN:* Budd-Chiari syndrome; Budd syndrome; Chiari-Budd syndrome; Chiari disease; Rokitansky disease (2)

Chiari II syndrome – elongation of medulla and cerebellar tonsils and vermis with displacement through the foramen magnum into the upper spinal canal.

Chiari, Johann B., German obstetrician, 1817-1854.

Chiari-Frommel syndrome – unphysiological lactation and amenorrhea following pregnancy, but not caused by infant's nursing. *SYN:* Frommel-Chiari syndrome

Frommel-Chiari syndrome – *SYN:* Chiari-Frommel syndrome

Chido, surname of patient in whom this specific antigen was first seen.

Chido blood group – found in red cells and plasma in 98% of population.

Chievitz, Johan H., Danish anatomist, 1850-1901.

Chievitz layer – in the developing retina of an embryo, a transitory zone between the inner and outer neuroblastic layers that is devoid of nuclei.

NOTES

Chievitz organ – a normal epithelial structure, possibly a neurotransmitter, found at the angle of the mandible with branches of the buccal nerve.

Chilaiditi, Demetrius, Austrian radiologist, *1883.
Chilaiditi syndrome – interposition of the colon between the liver and the diaphragm.

Chinese restaurant, a dining establishment that serves Chinese food.
Chinese restaurant syndrome – chest pain, facial pressure, and burning sensation that develops after persons sensitive to monosodium glutamate ingest this food additive. *SYN:* Kwok quease

Cholewa, Erasmus R., German physician, 1845-1931.
Cholewa-Itard sign – *SYN:* Itard-Cholewa sign
Itard-Cholewa sign – see under Itard

Chopart, François, French surgeon, 1743-1795.
Chopart amputation – amputation through the midtarsal joint. *SYN:* mediotarsal amputation
Chopart ankle dislocation
Chopart articulation
Chopart brace
Chopart fracture
Chopart joint – the synovial joints which act as a unit in allowing the front of the foot to pivot relative to the back of the foot about the longitudinal axis of the foot. *SYN:* transverse tarsal joint
Chopart osseous joint injury
Chopart partial foot prosthesis

Chotzen, F., 20th century German physician.
Chotzen syndrome – syndactyly, mild mental retardation, hypertelorism, and occasional ptosis. *SYN:* Saethre-Chotzen syndrome
Saethre-Chotzen syndrome – *SYN:* Chotzen syndrome

Christ, Josef, German physician and dentist, 1871-1948.
Christ-Siemens-Touraine syndrome – congenitally defective or absent sweat glands, smooth, finely wrinkled skin, sunken nose, malformed and missing teeth, sparse fragile hair, and associated with deformed nails, absent breast tissue, mental retardation, or syndactyly. *SYN:* anhidrotic ectodermal dysplasia

Christensen, Erna, Danish pathologist, 1906-1967.
Christensen-Krabbe disease – familial progressive spastic paresis of extremities with destruction and disorganization of nerve cells of the cerebral cortex. *SYN:* poliodystrophia cerebri progressiva infantalis

Christian, Henry Asbury, U.S. internist, 1876-1951.
 Christian disease – (1) *SYN:* Hand-Schüller-Christian disease; (2) *SYN:*
  Weber-Christian disease
 Christian syndrome – *SYN:* Hand-Schüller-Christian disease
 Hand-Schüller-Christian disease – see under Hand
 Weber-Christian disease – see under Weber, Frederick Parkes

Christian, Joe C., U.S. geneticist.
 Christian syndrome – (1) autosomal recessive trait causing
  craniosynostosis, arthrogryposis, cleft palate, microcephaly, and other
  musculoskeletal abnormalities. *SYN:* adducted thumbs syndrome; (2) X-
  linked trait causing short stature, cervical vertebral fusion, scoliosis;
  sometimes associated with glucose intolerance and imperforate anus.

Christison, Sir Robert, Scottish physician, 1797-1882.
 Christison formula – *SYN:* Häser formula

Christmas, Stephen, patient with the first case of this disease studied in
detail.
 Christmas disease – a clotting disorder caused by hereditary deficiency
  of factor IX. *SYN:* hemophilia B
 Christmas factor – *SYN:* factor IX coagulation factor

Churchill, E.D., U.S. thoracic surgeon, *1895.
 Churchill-Cope reflex – distention of pulmonary vascular bed results in
  increase in respiratory rate.

Churg, Jacob, Polish-born U.S. pathologist, *1910.
 Churg-Strauss syndrome – asthma, fever, eosinophilia, and varied
  symptoms and signs of vasculitis, primarily affecting small arteries, with
  vascular and extravascular granulomas. *SYN:* allergic granulomatosis;
  allergic granulomatous angiitis; Strauss-Churg-Zak syndrome

Churilov, A.V., Russian physician.
 Churilov disease – one of several acute, hemorrhagic infectious diseases
  caused by members of the hantaviruses.

NOTES

Chutorian, Abe, U.S. physician.
Rosenberg-Chutorian syndrome – see under Rosenberg, Roger N.

Chvostek, Franz, Austrian surgeon, 1834-1884.
Chvostek sign – facial irritability in tetany, unilateral spasm of the orbicularis oculi or oris muscle being excited by a slight tap over the facial nerve just anterior to the external auditory meatus. *SYN:* Chvostek tremor; Schultze-Chvostek sign; Schultze sign; Weiss sign
Chvostek tremor – *SYN:* Chvostek sign
Schultze-Chvostek sign – *SYN:* Chvostek sign

Ciaccio, Carmelo, Italian pathologist, 1877-1956.
Ciaccio fluid
Ciaccio method
Ciaccio stain – a method for demonstrating complex insoluble intracellular lipids.

Ciaccio, Giuseppe V., Italian anatomist, 1824-1901.
Ciaccio glands – *SYN:* accessory lacrimal glands

Cimino, James E., U.S. nephrologist, *1928.
Brescia-Cimino fistula – see under Brescia

Cinderella, fairy-tale character oppressed by her stepfamily until she magically attends a ball and ultimately marries a prince.
Cinderella complex – fear of being independent causes unconscious desire to be taken care of by others.
Cinderella dermatosis – skin disease characterized by ash-gray macules occurring most often on palms, extremities, buttocks, and scalp.
Cinderella stepmother syndrome – overcompensation by a stepmother in an effort to be accepted into new family.
Cinderella syndrome – false accusations made by adopted children of being mistreated or neglected by their stepmothers.

Citelli, Salvatore, Italian laryngologist, 1875-1947.
Citelli syndrome – nasopharyngeal obstruction caused by adenoid tissue and associated with mental retardation, sinus infection, and inability to concentrate.

Civatte, Achille, French dermatologist, 1877-1956.
Civatte bodies – eosinophilic hyaline spherical bodies seen in or just beneath the epidermis, particularly in lichen planus, formed by necrosis of individual basal cells. *SYN:* colloid bodies
Civatte disease – *SYN:* poikiloderma of Civatte

poikiloderma of Civatte – reticulated pigmentation and telangiectasia of the sides of the cheeks and neck; common in middle-aged women. *SYN:* Civatte disease

Civinini, Filippo, Italian anatomist, 1805-1844.

Civinini canal – a canal in the petrotympanic or glaserian fissure near its posterior edge through which the chorda tympani nerve issues from the skull. *SYN:* anterior canaliculus of chorda tympani

Civinini ligament – a membranous ligament extending from the spine of the sphenoid to the upper part of the posterior border of the lateral pterygoid lamina. *SYN:* pterygospinous ligament

Civinini process – a sharp projection from the posterior edge of the lateral pterygoid plate of the sphenoid bone. *SYN:* pterygospinous process

Clado, Spiro, French gynecologist, 1856-1905.

Clado anastomosis – anastomosis in the right suspensory ligament of the ovary between the appendicular and ovarian arteries.

Clado band – the suspensory ligament of the ovary.

Clado ligament – a mesenteric fold running from the broad ligament on the right side to the appendix.

Clado point – a point at the lateral border of the rectus abdominis muscle where marked tenderness on pressure is felt in some cases of appendicitis.

Clapton, Edward, English physician, 1830-1909.

Clapton line – a greenish discoloration of the marginal gingiva in cases of chronic copper poisoning.

Clara, Max, Austrian anatomist, *1899.

Clara cell – a rounded, club-shaped, nonciliated cell protruding between ciliated cells in bronchiolar epithelium; believed to be secretory in function. *SYN:* bronchiolar exocrine cell

Clara hematoxylin

Clark, Alonzo, U.S. pharmacologist, 1807-1887.

Clark sign – absence of liver dullness in the presence of peritonitis.

NOTES

Clark weight rule – an obsolete rule for an approximate child's dose.

Clark, Earl Perry, U.S. biochemist, *1892.
Clark-Collip method – method for detecting calcium and urea in serum and blood.

Clark, Eliot R., U.S. anatomist, 1881-1963.
Sandison-Clark chamber – see under Sandison

Clark, Leland, Jr., U.S. biochemist, *1918.
Clark electrode – used to measure oxygen pressure in arterial blood samples.

Clark, Wallace H., Jr., U.S. dermatopathologist, 1924-1997.
Clark level – the level of invasion of primary malignant melanoma of the skin, recorded by Roman numerals I, II, III, IV, V.

Clarke, Cecil, 20th century English physician.
Clarke-Hadfield syndrome – a congenital metabolic disorder in which secretions of exocrine glands are abnormal. *SYN:* cystic fibrosis

Clarke, Jacob A.L., English anatomist, 1817-1880.
Clarke column – a column of large neurons that gives rise to the dorsal spinocerebellar tract. *SYN:* Clarke nucleus; dorsal nucleus; stilling column; stilling nucleus; thoracic nucleus
Clarke nucleus– *SYN:* Clarke column

Clarke, Sir Charles Mansfield, English physician, 1782-1857.
Clarke ulcer – uterine neck ulceration.

Clauberg, Karl W., German bacteriologist, *1893.
Clauberg test – a test for progestational activity.
Clauberg unit

Claude, Albert, *1879, co-winner of the 1974 Nobel Prize for work related to cell structure and organization.

Claude, Henri, French psychiatrist, 1869-1945.
Claude syndrome – midbrain syndrome with oculomotor palsy on the side of the lesion and incoordination on the opposite side.

Claudius, Friedrich M., German anatomist, 1822-1869.
Claudius cells – columnar cells on the floor of the ductus cochlearis external to the organ of Corti.
Claudius fossa – a depression in the parietal peritoneum of the pelvis that lodges the ovary. *SYN:* ovarian fossa

Clausen, J., Danish physician.
Dyggve-Melchoir-Clausen syndrome – see under Dyggve

Claybrook, Edwin B., U.S. surgeon, 1871-1931.
  Claybrook sign – in rupture of abdominal viscus, transmission of breath and heart sounds through the abdominal wall.

Cleemann, Richard Alsop, U.S. physician, 1840-1912.
  Cleemann sign – in fracture of the femur with overriding of the fragments, wrinkling of the skin occurs directly above the patella.

Cleland, John, Scottish anatomist, 1835-1925.
  Cleland ligaments – digital ligaments.

Cleland, W. Wallace, U.S. biochemist, *1930.
  Cleland reagent – a substance used to reduce disulfide bonds in proteins. *SYN:* dithiothreitol

Cleopatra, queen and pharaoh of Egypt between 51 and 30 B.C.
  Cleopatra view – mammographic projection. *SYN:* exaggerated craniocaudal projection and axillary tail view

Clérambault, C.G., see under de Clérambault

Cléret, M., 20th century French physician.
  Launois-Cléret syndrome – *SYN:* Fröhlich syndrome

Clevenger, Shobal V., U.S. neurologist, 1843-1920.
  Clevenger fissure – the sulcus on the basal aspect of the temporal lobe that separates the fusiform gyrus from the inferior temporal gyrus on its lateral side. *SYN:* inferior temporal sulcus

Clias, Phokion Heinrich, U.S. therapist, 1780-1854.
  Clias exercises – basic exercises for younger individuals. *SYN:* Clias method
  Clias method – *SYN:* Clias exercises

Cloquet, Hippolyte, French anatomist, 1787-1840.
  Cloquet space – a space between the ciliary zonule and the vitreous body.

NOTES

Cloquet, Jules G., French anatomist, 1790-1883.
  Cloquet canal – a minute canal running through the vitreous from the discus nervi optici to the lens. *SYN:* hyaloid canal
  Cloquet canal remnants
  Cloquet hernia – a femoral hernia perforating the aponeurosis of the pectineus and insinuating itself between this aponeurosis and the muscle, therefore lying behind the femoral vessels.
  Cloquet septum – the delicate fibrous membrane that closes the femoral ring at the base of the femoral canal. *SYN:* femoral septum
  node of Cloquet – one of the deep inguinal lymph nodes located in or adjacent to the femoral canal. *SYN:* Rosenmüller gland; Rosenmüller node

Closs, Karl Philipp, Norwegian dermatologist, *1904.
  Danbolt-Closs syndrome – *SYN:* Brandt syndrome

Cloudman, Arthur M., U.S. zoologist and pathologist, *1901.
  Cloudman melanoma – a transplantable melanoma that arose spontaneously in a mouse of DBA strain and which grows and metastasizes in mice of related strains.

Clouston, H.R., Canadian pediatrician, 1889-1950.
  Clouston syndrome – autosomal dominant trait resulting in congenital dystrophy of hair and nails. *SYN:* hidrotic ectodermal dysplasia

Clutton, Henry Hugh, English surgeon, 1850-1909.
  Clutton joints – symmetrical arthrosis, especially of the knee joints, in cases of congenital syphilis.

Coanda, Henri-Marie, Romanian aerodynamicist, 1885-1972.
  Coanda effect – a stream of air or fluid emerging from a nozzle follows a nearby curved surface if the angle of curve is not too sharp.

Coats, George, English ophthalmologist, 1876-1915.
  Coats disease – a chronic abnormality characterized by deposition of cholesterol in outer retinal layers and subretinal space. *SYN:* exudative retinitis

Cobb, Stanley, U.S. neuropathologist, 1887-1968.
  Cobb chisel
  Cobb curette
  Cobb gouge
  Cobb method
  Cobb osteotome
  Cobb periosteal elevator

Cobb retractor

Cobb spinal elevator

Cobb syndrome – cutaneous angiomas, usually in a dermatomal distribution on the trunk, associated with vascular abnormality of the spinal cord and resulting neurologic symptoms. *SYN:* cutaneomeningospinal angiomatosis

Cobb technique

Cock, E., English surgeon, 1805-1892.

Cock tumor – *SYN:* infected sebaceous cyst

Cockayne, Edward Alfred, English physician, 1880-1956.

Cockayne disease – *SYN:* Cockayne syndrome

Cockayne syndrome – dwarfism, senile appearance, pigmentary degeneration of the retina, optic atrophy, deafness, sensitivity to sunlight, and mental retardation. *SYN:* Cockayne disease

Weber-Cockayne syndrome – see under Weber, Frederick Parkes

Cockett, Frank Bernard, English surgeon.

Cockett and Dodd operation – varicose vein surgery.

Codman, Ernest Amory, U.S. surgeon, 1869-1940.

Codman angle

Codman cartilage clamp

Codman classification

Codman drill

Codman exercises

Codman incision

Codman saber-cut shoulder approach

Codman shunt

Codman sign – in the absence of rotator cuff function, hunching of the shoulder occurs when the deltoid muscle contracts.

Codman sponge

NOTES

Codman triangle – in radiology, the interface between growing bone tumor and normal bone, presenting as an incomplete triangle formed by periosteum.

Codman tumor – chondroblastoma of the proximal humerus.

Codman vein stripper

Codman wire-passing drill

Coffey, Robert, U.S. surgeon, 1869-1933.

Coffey incision

Coffey suspension – an operative technique following partial excision of the cornu, as in salpingectomy, whereby the broad and the round ligaments are sutured over the cornual wound to restore continuity of the peritoneum and to suspend the uterus on the operated side.

Coffey ureterointestinal anastomosis

Coffin, Grange S., U.S. pediatrician, *1923.

Coffin-Lowry syndrome – *SYN:* Coffin-Siris syndrome

Coffin-Siris syndrome – mental retardation with wide bulbous (pugilistic) nose, low nasal bridge, moderate hirsutism, and digital anomalies. *SYN:* Coffin-Lowry syndrome

Cogan, David G., U.S. ophthalmologist, 1908-1993.

Cogan-Reese syndrome – syndrome of glaucoma, iris atrophy, decreased corneal endothelium, anterior peripheral synechia, and multiple iris nodules. *SYN:* iridocorneal endothelial syndrome

Cogan syndrome – a nonsyphilitic interstitial keratitis with vertigo and tinnitus, followed by deafness. *SYN:* oculovestibulo-auditory syndrome

Cohen, M. Michael, Jr., U.S. pathologist.

Cohen syndrome – probable inherited autosomal recessive trait causing obesity, hypotonia, and mental deficiency.

Cohen, Stanley, *1922, co-winner of 1986 Nobel Prize for work related to growth factors.

Cohnheim, Julius F., German histologist, pathologist, and physiologist, 1839-1884.

Cohnheim area – a shrinkage artifact of fixation. *SYN:* Cohnheim field

Cohnheim field – *SYN:* Cohnheim area

Cohnheim theory – that neoplasms originate from various cell rests. *SYN:* emigration theory

Coiter, Volcher, Dutch surgeon and anatomist, 1534-1600.

Coiter muscle – draws medial end of eyebrow downward and wrinkles forehead vertically. *SYN:* corrugator supercilii muscle

Cole, Laurent, French pathologist, *1903.
  Benedict-Hopkins-Cole reagent – see under Benedict, Stanley R.

Cole, Warren H., U.S. physician and professor, d. 1990.
  Graham-Cole test – see under Graham, Evarts Ambrose

Coleman, Claude C., U.S. physician, 1879-1953.
  Coleman syndrome – injury to the cervical spine caused by head and
    shoulder trauma.

Coley, W.B., U.S. surgeon, 1862-1936.
  Coley fluid – *SYN:* Coley toxin
  Coley toxin – injection with this bacterial toxin causes a febrile reaction
    and reduction in size of tumor mass. *SYN:* Coley fluid

Colles, Abraham, Irish surgeon, 1773-1843.
  Colles fascia – *SYN:* superficial fascia of perineum
  Colles fracture – a fracture of the lower end of the radius with
    displacement of the distal fragment dorsally.
  Colles ligament – a triangular fibrous band extending from the
    aponeurosis of the external oblique to the pubic tubercle of the opposite
    side. *SYN:* reflected inguinal ligament
  Colles operation
  Colles sling
  Colles space – *SYN:* superficial perineal space
  Colles splint

Collet, Frédric-Justin, French otolaryngologist, *1870.
  Collet-Sicard syndrome – unilateral lesions of cranial nerves IX, X, XI,
    and XII, producing Vernet syndrome and paralysis of the tongue on the
    same side.

Collier, James S., English physician, 1870-1935.
  Collier sign – unilateral or bilateral lid retraction due to midbrain lesion.
    SYN: Collier tucked lid sign

NOTES

Collier tract – a longitudinal bundle of fibers extending from the upper border of the mesencephalon into the cervical segments of the spinal cord. *SYN:* medial longitudinal fasciculus

Collier tucked lid sign – *SYN:* Collier sign

Collins, Edward Treacher, English ophthalmologist, 1862-1919.

Treacher Collins syndrome – mandibulofacial dysostosis, when limited to the orbit and malar region. *SYN:* Nager-de Reynier syndrome

Collip, James B., Canadian endocrinologist, 1892-1965.

Anderson-Collip test – see under Anderson, Evelyn

Clark-Collip method – see under Clark, Earl Perry

Collip unit – dosage of parathyroid extract.

Noble-Collip procedure – see under Noble, Robert L.

Collis, John Leighton, English thoracic surgeon, *1911.

Collis antireflux operation

Collis forceps

Collis gastroplasty – a technique for lengthening the esophagus.

Collis mouth gag

Collis repair

Collis spirometer

Collis technique

Colonna, Paul Crenshaw, U.S. surgeon, 1892-1966.

Colonna arthroplasty

Colonna hip fracture classification

Colonna operation – procedure for correction of congenital hip dislocation.

Colonna reconstruction

Comby, Jules, French pediatrician, 1853-1947.

Comby sign – an early sign of measles, consisting of thin whitish patches on the gums and buccal mucous membrane, formed of desquamating epithelial cells.

Comèl, M., Italian dermatologist and angiologist, 1902-1995.

Comèl-Netherton syndrome – *SYN:* Netherton syndrome

Rille-Comèl disease – see under Rille

Comly, Hunter Hall, U.S. physician, *1919.

Comly syndrome – potentially fatal syndrome characterized by inability of red blood cells to carry oxygen to body tissues.

Comolli, Antonio, Italian pathologist, *1879.
  Comolli sign – in cases of fracture of the scapula, a typical triangular cushion-like swelling appears, corresponding to the outline of the scapula.

Compton, Arthur H., U.S. physicist, 1892-1962, winner of the 1927 Nobel Prize for his work in physics.
  Compton effect – in electromagnetic radiations of medium energy, a decrease in energy of the bombarding photon with the dislodgement of an orbital electron, usually from an outer shell. *SYN:* Compton scattering
  Compton scattering – *SYN:* Compton effect

Concato, Luigi M., Italian physician, 1825-1882.
  Concato disease – chronic inflammation with effusions in several serous cavities resulting in fibrous thickening of the serosa and constrictive pericarditis. *SYN:* polyserositis

Conn, Harold J., U.S. microbiologist, 1886-1975.
  Hucker-Conn stain – a crystal violet-ammonium oxalate mixture used in Gram stain.

Conn, Jerome, U.S. physician, 1907-1981.
  Conn syndrome – an adrenocortical disorder caused by excessive secretion of aldosterone. *SYN:* primary aldosteronism

Connell, F. Gregory, U.S. surgeon, 1875-1968.
  Connell airway
  Connell breathing tube
  Connell ether vapor tube
  Connell incision
  Connell operation
  Connell suture – a continuous suture used for inverting the gastric or intestinal walls in performing an anastomosis.

NOTES

Conradi, Andrew, Norwegian physician, 1809-1869.
  Conradi line – a line corresponding approximately to the lower edge of the cardiac area.

Conradi, Erich, German physician, *1882.
  Conradi disease – congenital shortening of the humerus and femur, with stippled epiphyses, high-arched palate, cataracts, erythroderma in the newborn, and scaling followed by follicular atrophoderma. *SYN:* chondrodystrophia congenita punctata; Conradi-Hunermann disease; Conradi syndrome
  Conradi-Hunermann disease – *SYN:* Conradi disease
  Conradi syndrome – *SYN:* Conradi disease

Conradi, Heinrich, German bacteriologist, *1876.
  Conradi-Drigalski agar – a selective, nutrient medium for isolation of *Salmonella typhi* and other intestinal pathogens from fecal specimens. *SYN:* Drigalski-Conradi agar
  Drigalski-Conradi agar – *SYN:* Conradi-Drigalski agar

Contarini, Francesco, Venetian nobleman, d. 1625.
  Contarini condition – bilateral pleural effusions in cancer and leukemic patients with symptoms similar to those first observed in Contarini. *SYN:* Contarini syndrome
  Contarini syndrome – *SYN:* Contarini condition

Contino, Antonino, Italian ophthalmologist, 1878-1951.
  Contino epithelioma – papilloma of the eye.
  Contino glaucoma

Converse, John M., U.S. plastic surgeon, 1909-1981.
  Converse alar elevator
  Converse alar retractor
  Converse bistoury
  Converse curette
  Converse hinged skin hook
  Converse knife
  Converse method – earlobe reconstruction procedure.
  Converse nasal chisel
  Converse nasal retractor
  Converse nasal rongeur
  Converse nasal root rongeur
  Converse nasal saw
  Converse nasal speculum
  Converse nasal tip scissors

Converse needle holder
Converse operation
Converse osteotome
Converse rasp
Converse raspatory
Converse splint

Cooke, A. Bennett, U.S. physician, *1869.
   Cooke speculum – a three-pronged speculum for rectal examinations and operations.

Cooley, Denton, 20th century U.S. surgeon.
   Cooley anastomosis
   Cooley anastomosis clamp
   Cooley anastomosis forceps
   Cooley aortic aneurysm clamp
   Cooley aortic clamp
   Cooley aortic retractor
   Cooley aortic vent needle
   Cooley arterial occlusion forceps
   Cooley arteriotomy scissors
   Cooley atrial retractor
   Cooley auricular appendage forceps
   Cooley bronchial clamp
   Cooley bulldog clamp
   Cooley cardiac tucker
   Cooley cardiovascular forceps
   Cooley cardiovascular scissors
   Cooley cardiovascular suction tube
   Cooley caval occlusion clamp
   Cooley chisel
   Cooley coarctation clamp
   Cooley coarctation forceps

C

NOTES

Cooley coronary dilator
Cooley curved forceps
Cooley dilator
Cooley double-angled jaw forceps
Cooley first-rib shears
Cooley graft clamp
Cooley graft forceps
Cooley iliac clamp
Cooley iliac forceps
Cooley intrapericardial anastomosis
Cooley microvascular needle holder
Cooley neonatal retractor
Cooley neonatal vascular clamp
Cooley partial occlusion clamp
Cooley patent ductus clamp
Cooley patent ductus forceps
Cooley pediatric aortic forceps
Cooley pediatric clamp
Cooley pediatric dilator
Cooley peripheral vascular forceps
Cooley probe-point scissors
Cooley renal clamp
Cooley reverse-cut scissors
Cooley rib contractor
Cooley rib retractor
Cooley sternotomy retractor
Cooley suction tube
Cooley sump tube
Cooley tangential pediatric forceps
Cooley tissue forceps
Cooley U-sutures
Cooley valve dilator
Cooley vascular forceps
Cooley vascular tissue forceps
Cooley vena cava catheter clamp
Cooley vena cava clamp

Cooley, Thomas B., U.S. pediatrician, 1871-1945.
Cooley anemia – the syndrome of severe anemia with multiple organ disorders. *SYN:* thalassemia major
Cooley trait – *SYN:* thalassemia minor

Coolidge, William D., U.S. physicist, 1873-1974.
  Coolidge tube – a kind of x-ray tube.

Coombs, Carey F., English physician, 1879-1932.
  Carey Coombs murmur – *SYN:* Coombs murmur
  Coombs murmur – a blubbering apical mid-diastolic murmur occurring in the acute stage of rheumatic mitral valvulitis and disappearing as the valvulitis subsides. *SYN:* Carey Coombs murmur

Coombs, Robin R.A., English veterinarian and immunologist, *1921.
  Coombs serum – serum from a rabbit or other animal previously immunized with purified human globulin to prepare antibodies directed against IgG and complement. *SYN:* antihuman globulin
  Coombs test – a test for antibodies, the so-called antihuman globulin test, using either the direct or indirect Coombs tests. *SYN:* antiglobulin test
  direct Coombs test – a test for detecting sensitized erythrocytes in erythroblastosis fetalis and in cases of acquired immune hemolytic anemia.
  Gell and Coombs reaction – see under Gell
  indirect Coombs test – a test routinely performed in cross-matching blood or in the investigation of transfusion reaction.

Coons, A.H., U.S. immunologist, *1912.
  Coons fluorescent antibody method – method used to localize cell antigens.

Cooper, Sir Astley Paston, English anatomist and surgeon, 1768-1841.
  Cooper fascia – one of the coverings of the spermatic cord, formed of delicate connective tissue and of muscular fibers derived from the internal oblique muscle (cremaster muscle). *SYN:* cremasteric fascia
  Cooper hernia – a femoral hernia with two sacs. *SYN:* bilocular femoral hernia; Hey hernia
  Cooper herniotome – a slender bistoury with short cutting edge for dividing the constricting tissues at the neck of a hernial sac.
  Cooper ligament repair

NOTES

Cooper ligaments – (1) suspensory ligaments of breast. *SYN:* suspensory ligaments of Cooper; (2) pectineal ligament; (3) transverse ligament of elbow.

Cooper neuralgia – *SYN:* mastodynia

Cooper testis – neuralgia of the testicles.

suspensory ligaments of Cooper – *SYN:* Cooper ligaments (1)

Cooperman, H.N., U.S. dentist.

Cooperman-Miura syndrome – retrusion of the mandible causing tongue-uvula impingement; symptoms include respiratory disorders, headache, temporomandibular joint dysfunction. *SYN:* Miura-Cooperman syndrome; uvula-tongue malposture

Miura-Cooperman syndrome – *SYN:* Cooperman-Miura syndrome

Coopernail, George P., U.S. surgeon, 1876-1962.

Coopernail sign – in fracture of the pelvis, occurrence of ecchymosis of the perineum and scrotum, or labia.

Cope, O.J., U.S. surgeon, *1902.

Churchill-Cope reflex – see under Churchill

Cope, Sir Vincent Z., English surgeon, 1881-1974.

Cope biopsy needle

Cope clamp – a clamp used in excision of colon and rectum.

Cope double-ended retractor

Coplin, W.M.I., U.S. physician, 1864-1928.

Coplin jar – glass jar used to hold staining slides.

Coppet, Louis de, French physicist, 1841-1911.

Coppet law – solutions having the same freezing point have equal concentrations of dissolved substances.

Corbus, Budd Clarke, U.S. urologist, 1876-1954.

Corbus disease – spirochete causing infection that erodes the glans penis. *SYN:* balanitis gangrenosa

Cords, Richard, German ophthalmologist, *1861.

Cords angiopathy – thrombosis of a retinal vein that can eventually lead to visual field reduction; occurs in children.

Corey, R.B., U.S. chemist, 1897-1971.

Pauling-Corey helix – see under Pauling

Cori, Carl F., Czech-U.S. biochemist and Nobel laureate, 1896-1984.

Cori cycle – the phases in the metabolism of carbohydrate.

Cori ester – an important intermediate in glycogenesis and glycogenolysis. *SYN:* D-glucose 1-phosphate

Cori, Gerty Theresa, Czech-U.S. biochemist and Nobel laureate, 1896-1957.
   Cori disease – glycogenosis due to amylo-1,6-glucosidase deficiency, resulting in accumulation of abnormal glycogen with short outer chains in liver and muscle. *SYN:* type 3 glycogenosis
   Cori syndrome – *SYN:* McArdle syndrome

Cormack, Alan M., joint winner of 1979 Nobel Prize for work related to CT scan.

Cornell, William Mason, U.S. psychiatrist, 1802-1895.
   Cornell Medical Index – psychological test designed to screen for potential instability in World War II soldiers.
   Cornell Word Form – word-association test.

Corner, Edred M., English surgeon, 1873-1950.
   Corner tampon – a plug of omentum stuffed into a wound of the stomach or intestine as a temporary tampon.

Corner, George W., U.S. anatomist, 1889-1981.
   Corner-Allen test – a test for progestational activity.
   Corner-Allen unit – a unit of progestational activity, measured in rabbits.

Cornet, Georg, German bacteriologist, 1858-1915.
   Cornet forceps

Cornil, L.
   Roussy-Cornil syndrome – see under Roussy

Coroli, J., French gastroenterologist.
   Coroli syndrome – intrahepatic biliary tract cystic dilatation often accompanied by bile stones and increased incidence of adenocarcinoma in the intrahepatic bile ducts.

Corrigan, Sir Dominic John, Irish pathologist and clinician, 1802-1880.
   Corrigan disease – reflux of blood through an incompetent aortic valve into the left ventricle during ventricular diastole. *SYN:* aortic regurgitation

NOTES

Corrigan pulse – the collapsing or water-hammer-type pulse in aortic regurgitation or peripheral arterial dilation, characterized by an abrupt rise and rapid fall away.

Corti, Marquis Alfonso, Italian anatomist, 1822-1888.

Corti arch – the arch formed by the junction of the heads of Corti inner and outer pillar cells.

Corti auditory teeth – tooth-shaped formations or ridges occurring on the vestibular lip of the limbus lamina spiralis of the cochlear duct. *SYN:* auditory teeth

Corti canal – *SYN:* Corti tunnel

Corti cells – sensory cells in the organ of Corti in synaptic contact with sensory as well as efferent fibers of the cochlear (auditory) nerve. *SYN:* cochlear hair cells

Corti ganglion – an elongated ganglion of bipolar sensory nerve cell bodies on the cochlear part of the vestibulocochlear nerve in the spiral canal of the modiolus. *SYN:* spiral ganglion of cochlea

Corti membrane – a gelatinous membrane that overlies the spiral organ (Corti) in the inner ear. *SYN:* tectorial membrane of cochlear duct

Corti organ – a prominent ridge of highly specialized epithelium in the floor of the cochlear duct. *SYN:* spiral organ

Corti pillars – cells forming the outer and inner walls of the tunnel in the organ of Corti. *SYN:* Corti rods; pillar cells; pillar cells of Corti;

Corti rods – *SYN:* Corti pillars

Corti tunnel – the spiral canal in the organ of Corti, filled with fluid and occasionally crossed by nonmedullated nerve fibers. *SYN:* Corti canal

pillar cells of Corti – *SYN:* Corti pillars

Corvisart des Marets, Baron Jean N., French clinician, 1755-1821.

Corvisart disease

Corvisart facies – the characteristic facies seen in cardiac insufficiency or aortic regurgitation.

Costa, O.G., 20th century Brazilian dermatologist.

acrokeratoelastoidosis of Costa – *SYN:* Costa disease

Costa disease – cornified papules occurring on the borders of the hands and feet. *SYN:* acrokeratoelastoidosis of Costa

Costello, J.M., New Zealand physician.

Costello syndrome – syndrome of postnatal growth deficiency, mental subnormality, depressed nasal bridge, curly hair, short neck, cardiomyopathy, and other abnormalities.

Costen, James B., U.S. otolaryngologist, 1895-1962.
  Costen syndrome – a symptom complex of loss of hearing, otalgia, tinnitus, dizziness, headache, and burning sensation of the throat, tongue, and side of the nose.

Cotard, Jules, French neurologist, 1840-1887.
  Cotard syndrome – psychotic depression involving delusion of the existence of one's body, along with ideas of negation and suicidal impulses.

Cotte, Gaston, French surgeon, 1879-1951.
  Cotte operation – cutting of the presacral nerve to relieve severe dysmenorrhea. *SYN:* presacral neurectomy

Cotting, Benjamin E., U.S. surgeon, 1812-1898.
  Cotting operation – repair of ingrown toenail.

Cotton, Frank A., U.S. chemist, *1930.
  Cotton effect – a change in the sign of optical rotation of a specimen as the wavelength of observation is changed.

Cotton, Frederick J., U.S. physician, 1869-1938.
  Cotton fracture – tibial fracture.

Cotugno, var. of Cotunnius

Cotunnius, (Cotugno), Domenico Felice Antonio, Italian anatomist, 1736-1822.
  aqueductus cotunnii – a bony canal of the petrous portion of the temporal bone, giving passage to the endolymphatic duct and a small vein.
    SYN: aqueduct of vestibule; Cotunnius aqueduct; Cotunnius canal
  Cotunnius aqueduct – *SYN:* aqueductus cotunnii
  Cotunnius canal – *SYN:* aqueductus cotunnii
  Cotunnius disease – pain in the lower back and hip radiating down the back of the thigh into the leg now known to usually be due to herniated lumbar disk compromising the L5 or S1 root. *SYN:* sciatica

NOTES

Cotunnius liquid – the fluid contained within the osseus labyrinth.
  SYN: liquor cotunnii; perilymph
Cotunnius space – the dilated blind extremity of the endolymphatic duct.
  SYN: endolymphatic sac
liquor cotunnii – *SYN:* Cotunnius liquid

Councilman, William T., U.S. pathologist, 1854-1933.
  Councilman body – an eosinophilic globule seen in the liver in yellow
    fever, derived from necrosis of a single hepatic cell. *SYN:* Councilman cell;
    Councilman lesion
  Councilman cell – *SYN:* Councilman body
  Councilman lesion – *SYN:* Councilman body

Cournand, André F., French-U.S. physiologist, *1895, joint winner of 1956
Nobel Prize for work related to circulation and cardiac catheterization.
  Cournand arterial needle
  Cournand catheter
  Cournand needle

Courvoisier, Ludwig G., French surgeon, 1843-1918.
  Courvoisier gallbladder – an enlarged, often palpable, gallbladder in a
    patient with carcinoma of the head of the pancreas.
  Courvoisier law – enlargement of the gallbladder with jaundice is likely to
    result from carcinoma of the head of the pancreas and not from a stone
    in the common duct. *SYN:* Courvoisier sign
  Courvoisier sign – *SYN:* Courvoisier law

Couto, Miguel, South American physician, 1864-1934.
  Couto disease – visceral organ fatty degeneration.

Couvelaire, Alexandre, French obstetrician, 1873-1948.
  Couvelaire uterus – extravasation of blood into the uterine musculature
    and beneath the uterine peritoneum in association with severe forms of
    abruptio placentae. *SYN:* uteroplacental apoplexy

Cowden, Rachel, the first patient to be described with this condition in 1963.
  Cowden syndrome – an autosomal dominant syndrome characterized by
    multiple trichilemmomas occurring around the mouth, nose, and ears.

Cowdry, Edmund Vincent, U.S. cytologist, 1888-1975.
  Cowdry type A inclusion bodies – droplet-like masses of acidophilic
    material surrounded by clear halos within nuclei, with margination of
    chromatin on the nuclear membrane.

Cowdry type B inclusion bodies – droplet-like masses of acidophilic material surrounded by clear halos within nuclei, without other nuclear changes during early stages of development of the inclusion.

Cowen, J.P., 20th century U.S. ophthalmologist.
Cowen sign – sign of Graves disease.

Cowper, William, English anatomist, 1666-1709.
Cowper cyst – a retention cyst of a bulbourethral gland.
Cowper gland – *SYN:* bulbourethral gland
cowperitis – inflammation of Cowper gland.
Cowper ligament – the part of the fascia lata which is anterior to and provides origin for fibers of the pectineus muscle.

Coxsackie, city in New York where virus was first isolated.
coxsackie encephalitus – a viral encephalitis caused by Enterovirus human coxsackie B.
coxsackievirus – a group of picornaviruses. *SYN:* coxsackie virus
coxsackie virus – *SYN:* coxsackievirus

Crabtree, Herbert G., 20th century English physician and biochemist.
Crabtree effect – inhibition of cellular respiration of isolated systems by high concentrations of glucose.

Crafoord, Clarence, Swedish surgeon, *1899.
Crafoord aortic clamp
Crafoord bronchial forceps
Crafoord clamp – a clamp used in heart, lung, and vascular operations.
Crafoord coarctation clamp
Crafoord coarctation forceps
Crafoord forceps
Crafoord hemostat
Crafoord lobectomy scissors
Crafoord operation
Crafoord pulmonary forceps
Crafoord thoracic scissors

NOTES

Crafts, Leo M., U.S. neurologist, 1863-1938.
   Crafts test – test related to organic disease of pyramidal tract.

Craig, name of a rehabilitation hospital in Englewood, CO.
   Scott-Craig orthosis – see under Scott, Bruce A.

Craig, Jenny, 20th century businesswoman, founder of weight-loss program that bears her name.
   Jenny Craig diet – program that focuses on healthy eating, activity, and one-on-one consultations to achieve goal weight.

Cramer, Friedrich, German surgeon, 1847-1903.
   Cramer wire splint – a flexible splint consisting of two stout parallel wires with finer cross wires. *SYN:* ladder splint

Crampton, Charles Ward, U.S. physician, *1877.
   Crampton test – a test for physical condition and resistance.

Crampton, Sir Philip, Irish surgeon, 1777-1858.
   Crampton line – a guide to the common iliac artery.
   Crampton muscle – *SYN:* Brücke muscle

Crandall, Barbara F., U.S. pediatrician.
   Crandall syndrome – recessive trait causing deafness, baldness, and hypogonadism.

Crawford, Brian H., English physicist, *1906.
   Stiles-Crawford effect – see under Stiles

Credé, Karl S.F., German obstetrician and gynecologist, 1819-1892.
   Credé maneuver – *SYN:* Credé method (3)
   Credé method – (1) instillation of 0.1% silver nitrate in eyes of neonates; (2) resting the hand on the fundus uteri from the moment of the expulsion of the fetus; (3) use of manual pressure on a bladder to express urine. *SYN:* Credé maneuver

Creutzfeldt, Hans Gerhard, German neuropsychiatrist, 1885-1964.
   Creutzfeldt-Jakob disease – a form of subacute spongiform encephalopathy caused by a transmissible agent that has not been completely defined. *SYN:* Jakob-Creutzfeldt disease; mad cow disease; transmissible dementia
   Jakob-Creutzfeldt disease – *SYN:* Creutzfeldt-Jakob disease

Creveld, Simon van, see under van Creveld

Crichton-Browne, Sir James, English physician, 1840-1938.
   Crichton-Browne sign – a slight tremor at the angles of the mouth and at the outer canthus of each eye in general paresis.

Crick, Francis H.C., English biochemist and Nobel laureate, *1916.
  Watson-Crick helix – see under Watson, James Dewey

Crigler, John F., U.S. physician, *1919.
  Crigler-Najjar disease – *SYN:* Crigler-Najjar syndrome
  Crigler-Najjar syndrome – a rare defect in ability to form bilirubin
    glucuronide due to deficiency of bilirubin-glucuronide
    glucuronosyltransferase. *SYN:* Arias syndrome; Crigler-Najjar disease

Crile, George Washington, U.S. surgeon, 1864-1943.
  Crile appendiceal clamp
  Crile arterial forceps
  Crile blade
  Crile clamp – a clamp for temporary stoppage of blood flow.
  Crile dissector
  Crile gall duct forceps
  Crile gall hemostats
  Crile needle holder
  Crile single hook
  Crile spatula
  Crile vagotomy stripper

Crocker, Henry Radcliffe, English physician, 1845-1909.
  Crocker disease – dermatitis characterized by bullae and vesicles
    occurring predominantly on the upper extremities. *SYN:* dermatitis repens

Crocq, Jean, Belgian physician, 1868-1925.
  Crocq disease – a circulatory disorder. *SYN:* acrocyanosis

Crohn, Burrill Bernard, U.S. gastroenterologist, 1884-1983.
  Crohn disease – a subacute chronic enteritis. *SYN:* regional enteritis

Cronin, Thomas D., U.S. plastic surgeon, *1906.
  Cronin cheiloplasty
  Cronin cleft palate elevator
  Cronin implant

NOTES

Cronin mammary implant
Cronin method – nasal tip operation.
Cronin palate elevator
Cronin palate knife
Cronin Silastic mammary prosthesis

Cronkhite, Leonard W., Jr., U.S. physician, *1919.
  Cronkhite-Canada syndrome – a sporadically occurring syndrome of gastrointestinal polyps with diffuse alopecia and nail dystrophy.

Crooke, Arthur Carleton, English pathologist, *1905.
  Crooke granules – lumpy masses of basophilic material in the pituitary associated with Cushing disease or following the administration of ACTH.
  Crooke hyaline change – replacement of cytoplasmic granules of basophil cells of the anterior pituitary by homogenous hyaline material. *SYN:* Crooke hyaline degeneration
  Crooke hyaline degeneration – *SYN:* Crooke hyaline change

Crookes, Sir William, English physicist and chemist, 1832-1919.
  Crookes glass – a spectacle lens combined with metallic oxides to absorb ultraviolet or infrared rays.

Crosby, William Holmes, Jr., U.S. physician, *1914.
  Crosby capsule – an attachment to the end of a flexible tube used for peroral biopsy of the small intestine.
  Crosby syndrome – recessive trait causing hemolytic anemia.

Cross, Harold E., U.S. ophthalmologist, *1937.
  Cross-McKusick-Breen syndrome – *SYN:* Cross syndrome
  Cross syndrome – autosomal recessive trait resulting in corneal opacity and albinism, mental retardation.
  McKusick-Cross syndrome – *SYN:* McKusick syndrome

Crosti, A., Italian dermatologist, 1896-1988.
  Gianotti-Crosti syndrome – see under Gianotti

Crouzon, Octave, French physician, 1874-1938.
  Crouzon-Apert disease – *SYN:* Apert syndrome
  Crouzon disease – craniostosis with widening of the skull and high forehead, ocular hypertelorism, exophthalmos, beaked nose, and hypoplasia of the maxilla. *SYN:* craniofacial dysostosis

Crowe, Samuel J., U.S. physician, 1883-1955.
  Crowe-Davis mouth gag – *SYN:* Davis-Crowe mouth gag

Crowe sign – in the presence of lateral sinus thrombosis, internal jugular vein compression resulting in engorgement of retinal vessels.
Davis-Crowe mouth gag – see under Davis

Crozat, George B., U.S. dentist, *1876.
Crozat appliance – orthodontic appliance.
Crozat clasp – dental appliance clasp.
Crozat dental orthopedics
Crozat philosophy
Crozat removable orthodontic appliance
Crozat therapy

Cruchet, Jean R., French physician.
Cruchet disease – *SYN:* torticollis

Crutchfield, William G., U.S. neurosurgeon, *1900.
Crutchfield clamp
Crutchfield drill
Crutchfield operation
Crutchfield reduction technique
Crutchfield skeletal traction
Crutchfield skull-tip pin
Crutchfield tongs
Crutchfield tongs prosthesis
Crutchfield traction
Crutchfield traction bow
Crutchfield traction tongs

Cruveilhier, Jean, French pathologist and anatomist, 1791-1874.
Cruveilhier atrophy
Cruveilhier-Baumgarten disease – *SYN:* Cruveilhier-Baumgarten syndrome
Cruveilhier-Baumgarten murmur – a venous murmur heard over collateral veins, connecting portal and caval venous systems, on the abdominal wall.

NOTES

Cruveilhier-Baumgarten sign – a murmur over the umbilicus often in the presence of caput medusae.

Cruveilhier-Baumgarten syndrome – cirrhosis of the liver with patent umbilical or paraumbilical veins and varicose periumbilical veins (caput medusae). *SYN:* Cruveilhier-Baumgarten disease

Cruveilhier disease – *SYN:* Lou Gehrig disease

Cruveilhier fascia – *SYN:* superficial fascia of perineum

Cruveilhier fossa – a longitudinal hollow on the posterior surface of the superior portion (root) of the medial pterygoid plate. *SYN:* fossa navicularis Cruveilhier; scaphoid fossa

Cruveilhier joint – a pivot synovial joint between the dens of the axis and the ring formed by the anterior arch and the transverse ligament of the atlas. *SYN:* median atlantoaxial joint

Cruveilhier ligaments – the counterparts in the foot of the palmar ligaments in the hand. *SYN:* plantar ligaments

Cruveilhier nodules

Cruveilhier palsy – *SYN:* Lou Gehrig disease

Cruveilhier plexus – a nerve plexus formed by communications between the dorsal primary rami of the first three cervical nerves.

Cruveilhier sign – palpable groin swelling noted when patient coughs.

Cruveilhier tumor

Cruveilhier ulcer

fossa navicularis Cruveilhier – *SYN:* Cruveilhier fossa

Cruz, G. Oswaldo, Brazilian physician, 1872-1917.

Chagas-Cruz disease – *SYN:* Chagas disease

Cruz phenomenon – *SYN:* Kernohan-Woltman syndrome

Cruz trypanosomiasis – *SYN:* Chagas disease

Oswaldocruzia – genus of parasite which reside in the intestines and lungs of amphibians and reptiles.

Cryer, Matthew H., U.S. surgeon, 1840-1921.

Cryer elevator – dental elevator.

Csillag, J.

Csillag disease – chronic atrophic and lichenoid dermatitis.

Cuba, island 90 miles off the coast of Florida.

Cuban epidemic optic neuropathy – in 1993, malnutrition caused by food rationing and additional exposure to toxins led to an optic neuropathy outbreak affecting 50,000 Cubans.

Cuignet, Ferdinand L.J., 19th century French ophthalmologist.

Cuignet method – skiascopy. *SYN:* retinoscopy

Cullen, Thomas S., U.S. gynecologist, 1868-1953.
   Cullen sign – periumbilical darkening of the skin from blood, a sign of intraperitoneal hemorrhage, especially in ruptured ectopic pregnancy.

Culp, Ormond S., U.S. urologist, 1910-1977.
   Culp biopsy needle
   Culp pyeloplasty – a reconstructive technique for correction of uteropelvic obstruction.
   Culp ureteropelvioplasty

Cummer, William E., Canadian dentist, 1879-1942.
   Cummer classification – a listing of several types of removable partial dentures in accordance with the distribution of direct retainers.
   Cummer guideline – a line which serves as a guide in the proper location of various parts of a clasp assembly for a removable partial denture. *SYN:* survey line

Cupid, in Roman mythology, the god of love.
   arch of Cupid
   Cupid bow
   Cupid bow peak

Cureton, Thomas Kirk, U.S. physical educator, 1901-1976.
   Cureton exercises – a physical education system.

Curie, Marie, French physicist, 1867-1934.
   curie – a unit of measurement of radioactivity.

Curie, Pierre, French physicist, 1859-1906.
   curie – a unit of measurement of radioactivity.

Curling, Thomas B., English surgeon, 1811-1888.
   Curling ulcer – an ulcer of the duodenum in a patient with extensive superficial burns, intracranial lesions, or severe bodily injury. *SYN:* stress ulcers

NOTES

Currarino, Guido, U.S. radiologist born in Italy, *1920.
    Currarino-Silverman syndrome – growth abnormality of the sternum.
      SYN: Silverman syndrome
    Currarino syndrome – *SYN:* Currarino triad
    Currarino triad – complex of anococcygeal congenital anomalies.
      SYN: Currarino syndrome

Curschmann, Heinrich, German physician, 1846-1910.
    Curschmann-Batten-Steinert syndrome – rare hereditary condition
      resulting in atrophy of testicles in addition to muscle membrane
      abnormality which causes myotonia. *SYN:* myotonia dystrophia
    Curschmann disease – hyaloserositis of the liver. *SYN:* frosted liver
    Curschmann spirals – spirally twisted masses of mucus occurring in the
      sputum in bronchial asthma.

Curtis, Arthur H., U.S. gynecologist, 1881-1955.
    Fitz-Hugh and Curtis syndrome – see under Fitz-Hugh

Curtius, Friedrich, German physician, 1896-1975.
    Curtius syndrome – hypertrophy of a part or system of the body with
      various associated disorders. *SYN:* hemihypertrophy; ovarian
      insufficiency with various associated disorders

Cushing, Harvey Williams, U.S. neurosurgeon, 1869-1939.
    Cushing basophilism – *SYN:* Cushing syndrome
    Cushing bone rongeur
    Cushing brain depressor
    Cushing brain forceps
    Cushing brain spatula
    Cushing cranial bur
    Cushing cranial rongeur forceps
    Cushing disease – adrenal hyperplasia (Cushing syndrome) caused by
      an ACTH-secreting basophil adenoma of the pituitary. *SYN:* Cushing
      pituitary basophilism
    Cushing dressing forceps
    Cushing dural hook
    Cushing dural hook knife
    Cushing effect – *SYN:* Cushing phenomenon
    Cushing Gigli-saw guide
    Cushing nerve retractor
    Cushing perforator
    Cushing perforator drill
    Cushing periosteal elevator

Cushing phenomenon – a rise in systemic blood pressure when the intracranial pressure acutely increases. *SYN:* Cushing effect; Cushing response

Cushing pituitary basophilism – *SYN:* Cushing disease

Cushing response – *SYN:* Cushing phenomenon

Cushing self-retaining retractor

Cushing straight retractor

Cushing syndrome – a disorder resulting from increased adrenocortical secretion of cortisol. *SYN:* adrenalism; Cushing basophilism; Gallais syndrome; Itsenko-Cushing syndrome

Cushing syndrome medicamentosus – a variable number of the signs and symptoms of Cushing syndrome.

Cushing ulcer

Itsenko-Cushing syndrome – *SYN:* Cushing syndrome

Cushing, Hayward W., U.S. surgeon, 1854-1934.

Cushing suture – a running horizontal mattress suture used to approximate two adjacent surfaces.

Cuvier, Baron Georges L.C.F.D. de la, French scientist, 1769-1832.

Cuvier ducts – obsolete term for the common cardinal veins.

Cuvier veins – the common cardinal vein of the embryo.

Cyon, Elie de, Russian physiologist, 1843-1912.

Cyon nerve – a branch of the vagus that ends in the aortic arch and base of the heart. *SYN:* aortic nerve

Cyriax, Edward F., 20th century English orthopedic surgeon.

Cyriax syndrome – costal cartilage lesions cause a "slipping" sensation of the ribs; pain radiates to shoulder and arm and is often confused with angina pectoris.

Czapek, Friedrich J.F., Czech botanist, 1868-1921.

Czapek-Dox medium – *SYN:* Czapek solution agar

NOTES

Czapek solution agar – a culture medium used for the cultivation of fungus species and for identification of *Aspergillus* and *Penicillium* species. *SYN:* Czapek-Dox medium

Czapski, Sigfried, German optician, *1861.
Czapski microscope – ophthalmologic microscope.

Czerny, Vincenz, German surgeon, 1842-1916.
Czerny herniorrhaphy
Czerny incision
Czerny-Lembert suture – an intestinal suture in two rows combining the Czerny suture (first) and the Lembert suture (second).
Czerny operation
Czerny rectal speculum
Czerny suture – the first row of the Czerny-Lembert intestinal suture.

Daae, Anders, Norwegian physician, 1838-1910.

Daae disease – an acute infectious disease usually occurring in epidemic form, characterized by paroxysms of pain and associated with strains of *Enterovirus* coxsackievirus type B. *SYN:* epidemic pleurodynia

Dabska, Maria, 20th century Polish pathologist.

Dabska tumor – rare, low-grade angiosarcoma that presents as slow-growing violaceous, pink, or blue-black intradermal nodule on the skin of children.

Dacie, Sir John Vivian, English physician.

Dacie syndrome – massive splenomegaly, etiology unknown.

DaCosta, Jacob M., U.S. surgeon, 1833-1900.

DaCosta disease

DaCosta syndrome – a syndrome of functional nervous and circulatory irregularities. *SYN:* neurocirculatory asthenia

Da Fano, Corrado D., Italian-U.S. anatomist, 1879-1927.

Da Fano stain – a silver stain that produces a blackening of Golgi elements after tissues are fixed in a mixture of nitrate and formalin.

Dagnini, Giuseppe, Italian physician, 1866-1928.

Aschner-Dagnini reflex – *SYN:* Aschner phenomenon

Dagnini, Guido, Italian physician, *1905.

Scaglietti-Dagnini syndrome – *SYN:* Erdheim syndrome

Dakin, Henry Drusdale, U.S. chemist, 1880-1952.

Dakin-Carrel treatment – *SYN:* Carrel treatment

Dakin catheter

Dakin dressing

Dakin fluid – *SYN:* Dakin solution

Dakin solution – a bactericidal wound irrigant. *SYN:* Dakin fluid

Dakin tube

NOTES

Dalcroze, Emile-Jacques, Swiss composer and educator, 1865-1950.
Dalcroze eurhythmics – a method of musical education used in therapy.

Dale, Sir Henry Hallett, English physiologist and Nobel laureate, 1875-1968.
Dale-Feldberg law – an identical chemical transmitter is liberated at all the functional terminals of a single neuron.
Dale reaction – *SYN:* Schultz-Dale reaction
Schultz-Dale reaction – see under Schultz, Werner

Dalen, Johan A., Swedish ophthalmologist, 1866-1940.
Dalen-Fuchs nodules – collections of epithelial cells lying between the Bruch membrane and the retinal pigment epithelium in sympathetic ophthalmia and rarely in other granulomatous intraocular inflammations.

Dalibour, J., French surgeon, d. 1735.
Dalibour water – an astringent solution, composed of copper sulfate 1% and zinc sulfate 1.5% in camphor water 2.5%; water to 100%.

Dalldorf, G.J., U.S. pathologist, *1900.
Dalldorf test – test for capillary fragility.

Dalrymple, John, English oculist, 1804-1852.
Dalrymple disease
Dalrymple sign – retraction of the upper eyelid in Graves disease, causing abnormal wideness of the palpebral fissure.

Dalton, John, English chemist, mathematician, and natural philosopher, 1766-1844.
Dalton-Henry law – in dissolving a mixture of gases, a liquid will absorb as much of each gas in the mixture as if that were the only gas dissolved.
Dalton law – each gas in a mixture of gases exerts a pressure proportionate to the percentage of the gas and independent of the presence of the other gases present. *SYN:* law of partial pressures

Dam, Carl P. Henrik, Danish biochemist, 1895-1976, winner of 1943 Nobel Prize for discovery of vitamin K.
Dam unit – a unit of activity of vitamin K.

Dana, Charles L., U.S. neurologist, 1852-1935.
Dana operation – section of posterior spinal root. *SYN:* posterior rhizotomy
Dana syndrome – degenerative disease of the spinal cord associated with pernicious anemia.
Putnam-Dana syndrome – see under Putnam

Danbolt, Niels Christian, Norwegian internist and dermatologist, 1900-1984.
Danbolt-Closs syndrome – *SYN:* Brandt syndrome
Danbolt syndrome – *SYN:* Brandt syndrome

Dance, Jean B.H., French physician, 1797-1832.
  Dance sign – *SYN:* signe de Dance
  signe de Dance – slight retraction in area of right iliac fossa sometimes seen in presence of intussusception. *SYN:* Dance sign

Dandy, Walter Edward, U.S. surgeon, 1886-1946.
  Dandy clamp
  Dandy forceps
  Dandy hemostat
  Dandy nerve hook
  Dandy neurosurgical scissors
  Dandy operation
  Dandy suction tube
  Dandy ventriculostomy
  Dandy-Walker syndrome – developmental anomaly of the fourth ventricle associated with atresia of the foramina of Luschka and Magendie that results in cerebellar hypoplasia, hydrocephalus, and posterior fossa cyst formation.

Dane, David S., 20th century English virologist.
  Dane method
  Dane particles – the larger spherical forms of hepatitis-associated antigens.

Danforth, William Clark, U.S. obstetrician-gynecologist, 1878-1949.
  Danforth sign – shoulder pain on inspiration, due to irritation of the diaphragm by a hemoperitoneum in ruptured ectopic pregnancy.

Danielli, J.F., English biologist, *1911.
  Davson-Danielli model – see under Davson

Danielssen, Daniel Cornelius, Norwegian physician, 1815-1894.
  Danielssen-Boeck disease – *SYN:* anesthetic leprosy
  Danielssen disease – *SYN:* anesthetic leprosy

NOTES

Danlos, Henri-Alexander, French dermatologist, 1844-1912.
Danlos phenomenon
Danlos syndrome
Ehlers-Danlos syndrome – see under Ehlers

Danysz, Jean, Polish pathologist in France, 1860-1928.
Danysz phenomenon – reduction of the neutralizing effect of an antitoxin when toxin is mixed with it in divided portions.

d'Arcet, Jean, French chemist, 1725-1801.
d'Arcet metal – an alloy of lead, bismuth, and tin used in dentistry.

Darier, Jean Ferdinand, Hungarian-born French dermatologist, 1856-1938.
Darier disease – a familial, autosomal dominant eruption of pruritic keratotic papules on the trunk, face, scalp, and axillae. *SYN:* keratosis follicularis
Darier sign – urtication on stroking of cutaneous lesions of urticaria pigmentosa (mastocytosis).

Darkschewitsch, (Darkshevich), Liverij Osipovich, Russian neurologist, 1858-1925.
nucleus of Darkschewitsch – an ovoid cell group in the ventral central gray substance rostral to the oculomotor nucleus.

Darkshevich, var. of Darkschewitsch

Darling, Samuel Taylor, U.S. physician in Panama, 1872-1925.
Darling disease – a widely distributed infectious disease caused by *Histoplasma capsulatum* and manifested by a primary benign pneumonitis. *SYN:* histoplasmosis

Darrow, D.C., U.S. pediatrician, 1895-1965.
Darrow solution – potassium-containing electrolyte solution.

d'Arsonval, Jacques Arsène, French biophysicist, 1851-1940.
d'Arsonval current – an alternating electric current having a frequency of 10,000 or more per second. *SYN:* high-frequency current
d'Arsonval galvanometer – a sensitive galvanometer consisting of a moving coil suspended in a permanent magnetic field between delicate metallic wires.

Darwin, Charles R., English biologist and evolutionist, 1809-1882.
darwinian ear – an auricle in which the upper border is not rolled over to form the helix, but projects upward as a flat, sharp edge.
darwinian reflex – the tendency of young infants to grasp a bar and hang suspended.

darwinian theory – the theory of the origin of species and of the development of higher organisms from lower forms through natural selection.

darwinian tubercle – a small projection from the upper end of the posterior portion of the incurved free margin of the helix. *SYN:* auricular tubercle

Daubenton, Louis J.M., French physician, 1716-1799.

Daubenton angle – an angle formed by the junction of lines coming from the basion and from the projection in the median plane of the lower border of the orbits. *SYN:* angulus occipitalis ossis parietalis; occipital angle of parietal bone

Daubenton line – the line passing between the opisthion and the basion.

Daubenton plane – the plane of the foramen magnum.

Dausset, Jean, joint winner of 1980 Nobel Prize for work related to cell structures and regulation of immunological reactions.

David, Laurence M., U.S. physician.

David-Baker clamp – used in carbon dioxide laser blepharoplasty of the upper eyelid.

David, W. Walter, German physician, *1890.

David disease – hemorrhage of gingivae and mucous membranes due to ovarian hormone deficiency.

Davidoff, M. von, German histologist, d. 1904.

Davidoff cells – *SYN:* Paneth granular cells

Davidson, Edward C., U.S. surgeon, 1894-1933.

Davidson bur
Davidson clamp
Davidson collector
Davidson forceps
Davidson muscle clamp
Davidson periosteal elevator

Davidson retractor
Davidson syringe – a rubber tube intersected with a compressible bulb designed to take up fluid.
Davidson trocar

Daviel, Jacques, French oculist, 1696-1762.
Daviel cataract extraction
Daviel chalazion knife
Daviel knife
Daviel lens loupe
Daviel lens spoon
Daviel operation – extracapsular cataract extraction.
Daviel scoop
Daviel spoon – a small oval-shaped instrument for removing the remains of a cataract after discission.

Davies, J.N.P., U.S. pathologist, *1915.
Davies disease – thickening of the ventricular endocardium by fibrosis leading to progressive right and left ventricular failure with mitral and tricuspid insufficiency. *SYN:* endomyocardial fibrosis

Davis, John Staige, U.S. surgeon, 1872-1946.
Crowe-Davis mouth gag – *SYN:* Davis-Crowe mouth gag
Davis-Crowe mouth gag – instrument used for opening the mouth, depressing the tongue, maintaining the airway, and transmitting volatile anesthetics during tonsillectomy or other oropharyngeal surgery. *SYN:* Crowe-Davis mouth gag
Davis graft – small pieces (2 to 3 mm) of full-thickness skin. *SYN:* pinch graft

Davson, H., English physiologist.
Davson-Danielli model – model of cell membrane.

Dawbarn, Robert Hugh Mackay, U.S. surgeon, 1860-1915.
Dawbarn sign – pain of subacromial bursitis disappears when the arm is abducted.

Dawson, James R., U.S. pathologist, *1908.
Dawson encephalitis – a rare chronic, progressive encephalitis caused by the measles virus. *SYN:* subacute sclerosing panencephalitis

Day, Richard H., U.S. physician, 1813-1892.
Day test – a test for blood.

Day, Richard Lawrence, U.S. pediatrician, 1905-1989.
Riley-Day syndrome – see under Riley, Conrad Milton

Dean, Henry Trendley, U.S. dentist and epidemiologist, 1893-1962.
Dean fluorosis index – an index that measures the degree of mottled enamel (fluorosis) in teeth.
Dean periosteal elevator

Deaver, George G., U.S. physiatrist, 1890-1973.
Deaver method – a method of motor reeducation.

Deaver, John B., U.S. surgeon, 1855-1931.
Deaver blade
Deaver clamp
Deaver hemostat
Deaver incision – an incision in the right lower abdominal quadrant, with medial displacement of the rectus muscle.
Deaver operating scissors
Deaver retractor
Deaver skin incision
Deaver T-tube

De Azua y Suarez, Juan, Spanish dermatologist, 1859-1922.
Azua pseudoepithelioma – *SYN:* De Azua pseudoepithelioma
De Azua pseudoepithelioma – a form of pyoderma with histology similar to that of epithelioma. *SYN:* Azua pseudoepithelioma

DeBakey, Michael Ellis, U.S. heart surgeon, *1908.
DeBakey aortic aneurysm clamp
DeBakey arterial clamp
DeBakey Atraugrip forceps
DeBakey ball-valve prosthesis
DeBakey Beaver blade
DeBakey bulldog clamp
DeBakey chest retractor
DeBakey classification – three types of dissections of the aorta: type I, type II, type III, type IIIA.
DeBakey coarctation clamp

D

NOTES

DeBakey dissecting forceps
DeBakey endarterectomy scissors
DeBakey forceps – nontraumatic forceps used to pick up blood vessels.
DeBakey graft
DeBakey heart valve
DeBakey implant
DeBakey needle
DeBakey patent ductus clamp
DeBakey scissors
DeBakey stripper
DeBakey tangential occlusion clamp
DeBakey tunneler
DeBakey valve prosthesis
DeBakey vascular dilator
DeBakey Vasculour-II vascular prosthesis

De Blasio, P., U.S. ophthalmologist.
De Blasio LASIK marker

Debler, K., German physician.
Debler anemia – inherited form of hemolytic anemia.

de Bordeau, Théophile, see under Bordeau

Debove, George M., French physician, 1845-1920.
Debove disease – splenomegaly.

Debré, Robert, French pediatrician and bacteriologist, 1882-1978.
Debré-De Toni-Fanconi syndrome – *SYN:* Fanconi syndrome (2)
Debré-Fibiger syndrome – pyloric pseudospasm causing vomiting and dehydration and which can lead to death. *SYN:* Fibiger-Debré-von Gierke syndrome; Pirie syndrome
Debré-Marie syndrome – (1) infectious edematous polyneuropathy; (2) dwarfism and underdevelopment of sexual organs.
Debré phenomenon – in measles, the failure of the rash to develop at the site of immune serum injection.
Debré-Semelaigne syndrome – *SYN:* Kocher-Debré-Semelaigne syndrome
Fibiger-Debré-von Gierke syndrome – *SYN:* Debré-Fibiger syndrome
Kocher-Debré-Semelaigne syndrome – see under Kocher

Dechaume, Jean, French physician, 1896-1968.
Bonnet-Dechaume-Blanc syndrome – see under Bonnet, Paul

de Clérambault, G.G., French psychiatrist, 1872-1934.

Clérambault-Kandinsky complex – psychosis in which patient believes his mind is controlled by a source outside himself. *SYN:* Clérambault-Kandinsky syndrome

Clérambault-Kandinsky syndrome – *SYN:* Clérambault-Kandinsky complex

Clérambault syndrome – psychosis primarily affecting females in which patient believes she is loved by someone of high status. *SYN:* de Clérambault syndrome

de Clérambault syndrome – *SYN:* Clérambault syndrome

De Duve, Christian, joint winner of 1974 Nobel Prize for work related to cell structure and organization.

Deen, Izaak A. van, see under van Deen

Deetjen, Hermann, German physician, 1867-1915.

Deetjen bodies – a disklike cytoplasmic fragment found in the peripheral blood where it functions in clotting. *SYN:* platelet

de Gimard, see under Martin de Gimard

Degos, Robert, French dermatologist, 1904-1987.

Degos acanthoma – obsolete term for clear cell acanthoma.

Degos disease – a cutaneovisceral syndrome characterized by pathognomonic umbilicated porcelain-white papules followed by peritonitis, progressive neurological disability, and death. *SYN:* Degos syndrome; malignant atrophic papulosis

Degos syndrome – *SYN:* Degos disease

Kohlmeier-Degos syndrome – see under Kohlmeier

Dehio, Karl K., Russian physician, 1851-1927.

Dehio test – a test to determine the cause of bradycardia. *SYN:* atropine test

D

NOTES

Deiters, Otto F.K., German anatomist, 1834-1863.

Deiters cells – the supporting cells of the organ of Corti; one of the large neuroglia cells of nervous tissue. *SYN:* astrocyte; phalangeal cell

Deiters nucleus – lateral vestibular nucleus.

Deiters terminal frames – platelike structures in the organ of Corti uniting the outer phalangeal cells with Hensen cells.

Dejerine, Joseph J., Paris neurologist, 1849-1917.

Dejerine anterior bulbar syndrome – occlusion of anterior spinal arteries with involvement of cortical spinal tract, hypoglossal nerves, and medial lemnisci.

Dejerine cortical sensory syndrome – (1) radiculitis; (2) bulbar syndrome caused by medullar lesion and resulting in cranial nerve paralysis in the area; (3) polyneuropathy resulting in depression of deep sensation; tactile sensation remains normal.

Dejerine disease – *SYN:* Dejerine-Sottas disease

Dejerine hand phenomenon – clonic contractions of the flexors of the hand (wrist) on tapping the dorsum of the hand or the volar side of the forearm near the wrist, exaggerated in pyramidal tract lesions. *SYN:* Dejerine reflex

Dejerine-Landouzy dystrophy – *SYN:* Landouzy-Dejerine dystrophy

Dejerine-Landouzy myopathy – *SYN:* Landouzy-Dejerine dystrophy

Dejerine-Lichtheim phenomenon – *SYN:* Lichtheim sign

Dejerine reflex – *SYN:* Dejerine hand phenomenon

Dejerine-Roussy syndrome – infraction of posteroinferior thalamus causing transient hemiparesis, severe loss of superficial and deep sensation with preservation of crude pain in the limbs with decreased sensation; the limbs frequently have vasomotor or trophic disturbances. *SYN:* thalamic syndrome

Dejerine sign – aggravation of symptoms of radiculitis by the acts of coughing, sneezing, or straining to defecate.

Dejerine-Sottas disease – a familial type of demyelinating sensorimotor polyneuropathy that begins in early childhood and is slowly progressive. *SYN:* Dejerine disease; Dejerine-Sottas neuropathy; progressive hypertrophic polyneuropathy

Dejerine-Sottas neuropathy – *SYN:* Dejerine-Sottas disease

Landouzy-Dejerine dystrophy – see under Landouzy

Dejerine-Klumpke, Augusta, French neurologist, 1859-1927.

Dejerine-Klumpke palsy – *SYN:* Klumpke palsy

Dejerine-Klumpke syndrome – *SYN:* Klumpke palsy

Klumpke palsy – a type of brachial birth palsy in which there is paralysis of the muscles of the distal forearm and hand. *SYN:* Dejerine-Klumpke palsy; Dejerine-Klumpke syndrome; Klumpke paralysis

Klumpke paralysis – *SYN:* Klumpke palsy

Delafield, Francis, U.S. physician and pathologist, 1841-1915.

Delafield hematoxylin – an alum type of hematoxylin used in histology.

de Lange, Cornelia, Dutch pediatrician, 1871-1950.

Cornelia de Lange syndrome – *SYN:* de Lange syndrome

de Lange syndrome – a congenital anomaly characterized by impaired development, mental retardation, characteristic facies with synophrys and hairline well down on forehead, depressed bridge of nose with uptilted tip of nose, small head with low-set ears, and flat spadelike hands with simian crease and short tapering fingers. *SYN:* Amsterdam syndrome; Cornelia de Lange syndrome

Delbet, Pierre, French surgeon, 1861-1925.

Delbet sign – in a case of aneurysm of a main artery, efficient collateral circulation if the nutrition of the part below is well maintained, despite the fact that the pulse has disappeared.

Delbet splint for heel fracture

Delbrück, Max, joint winner of 1969 Nobel Prize for work related to viruses.

del Castillo, E.B., 20th century Argentinian physician.

Ahumada-del Castillo syndrome – see under Ahumada

Argonz-del Castillo syndrome – *SYN:* Ahumada-del Castillo syndrome

del Castillo syndrome – *SYN:* Sertoli-cell-only syndrome

DeLee, Joseph B., U.S. obstetrician and gynecologist, 1869-1942.

DeLee catheter

DeLee forceps

DeLee-Hillis stethoscope

DeLee infant catheter

D

NOTES

DeLee maneuver – a method by which obstetrical forceps are used to rotate the fetal head. *SYN:* key-in-lock maneuver
DeLee obstetrical forceps
DeLee ovum forceps
DeLee pelvimeter
DeLee trap meconium aspirator
DeLee uterine packing forceps

Delleman, J.W., 20th century Dutch ophthalmologist and geneticist.
Delleman-Oorthuys syndrome – *SYN:* Delleman syndrome
Delleman syndrome – rare malformation syndrome characterized by orbital cysts, microphthalmia, and cerebral malformations. *SYN:* Delleman-Oorthuys syndrome

Delmege, Jean A., 20th century French physician.
Delmege sign – early tuberculosis sign.

DeLorme, Thomas L., U.S. orthopedic surgeon.
DeLorme exercises – progressive resistance exercise system.
DeLorme table – an exercise table with adjustable parts.

Delsarte, Francois-Alexandre-Nicolas, 1811-1871.
Delsarte exercises – *SYN:* Delsarte system
Delsarte system – a method of breathing, speaking, posture, etc. *SYN:* Delsarte exercises; delsartism
delsartism – *SYN:* Delsarte system

Demarquay, Jean N., French surgeon, 1811-1875.
Demarquay symptom – absence of elevation of the larynx during deglutition, said to indicate syphilitic induration of the trachea.

De Martini, A., Italian physician.
De Martini-Balestra syndrome – *SYN:* Burke syndrome

Demoivre, Abraham, English mathematician, 1667-1754.
Demoivre formula – an obsolete formula for calculating life expectancy.

Demons, Albert Jean Octave, French physician, 1842-1920.
Demons-Meigs syndrome – *SYN:* Meigs syndrome

De Morgan, Campbell, English physician, 1811-1876.
Campbell De Morgan spots – congenital anomaly in which proliferation of blood vessels leads to a mass resembling a neoplasm; primarily seen on skin and in subcutaneous tissue; incidence increases with age. *SYN:* cherry angioma; De Morgan spots; senile hemangioma
De Morgan spots – *SYN:* Campbell De Morgan spots

de Morsier, G., 20th century Swiss neurologist.
   de Morsier syndrome – congenital optic nerve hypoplasia associated with midline cerebral anomalies. *SYN:* septooptic dysplasia

Dempsey, Sister Mary Joseph, see under Sister Mary Joseph Dempsey

de Musset, L.C. Alfred, see under Musset

de Mussey, see under Guéneau de Mussey

Denis Browne, see under Browne, Sir Denis John

Denman, Thomas, English obstetrician, 1733-1815.
   Denman spontaneous evolution – a mechanism of spontaneous molding of the fetus and impaction of the shoulder with prolapse of the arm noted in some cases of transverse lie.

Dennie, C.C., U.S. dermatologist, 1883-1971.
   Dennie-Marfan syndrome – juvenile spastic paraplegia and mental retardation due to congenital syphilis.

Denny-Brown, Derek E., New Zealand neurologist in England and U.S., 1901-1981.
   Denny-Brown syndrome – bronchogenic carcinoma.

Denonvilliers, Charles P., French surgeon, 1808-1872.
   Denonvilliers aponeurosis – a fascial layer that extends superiorly from the central tendon of the perineum to the peritoneum between the prostate and rectum. *SYN:* rectovesical septum
   Denonvilliers blepharoplasty
   Denonvilliers fascia
   Denonvilliers ligament – the localized thickening of the superior fascia of the pelvic diaphragm anteriorly that anchors the prostate and neck of the bladder to the pubis on each side. *SYN:* puboprostatic ligament
   Denonvilliers space

NOTES

Denucé, Jean L.P., French surgeon, 1824-1889.
    Denucé ligament – fibers that pass from the distal margin of the radial notch of the ulna to the neck of the radius. *SYN:* quadrate ligament

Denver, city in Colorado.
    Denver classification – a classification of chromosomes first discussed at a meeting in Denver, Colorado.

Denys, Joseph, Belgian bacteriologist, 1857-1932.
    Denys-Leclef phenomenon – enhanced phagocytosis by leukocytes of microorganisms in the presence of immune serum.

de Pezzer, Oscar M.B., French surgeon, 1853-1917.
    de Pezzer catheter – a self-retaining catheter with a bulbous extremity.
    de Pezzer mushroom-tipped catheter
    de Pezzer self-retaining catheter
    Pezzer catheter
    Pezzer drain

de Quervain, Fritz, Swiss surgeon, 1868-1940.
    de Quervain disease – fibrosis of the sheath of a tendon of the thumb. *SYN:* radial styloid tendovaginitis
    de Quervain fracture – fracture of navicular bone with dislocation of lunar bone.
    de Quervain incision
    de Quervain release
    de Quervain tenolysis
    de Quervain tenosynovitis
    de Quervain thyroiditis – thyroiditis with round cell infiltration, destruction of thyroid cells, epithelial giant cell proliferation, and evidence of regeneration. *SYN:* subacute granulomatous thyroiditis
    Quervain abdominal retractor
    Quervain cranial forceps
    Quervain elevator
    Quervain forceps
    Quervain incision
    Quervain release
    Quervain rongeur

Dercum, Francis Xavier, U.S. neurologist, 1856-1931.
    Dercum disease – a condition characterized by a deposit of symmetrical nodular or pendulous masses of fat in various regions of the body, with discomfort or pain. *SYN:* adiposis dolorosa

De Sanctis, Carlo, Italian psychiatrist, *1888.

De Sanctis-Cacchione syndrome – xeroderma pigmentosum with mental deficiency, dwarfism, and gonadal hypoplasia.

Desault, Pierre J., French surgeon, 1744-1795.
Desault bandage – a bandage for fracture of the clavicle.
Desault ligature – a ligature of the femoral artery in the adductor muscle, for treatment of popliteal aneurysm.
Desault sign
Desault wrist bandage
Desault wrist dislocation

Descartes, René, French philosopher, mathematician, physiologist, 1596-1650.
cartesian – relating to Cartesius, latinized form of Descartes.
Descartes law – for two given media, the sine of the angle of incidence bears a constant relation to the sine of the angle of refraction. *SYN:* law of refraction

Descemet, Jean, French physician, 1732-1810.
Descemet membrane – a transparent homogeneous acellular layer between the substantia propria and the endothelial layer of the cornea. *SYN:* posterior limiting layer of cornea

Deschamps, Joseph F., French surgeon, 1740-1824.
Deschamps needle – a needle with a long shaft for passing sutures in the deep tissues.

Desmarres, Louis A., French ophthalmologist, 1810-1882.
Desmarres dacryoliths – *SYN:* Nocardia dacryoliths
Desmarres fixation pick
Desmarres lid elevator
Desmarres marker
Desmarres refractor

Desmons, F., French dermatologist.

Desmons syndrome – autosomal recessive syndrome featuring keratitis, ichthyosis, and deafness. *SYN:* keratitis, ichthyosis, and deafness syndrome (KIDS)

De Souza, A.R.
De Souza syndrome – bullous cutaneous amyloidosis, reported in one family.

D'Éspine, Jean H.A., French physician, 1846-1930.
D'Éspine sign – bronchophony over the spinous processes heard at a lower level than in health, in pulmonary tuberculosis.

Determann, Hermann, German physician, *1865.
Determann syndrome – intermittent muscle myasthenia caused by arteriosclerosis.

De Toni, Giovanni, Italian pediatrician, 1895-1973.
Debré-De Toni-Fanconi syndrome – *SYN:* Fanconi syndrome (2)
De Toni-Fanconi syndrome – the most common of a group of diseases with characteristic renal tubular dysfunction disorders. *SYN:* cystinosis

Deutschländer, Carl E.W., German surgeon, 1872-1942.
Deutschländer disease – tumor of one of the metatarsal bones; a fatigue fracture of one of the metatarsals. *SYN:* march fracture

Deventer, Hendrik van, Dutch obstetrician, 1651-1724.
Deventer pelvis – a pelvis with shortened anteroposterior diameter.

Devic, Eugène, French physician, 1869-1930.
Devic disease – a demyelinating disorder consisting of a transverse myelopathy and optic neuritis. *SYN:* neuromyelitis optica

Devine, Sir Hugh B., Australian surgeon, 1878-1959.
Devine exclusion – exclusion of the lower part of the stomach, followed by gastrojejunostomy, for treatment of duodenal ulcer.

Devonshire, city in England.
Devonshire colic – colic which was first discovered in the city of Devonshire; caused by drinking cider made in lead-lined presses. *SYN:* lead poisoning

De Vries, Andre, Israeli physician.
De Vries syndrome – congenital disorder associated with bleeding tendency and syndactyly.

Dew, Sir Harold Robert, Australian physician, 1891-1962.
Dew sign – an area of resonance which moves caudally when patient is on hands and knees, related to diaphragmatic hydatid abscess.

DeWall, Richard A., U.S. physician.
Lillehei-DeWall oxygenator – see under Lillehei

Dewar, Sir James, English chemist, 1842-1923.
Dewar flask – a glass vessel with two walls, the space between which is evacuated. *SYN:* vacuum flask

de Wecker, Louis H., French physician, 1832-1906.
de Wecker cannula
de Wecker eye implant
de Wecker forceps
de Wecker iridectomy scissors
de Wecker iris scissors
de Wecker iris spatula
de Wecker operation
de Wecker scissors – a small scissors with sharp points for intraocular cutting of the iris and lens capsule.
de Wecker sclerotomy
de Wecker syringe cannula

d'Herelle, Felix H., Canadian physician and bacteriologist, 1873-1949.
d'Herelle phenomenon – *SYN:* Twort-d'Herelle phenomenon
Twort-d'Herelle phenomenon – see under Twort

Diamond, Louis Klein, U.S. physician, 1902-1999
Diamond-Blackfan anemia – autosomal recessive normocytic normochromic anemia. *SYN:* congenital hypoplastic anemia; Diamond-Blackfan syndrome
Diamond-Blackfan syndrome – *SYN:* Diamond-Blackfan anemia
Gardner-Diamond syndrome – see under Gardner, Frank H.
Shwachman-Diamond syndrome – *SYN:* Shwachman syndrome

Diana, Roman goddess of the hunt.
Diana complex – the adoption of masculine traits and behavior by a female.

D

NOTES

Dick, George Frederick, U.S. internist, 1881-1967, and Gladys R.H., U.S. internist, 1881-1963.

  Dick method – *SYN:* Dick test

  Dick test – an intracutaneous test of susceptibility to the erythrogenic toxin of *Streptococcus pyogenes* responsible for the rash and other manifestations of scarlet fever. *SYN:* Dick method

  Dick test toxin – a test for scarlet fever antibodies. *SYN:* streptococcus erythrogenic toxin

Dickens, Frank, English biochemist, *1899.

  Dickens shunt – a secondary pathway for the oxidation of d-glucose (not occurring in skeletal muscle), generating reducing power in the cytoplasm outside the mitochondria and synthesizing pentoses and a few other sugars. *SYN:* pentose phosphate pathway; Warburg-Lipmann-Dickens-Horecker shunt

  Warburg-Lipmann-Dickens-Horecker shunt – *SYN:* Dickens shunt

Dick-Read, Grantley, English physician, 1890-1959.

  Read method – psychoprophylactic method of prepared childbirth.

Dieffenbach, Johann F., German surgeon, 1792-1847.

  Dieffenbach method – plastic surgery for covering a defect by sliding a flap with broad pedicle.

Diego, Venezuelan patient in whom a blood group antigen was originally found.

  Diego antigen – dominant inherited blood group antigen presumably of Mongolian origin.

Dieker, H., U.S. physician.

  Miller-Dieker syndrome – see under Miller, James Q.

Diels, Otto, German chemist and Nobel laureate, 1876-1954.

  Diels hydrocarbon – a phenanthrene derivative obtained by the dehydrogenation of various steroids.

Dieterle, R.R.

  Dieterle stain – a silver impregnation method for staining *Legionella* and other organisms.

Dietl, Józef, Polish physician, 1804-1878.

  Dietl crisis – paroxysmal attacks of lumbar and abdominal pain with nausea and vomiting, resulting from kinking of the ureter in persons with floating kidney. *SYN:* incarceration symptom

Dietlen, Hans, German physician, 1879-1955.

Dietlen syndrome – syndrome characterized by cardiac flutter and tension of the diaphragm on inspiration and associated with cardiac adhesions.

Dieulafoy, Georges, French physician, 1839-1911.
Dieulafoy disease – *SYN:* Dieulafoy erosion
Dieulafoy erosion – acute ulcerative gastroenteritis complicating pneumonia, possibly caused by overproduction of adrenal steroid hormones. *SYN:* Dieulafoy disease
Dieulafoy lesion
Dieulafoy theory – an obsolete theory that appendicitis is always the result of the transformation of the appendicular canal into a closed cavity.
Dieulafoy vascular malformation of the stomach

DiGeorge, Angelo Mario, U.S. pediatrician.
DiGeorge syndrome – a condition arising from developmental failure of the third and fourth pharyngeal pouches, associated with facial deformity, hypoparathyroidism, and deficiency in cellular (T-lymphocyte) immunity. *SYN:* congenital aplasia of thymus; immunodeficiency with hypoparathyroidism; pharyngeal pouch syndrome; third and fourth pharyngeal pouch syndrome

Dighton, C.A.C., English otolaryngologist, *1885.
Dighton syndrome – genetic trait causing abnormal fragility and plasticity of bone and deafness.

Di Guglielmo, Giovanni, Italian hematologist, 1886-1961.
Di Guglielmo disease – (1) variant of acute myeloblastic leukemia. *SYN:* Di Guglielmo syndrome; (2) prolonged bleeding time in spite of permanent increase in platelet count; may occur as a complication of leukemia, polycythemia, or splenomegaly. *SYN:* Mortensen syndrome (obsolete term)
Di Guglielmo syndrome – *SYN:* Di Guglielmo disease (1)

Dillwyn Evans, see under Evans, Dillwyn

NOTES

Di Mauro, Salvatore, U.S. physician.
   Di Mauro disease – disorder related to lipid metabolism in muscle tissue.

Dimmer, Friedrich, Austrian ophthalmologist, 1855-1926.
   Dimmer keratitis – coin-shaped or round, discrete, grayish areas 0.5 to
   1.5 mm in diameter scattered throughout the various layers of the
   cornea. *SYN:* keratitis nummularis

Diogenes, of Sinope, Greek philosopher, 412-323 B.C.
   Diogenes cup – the palm of the hand when contracted and deepened by
   the action of the muscles on either side. *SYN:* poculum diogenis
   Diogenes syndrome – condition of self-neglect generally observed in
   older individuals, associated with deficiencies in nutrition.
   poculum diogenis – *SYN:* Diogenes cup

Dische, Zacharias, Austrian-U.S. biochemist, *1895.
   Dische reaction – the assay of DNA by means of the blue color formed
   with diphenylamine in acid (Dische reagent).
   Dische reagent – acid used in assay of DNA.
   Dische-Schwarz reagent – reagent used in the colorimetric detection of
   RNA.

Dishler, Jon G., U.S. ophthalmologist.
   Dishler Excimer Laser System for LASIK
   Dishler-type LASIK irrigating cannula

Disse, Josef, German anatomist, 1852-1912.
   Disse space – the potential extravascular space between the liver
   sinusoids and liver parenchymal cells. *SYN:* perisinusoidal space

Dittrich, Franz, German pathologist, 1815-1859.
   Dittrich plugs – minute, dirty-grayish, foul-smelling masses of bacteria
   and fatty acid crystals in the sputum in pulmonary gangrene and fetid
   bronchitis. *SYN:* Traube plugs
   Dittrich stenosis – narrowing of the outflow tract of the right ventricle
   below the pulmonic valve. *SYN:* infundibular stenosis

Divry, Paul, Belgian neurologist, *1889.
   Divry-van Bogaert disease – multiple angiomas of skin and cerebral
   meninges with progressive loss of myelin in white matter.

Dixon Mann, see under Mann, John Dixon

Dobrin, Robert S., U.S. physician.
   Dobrin syndrome – acute eosinophilic interstitial nephritis with uveitis,
   renal failure, and granulomas of bone marrow and lymph nodes.

d'Ocagne, Philbert M., French mathematician, 1862-1938.
   d'Ocagne nomogram – an alignment chart.

Dodd, Harold C., English surgeon.
   Cockett and Dodd operation – see under Cockett

Döderlein, Albert S.G., German obstetrician, 1860-1941.
   Döderlein bacillus – a large, gram-positive bacterium occurring in normal vaginal secretions.

Doehle, var. of Döhle

Doerfler, Leo, U.S. audiologist, *1919.
   Doerfler-Stewart test – used in differentiating between functional and organic hearing loss. *SYN:* D-S test

Dogiel, Alexander S., Russian histologist, 1852-1922.
   Dogiel corpuscle – an encapsulated sensory nerve ending.

Dogiel, Jan von, Russian anatomist and physiologist, 1830-1905.
   Dogiel cells – the different cell types in cerebrospinal ganglia.

Doherty, Peter C., joint winner of 1996 Nobel Prize for work related to immunity.

Dohi, Keizo, Japanese dermatologist, 1866-1931.
   Dohi acropigmentation – pigment disorder, likely autosomal dominant, reported mainly from Japan, with mottled pigmentation and hypopigmentation on the hands and feet, beginning in infancy or early childhood.

Döhle, (Doehle), Karl G.P., German histologist and pathologist, 1855-1928.
   Döhle bodies – found in neutrophils of patients with infections, burns, trauma, pregnancy, or cancer. *SYN:* Döhle inclusions; leukocyte inclusions
   Döhle-Heller aortitis – a common manifestation of tertiary syphilis, involving the thoracic aorta, where destruction of elastic tissue in the media results in dilation and aneurysm formation. *SYN:* syphilitic aortitis
   Döhle inclusions – *SYN:* Döhle bodies

D

NOTES

Doisy, Edward A., U.S. biochemist and Nobel laureate, 1893-1986.
  Allen-Doisy test – see under Allen, Edgar
  Allen-Doisy unit – see under Allen, Edgar

Dollinger, Albert, German physician, *1888.
  Bielschowsky-Dollinger syndrome – *SYN:* Dollinger-Bielschowsky
  syndrome
  Dollinger-Bielschowsky syndrome – genetic disorder with onset
  between three and four years of age, resulting in mental deterioration,
  hearing and visual disorders. *SYN:* Bielschowsky-Dollinger syndrome;
  Bielschowsky syndrome

Domagk, Gerhard, winner of 1939 Nobel Prize for work related to prontosil.

D'Ombrain, Ernest Arthur, Irish-born Australian ophthalmologist, 1867-1944.
  D'Ombrain operation

Donaldson, Susanne W., U.S. nurse.
  Donaldson scale – a scale used to score a patient's activities of daily
  living.

Donath, Julius, German physician, 1870-1950.
  Donath-Landsteiner cold autoantibody – an autoantibody of the IgG
  class responsible for paroxysmal cold hemoglobinuria. *SYN:* cold
  hemolysin
  Donath-Landsteiner phenomenon – the hemolysis which results in a
  sample of blood of a subject of paroxysmal hemoglobinuria when the
  sample is cooled to around 5°C and then warmed again.
  Landsteiner-Donath test

Donders, Franz C., Dutch ophthalmologist, 1818-1889.
  Donders glaucoma – obsolete term for open-angle glaucoma.
  Donders law – rotation of the eyeball is determined by the distance of an
  object from the median plane and the line of the horizon.
  Donders pressure – an increase of about 6 mmHg shown by a
  manometer connected with the trachea when the thorax of the corpse is
  opened, caused by the collapse of the lungs when air is admitted to the
  thorax.
  Donders rings – an obsolete term for the iridescent rings or halos
  observed in a cloudy cornea due to acute glaucoma.
  space of Donders – the space between the dorsum of the tongue and the
  hard palate when the mandible is in rest position following the expiratory
  cycle of respiration.

Donnan, Frederick G., English physical chemist, 1870-1956.

Donnan equilibrium – the equilibrium of small ions between a solution with charged macromolecules, and one without. *SYN:* Gibbs-Donnan equilibrium

Gibbs-Donnan equilibrium – *SYN:* Donnan equilibrium

Donné, Alfred, French physician, 1801-1878.

Donné corpuscle – one of numerous bodies present in the colostrum, supposed to be modified leukocytes containing fat droplets. *SYN:* colostrum corpuscle

Donohue, William Leslie, Canadian pathologist, 1906-1985.

Donohue disease – a congenital form of dwarfism. *SYN:* Donohue syndrome; leprechaunism

Donohue syndrome – *SYN:* Donohue disease

Donovan, Charles, English surgeon, 1863-1951.

Donovan bodies – clusters of blue or black staining, bipolar chromatin condensations in large mononuclear cells in granulation tissue infected with *Calymmatobacterium granulomatis*.

Leishman-Donovan body – see under Leishman

Doose, H., 20th century German pediatrician and epileptologist.

Doose syndrome – a rare familial type of primary generalized myoclonic astatic epilepsy.

Doppler, Christian J., Austrian mathematician and physicist in U.S., 1803-1853.

Doppler bidirectional test

Doppler echocardiography – use of Doppler ultrasonography techniques to augment two-dimensional echocardiography by allowing velocities to be registered within the echocardiographic image. *SYN:* duplex echocardiography

Doppler effect – a change in frequency is observed when the sound and observer are in relative motion away from or toward each other. *SYN:* Doppler phenomenon; Doppler principle

NOTES

Doppler flow test

Doppler measurement

Doppler phenomenon – *SYN:* Doppler effect

Doppler principle – *SYN:* Doppler effect

Doppler probe

Doppler pulse evaluation

Doppler scope

Doppler shift – the magnitude of the frequency change in hertz when sound and observer are in relative motion away from or toward each other.

Doppler ultrasonography – application of the Doppler effect in ultrasound to detect movement of scatterers (usually red blood cells) by the analysis of the change in frequency of the returning echoes.

Doppler ultrasound flowmeter

Doppler ultrasound segmental blood pressure testing

Dorello, Primo, Italian anatomist, *1872.

Dorello canal – a bony canal sometimes found at the tip of the temporal bone enclosing the abducens nerve and inferior petrosal sinus.

Dorendorf, Hans, German physician, 1866-1953.

Dorendorf sign – fullness of one supraclavicular groove in an aneurysm of the aortic arch.

Dorfman, Maurice L., 20th century Israeli dermatologist.

Dorfman-Chanarin syndrome – congenital ichthyosis, leukocyte vacuoles, and variable involvement of other organ systems. *SYN:* neutral lipid storage disease

Dorfman, Ronald F.

Rosai-Dorfman syndrome– see under Rosai

Döring, G., German neurologist.

Pette-Döring disease – see under Pette

Dormia, Enrico, Italian professor of urology.

Dormia basket – device used to remove calculi from ureter.

Dormia biliary stone basket

Dormia dislodger

Dormia extracorporeal shockwave lithotripsy system

Dormia gallstone lithotriptor

Dormia lithotriptor

Dormia stone basket

Dormia stone basket catheter

Dormia stone dislodger

Dormia ureteral basket
Dormia ureteral stone dislodger
Dormia waterbath lithotriptor

Dorno, Carl, Swiss climatologist, 1865-1942.
Dorno rays – the biologically active ultraviolet rays.

Dorothy Reed, see under Reed, Dorothy

Dorset, Marion, U.S. bacteriologist, 1872-1935.
Dorset culture egg medium – a medium for cultivating *Mycobacterium tuberculosis.*

Douglas, Beverly, U.S. surgeon, *1891.
Douglas graft – obsolete term for sieve graft.

Douglas, Claude G., English physiologist, 1882-1963.
Douglas bag – a large bag in which expired gas is collected for several minutes to determine oxygen consumption in humans under conditions of actual work.

Douglas, James, Scottish anatomist in London, 1675-1742.
cavum douglasi – *SYN:* Douglas cul-de-sac
Douglas abscess – suppuration in Douglas pouch.
Douglas cul-de-sac – a pocket formed by the deflection of the peritoneum from the rectum to the uterus. *SYN:* cavum douglasi; Douglas pouch; rectouterine pouch
Douglas fold – a fold of peritoneum, containing the rectouterine muscle, forming the lateral boundary of the rectouterine (Douglas) pouch. *SYN:* sacrouterine fold
Douglas line – a crescentic line that marks the lower limit of the posterior layer of the sheath of the rectus abdominis muscle. *SYN:* arcuate line of rectus sheath
Douglas pouch – *SYN:* Douglas cul-de-sac

D

NOTES

Douglas, John C., Irish obstetrician, 1777-1850.
Douglas mechanism – mechanism of spontaneous evolution in transverse lie.
Douglas spontaneous evolution – a mechanism whereby molding of the fetus and impaction of the shoulder and prolapsed arm occurs in transverse lie, allowing vaginal delivery with the lateral aspect of the thorax following the prolapsed shoulder.

Dover, Thomas, English physician, 1660-1742.
Dover powder – a sedative.

Dowling, Geoffrey B., English dermatologist, 1892-1976.
Dowling-Meara syndrome – type of epidermolysis bullosa simplex.

Down, John Langdon H., English physician, 1828-1896.
Down syndrome – a chromosomal dysgenesis syndrome consisting of a variable constellation of abnormalities, caused by triplication or translocation of chromosome 21. *SYN:* Langdon Down syndrome; trisomy 21 syndrome
Langdon Down syndrome – *SYN:* Down syndrome

Downey, H., U.S. hematologist, 1877-1959.
Downey cell – the atypical lymphocyte of infectious mononucleosis.

Downey, June Etta, U.S. psychologist, 1875-1932.
Downey Will-Temperament Tests – use of handwriting tasks to measure differences in temperament and/or personality.

Downs, William B., U.S. orthodontist, 1899-1966.
Downs analysis – a series of cephalometric criteria used as an aid in orthodontic diagnosis.

Dox, Arthur W., U.S. chemist, *1882.
Czapek-Dox medium – *SYN:* Czapek solution agar

Doyère, Louis, French physiologist, 1811-1863.
Doyère eminence – the slightly elevated area of the striated muscle fiber surface that corresponds to the site of the motor endplate.

Doyle, J.B., U.S. gynecologist, *1907.
Doyle operation – paracervical uterine denervation.

Doyne, Robert Walter, English ophthalmologist, 1857-1916.
Doyne choroiditis – genetic trait resulting in retinal degeneration and retinal drusen.
Doyne honeycomb choroidopathy – obsolete term for macular drusen.
Doyne iritis – grey precipitate found on iris.

Dragendorff, Georg J.N., German physician and pharmaceutical chemist, 1836-1898.
    Dragendorff solution
    Dragendorff test – a qualitative test for bile.

Drager, Glenn A., U.S. neurologist, *1917.
    Shy-Drager syndrome – see under Shy

Dräger, Heinrich, German manufacturer of industrial and diving respiratory apparatus, *1898.
    Dräger respirometer – an inferential meter to measure tidal and minute volume.

Dragstedt, L.R., U.S. surgeon, 1893-1975.
    Dragstedt operation – procedure for repair of duodenal ulcer.

Draper, John W., English chemist, 1811-1882.
    Draper law – a chemical change is produced in a photochemical substance only by those light rays that are absorbed by that substance.

Drash, Allan, U.S. physician, *1931.
    Drash syndrome – pseudohermaphroditism.

Dresbach, Melvin, U.S. physician, 1874-1946.
    Dresbach anemia – inherited blood disorder resulting in elliptical red cells.
    Dresbach syndrome

Drescher, Edward, Polish physician.
    Murray-Puretic-Drescher syndrome – see under Murray, John

Dressler, William, U.S. physician, 1890-1969.
    Dressler beat – presence of Dressler beats strongly supporting the diagnosis of ventricular tachycardia by interruption of it.
    Dressler syndrome – *SYN:* pericarditis

D

NOTES

Dreuw, H.

    Dreuw disease – outbreak in children of alopecia of unknown cause, with 1- to 2-cm patches of hair loss, which usually regrow in several weeks without scarring.

Dreyer, Georges, English pathologist, 1873-1934.

    Dreyer formula – an obsolete formula indicating relationship between vital capacity and body surface area.

Driesch, H.A.E., German biologist, 1867-1941.

    Driesch law of constant volume – number of cells determines total mass of an organ.

Drigalski, Wilhelm von, German bacteriologist, 1871-1950.

    Conradi-Drigalski agar – see under Conradi, Heinrich

    Drigalski-Conradi agar – *SYN:* Conradi-Drigalski agar

Drinker, Philip, U.S. industrial hygienist, 1894-1972.

    Drinker respirator – a mechanical respirator in which the body below the head is encased within a metal tank, which is sealed at the neck with an airtight gasket. *SYN:* iron lung; tank respirator

Drummond, Sir David, English physician, 1852-1932.

    artery of Drummond – artery formed by anastomoses between the right and left colic arteries. *SYN:* marginal artery of colon

    Drummond sign – in certain cases of aortic aneurysm, a puffing sound synchronous with cardiac systole, heard from the nostrils when the mouth is closed.

Duane, Alexander, U.S. ophthalmologist, 1858-1926.

    Duane syndrome – a retraction of the globe and pseudoptosis on attempted adduction. *SYN:* retraction syndrome

Dubin, I. Nathan, U.S. pathologist, 1913-1980.

    Dubin-Johnson syndrome – chronic idiopathic jaundice. *SYN:* Sprinz-Dubin syndrome; Sprinz-Nelson syndrome

    Sprinz-Dubin syndrome – *SYN:* Dubin-Johnson syndrome

Dubini, Angelo, Italian physician, 1813-1902.

    Dubini disease – infection of the central nervous system resulting in usually fatal form of chorea. *SYN:* electrolepsy

DuBois, Eugene F., U.S. physiologist, 1882-1959.

    Aub-DuBois table – see under Aub

    DuBois formula – a formula for predicting a person's surface area from weight and height.

    Meeh-DuBois formula – see under Meeh

Dubois, Paul, French obstetrician, 1795-1871.
Dubois abscess – small cyst of the thymus reported in congenital syphilis but also found in the absence of syphilis. *SYN:* Dubois disease; thymic abscess
Dubois disease – *SYN:* Dubois abscess

Du Bois-Reymond, Emil H., German physiologist, 1818-1896.
Du Bois-Reymond law – a motor nerve responds, not to the absolute value, but to the alteration of value from moment to moment, of the electric current. *SYN:* law of excitation

Duboscq, Jules, French optician, 1817-1886.
Duboscq colorimeter – an apparatus for measuring the depth of tint in a fluid.

Dubowitz, Victor, South African-English pediatrician, *1931.
Dubowitz score – a method of clinical assessment of gestational age in the newborn.
Dubowitz syndrome – congenital dwarfism.

Dubreuil-Chambardel, Louis, French dentist, 1879-1927.
Dubreuil-Chambardel syndrome – simultaneous caries of the upper incisor teeth occurring in either sex between the ages of 14 and 17.

Dubreuilh, M. William, French dermatologist, 1857-1935.
precancerous melanosis of Dubreuilh – obsolete term for lentigo maligna.

Duchenne, Guillaume B.A., French neurologist, 1806-1875.
Aran-Duchenne disease – *SYN:* Lou Gehrig disease
Aran-Duchenne dystrophy – *SYN:* Lou Gehrig disease
Duchenne-Aran disease – *SYN:* Lou Gehrig disease
Duchenne attitude – paralysis of trapezius resulting in shoulder lowering on external rotation.
Duchenne disease – (1) *SYN:* Duchenne dystrophy; (2) progressive bulbar paralysis.

NOTES

Duchenne dystrophy – the most common childhood muscular dystrophy, with onset usually before age 6. *SYN:* childhood muscular dystrophy; Duchenne disease (1); Duchenne-Griesinger disease; pseudohypertrophic muscular dystrophy

Duchenne-Erb paralysis – *SYN:* Erb palsy

Duchenne-Erb syndrome – *SYN:* Erb palsy

Duchenne-Griesinger disease – *SYN:* Duchenne dystrophy

Duchenne paralysis – brachial birth palsy in which there is paralysis of upper arm and shoulder girdle muscles due to lesion of upper trunk of brachial plexus or roots of fifth and sixth cervical roots.

Duchenne sign – falling in of the epigastrium during inspiration in paralysis of the diaphragm.

Duchenne syndrome – subacute or chronic anterior spinal paralysis combined with multiple neuritis.

Erb-Duchenne paralysis – *SYN:* Erb palsy

Duckworth, Sir Dyce, English physician, 1840-1928.

Duckworth phenomenon – respiratory arrest before cardiac arrest as a result of intracranial disease.

Ducrey, Augusto, Italian dermatologist, 1860-1940.

Ducrey bacillus – a species which causes soft chancre (chancroid). *SYN: Haemophilus ducreyi*

Ducrey test – an intradermal test, using inactivated *Haemophilus ducreyi*, for diagnosis of chancroid. *SYN:* Ito-Reenstierna test

Duddell, Benedict, 18th century English oculist.

Duddell membrane – considered to be a highly developed basement membrane. *SYN:* posterior limiting layer of cornea

Duffy, surname of the patient in whom this antigen was first found in 1950.

Duffy antigen – may be related to resistance to malarial infection.

Duffy blood group

Dugas, Louis A., U.S. physician, 1806-1884.

Dugas test – in the case of an injured shoulder, if the elbow cannot be made to touch the chest while the hand rests on the opposite shoulder, the injury is a dislocation and not a fracture of the humerus.

Duhot, Robert, 19th century Belgian urologist and dermatologist.

Duhot line – line from the superior iliac spine to the sacral apex.

Duhring, Louis Adolphus, U.S. dermatologist, 1845-1913.
  Duhring disease – a chronic skin disease marked by a symmetric itching eruption of vesicles and papules that occur in groups. *SYN:* dermatitis herpetiformis

Dührssen, Alfred, German obstetrician-gynecologist, 1862-1933.
  Dührssen incisions – three surgical incisions of an incompletely dilated cervix used as a means of effecting immediate delivery of the fetus.
  Dührssen operation
  Dührssen tampon
  Dührssen vaginal fixation

Duke, William Waddell Duke, U.S. pathologist, 1883-1945.
  Duke bleeding time test – a bleeding time test in which an incision is made in the earlobe and the time until bleeding stops is measured.

Dukes, Clement, English physician, 1845-1925.
  Dukes disease – *SYN:* Filatov-Dukes disease
  Filatov-Dukes disease – see under Filatov, Nil

Dukes, Cuthbert E., English pathologist, 1890-1977.
  Dukes classification – a classification of the extent of operable adenocarcinoma of the colon or rectum: Dukes A, Dukes B, Dukes B_2, Dukes C_1, Dukes C_2.

Dulbecco, Renato, joint winner of 1975 Nobel Prize for work related to tumor viruses and cell material.

Dulong, Pierre L., French chemist, 1785-1838.
  Dulong-Petit law – the specific heats of many solid elements are inversely proportional to their atomic weights.

Dumontpallier, Alphonse, French physician, 1827-1899.
  Dumontpallier pessary – *SYN:* Mayer pessary

Duncan, surname of one of the first individuals to carry a recessive trait that causes propensity to B-cell malignant lymphoproliferative disease.

NOTES

Duncan disease – immunodeficiency disease with propensity to B-cell malignant lymphoproliferative disease in the presence of Epstein-Barr virus, leading to death. *SYN:* Duncan syndrome
Duncan syndrome – *SYN:* Duncan disease

Duncan, David Beattie, Australian-U.S. statistician, *1916.
Duncan multiple-range test – a test designed to compare various means.

Duncan, James M., Scottish gynecologist, 1826-1890.
Duncan curette
Duncan endometrial biopsy curette
Duncan endometrial curette
Duncan fold – the folds on the peritoneal surface of the uterus immediately after delivery.
Duncan mechanism – passage of the placenta from the uterus with the rough side foremost.
Duncan position
Duncan ventricle – a slitlike, fluid-filled space of variable width between the left and right transparent septum, which may communicate with the third ventricle. *SYN:* cavity of septum pellucidum

Dungy, Claiborne I., U.S. pediatrician.
McKusick-Dungy-Kaufman syndrome – *SYN:* McKusick-Kaufman syndrome

Dunlop, John, U.S. orthopedic surgeon, *1876.
Dunlop elbow traction
Dunlop sleeve
Dunlop stripper
Dunlop thrombus stripper
Dunlop traction

Dunn, R.L.
Lison-Dunn stain – see under Lison, Lucien

Du Pan, C. Martin, Swiss orthopedic surgeon.
Du Pan syndrome – fibular hypoplasia and complex brachydactyly, thought to be an inherited autosomal recessive trait.

Duplay, Emanuel Simon, French surgeon, 1836-1924.
Duplay disease – *SYN:* subacromial bursitis
Duplay syndrome

Dupré, 17th century Paris surgeon and anatomist.
Dupré muscle – *SYN:* articularis genu muscle

Dupuy-Dutemps, Louis, French ophthalmologist, 1871-1946.
  Dupuy-Dutemps operation – a modified dacryocystorhinostomy for stenosis of the lacrimal duct.

Dupuytren, Baron Guillaume, French surgeon and surgical pathologist, 1777-1835.
  Dupuytren amputation – amputation of the arm at the shoulder joint.
  Dupuytren canal – one of the veins in the diploë of the cranial bones. *SYN:* diploic vein
  Dupuytren contracture – a disease of the palmar fascia resulting in thickening and shortening of fibrous bands on the palmar surface of the hand and fingers.
  Dupuytren diathesis
  Dupuytren disease of the foot – nodular fibroblastic proliferation in plantar fascia of one or both feet. *SYN:* plantar fibromatosis
  Dupuytren enterotome
  Dupuytren exostosis
  Dupuytren fascia – the thickened, central portion of the fascia ensheathing the hand. *SYN:* palmar aponeurosis
  Dupuytren fracture – fracture of lower part of fibula, with dislocation of ankle. *SYN:* Pott I syndrome
  Dupuytren hydrocele – bilocular hydrocele in which the sac fills the scrotum and also extends into the abdominal cavity beneath the peritoneum.
  Dupuytren knife
  Dupuytren operation
  Dupuytren sign – (1) in congenital dislocation, free up-and-down movement of the head of the femur occurring upon intermittent traction; (2) a crackling sensation on pressure over the bone in certain cases of sarcoma.
  Dupuytren splint
  Dupuytren suture – a continuous Lembert suture.

NOTES

Dupuytren tourniquet – an instrument for compression of the abdominal aorta.

Durand, Paul, Italian physician.
Durand disease – *Chlamydia trachomatis* infection which may present as venereal disease or in nonvenereal form. *SYN:* Favre-Durand-Nicolas disease; venereal lymphogranuloma
Favre-Durand-Nicolas disease – *SYN:* Durand disease

Duran-Reynals, Francisco, U.S. bacteriologist, 1899-1958.
Duran-Reynals permeability factor – a soluble enzyme product prepared from mammalian testes. *SYN:* hyaluronidase

Durante, Gustave, French physician, 1865-1934.
Durante disease – abnormal fragility and plasticity of bone. *SYN:* osteogenesis imperfecta

Dürck, Hermann, German pathologist, 1869-1941.
Dürck nodes – perivascular chronic inflammatory infiltrates in the brain, occurring in human trypanosomiasis.

Duret, Henri, French neurosurgeon, 1849-1921.
Duret hemorrhage – small brainstem hemorrhage resulting from brainstem distortion secondary to transtentorial herniation.
Duret lesion – small hemorrhage(s) in the floor of the fourth ventricle or beneath the aqueduct of Sylvius.

Durham, Arthur E., English surgeon, 1834-1895.
Durham needle
Durham operation
Durham tracheostomy tube
Durham tracheotomy trocar
Durham trocar
Durham tube – a jointed tracheotomy tube.

Durkheim, Emile, French sociologist, 1858-1917.
Durkheim theory of suicide – societal factors influence individual risk for suicide, and there are three categories of suicide.

Duroziez, Paul L., French physician, 1826-1897.
Duroziez disease – congenital stenosis of the mitral valve.
Duroziez murmur – a two-phase murmur over peripheral arteries, especially the femoral artery, due to rapid ebb and flow of blood during aortic insufficiency. *SYN:* Duroziez sign
Duroziez sign – *SYN:* Duroziez murmur

Dusart, surname of individuals in which syndrome was discovered.
    Dusart syndrome – autosomal dominant disorder of qualitatively abnormal fibrinogens; causes inadequate lysis of fibrin with probable thrombotic tendency.

Dutcher, Thomas F., U.S. pathologist, *1923.
    Dutcher body – a type of cytoplasm found in benign and malignant conditions.

Dutton, Joseph Everett, English physician, 1877-1905.
    Dutton disease – African tick-borne relapsing fever caused by *Borrelia duttonii* and spread by the soft tick, *Ornithodoros moubata*. *SYN:* Dutton relapsing fever
    Dutton relapsing fever – *SYN:* Dutton disease

Duverney, Joseph G., French anatomist, 1648-1730.
    Duverney fissures – (usually) two vertical fissures in the anterior portion of the cartilage of the external auditory meatus, filled by fibrous tissue. *SYN:* notches in cartilage of external acoustic meatus
    Duverney foramen – the passage, below and behind the portal hepatis, connecting the two sacs of the peritoneum. *SYN:* epiploic foramen
    Duverney gland – one of two mucoid-secreting tubuloalveolar glands on either side of the lower part of the vagina, the equivalent of the bulbourethral glands in the male. *SYN:* greater vestibular gland
    Duverney muscle – *SYN:* lacrimal part of orbicularis oculi muscle

Dwyer, Allan Frederick, Australian orthopedic surgeon, 1920-1975.
    Dwyer fusion – method of spinal fusion.
    Dwyer instrumentation

Dwyer, Frederick Charles, English orthopedic surgeon.
    Dwyer osteotomy – a procedure for clubfoot.

Dyggve, H.V., Danish physician.
    Dyggve-Melchoir-Claussen syndrome – a type of dwarfism and mental retardation including multiple anomolies.

D

NOTES

Eagle, Harry, U.S. physician and cell biologist, 1905-1992.
Eagle basal medium – a solution of various salts used as a tissue culture medium.
Eagle minimum essential medium – a tissue culture medium similar to Eagle basal medium but with different amounts and a few exclusions (e.g., antibiotics and phenol red).

Eagle, J.F., Jr., 20th century U.S. physician.
Eagle-Barrett syndrome – *SYN:* prune belly syndrome

Eagle, W., 20th century U.S. otolaryngologist.
Eagle syndrome – facial pain due to an elongated styloid process.

Eales, Henry, English ophthalmologist, 1852-1913.
Eales disease – peripheral retinal periphlebitis causing recurrent retinal or intravitreous hemorrhages in young adults.

Earle, Wilton R., U.S. pathologist, 1902-1962.
Earle L fibrosarcoma – a transplantable fibrosarcoma derived from subcutaneous tissue of a mouse of C3H strain, grown in tissue culture to which 20-methylcholanthrene had been added.
Earle medium
Earle solution

Eaton, Lee M., U.S. neurologist, 1905-1958.
Eaton-Lambert syndrome – *SYN:* Lambert-Eaton syndrome
Lambert-Eaton syndrome – see under Lambert, Edward H.

Eaton, Monroe D., U.S. microbiologist, 1904-1958.
Eaton agent – a species causing primary atypical pneumonia. *SYN:* Eaton virus; *Mycoplasma pneumoniae*

Eaton agent pneumonia – an acute systemic disease with involvement of the lungs, caused by *Mycoplasma pneumoniae*. *SYN:* primary atypical pneumonia

Eaton virus – *SYN:* Eaton agent

Ebbinghaus, Hermann, German psychologist, 1850-1909.
   Ebbinghaus test – a psychological test in which the patient is asked to complete certain sentences from which several words have been left out.

Ebers, Georg M., German Egyptologist, 1837-1898.
   Ebers papyrus – Egyptian papyrus from the 16th century B.C., which covered many aspects of medicine, including diabetes mellitus, trachoma, different forms of arthritis; many remedies were discussed as well.

Eberth, Karl J., German physician, 1835-1926.
   Eberth bacillus – a species that causes typhoid fever and is transmitted in contaminated water and food. *SYN: Salmonella typhi*; typhoid bacillus
   Eberth lines – lines appearing between the cells of the myocardium when stained with silver nitrate.
   Eberth perithelium – an incomplete layer of connective tissue cells encasing the blood capillaries.

Ebner, Victor von, see under von Ebner

Ebola, river in Zaire, Africa.
   Ebola hemorrhagic fever– *SYN:* Ebola virus
   Ebola virus – filovirus discovered in 1976, level 4 pathogen; severity of illness can run from mild to fatal in host. *SYN:* Ebola hemorrhagic fever

Ebstein, Wilhelm, German physician, 1836-1912.
   Armanni-Ebstein change – see under Armanni
   Armanni-Ebstein kidney – *SYN:* Armanni-Ebstein change
   Armanni-Ebstein nephropathy – see under Armanni
   Ebstein anomaly – congenital downward displacement of the tricuspid valve into the right ventricle. *SYN:* Ebstein disease; Ebstein malformation
   Ebstein disease – *SYN:* Ebstein anomaly
   Ebstein malformation – *SYN:* Ebstein anomaly
   Ebstein sign – in pericardial effusion, obtuseness of the cardiohepatic angle on percussion.
   Murchison-Pel-Ebstein syndrome – see under Murchison
   Pel-Ebstein disease – *SYN:* Pel-Ebstein fever
   Pel-Ebstein fever – see under Pel

Eccles, Sir John Carew, joint winner of 1963 Nobel Prize for work related to nerve cell membrane.

Eck, Nikolai V., Russian physiologist, 1849-1917.
> **Eck fistula** – transposition of the portal circulation to the systemic by making an anastomosis between the vena cava and portal vein.
> **reverse Eck fistula** – side-to-side anastomosis of the portal vein with the inferior vena cava and ligation of the latter above the anastomosis but below the hepatic veins.

Ecker, Alexander, German anatomist, 1816-1887.
> **Ecker fissure** – a fissure between the petrous part of the temporal bone and the basilar part of the occipital bone that extends anteromedially from the jugular foramen. *SYN:* petrooccipital fissure

Ecker, Enrique E., U.S. bacteriologist, 1887-1966.
> **Ecker fluid** – dilating fluid.
> **Rees-Ecker fluid** – see under Rees, H. Maynard

Ecklin, Theophil, Swiss physician.
> **Ecklin anemia** – a generally fatal form of anemia of the newborn.

Economo, Constantin von, see under von Economo

Eddowes, A., English dermatologist, 1850-1946.
> **Eddowes disease** – osteogenesis imperfecta. *SYN:* Eddowes syndrome
> **Eddowes syndrome** – *SYN:* Eddowes disease

Edelman, Gerald M., U.S. biochemist, *1929, co-winner of the 1972 Nobel Prize for his work in identifying and separating heavy and light chains in antibody molecules.

Edelmann, Adolf, Polish physician, 1885-1939.
> **Edelmann syndrome** – (1) chronic infectious anemia; (2) chronic pancreatitis.

E

NOTES

Edinburgh University, institution of higher learning in Edinburgh, Scotland.
 Edinburgh University solution – antiseptic wound irrigation solution.
  SYN: Eusol
 Eusol – *SYN:* Edinburgh University solution

Edinger, Ludwig, German anatomist, 1855-1918.
 Edinger-Westphal nucleus – a small group of preganglionic parasympathetic motor neurons in the midline near the rostral pole of the oculomotor nucleus of the midbrain.

Edlefsen, Gustav J.F., German physician, 1842-1910.
 Edlefsen reagent – an alkaline permanganate solution used in the determination of sugar in the urine.

Edman, Pehr, Australian scientist, 1916-1977.
 Edman method – a method of identifying N-terminal amino acids.
 Edman reagent – used in the Edman method of identifying N-terminal amino acids. *SYN:* phenylisothiocyanate

Edridge-Green, Frederick W., English ophthalmologist, 1863-1953.
 Edridge-Green lamp – a test for color blindness, now seldom used.

Edsall, David L., U.S. physician, 1869-1945.
 Edsall disease – heat cramp. *SYN:* myalgia thermica

Edwards, James Hilton, English physician and medical geneticist, *1928.
 Edwards Personal Preferences Schedule – personality inventory test.
 Edwards syndrome – characterized by mental retardation, abnormal skull shape, low-set and malformed ears, small mandible, cardiac defects, short sternum, diaphragmatic or inguinal hernia, Meckel diverticulum, abnormal flexion of fingers, and dermatoglyphic anomalies. *SYN:* trisomy 18 syndrome

Edwards, Miles Lowell, U.S. physician, *1906.
 Carpentier-Edwards aortic valve prosthesis
 Carpentier-Edwards bioprosthesis
 Carpentier-Edwards bioprosthetic valve
 Carpentier-Edwards mitral annuloplasty valve
 Carpentier-Edwards pericardial valve
 Carpentier-Edwards porcine prosthetic valve
 Carpentier-Edwards valve
 Starr-Edwards aortic valve prosthesis
 Starr-Edwards ball-cage valve
 Starr-Edwards ball valve prosthesis
 Starr-Edwards disk valve prosthesis

Starr-Edwards heart valve
Starr-Edwards mitral prosthesis
Starr-Edwards pacemaker
Starr-Edwards prosthesis
Starr-Edwards prosthetic aortic valve
Starr-Edwards prosthetic mitral valve
Starr-Edwards Silastic valve
Starr-Edwards silicone rubber ball valve
Starr-Edwards valve – see under Starr

Efron, M.L.
Paine-Efron syndrome – see under Paine

Egger, Fritz, Swiss internist, 1863-1938.
Egger line – seldom-used term for the circular line of adhesion between the vitreous and posterior lens.

Eggers, George William Nordholtz, U.S. orthopedic surgeon, 1896-1963.
Eggers bone plate
Eggers contact splint
Eggers neurectomy
Eggers plate – orthopedic fixation plate.
Eggers screw
Eggers tendon transfer
Eggers tenodesis

Eggleston, Cary, U.S. physician, 1884-1966.
Bradbury-Eggleston syndrome – see under Bradbury
Eggleston-Bradbury syndrome – *SYN:* Bradbury-Eggleston syndrome
Eggleston method – obsolete term for rapid digitalization by means of large doses of digitalis leaf or tincture frequently repeated.

Egypt, Middle-Eastern country that is home to 66.5 million people.
Egyptian splenomegaly – massive enlargement of the spleen caused by *Schistosoma mansoni*; often found in rural areas of Egypt.

E

Ehlers, Edvard L., Danish dermatologist, 1863-1937.

Ehlers-Danlos syndrome – a group of inherited generalized connective tissue diseases. *SYN:* Meekeren-Ehlers-Danlos syndrome

Ehrenfried, Albert, U.S. physician, 1880-1951.

Ehrenfried disease – autosomal dominant trait characterized by bone dysplasia. *SYN:* multiple cartilaginous exostoses syndrome

Ehrenritter, Johann, Austrian anatomist, d. 1790.

Ehrenritter ganglion – the upper and smaller of two ganglia on the glossopharyngeal nerve as it traverses the jugular foramen. *SYN:* superior ganglion of glossopharyngeal nerve

Ehret, Heinrich, German physician, *1870.

Ehret phenomenon – a sudden throb felt by the finger on the brachial artery, said to indicate fairly accurately the diastolic pressure.

Ehret syndrome – efforts to compensate for pain by assuming the least painful posture resulting in contractures and muscle atrophy.

Ehrlich, Paul, German bacteriologist, immunologist, and Nobel laureate, 1854-1915.

Ehrlich anemia – anemia resulting from hypoplastic or aplastic bone marrow. *SYN:* aplastic anemia

Ehrlich diazo reagent – two solutions, one of sodium nitrite, the other of acidified sulfanilic acid, used in bringing about diazotization. *SYN:* diazo reagent

Ehrlichia – a genus of small, often pleomorphic, coccoid to ellipsoidal, nonmotile, gram-negative bacteria (order Rickettsiales) that are the etiologic agents of ehrlichiosis and are transmitted by ticks.

Ehrlich inner body – a round oxyphil body found in the red blood cell in case of hemocytolysis due to a specific blood poison. *SYN:* Heinz-Ehrlich body

Ehrlich phenomenon – the difference between the amount of diphtheria toxin that will exactly neutralize one unit of antitoxin.

Ehrlich postulate – that cells contain surface extensions or side chains (haptophores) that bind to the antigenic determinants of a toxin (toxophores). *SYN:* Ehrlich theory; side-chain theory

Ehrlich test – urobilinogen test using Ehrlich reagent.

Ehrlich theory – *SYN:* Ehrlich postulate

Ehrlich tumor – solid or ascitic transplantable tumor derived from breast carcinoma in mice.

Ehrlich-Türk line – seldom-used term for the thin vertical deposition of material on the posterior surface of the cornea seen in uveitis.

Ehrlich unit

Heinz-Ehrlich body – *SYN:* Ehrlich inner body

Eichhorst, Hermann L., Swiss physician, 1849-1921.

Eichhorst corpuscles – the globular forms sometimes occurring in the poikilocytosis of pernicious anemia.

Eichhorst neuritis – inflammation of the connective tissue framework of a nerve. *SYN:* interstitial neuritis

Eicken, Karl von, German laryngologist, 1873-1960.

Eicken method – facilitation of hypopharyngoscopy by means of forward traction on the cricoid cartilage by a laryngeal probe.

Eijkman, Christiaan, Dutch physiologist, 1858-1930, co-winner of the 1929 Nobel Prize for the discovery of thiamine, an antineuritic vitamin.

Eimer, Gustav Heinrich Theodor, German zoologist, 1843-1898.

Eimeria – the largest, most economically important, and most widespread genus of the coccidial protozoa (family Eimeriidae, class Sporozoea).

Einthoven, Willem, Dutch physiologist and Nobel laureate, 1860-1927.

Einthoven equation – *SYN:* Einthoven law

Einthoven law – in the electrocardiogram the potential of any wave or complex in lead II is equal to the sum of its potentials of leads I and III. *SYN:* Einthoven equation

Einthoven string galvanometer – the original instrument on which Einthoven developed the first electrocardiogram.

Einthoven triangle – an imaginary equilateral triangle with the heart at its center, its equal sides representing the three standard limb leads of the electrocardiogram.

Eisenlohr, Carl, German physician, 1847-1896.

Eisenlohr syndrome – numbness and weakness in the extremities; paralysis of the lips, tongue, and palate; and dysarthria.

E

NOTES

Eisenmenger, Victor, German physician, 1864-1932.
  Eisenmenger complex – the combination of ventricular septal defect with pulmonary hypertension and consequent right-to-left shunt through the defect, with or without an associated overriding aorta. *SYN:* Eisenmenger defect; Eisenmenger disease; Eisenmenger tetralogy
  Eisenmenger defect – *SYN:* Eisenmenger complex
  Eisenmenger disease – *SYN:* Eisenmenger complex
  Eisenmenger syndrome – cardiac failure usually due to the Eisenmenger complex, a ventricular septal defect.
  Eisenmenger tetralogy – *SYN:* Eisenmenger complex

Eisenmenger, William J., U.S. physician.
  Bongiovanni-Eisenmenger syndrome – see under Bongiovanni

Eisenson, Jon, U.S. speech pathologist.
  Eisenson test – a test for aphasia.

Ejrup, Erick, 20th century Swedish internist.
  Ejrup maneuver – demonstration of collateral circulation by reduction in the prominence of activity of the greater arteries and reduced pulse volume following muscular activity.

Ekbom, Karl-Axel, Swedish neurologist, *1907.
  Ekbom syndrome – *SYN:* restless legs syndrome

Ekman, Olof J., Swedish physician, 1764-1839.
  Ekman syndrome – abnormal fragility and plasticity of bone. *SYN:* osteogenesis imperfecta

Elaut, Leon J.S., 20th century Belgian pathologist.
  Elaut triangle – triangle formed by the iliac arteries and the promontory of the sacrum.

Elejalde, Rafael, U.S. geneticist.
  Elejalde syndrome – a rare autosomal recessive disease characterized by silvery hair, severe central nervous system dysfunction, bronze skin observed after sun exposure, ophthalmologic abnormalities, and neurologic involvement, including seizures and mental retardation.

Elion, Gertrude B., joint winner of 1988 Nobel Prize for work related to drug treatment.

Ellenberg, Max, U.S. physician.
  Ellenberg syndrome – peripheral neuropathy associated with diabetes mellitus; spontaneous recovery has been noted.

Ellik, Milo, U.S. urologist, *1905.
   Ellik bladder evacuator
   Ellik evacuator – an instrument used to evacuate tissue fragments, blood
      clots, or calculi from the urinary bladder.
   Ellik kidney stone basket
   Ellik loop stone dislodger
   Ellik meatotome
   Ellik sound

Elliot, John W., U.S. surgeon, 1852-1925.
   Elliot position – a supine position used to facilitate abdominal section.

Elliot, Robert H., English ophthalmologist, 1864-1936.
   Elliot corneal trephination
   Elliot operation – trephining of the eyeball at the corneoscleral margin to
      relieve tension caused by glaucoma.

Elliott, Thomas R., English physician, 1877-1961.
   Elliot law – adrenaline acts on those structures innervated by sympathetic
      nerve fibers.
   Elliott treatment regulator – a regulator used to control heat, circulation,
      and pressure of water through Elliott applicators.

Ellis, Calvin, U.S. physician, 1826-1883.
   Ellis sign – line of dullness related to pleuritic exudate resorption.

Ellis, Richard White Bernhard, English physician, 1902-1966.
   Ellis-van Creveld syndrome – triad of chondrodysplasia, ectodermal
      dysplasia, and polydactyly, with congenital heart defects in over half of
      patients. *SYN:* chondroectodermal dysplasia

Ellison, Edwin Homer, U.S. physician, 1918-1970.
   Zollinger-Ellison syndrome – see under Zollinger
   Zollinger-Ellison tumor – see under Zollinger

NOTES

Ellsworth, Read McLane, U.S. physician, 1899-1970.
   Ellsworth-Howard test – used in the diagnosis of
      pseudohypoparathyroidism.

Eloesser, Leo, U.S. thoracic surgeon, 1881-1976.
   Eloesser flap
   Eloesser procedure – transposition of a tonguelike skin flap pedicle from
      the chest wall into the depths of an incision that communicates with an
      empyema or peripheral lung abscess.

Elsberg, C.A., U.S. physician.
   Elsberg syndrome – acute urinary retention in women, often associated
      with genital herpes.

Elschnig, Anton, German ophthalmologist, 1863-1939.
   Elschnig blepharorrhaphy
   Elschnig bodies
   Elschnig canthorrhaphy
   Elschnig capsular forceps
   Elschnig cataract knife
   Elschnig corneal knife
   Elschnig cyclodialysis spatula
   Elschnig extrusion needle
   Elschnig eye spoon
   Elschnig iridectomy
   Elschnig lens scoop
   Elschnig lid retractor
   Elschnig pearls – the proliferated anterior capsule of the lens of the eye
      after surgical capsulotomy or injury.
   Elschnig pterygium knife
   Elschnig refractor
   Elschnig spots – isolated choroidal bright yellow or red spots with black
      pigment flecks at their borders, seen by ophthalmoscope in advanced
      hypertensive retinopathy.
   Elschnig syndrome – ocular deformities often associated with cleft palate.
   Elschnig trephine
   Koerber-Salus-Elschnig syndrome – *SYN:* Parinaud I syndrome

Elsner, Christoph F., German physician, 1749-1820.
   Elsner asthma – chest pain caused by oxygen deficiency in the heart
      muscle, often precipitated by stress, associated with pathological heart
      conditions.

Ely, L.W., U.S. orthopedic surgeon, 1868-1944.

Ely sign – discomfort indicative of his lesion or psoas muscle irritation on testing.

Ely test – a test for hip extension.

Embden, Gustav G., German biochemist, 1874-1933.

Embden ester – significant in the understanding of sugar metabolism. *SYN:* Robison-Embden ester; Robison ester

Embden-Meyerhof-Parnas pathway – *SYN:* Embden-Meyerhof pathway

Embden-Meyerhof pathway – the anaerobic glycolytic pathway by which D-glucose is converted to lactic acid. *SYN:* Embden-Meyerhof-Parnas pathway

Robison-Embden ester – *SYN:* Embden ester

Emmet, Thomas A., U.S. gynecologist, 1828-1919.

Emmet forceps

Emmet hemostatic bag

Emmet needle – a needle that is used to pass a ligature around an undissected structure.

Emmet operation – suture repair of a cervix uteri laceration. *SYN:* trachelorrhaphy

Emmet ovarian trocar

Emmet probe

Emmet tenaculum

Emmet uterine probe

Emmet uterine scissors

Enders, John F., U.S. microbiologist, 1897-1985, co-winner of the 1954 Nobel Prize for the discovery that some viruses can be grown, studied, and isolated, making vaccine production possible.

Endo, Shigeru, Japanese bacteriologist, 1869-1937.

Endo agar – a medium useful in the bacteriological examination of water. *SYN:* Endo medium

E

NOTES

Endo fuchsin agar – nutrient agar used as a culture medium to differentiate *Salmonella typhi* from coliform bacteria. *SYN:* fuchsin agar
Endo medium – *SYN:* Endo agar

Engelmann, Guido, German surgeon, *1876.
Camurati-Engelmann syndrome – *SYN:* Engelmann disease
Engelmann disease – progressive, symmetrical fusiform enlargement of the shafts of long bones. *SYN:* Camurati-Engelmann syndrome; diaphysial dysplasia

Engelmann, Theodor W., German physiologist, 1843-1909.
Engelmann basal knobs – obsolete term for blepharoplast.

Englisch, Josef, Austrian physician, 1835-1915.
Englisch sinus – a paired dural venous sinus running in the groove on the petrooccipital fissure connecting the cavernous sinus with the superior bulb of the internal jugular vein. *SYN:* inferior petrosal sinus

Engman, Martin Feeney, U.S. dermatologist, 1869-1953.
Engman disease – a pattern of dermatitis with features of eczema and impetigo.
Engman syndrome – *SYN:* Zinsser-Engman-Cole syndrome
Zinsser-Engman-Cole syndrome – see under Zinsser

Enroth, Emil, Finnish ophthalmologist, 1879-1953.
Enroth sign – in Graves disease, edema of the eyelids, especially of the upper eyelid near the supraorbital margin.

Entebbe, city in Uganda, Africa.
Entebbe bat virus – a group B arbovirus.

Epple, associate of Leonard S. Fosdick.
Fosdick-Hansen-Epple test – see under Fosdick

Epstein, A.A., U.S. physician, 1880-1965.
Epstein syndrome – symptoms include edema, protein concentration in urine, low concentration of albumin in the blood, and hyperlipidemia. *SYN:* nephrotic syndrome

Epstein, Alois, Czech pediatrician working in Austria, 1849-1918.
Epstein disease – one of a group of local infections suggesting diphtheria, but caused by microorganisms other than *Corynebacterium diphtheriae*. *SYN:* diphtheroid
Epstein pearls – multiple small white epithelial inclusion cysts found in the midline of the palate in newborn infants.

Epstein sign – lid retraction in an infant, giving it a frightened expression and a wild glance.
Epstein symptom

Epstein, E., German physician.
Epstein-Goedel syndrome – hematological disorder resulting in prolonged bleeding time despite increased platelets; accompanied by splenomegaly, hematemesis, and thrombosis.

Epstein, Michael Anthony, English virologist, *1921.
Epstein-Barr virus – a herpesvirus that causes infectious mononucleosis. *SYN:* EB virus

Eranko, Eino, Finnish anatomist, *1924.
Eranko fluorescence stain – exposure of frozen sections to formaldehyde, which produces a strong yellow-green fluorescence from cells containing norepinephrine.

Erasmus, L.D., South African physician.
Erasmus syndrome – scleroderma with silicosis, associated with pulmonary symptoms.

Erb, Wilhelm Heinrich, German neurologist, 1840-1921.
Duchenne-Erb paralysis – *SYN:* Erb palsy
Duchenne-Erb syndrome – *SYN:* Erb palsy
Erb atrophy – a form of progressive muscular atrophy in which the disease begins in the muscle and not in the spinal centers. *SYN:* progressive muscular dystrophy
Erb-Charcot disease – a type of cerebral palsy. *SYN:* spastic diplegia; spastic paraplegia
Erb disease – progressive weakness and atrophy of the muscles of the tongue, lips, palate, pharynx, and larynx, most often caused by motor neuron disease. *SYN:* progressive bulbar paralysis
Erb-Duchenne paralysis – *SYN:* Erb palsy
Erb formula – the portion of the brachial plexus that can be stimulated through intact skin.

E

NOTES

Erb-Goldflam disease – *SYN:* Goldflam disease

Erb palsy – a type of brachial birth palsy in which there is paralysis of the muscles of the upper arm and shoulder girdle. *SYN:* Duchenne-Erb paralysis; Duchenne-Erb syndrome; Erb-Duchenne paralysis; Erb paralysis

Erb paralysis – *SYN:* Erb palsy

Erb sign – *SYN:* Erb-Westphal sign

Erb spinal paralysis – chronic myelitis of syphilitic origin.

Erb-Westphal sign – abolition of the patellar tendon reflex in certain diseases of the spinal cord and occasionally in brain disease. *SYN:* Erb sign; Westphal-Erb sign; Westphal phenomenon; Westphal sign

Nievergelt-Erb syndrome – *SYN:* Nievergelt syndrome

Westphal-Erb sign – *SYN:* Erb-Westphal sign

Erben, Siegmund, Austrian neurologist, *1863.

Erben phenomenon – vagal stimulation slowing of the pulse when head and trunk are flexed. *SYN:* Erben reflex; Erben sign

Erben reflex – *SYN:* Erben phenomenon

Erben sign – *SYN:* Erben phenomenon

Erdheim, Jakob, Austrian physician, 1874-1937.

Erdheim disease – a disease of unknown cause that may be inherited and that predisposes to dissecting aneurysms. *SYN:* cystic medial necrosis

Erdheim syndrome – acromegaly causing cervical stiffening and often associated with clavicular hypertrophy. *SYN:* Scaglietti-Dagnini syndrome

Erdheim tumor – a suprasellar neoplasm, usually cystic, that develops from the nests of epithelium derived from Rathke pouch. *SYN:* craniopharyngioma

Erdmann, Hugo, German chemist, 1862-1910.

Erdmann reagent – a mixture of sulfuric and nitric acids, used in testing alkaloids.

Erhardt, Werner, 20th century salesman and founder of EST training seminars.

Erhardt Seminar Training (EST) – weekend-long training sessions designed to remove inhibitions and open the mind.

Erichsen, Sir John, English surgeon, 1818-1896.

Erichsen disease – neurosis following spinal injury. *SYN:* railway spine

Erichsen sign – in sacroiliac disease, pain when sudden pressure approximates the iliac bones.

Erlanger, Joseph, U.S. physiologist, 1874-1965, joint winner of 1944 Nobel Prize for work related to nerve fibers.

Erlenmeyer, Emil, German chemist, 1825-1909.
> **Erlenmeyer flask** – shaped so that its liquid content can be shaken laterally without spilling.
> **Erlenmeyer flask deformity** – a deformity at the distal end of the femur with the result that the bone is wide for a much longer distance up the shaft than normal.

Ernst, Paul, German pathologist, 1859-1937.
> **Babès-Ernst bodies** – see under Babès
> **Babès-Ernst granules** – *SYN:* Babès-Ernst bodies
> **Ernst-Babès granules** – *SYN:* Babès-Ernst bodies

Esbach, Georges H., French physician, 1843-1890.
> **Esbach reagent** – picric acid, citric acid, and water (in the proportions 1, 2, and 97) used for the detection of albumin in the urine.

Escamilla, Roberto Francisco, Mexican-U.S. physician, *1905.
> **Escamilla-Lisser-Shepardson syndrome**
> **Escamilla-Lisser syndrome** – adult hypothyroidism.

Escat, Etienne, French physician, 1865-1948.
> **Escat phlegmon** – abscess of connective tissue in the region of tonsils.

Escherich, Theodor, German physician, 1857-1911.
> *Escherichia coli* – a species that occurs normally in the intestines of humans and is a frequent cause of infections of the urogenital tract and of diarrhea in infants. *SYN:* colibacillus; colon bacillus
> **Escherich sign** – in hypoparathyroidism (latent tetany) tapping the skin at the angle of the mouth causes protrusion of the lips.

Escobar, Victor, 20th century U.S. physician.
> **Escobar syndrome** – syndrome manifested by orthopedic and cranial anomalies due to recessive trait. *SYN:* multiple pterygium syndrome

Eshmun, Phoenician deity of vegetation who castrated himself to avoid the advances of the goddess Astronae.
> **Eshmun complex** – autocastration. *SYN:* genital self-mutilation

E

NOTES

Esmarch, Johann F.A. von, German surgeon, 1823-1908.
    Esmarch bandage – *SYN:* Esmarch tourniquet
    Esmarch operation
    Esmarch probe
    Esmarch roll dressing
    Esmarch scissors
    Esmarch shears
    Esmarch tin bullet probe
    Esmarch tourniquet – a narrow hard rubber tourniquet with a chain
        fastener. *SYN:* Esmarch bandage
    Esmarch tube

Esser, Johannes F.S., Dutch surgeon, 1877-1946.
    Esser eyelid operation
    Esser graft – a skin graft wrapped (raw side out) around a bolus of dental
        compound and inserted into a prepared surgical pocket. *SYN:* inlay graft
    Esser implant
    Esser operation
    Esser prosthesis

Essick, C., 20th century U.S. anatomist.
    Essick cell bands – groups of cells in the developing rhombencephalon
        which migrate in two bands, one of which eventually forms the inferior
        olivary nucleus and the arcuate nucleus, and the other the pontine
        nuclei.

Esterly, Nancy Burton, U.S. pediatrician and dermatologist, *1935.
    Esterly-McKusick syndrome – rare disorder characterized by stony hard
        skin (especially over buttocks and upper thighs), mild hirsutism, and
        limitation of joint mobility.

Estes, William L., Jr., U.S. surgeon, 1885-1940.
    Estes operation – an operation for sterility in which a portion of an ovary is
        implanted on one uterine cornu.

Estlander, Jakob A., Finnish surgeon, 1831-1881.
    Abbe-Estlander cheiloplasty
    Estlander cheiloplasty
    Estlander flap – a full-thickness flap of the lip, transferred from the side of
        one lip to the same side of the other lip.
    Estlander operation – use of an Estlander flap in plastic surgery of the
        lips.

Eulenburg, Albert, German neurologist, 1840-1917.
    Eulenburg disease – a nonprogressive myotonia induced by exposure of muscles to cold. *SYN:* congenital paramyotonia

Euler, Ulf Von, Swedish physiologist, 1905-1983, joint winner of 1970 Nobel Prize for work related to neural transmitters.

Eustace Smith, see under Smith, Eustace

Eustachio, Bartolommeo E., Italian anatomist, 1524-1574.
    eustachian catheter – a catheter used for catheterization of the middle ear through the eustachian tube.
    eustachian cushion – a ridge in the nasopharyngeal wall posterior to the opening of the eustachian tube. *SYN:* torus tubarius
    eustachian tonsil – a collection of lymphoid nodules near the pharyngeal opening of the auditory tube. *SYN:* tubal tonsil
    eustachian tube – a tube leading from the tympanic cavity to the nasopharynx. *SYN:* auditory tube; tuba eustachiana; tuba eustachii
    eustachian tuber – a slight projection from the labyrinthine wall of the middle ear below the fenestra vestibuli (ovalis).
    eustachian valve – an endocardial fold extending from the anterior inferior margin of the inferior vena cava to the anterior part of the limbus fossa ovalis. *SYN:* valve of inferior vena cava
    tuba eustachiana – *SYN:* eustachian tube
    tuba eustachii – *SYN:* eustachian tube

Evans, Dillwyn, Welsh orthopedic surgeon, 1910-1974.
    Dillwyn Evans procedure – procedure related to clubfoot.

Evans, H.M., U.S. anatomist and physiologist, 1882-1971.
    Evans blue – a diazo dye used as a vital stain for following diffusion through blood vessel walls. *SYN:* azovan blue

Evans, Robert S., U.S. physician, 1912-1974.
    Evans syndrome – acquired hemolytic anemia and thrombocytopenia.

E

NOTES

Evans, William, English physician, *1895.
    Evans disease – familial form of cardiomegaly often accompanied by intracardiac thrombosis; sudden death may occur. *SYN:* familial cardiomegaly

Everett, Charles E., a patient at the Georgia Warm Springs Foundation for whom the crutch was made.
    Everett crutch – aluminum variety of crutch. *SYN:* metal triceps crutch; Warm Springs crutch

Everglades, subtropical swamp area located in southern Florida.
    Everglades virus – virus producing symptoms from mild influenza-like illness to encephalitis syndrome; found only in the state of Florida.

Eversbusch, Oskar, German ophthalmologist, 1853-1912.
    Eversbusch operation – correction of upper eyelid ptosis.

Ewart, William, English physician, 1848-1929.
    Ewart procedure – elevation of the larynx between the thumb and forefinger to elicit tracheal tugging.
    Ewart sign – in large pericardial effusions, an area of dullness with bronchial breathing and bronchophony below the angle of the left scapula. *SYN:* Pins sign

Ewing, James, U.S. pathologist, 1866-1943.
    Ewing sarcoma – *SYN:* Ewing tumor
    Ewing tumor – a malignant neoplasm that involves bones of the extremities, including the shoulder girdle, with a predilection for the metaphysis. *SYN:* endothelial myeloma; Ewing sarcoma

Ewing, James H., pathologist, 1798-1827.
    Ewing sign – dullness on percussion to the inner side of the angle of the left scapula, denoting an accumulation of fluid in the pericardium behind the heart.

Exner, Siegmund, Austrian physiologist, 1846-1926.
    Call-Exner bodies – see under Call
    Exner plexus – a plexus formed by tangential nerve fibers in the superficial plexiform or molecular layer of the cerebral cortex.

Exton, William G., U.S. physician, 1876-1943.
    Exton reagent – a test for albumin.

Eysenck, Hans Jurgen, German-English psychologist, *1916.
    Eysenck Personality Inventory

Faber, Knud H., Danish physician, 1862-1956.

Faber anemia – a form of chronic hypochromic microcytic anemia associated with achlorhydria or achylia gastrica. *SYN:* achlorhydric anemia; Faber syndrome

Faber syndrome – *SYN:* Faber anemia

Fabricius, Girolamo (Hieronymus ab Aquapendente), Italian anatomist and embryologist, 1537-1619.

bursa fabricii – in poultry, a blind saclike structure located on the posterodorsal wall of the cloaca. *SYN:* bursa of Fabricius

bursa of Fabricius – *SYN:* bursa fabricii

Fabricius ship – the outlines of the sphenoid, occipital, and frontal bones, from their fancied resemblance to the hull of a ship.

Fabry, Johannes, German dermatologist, 1860-1930.

Anderson-Fabry disease – *SYN:* Fabry disease

Fabry disease – an X-linked recessive disorder of glycosphingolipid metabolism. *SYN:* Anderson-Fabry disease; diffuse angiokeratoma; glycolipid lipidosis

Fadhil, Mahmoud, Lebanese physician.

Fadhil syndrome – autosomal recessive ectodermal dysplasia, characterized by hyperhidrosis, hyperkeratosis of palms and soles, dry and sparse hair, facial erythema, and teeth abnormalities.

Faget, Jean C., French physician, 1818-1884.

Faget sign – a slow pulse with an elevated temperature, often seen in yellow fever.

Fahr, Theodore, German physician, 1877-1945.

Fahr disease – progressive calcific deposition in the walls of blood vessels of the basal ganglia, occasionally associated with mental retardation and extrapyramidal symptoms.

NOTES

Fahraeus, Robert (Robin) Sanno, Swedish pathologist, 1888-1968.
  Fahraeus-Lindqvist effect – decrease in apparent viscosity that occurs when a suspension, such as blood, is made to flow through a tube of smaller diameter.
  Fahraeus method

Fahrenheit, Gabriel D., German-Dutch physicist, 1686-1736.
  Fahrenheit scale – a thermometer scale in which the freezing point of water is 32°F and the boiling point of water 212°F.

Fairbank, Sir Thomas, English physician.
  Fairbank disease – *SYN:* hyperostosis generalisata

Fairley, K.F., Australian physician, *1927.
  Fairley test – test to identify site of infection within the bladder.

Fallopius, Gabriele, Italian anatomist, 1523-1562.
  fallopian aqueduct – the bony passage in the temporal bone through which the facial nerve passes. *SYN:* facial canal; fallopian canal
  fallopian arch – *SYN:* fallopian ligament
  fallopian artery
  fallopian canal – *SYN:* fallopian aqueduct
  fallopian cannula
  fallopian catheter
  fallopian hiatus – the opening on the anterior aspect of the petrous part of the temporal bone which leads to the facial canal and gives passage to the greater petrosal nerve. *SYN:* hiatus of facial canal
  fallopian ligament – forms the floor of the inguinal canal and gives origin to lowermost fibers of internal oblique and transversus abdominis muscles. *SYN:* fallopian arch; inguinal ligament
  fallopian neuritis – *SYN:* facial paralysis
  fallopian pregnancy – *SYN:* tubal pregnancy
  fallopian tube – one of the tubes leading on either side from the upper or outer extremity of the ovary to the fundus of the uterus. *SYN:* tuba fallopiana; tuba fallopii; uterine tube
  tuba fallopiana – *SYN:* fallopian tube
  tuba fallopii – *SYN:* fallopian tube

Fallot, Étienne-Louis A., French physician, 1850-1911.
  Fallot tetrad – *SYN:* tetralogy of Fallot
  Fallot tetralogy – *SYN:* tetralogy of Fallot
  Fallot triad – *SYN:* trilogy of Fallot
  pentalogy of Fallot – Fallot tetralogy with, in addition, a patent foramen ovale or atrial septal defect.

tetralogy of Fallot – a set of congenital cardiac defects. *SYN:* Fallot tetrad; Fallot tetralogy

trilogy of Fallot – atrial septal defect associated with pulmonic stenosis and right ventricular hypertrophy. *SYN:* Fallot triad

Falls, Harold Francis, U.S. internist, *1911.
Rundles-Falls syndrome – see under Rundles

Falret, Jean-Pierre, French psychiatrist, 1794-1870.
Falret disease – manic-depressive psychosis. *SYN:* circular insanity; cyclic insanity

Falta, Wilhelm, Austrian physician, 1875-1950.
Falta syndrome – insufficiency of the pituitary and other glands.

Fañanás, J., Spanish physician.
Fañanás cell – a specialized astrocyte found in the cerebellar cortex.

Fanconi, Guido, Swiss pediatrician, 1892-1979.
Debré-De Toni-Fanconi syndrome – *SYN:* Fanconi syndrome (2)
De Toni-Fanconi syndrome – see under De Toni
Fanconi-Albertini-Zellweger syndrome – syndrome characterized by multiple conditions including congenital heart defect, microdontia, metabolic acidosis, and bone-related problems as well as growth retardation.
Fanconi anemia – a type of idiopathic refractory anemia characterized by pancytopenia, hypoplasia of the bone marrow, and congenital anomalies. *SYN:* congenital aplastic anemia; congenital pancytopenia; Fanconi pancytopenia; Fanconi syndrome (1)
Fanconi pancytopenia – *SYN:* Fanconi anemia
Fanconi syndrome – (1) *SYN:* Fanconi anemia; (2) a group of conditions with characteristic disorders of renal tubular function. *SYN:* Debré-De Toni-Fanconi syndrome
Lignac-Fanconi syndrome – see under Lignac
Wissler-Fanconi syndrome – see under Wissler

F

NOTES

Farabeuf, Louis H., French surgeon, 1841-1910.
  Farabeuf amputation – amputation of the leg or of the foot.
  Farabeuf bone-holding forceps
  Farabeuf double-ended retractor
  Farabeuf elevator
  Farabeuf forceps
  Farabeuf raspatory
  Farabeuf retractor
  Farabeuf saw
  Farabeuf triangle – the triangle formed by the internal jugular and facial veins and the hypoglossal nerve.

Faraday, Michael, English physicist and chemist, 1791-1867.
  farad – a practical unit of electrical capacity.
  faraday – 96,485.309 coulombs per mole, the amount of electricity required to reduce one equivalent of silver ion.
  Faraday cage – cage designed to enclose and protect an electric instrument from outside electric interference.
  Faraday constant
  Faraday laws – the amount of an electrolyte decomposed by an electric current is proportional to the amount of the current.
  faradic bath – water bath in which there is faradic current.
  faradic current – current that stimulates muscle through its nerve.
  faradism – *SYN:* faradization
  faradization – use of the faradic current. *SYN:* faradism

Farber, Sidney, U.S. pediatric pathologist, 1903-1973.
  Farber disease – a form of mucolipidosis, developing soon after birth because of deficiency of ceramidase. *SYN:* disseminated lipogranulomatosis; Farber syndrome
  Farber syndrome – *SYN:* Farber disease

Farnsworth, Dean, U.S. naval officer, 1902-1959.
  Farnsworth-Munsell color test – a test for color perception.

Farr, William, English medical statistician, 1807-1883.
  Farr law – the curve of cases of an epidemic rises rapidly at first, then climbs slowly to a peak from which the fall is steeper than the previous rise.

Farre, Arthur, English obstetrician and gynecologist, 1811-1887.
  Farre line – a whitish line marking the insertion of the mesovarium at the hilum of the ovary.

Farre, John R., English physician, 1775-1862.
Farre tubercles – masses beneath the liver capsule, sometimes associated with hepatic carcinoma.

Fauchard, Pierre, French dentist, 1678-1761.
Fauchard disease – marginal periodontitis.

Faught, Francis A., 20th century U.S. chemist.
Faught sphygmomanometer

Fauvel, Sulpice Antoine, French epidemiologist, 1813-1884.
Fauvel granules – multiple abscesses of the peribronchial region.

Favre, Maurice Jules, French physician, 1876-1954.
Favre disease – (1) lymphogranuloma venereum; (2) venous insufficiency resulting in angiodermatitis of lower limbs.
Favre-Durand-Nicolas disease – *SYN:* Durand disease
Gamna-Favre bodies – see under Gamna
Nicolas-Favre disease – see under Nicolas

Fay, Temple S., U.S. neurosurgeon, 1895-1963.
Fay exercises – *SYN:* Fay reflex therapy
Fay method – *SYN:* Fay reflex therapy
Fay reflex therapy – exercise used for patients with neuromuscular disorders. *SYN:* Fay exercises; Fay method
Fay suction elevator
Fay suction tube

Fazio, E., Italian physician, 1849-1902.
Fazio-Londe atrophy – hereditary trait leading to muscular atrophy. *SYN:* Fazio-Londe disease
Fazio-Londe disease – *SYN:* Fazio-Londe atrophy

Fechner, Gustav T., German physicist, 1801-1887.
Fechner paradox – refers to apparent increase in brightness of a figure when viewed with one eye after first viewing with both eyes.
Fechner-Weber law – *SYN:* Weber-Fechner law

F

NOTES

Weber-Fechner law – see under Weber, Ernst Heinrich

Fede, Francesco, Italian physician, 1832-1913.
　Fede-Riga disease – *SYN:* Riga-Fede disease
　Riga-Fede disease – see under Riga

Federici, Cesare, Italian physician, 1838-1892.
　Federici sign – intestinal perforation causing cardiac sounds to be heard on auscultation of abdomen.

Feer, Emil, Swiss pediatrician, 1864-1955.
　Feer disease – pain in peripheral or acral parts of the body; caused almost exclusively by mercury poisoning in children. *SYN:* acrodynia; pink disease; Swift disease

Fegeler, Ferdinand, German dermatologist, *1920.
　Fegeler syndrome – neck injury causing capillary nevus.

Fehling, Hermann von, German chemist, 1812-1885.
　Fehling reagent – *SYN:* Fehling solution
　Fehling solution – an alkaline copper tartrate solution formerly used for detection of reducing sugars. *SYN:* Fehling reagent
　Fehling test – used to reduce substances in urine.

Feil, André, French physician, *1884.
　Feil-Klippel syndrome – *SYN:* Klippel-Feil syndrome
　Klippel-Feil syndrome – see under Klippel

Feingold, Benjamin, pediatrician and allergist.
　Feingold diet – diet which eliminates synthetic coloring, flavoring, salicylates, and various preservatives in the belief that they contribute to behavior disorders.

Feiss, Henry O., 20th century U.S. orthopedic surgeon.
　Feiss line – a line running from the medial malleolus to the plantar aspect of the first metatarsophalangeal joint.

Feldberg, Wilhelm, English physiologist, *1900.
　Dale-Feldberg law – see under Dale, Sir Henry Hallett

Feldenkrais, Moshe, Israeli physicist, 1904-1979.
　Feldenkrais exercises – system used to improve posture, movement, and body awareness.

Feldman, Harry Alfred, U.S. epidemiologist, *1914.
　Sabin-Feldman dye test – see under Sabin
　Sabin-Feldman syndrome – see under Sabin

Felix, Arthur, Polish bacteriologist, 1887-1956.
  Weil-Felix reaction – *SYN:* Weil-Felix test
  Weil-Felix test – see under Weil, Edmund

Felton, Lloyd D., U.S. physician, 1885-1953.
  Felton phenomenon – in laboratory animals, immunologic unresponsiveness or tolerance to pneumococcal polysaccharide on administration of large doses of antigen.

Felty, Augustus R., U.S. physician, 1895-1964.
  Felty syndrome – rheumatoid arthritis with splenomegaly and leukopenia.

Fendt, Heinrich, Austrian dermatologist, *1872.
  Spiegler-Fendt pseudolymphoma – see under Spiegler
  Spiegler-Fendt sarcoid – *SYN:* Spiegler-Fendt pseudolymphoma

Fenn, Wallace Osgood, U.S. physiologist, 1893-1971.
  Fenn effect – the increased liberation of heat in a stimulated muscle when it is allowed to do mechanical work.

Fenwick, Edwin Hurry, English urologist, 1856-1944.
  Fenwick-Hunner ulcer – *SYN:* Hunner ulcer

Fenwick, Samuel, English physician, 1821-1902.
  Fenwick disease – idiopathic gastric atrophy.

Féréol, Louis H.F., French physician, 1825-1891.
  Féréol node – subcutaneous nodes seen around joints in the presence of acute rheumatism.

Ferguson Smith, John, English physician, 1888-1978.
  Ferguson Smith epithelioma – squamous epithelioma, self-healing.

Fergusson, Sir William, Scottish surgeon, 1808-1877.
  Fergusson incision – an incision used in maxillectomy, along the junction of cheek and nose, to bisect the upper lip.

F

NOTES

Fernandez, J.M.M., Argentinian dermatologist and leprologist, 1902-1965.
Fernandez reaction – an intraepidermal injection of 0.1 ml of lepromin is read at 48 hours for erythema used in classifying leprosy into the various subtypes.

Fernbach, Auguste, French microbiologist, 1860-1939.
Fernbach flask – a flask used in microbial fermentations where a large surface area of the liquid substrate is required.

Ferrata, Adolfo, Italian physician, 1880-1946.
Ferrata cell – primitive cell believed to be capable of developing into all types of blood cells. *SYN:* hemohistioblast

Ferraton, L., French physician.
Perrin-Ferraton disease – see under Perrin

Ferrein, Antoine, French anatomist, 1693-1769.
Ferrein canal – a space between the closed lids and the eyeball through which the tears flow to the punctum lacrimale. *SYN:* rivus lacrimalis
Ferrein cords
Ferrein foramen – the opening on the anterior aspect of the petrous part of the temporal bone which leads to the facial canal and gives passage to the greater petrosal nerve. *SYN:* hiatus of facial canal
Ferrein ligament – the capsular ligament that passes obliquely down and backward across the lateral surface of temporomandibular joint. *SYN:* lateral temporomandibular ligament
Ferrein pyramid – the center of the renal lobule, which has the shape of a small, steep pyramid, consisting of straight tubular parts. *SYN:* medullary ray; processus ferreini
Ferrein tube – *SYN:* convoluted tubule of kidney
Ferrein vasa aberrantia – biliary canaliculi that are not connected with hepatic lobules.
processus ferreini – *SYN:* Ferrein pyramid

Ferry, Erwin S., U.S. physicist, 1868-1956.
Ferry-Porter law – the critical fusion is directly proportional to the logarithm of the light intensity.

Feuerstein, Frichard C., U.S. physician.
Feuerstein-Mims-Schimmelpenning syndrome –
SYN: Schimmelpenning-Feuerstein-Mims syndrome
Feuerstein-Mims syndrome – *SYN:* Schimmelpenning-Feuerstein-Mims syndrome
Schimmelpenning-Feuerstein-Mims syndrome – see under Schimmelpenning

Feulgen, Robert, German nucleic acid biochemist and cytochemist, 1884-1955, first to detect DNA in cells by a specific cytochemical test.
Feulgen reaction – DNA staining reaction.
Feulgen test
Kasten fluorescent Feulgen stain – see under Kasten

Fevold, Harry Leonard, U.S. biochemist, *1902.
Fevold test – a test to determine the chemical nature of a substance by means of reagents.

Fèvre, Marcel Paul Luis Edmond, French orthopedic surgeon, *1897.
Fèvre-Lanquepin syndrome – popliteal webbing associated with multiple anomalies. *SYN:* popliteal pterygium

Feyrter, Friedrich, Austrian physician, *1895.
Feyrter disease – plasmacytosis of pulmonary tissue in infants born prematurely.

Fiamberti, Adamo Mario, Italian psychiatrist, 1894-1970.
Fiamberti hypothesis – theory that schizophrenia results from acetylcholine deficiency due to infection or toxicity.

Fibiger, Johannes A.G., Danish pathologist, 1867-1928.
Debré-Fibiger syndrome – see under Debré
Fibiger-Debré-von Gierke syndrome – *SYN:* Debré-Fibiger syndrome
Fibiger tumor – gastric squamous cell carcinoma in rats caused by larvae of Spiroptera neoplastica nematode.

Fick, Adolf, German physician, 1829-1901.
Fick method – cardiac output can be calculated as the quotient of total body oxygen consumption divided by the difference in oxygen content of arterial blood and mixed venous blood. *SYN:* Fick principle
Fick principle – *SYN:* Fick method

Fiedler, Carl L.A., German physician, 1835-1921.
Fiedler disease

F

NOTES

Fiedler myocarditis – an acute interstitial myocarditis of unknown cause, the endocardium and pericardium being unaffected. *SYN:* acute isolated myocarditis

Fielding, George H., English anatomist, 1801-1871.
Fielding membrane – in neuroanatomy, a thin sheet of fibers in the lateral wall of the temporal and occipital horns of the lateral ventricle, continuous with the corpus callosum. *SYN:* tapetum

Fiessinger, Noël Armand, French bacteriologist, 1881-1946.
Fiessinger-Leroy-Reiter syndrome – *SYN:* Reiter syndrome

Figueira, Fernandes, Brazilian pediatrician, d. 1928.
Figueira syndrome – weakness of the neck muscles with slight spasticity of the muscles of the lower extremities and increased tendon reflexes.

Filatov, (Filatow), Nil Feodorovich, Russian pediatrician, 1847-1902.
Filatov disease – *SYN:* Filatov-Dukes disease
Filatov-Dukes disease – exanthem-producing infectious disease of childhood, etiology unknown. *SYN:* Dukes disease; Filatov disease; fourth disease; parascarlatina; scarlatinella
Filatov spots – *SYN:* Koplik spots

Filatov, (Filatow), Vladimir P., Russian ophthalmologist, 1875-1956.
Filatov flap – a flap in which the sides of the pedicle are sutured together to create a tube, with the entire surface covered by skin. *SYN:* Filatov-Gillies flap; Filatov-Gillies tubed pedicle; tubed flap
Filatov-Gillies flap – *SYN:* Filatov flap
Filatov-Gillies tubed pedicle – *SYN:* Filatov flap
Filatov operation – obsolete term for penetrating keratoplasty.

Filatow, var. of Filatov

Fildes, Sir Paul Gordon, English bacteriologist, *1882.
Fildes enrichment agar
McIntosh-Fildes jar – see under McIntosh

Filipovitch, Casimir, 19th century Polish physician.
Filipovitch sign – yellow discoloration of palms of hands and soles of feet due to typhoid.

Filmer, David L., U.S. biochemist, *1932.
Adair-Koshland-Némethy-Filmer model – *SYN:* Koshland-Némethy-Filmer model
Koshland-Némethy-Filmer model – see under Koshland

Fincher, Edgar F., U.S. physician.
Fincher syndrome – tumor of the cauda equina region associated with spinal subarachnoid hemorrhage, low back pain, and headache.

Finckh, Johann, German psychiatrist, *1873.
Finckh test – a psychological test.

Fink, R.P., 20th century U.S. anatomist.
Fink-Heimer stain – a method used for histologic demonstration of degenerating nerve fibers and terminals of the central nervous system.

Finkeldey, Wilhelm, 20th century German pathologist.
Finkeldey cells – *SYN:* Warthin-Finkeldey cells
Warthin-Finkeldey cells – see under Warthin

Finkelstein, Harry, U.S. surgeon, 1865-1939.
Finkelstein maneuver
Finkelstein test – test indicative of de Quervain tenosynovitis.

Finkelstein, Heinrich, German pediatrician, 1865-1942.
Finkelstein feeding – form of infant feeding based on decrease in milk sugar.

Finn, Huckleberry, a character created by Mark Twain; teenaged boy considered a misfit, who has adventures on the Mississippi River.
Huck Finn syndrome – *SYN:* Huckleberry Finn syndrome (1), (2)
Huckleberry Finn syndrome – (1) the neglecting of responsibilities; behavior arises from feelings of rejection. *SYN:* Huck Finn syndrome; persistent truancy syndrome; truancy syndrome; (2) maladjustment of normal or highly intelligent children of parents with retardation. *SYN:* Huck Finn syndrome

Finney, John M.T., U.S. surgeon, 1863-1942.
Finney gastroduodenostomy
Finney gastroenterostomy
Finney operation – gastroduodenostomy which creates, by the technique of closure, a large opening to ensure free emptying from the stomach.

F

NOTES

Finney pyloroplasty – operation to provide a wider opening between stomach and duodenum.

Finochietto, Enrique, Argentinian surgeon, 1881-1948.
Finochietto artery clamp
Finochietto clamp carrier
Finochietto forceps
Finochietto laminectomy retractor
Finochietto needle
Finochietto needle holder
Finochietto operation
Finochietto retractor
Finochietto rib retractor
Finochietto rib spreader
Finochietto scissors
Finochietto spreader
Finochietto stirrup – used for traction in leg fractures.
Finochietto thoracic forceps
Finochietto thoracic scissors

Finsen, Niels Ryberg, Danish physician, 1860-1904, winner of the 1903 Nobel Prize for work related to disease treatment, particularly lupus vulgaris.
finsen – *SYN:* finsen unit
Finsen bath – ultraviolet irradiation.
Finsen carbon arc light
Finsen lamp – carbon-arc lamp.
Finsen method – to treat by using concentrated ultraviolet rays.
SYN: Finsen therapy
Finsen retractor
Finsen therapy – *SYN:* Finsen method
finsen unit – erythemal flux density of irradiation. *SYN:* finsen

Fisch, L., English physician.
Fisch-Renwick syndrome – disorder resulting in congenital deafness, abnormal distance between paired organs, and white forelock. *SYN:* Renwick-Fisch syndrome
Renwick-Fisch syndrome – *SYN:* Fisch-Renwick syndrome

Fischer, Emil, German chemist and Nobel laureate, 1852-1919.
Fischer projection formulas of sugars – representations, by projection, of cyclic sugars, or derivatives thereof, in which the carbon chain is depicted vertically.
Kiliani-Fischer reaction – *SYN:* Kiliani-Fischer synthesis

Kiliani-Fischer synthesis – see under Kiliani

Fischer, Louis, U.S. pediatrician, 1864-1944.
  Fischer sign – an obsolete sign of tuberculosis. *SYN:* Fischer symptom
  Fischer symptom – *SYN:* Fischer sign

Fishberg, Arthur M., U.S. physician, 1898-1992.
  Fishberg concentration test – a test of renal water conservation.

Fisher, Miller, U.S. neurologist, *1910.
  Fisher syndrome – a syndrome characterized by ophthalmoplegia, ataxia, and areflexia; a form of polyneuroradiculitis.

Fisher, Ronald A., English statistician, 1890-1962.
  Fisher exact test – a statistical hypothesis test.

Fitz, Reginald Heber, U.S. physician, 1843-1913.
  Fitz syndrome – *SYN:* acute pancreatitis

Fitzgerald, (origin unknown).
  Fitzgerald-Gardner syndrome – genetic trait resulting in multiple tumors, osteomas of the skull, epidermoid cysts, fibromas, and multiple polyposis predisposing to carcinoma of the colon.
  Fitzgerald trait – defect resulting in prolongation of clotting tests but seldom causing hemostatic symptoms. *SYN:* Flaujeac and Williams trait; kallikrein deficiency

Fitz-Hugh, Thomas, Jr., U.S. physician, 1894-1963.
  Fitz-Hugh and Curtis syndrome – perihepatitis in women with a history of gonococcal or chlamydial salpingitis.

Fitzsimmons, J.S., English physician.
  Fitzsimmons syndrome – hereditary syndrome resulting in limb spasticity, mental retardation, and foot deformities.

Flack, Martin, English physiologist, 1882-1931.
  Flack node – *SYN:* Keith and Flack node
  Flack test – a cardiopulmonary test.

F

NOTES

Keith and Flack node – see under Keith

Flatau, Edward, Polish neurologist, 1869-1932.

Flatau law – a law concerning the eccentric position of the long spinal tracts.

Flatau-Schilder disease – *SYN:* Schilder disease

Flatau syndrome – recessive trait resulting in bizarre movements brought on by physical activity. *SYN:* torsion dystonia

Flaujeac, one of two patients in whom the trait was detected.

Flaujeac and Williams trait – *SYN:* Fitzgerald trait

Flechsig, Paul E., German neurologist, 1847-1929.

Flechsig areas – three divisions (anterior, lateral, posterior) of each lateral half of the medulla as seen on transverse section, marked off by the root fibers of the hypoglossal and vagus nerves.

Flechsig fasciculi – fasciculus anterior proprius and fasciculus lateralis proprius. *SYN:* Flechsig ground bundles

Flechsig ground bundles – *SYN:* Flechsig fasciculi

Flechsig tract – a compact bundle of heavily myelinated, thick fibers at the periphery of the dorsal half of the lateral funiculus of the spinal cord. *SYN:* posterior spinocerebellar tract

oval area of Flechsig

semilunar nucleus of Flechsig – the small ventral region of the ventral posteromedial nucleus of thalamus in which the fibers of the gustatory lemniscus and secondary trigeminal tracts terminate. *SYN:* arcuate nucleus of thalamus

Fleck, F., German dermatologist, 1909-1995.

Fleck syndrome – diabetes insipidus associated with hypohidrosis, hypotrichosis, anodontia syndactyly, coloboma, and abnormal hematopoiesis.

Fleck, L., Polish physician.

Fleck syndrome – aggregation of leukocytes into similar cytological groups in the presence of pregnancy, fever, inflammatory processes, and other pathological disorders. *SYN:* leukergy

Flegel, Heinz, German dermatologist, *1923.

Flegel disease – small keratotic papules on the dorsa of the feet and legs, and occasionally elsewhere, with pinpoint keratotic papules of the palms and soles. *SYN:* hyperkeratosis lenticularis perstans

Fleisch, Alfred, Swiss physician and physiologist, *1892.
  Fleisch pneumotachograph – a pneumotachograph that measures flow in terms of the proportional pressure drop across a resistance consisting of numerous capillary tubes in parallel.

Fleischer, Bruno, German ophthalmologist, 1874-1965.
  Fleischer corneal ring
  Fleischer lines
  Fleischer ring – an incomplete ring often present at the base of the keratoconus cone.
  Fleischer-Strümpell ring – *SYN:* Kayser-Fleischer ring
  Fleischer vortex – congenital whorl-like opacities in the cornea. *SYN:* cornea verticillata
  Kayser-Fleischer ring – see under Kayser

Fleischmann, Friedrich Ludwig, 19th century German anatomist.
  Fleischmann bursa – an inconstant serous bursa at the level of the frenulum linguae, between the surface of the genioglossus muscle and the mucous membrane of the floor of the mouth. *SYN:* bursa sublingualis; sublingual bursa

Fleischner, Felix, Austrian-U.S. radiologist, 1893-1969.
  Fleischner lines – coarse linear shadows on chest x-ray, indicating bands of subsegmental atelectasis.

Fleisher, Thomas A., U.S. physician.
  Fleisher syndrome – genetically transmitted syndrome related to growth hormone deficiency and immune system deficiencies.

Fleitmann, Theodore, 19th century German chemist.
  Fleitmann test – a test for arsenic.

Fleming, Sir Alexander, Scottish bacteriologist, 1881-1955, co-winner of the 1945 Nobel Prize for the discovery of penicillin.

Flemming, Walther, German anatomist, 1843-1905.
  Flemming fixative – a cytoplasmic and chromosomal fixative.

F

NOTES

Flemming triple stain – a stain comprised of safranin, methyl violet, and orange G.

germinal center of Flemming – the lightly staining center in a lymphatic nodule in which the predominant cells are large lymphocytes and macrophages. *SYN:* reaction center

intermediate body of Flemming – a dense stalk of residual interzonal spindle fibers (microtubules) and actin-containing filaments that is formed during anaphase of mitosis. *SYN:* midbody

Flesch, Rudolf, Austrian educator, *1911.

Flesch formula – a method of determining the difficulty of a written passage used in determining patient comprehension of hospital consent forms.

Fletcher, surname of the patient in whom the defect was first noted.

Fletcher defect – slow contact activation in coagulation of the blood.

Fletcher factor – factor found in coagulation studies, revealing a slow contact activation but not associated with bleeding abnormalities. *SYN:* prekallikrein

Flexner, Simon, U.S. pathologist, 1863-1946.

Flexner bacillus – *SYN: Shigella flexneri*

Shigella flexneri – see under Shiga

Flier, J.S.

Flier syndrome – insulin-resistant diabetes mellitus associated with acanthosis nigricans, hypertrichosis, lipodystrophy, and muscle cramps.

Flieringa, Henri J., Dutch ophthalmologist, *1891.

Flieringa fixation ring

Flieringa ring – a stainless steel ring sutured to the sclera to prevent collapse of the globe in difficult intraocular operations.

Flieringa scleral ring

Flinders Island, island off southern coast of Australia.

Flinders Island spotted fever – a form of spotted fever, treatable with antibiotics, transmitted to humans by ticks.

Flindt, N., Danish physician, 1843-1913.

Flindt spots – *SYN:* Koplik spots

Flint, Austin, U.S. physician, 1812-1886.

Austin Flint murmur – *SYN:* Flint murmur

Austin Flint phenomenon – *SYN:* Flint murmur

Austin Flint respiration

Flint murmur – a diastolic murmur, similar to that of mitral stenosis, heard best at the cardiac apex in some cases of free aortic insufficiency. *SYN:* Austin Flint murmur; Austin Flint phenomenon

Flint, Austin, Jr., U.S. physiologist, 1836-1915.
Flint arcade – a series of vascular arches at the bases of the pyramids of the kidney.

Flocks, Milton, U.S. ophthalmologist, *1914.
Harrington-Flocks test – see under Harrington, David O.

Flood, Valentine, Irish anatomist and surgeon, 1800-1847.
Flood ligament – a band of the coracohumeral ligament, attached to the lower part of the lesser tuberosity of the humerus.

Florence, Albert, French physician, 1851-1927.
Florence crystals – brown rhombic crystals formed at the interface between a drop of Lugol solution and a drop of fluid that contains semen.

Florey, Sir Howard W., Australian-English pathologist and Nobel laureate, 1898-1968.
Florey unit – 1 unit equals 0.6 mcg of crystalline sodium salt of penicillin. *SYN:* Oxford unit

Florschütz, Georg, German physician, *1859.
Florschütz formula – the correct relation of height to the abdominal circumference.

Flourens, Marie J.P., French physiologist, 1794-1867.
Flourens theory – that thought is a process depending on the action of the entire cerebrum.

Flower, Sir William H., English surgeon and anatomist, 1831-1899.
Flower bone – a sutural bone occasionally present at the pterion or junction of the parietal, frontal, greater wing of the sphenoid, and squamous portion of the temporal bones. *SYN:* epipteric bone

F

NOTES

Flower dental index – a system of numbers for indicating comparative size of the teeth. *SYN:* dental index

Flynn, P., 20th century U.S. neurologist.

Flynn-Aird syndrome – a familial syndrome characterized by muscle wasting, ataxia, dementia, skin atrophy, and ocular anomalies.

Flynn phenomenon – a pupillary response to light, the reverse of that expected. *SYN:* paradoxical pupillary reflex

Fobi, Mathias A.L., U.S. surgeon.

Fobi pouch – vertical gastric bypass banding procedure that reduces stomach size to a 15- to 30-ml capacity.

Fogarty, Thomas J., U.S. thoracic surgeon, *1934.

Fogarty arterial embolectomy

Fogarty biliary probe

Fogarty catheter – a catheter used to remove arterial emboli and thrombi from major veins. *SYN:* balloon-tip catheter

Fogarty clamp – a clamp with rubber-shod blades having serrated surfaces, to provide an atraumatic grip on tissues.

Fogarty forceps

Fogarty irrigation catheter

Fogarty venous thrombectomy catheter

Foix, Charles, French neurologist, 1882-1927.

Foix-Alajouanine myelitis – a disorder of the lower spinal cord in adult males resulting in progressive paraplegia. *SYN:* subacute necrotizing myelitis

Foix-Alajouanine syndrome – thrombophlebitis of spinal veins resulting in a subacute ascending painful flaccid paralysis from necrotic myelitis.

Foix-Cavany-Marie syndrome – constellation of faciopharyngoglossomasticatory diplegia, usually caused by bilateral large artery infarcts of the opercular cortex.

Foix syndrome – paralysis of cranial nerves III through VI resulting in proptosis and eyelid edema; trigeminal neuralgia may also be present.

Foley, Frederic E.B., U.S. urologist, 1891-1966.

Foley acorn-bulb catheter

Foley bag

Foley balloon catheter

Foley catheter – a catheter with a retaining balloon.

Foley cone-tip catheter

Foley forceps

Foley hemostatic bag

Foley operation – *SYN:* Foley Y-plasty pyeloplasty
Foley plate
Foley pyeloplasty
Foley three-way catheter
Foley ureteropelvioplasty
Foley vas isolation forceps
Foley Y-plasty pyeloplasty – a reconstructive procedure for correction of ureteropelvic obstruction. *SYN:* Foley operation
Foley Y-type ureteropelvioplasty
Foley Y-V pyeloplasty

Folin, Otto K.O., U.S. biochemist, 1867-1934.
Folin-Looney test – a test for tyrosine that gives a blue color in alkaline solution with a reagent consisting of sodium tungstate, phosphomolybdic acid, and phosphoric acid.
Folin reaction – the reaction of amino acids in alkaline solution with 1,2-naphthoquinone-4-sulfonate (Folin reagent) to yield a red color. *SYN:* Folin reagent
Folin reagent – *SYN:* Folin reaction
Folin test – a quantitative test for urea.
Lowry-Folin assay – *SYN:* Lowry protein assay

Folling, Ivar Asbjorn, Norwegian physician, 1888-1973.
Folling disease – congenital deficiency of phenylalanine 4-monooxygenase or occasionally of dihydropteridine reductase or of dihydrobiopterin synthetase that can cause brain damage and other neurologic abnormalities. *SYN:* phenylketonuria

Foltz, Jean C.E., French anatomist and ophthalmologist, 1822-1876.
Foltz valvule – *SYN:* Bochdalek valve

Fones, Alfred Civilion, U.S. dentist, 1869-1938.
Fones method of tooth brushing
Fones technique

F

NOTES

Fong, Edward Everett, U.S. radiologist, *1912.
    Fong lesion – genetic trait resulting in abnormality of thumb and great toe nails; may result in iliac bone abnormalities and abnormalities of the renal system. *SYN:* Fong syndrome; nail-patella syndrome; Österreicher-Fong syndrome
    Fong syndrome – *SYN:* Fong lesion

Fonio, Anton, Swiss physician, *1889.
    Fonio solution – a diluent with magnesium sulfate, used for stained smears of blood platelets.

Fontan, François, French thoracic surgeon, *1929.
    Fontan operation – *SYN:* Fontan procedure
    Fontan procedure – placement of a conduit (usually valved) from the right atrium to the main pulmonary artery as a bypass to a hypoplastic right ventricle, as in tricuspid atresia. *SYN:* Fontan operation

Fontana, Arturo, Italian dermatologist, 1873-1950.
    Fontana-Masson silver stain – *SYN:* Masson-Fontana ammoniacal silver stain
    Fontana stain – a traditional method for silver-impregnation of treponemes and other spirochetal forms.
    Masson-Fontana ammoniacal silver stain – see under Masson

Fontana, Felice, Italian physiologist, 1730-1805.
    Fontana canal – the vascular structure encircling the anterior chamber of the eye and through which the aqueous is returned to the blood circulation. *SYN:* sinus venosus sclerae
    Fontana spaces – irregularly shaped endothelium-lined spaces within the trabecular reticulum, through which the aqueous filters to reach the sinus venosus sclerae. *SYN:* spaces of iridocorneal angle

Foot, N.C., 20th century U.S. pathologist.
    Foot reticulin impregnation stain – a silver stain.

Forbes, Anne P., 20th century U.S. physician.
    Forbes-Albright syndrome – pituitary tumor in a patient without acromegaly, which secretes excessive amounts of prolactin and produces persistent lactation.

Forbes, Gilbert B., U.S. pediatrician, *1915.
    Forbes disease – (1) storage of excess amounts of glycogen; (2) glycogenosis due to amylo-1,6-glucosidase deficiency, resulting in accumulation of abnormal glycogen with short outer chains in liver and muscle. *SYN:* type 3 glycogenosis

Forbes, Thomas R.
   Hooker-Forbes test – see under Hooker

Forchheimer, Frederick, U.S. physician, 1853-1913.
   Forchheimer sign – the presence in German measles of a reddish maculopapular eruption on the soft palate.

Fordyce, John Addison, U.S. dermatologist, 1858-1925.
   Fordyce angiokeratoma – asymptomatic vascular papules of the scrotum.
   Fordyce disease – *SYN:* Fordyce spots
   Fordyce granules – *SYN:* Fordyce spots
   Fordyce lesion – scrotal angiomas of no significance.
   Fordyce spots – a condition marked by the presence of numerous small, yellowish-white bodies or granules on the inner surface and vermilion border of the lips. *SYN:* Fordyce disease; Fordyce granules; pseudocolloid of lips
   Fox-Fordyce disease – see under Fox, George Henry

Forel, Auguste H., Swiss neurologist, 1848-1931.
   campi foreli – *SYN:* fields of Forel
   fields of Forel – three circumscript, myelin-rich regions of the subthalamus. *SYN:* campi foreli; tegmental fields of Forel
   Forel commissure
   Forel decussation
   Forel space
   tegmental fields of Forel – *SYN:* fields of Forel

Forestier, Jacques, French rheumatologist, *1890.
   Forestier disease – a generalized spinal and extraspinal articular disorder characterized by calcification and ossification of ligaments. *SYN:* diffuse idiopathic skeletal hyperostosis

Formad, Henry, U.S. physician, 1847-1892.
   Formad kidney – an enlarged and deformed kidney, sometimes seen in chronic alcoholism.

F

NOTES

Forssell, Gösta, Swedish radiologist, 1876-1950.
Forssell sinus – mucosal folds surround this smooth space in the stomach wall.

Forssell, Jarl, Finish physician, 1912-1964.
Forssell syndrome – polycythemia.

Forssman, Hans, Swedish physician, *1912.
Börjeson-Forssman-Lehmann syndrome – see under Börjeson

Forssman, John, Swedish bacteriologist and pathologist, 1868-1947.
Forssman antibody – a heterogenetic antibody specific for the Forssman group of heterogenetic antigens. *SYN:* heterophil antibody; heterophile antibody
Forssman antigen – the antibody that develops in infectious mononucleosis reacts specifically with the Forssman antigen.
Forssman antigen-antibody reaction – the combination of Forssman antibody with heterogenetic antigen of the Forssman type. *SYN:* Forssman reaction
Forssman reaction – *SYN:* Forssman antigen-antibody reaction

Forssmann, Werner Theodor Otto, German surgeon, 1904-1979, co-winner of 1956 Nobel Prize for work related to circulation and heart catheterization.

Förster, Richard, German ophthalmologist, 1825-1902.
Förster eye forceps
Förster iris forceps
Förster photometer
Förster uveitis – syphilitic inflammation, with diffuse nodules involving the choroid and retinal vasculitis.

Fosdick, Leonard S., U.S. chemist, *1903.
Fosdick-Hansen-Epple test – a test for determining dental caries activity based on a solution of powdered human enamel in a saliva-glucose-enamel mixture.

Foshay, Lee, U.S. bacteriologist, 1896-1961.
Foshay test – an intradermal test for cat-scratch disease or tularemia, using material prepared from suppurative lymph nodes of persons known to have had the disease.

Foster Kennedy, see under Kennedy, Robert Foster

Fothergill, John, English physician, 1712-1780.
Fothergill disease – severe, paroxysmal bursts of pain in one or more branches of the trigeminal nerve. *SYN:* anginose scarlatina; Fothergill neuralgia; trigeminal neuralgia

Fothergill neuralgia – *SYN:* Fothergill disease

Fothergill sign – in rectus sheath hematoma, the hematoma produces a mass that does not cross the midline and remains palpable when the rectus muscle is tense.

Fothergill, William E., English gynecologist, 1865-1926.
Fothergill operation – *SYN:* Manchester operation
Fothergill suture

Fouchet, André, French physician, *1894.
Fouchet reagent – a test for bilirubin.
Fouchet stain – Fouchet reagent employed to demonstrate bile pigments.

Fountain, R.B., English physician.
Fountain syndrome – recessive trait related to mental retardation, bone abnormalities, and tissue swelling.

Fourier, J.B.J., French mathematician and administrator, 1768-1830.
Fourier analysis – used in reconstruction of images in computed tomography and magnetic resonance imaging in radiology and in analysis of any kind of signal for its frequency content. *SYN:* Fourier law; Fourier transform
Fourier law – *SYN:* Fourier analysis
Fourier transform – *SYN:* Fourier analysis

Fourneau, Ernest F.A., French chemist and pharmacologist, 1872-1949.
Fourneau 693 – a synthetic organic compound of antimony used in the treatment of several protozoal diseases and for the relief of pain in multiple myeloma. *SYN:* ethylstibamine
Fourneau 710 – a synthetic antimalarial agent.
Fourneau 933 – used as a diagnostic test for pheochromocytoma. *SYN:* piperoxan hydrochloride

Fournier, Jean Alfred, French syphilographer, 1832-1914.
Fournier disease – infective gangrene involving the scrotum. *SYN:* Fournier gangrene; syphiloma of Fournier

F

Fournier gangrene – *SYN:* Fournier disease
syphiloma of Fournier – *SYN:* Fournier disease

Foville, Achille L., French neurologist, 1799-1878.
   Foville fasciculus – a slender, compact fiber bundle that connects the amygdala with the hypothalamus and other basal forebrain regions. *SYN:* terminal stria
   Foville paralysis – *SYN:* Foville syndrome
   Foville syndrome – a form of alternating hemiplegia characterized by abducens paralysis on one side, paralysis of the extremities on the other. *SYN:* Foville paralysis

Fowler, Edson Brady, U.S. surgeon, 1865-1942.
   Fowler procedure – orthopedic procedure performed on metatarsal heads.

Fowler, George R., U.S. surgeon, 1848-1906.
   Fowler position – an inclined position obtained by raising the head of the bed about 60-90 cm to promote better dependent drainage after an abdominal operation.

Fowler, Thomas, English physician, 1736-1801.
   Fowler solution – solution of potassium arsenate used in treatment of leukemia.

Fox, George Henry, U.S. dermatologist, 1846-1937.
   Fox-Fordyce disease – a rare chronic pruritic eruption of dry papules and distended ruptured apocrine glands, with follicular hyperkeratosis of the nipples, axillae, and pubic and sternal regions. *SYN:* apocrine miliaria

Fox, Lewis, U.S. periodontist, *1903.
   Goldman-Fox knives – see under Goldman, Henry M.

Fraccaro, M., Italian physician.
   Schmid-Fraccaro syndrome – see under Schmid, W.

Fraenkel, (Fränkel), Albert, German physician, 1848-1916.
   Fraenkel pneumococcus – normal inhabitants of the respiratory tract and perhaps the most common cause of lobar pneumonia, they are relatively common causative agents of meningitis, sinusitis, and other infections. *SYN:* *Streptococcus pneumoniae*; Fraenkel-Weichselbaum pneumococcus
   Fraenkel-Weichselbaum pneumococcus – *SYN:* Fraenkel pneumococcus

Fraley, Elwin E., U.S. urologist, *1934.
   Fraley syndrome – dilation of the upper pole renal calices due to stenosis of the upper infundibulum.

Franceschetti, Adolphe, Swiss ophthalmologist, 1896-1968.
   Franceschetti-Jadassohn syndrome – *SYN:* Naegeli syndrome
   Franceschetti syndrome – mandibulofacial dysostosis, when complete or nearly complete.

Francis, C.A., English otolaryngologist, 1898-1951.
   Francis triad – aspirin sensitivity in conjunction with asthma and nasal polyps.

Francis, Edward, U.S. physician, 1872-1957.
   Francis disease – tularemia.

Francke, Karl E., German physician, 1859-1920.
   Francke needle – a small lancet-shaped, spring-activated needle, used to evacuate a small effusion of blood.

Franco, Pierre, French surgeon, 1500-1561.
   Franco operation – cystotomy.

François, Jules, Belgian ophthalmologist, 1907-1984.
   François syndrome – *SYN:* Hallermann-Streiff syndrome
   Hallermann-Streiff-François syndrome – *SYN:* Hallermann-Streiff syndrome

Frank, A.E., German physician, 1884-1957.
   Frank capillary toxicosis – purpura without any platelet count decrease. *SYN:* nonthrombocytopenic purpura

Frank, Otto, German physiologist, 1865-1944.
   Frank-Starling curve – *SYN:* Starling curve

Frank, Rudolf, Austrian surgeon, 1862-1913.
   Ssabanejew-Frank operation – see under Ssabanejew

Frank, Sanders T., U.S. thoracic physician, *1938.
   Frank sign – oblique earlobe fissure associated with hypertension, heart disease, and diabetes; acquired as opposed to congenital.

F

NOTES

Franke, Gustav, German physician, *1878.
   Franke syndrome – abnormalities of the palate, septal deviation, and enlarged adenoids leading to infections and breathing through the mouth rather than the nose. *SYN:* Franke triad
   Franke triad – *SYN:* Franke syndrome

Fränkel, var. of Fraenkel

Frankenhäuser, Ferdinand, German gynecologist, 1832-1894.
   Frankenhäuser ganglion – a gangliated autonomic plexus on each side of the cervix of the uterus, derived from the inferior hypogastric plexus. *SYN:* uterovaginal plexus

Franklin, Benjamin, U.S. physicist and statesman, 1706-1790.
   franklinic – denoting static or frictional electricity.
   Franklin spectacles – an early form of bifocal spectacles in which the lower half of the lens is for near vision, the upper half for distant vision. *SYN:* divided spectacles

Franklin, Edward C., U.S. physician, 1928-1982.
   Franklin disease – common features include anemia, lymphocytosis, eosinophilia, thrombocytopenia, hyperuricemia, lymphadenopathy, and hepatosplenomegaly. *SYN:* γ-heavy-chain disease

Fraser, Alexander, Canadian pathologist, 1869-1939.
   Fraser-Lendrum stain for fibrin – a multistaining procedure after Zenker fixative in which fibrin, keratin, and some cytoplasmic granules appear red, erythrocytes appear orange, and collagen appears green.

Fraser, George R., English geneticist, *1932.
   Fraser syndrome – an association of cryptophthalmus with multiple anomalies. *SYN:* cryptophthalmus syndrome
   Melnick-Fraser syndrome – see under Melnick, M.

Fraumeni, Joseph F., Jr., 20th century epidemiologist.
   Li-Fraumeni cancer syndrome – see under Li

Fraunhofer, Joseph von, German optician, 1787-1826.
   Fraunhofer lines – a number of the most prominent of the absorption lines of the solar spectrum.

Frazier, Charles H., U.S. surgeon, 1870-1936.
   Frazier dural guide
   Frazier incision
   Frazier needle – a needle for draining lateral ventricles of brain.
   Frazier-Spiller operation – division or section of a sensory root of the fifth cranial nerve, accomplished through a subtemporal approach.

Frazier stylet
Frazier suction tip
Frazier suction tube

Frechet, P.
Frechet extender – a thin silicone device with a row of hooks on two opposite ends used in scalp extension as part of hair restoration.
Frechet flap procedure – a flap procedure that improves the result of a midline scalp reduction.

Frederick, Maurice Hugh, joint winner of 1963 Nobel Prize for work related to nuclear acids.

Fredet, Pierre, French surgeon, 1870-1946.
Fredet-Ramstedt operation – *SYN:* Ramstedt operation

Freeman, Charles.
Freeman rule – a person is not responsible for crimes committed if that person has a condition which prevents him/her from knowing what he/she is doing.

Freeman, Ernest A., English orthopedic surgeon, 1900-1975.
Freeman-Sheldon syndrome – *SYN:* craniocarpotarsal dystrophy

Frei, Wilhelm Siegmund, German dermatologist, 1885-1943.
Frei disease – lymphogranuloma venereum.
Frei-Hoffmann reaction – *SYN:* Frei test
Frei test – an intracutaneous diagnostic test for lymphogranuloma venereum. *SYN:* Frei-Hoffmann reaction

Freiberg, Albert Henry, U.S. surgeon, 1869-1940.
Freiberg cartilage knife
Freiberg disease – epiphysial ischemic (aseptic) necrosis of the second metatarsal head.
Freiberg hip retractor
Freiberg infraction
Freiberg meniscectomy knife

F

NOTES

Freiberg traction
Freiberg tractor

Frejka, B., Czech orthopedist, *1890.
Frejka cast
Frejka hip pillow
Frejka jacket
Frejka orthosis
Frejka pillow splint – a pillow splint used for abduction and flexion of the femurs in treatment of congenital hip dysplasia or dislocation in infants.
Frejka splint
Frejka traction

Frenkel, Heinrich S., Swiss neurologist, 1860-1931.
Frenkel exercises – exercises designed for reeducating those with incoordination problems. *SYN:* Frenkel method
Frenkel method – *SYN:* Frenkel exercises
Frenkel tracks – a method of painting footprints or other marks on a floor to use as a guide for patients with ataxia in walking reeducation.

Frenkel, Henri, French ophthalmologist, 1864-1934.
Frenkel anterior ocular traumatic syndrome – an obsolete term for traumatic iridoplegia.

Frerichs, Friedrich T. von, German pathologist and clinician, 1819-1885.
Frerichs theory – that uremia represents a toxic condition caused by ammonium carbonate, which is formed as the result of the action of a plasma enzyme on the increased amounts of urea.

Fresnel, Augustin Jean, French physicist, 1788-1827.
Fresnel lens – a lens with a surface consisting of a concentric series of zones that duplicate the power of a lens or prism but with less thickness. *SYN:* Fresnel prism; lighthouse lens
Fresnel prism – *SYN:* Fresnel lens

Freud, Sigmund, Austrian neurologist and psychiatrist, 1856-1939, founder of psychoanalysis.
freudian – relating to or described by Freud.
freudian fixation
freudian psychoanalysis – the theory and practice of psychoanalysis and psychotherapy as developed by Freud.
freudian slip – a mistake in speech or deed which presumably suggests some underlying motive, often sexual or aggressive in nature.
Freud theory – a comprehensive theory of how personality is formed and develops in normal and emotionally disturbed individuals.

Freund, Emanuel, Austrian physician, *1869.
Freund dermatitis – application of cosmetics causes erythema at application site and later brown pigmentation when that area of skin is exposed to sunlight. *SYN:* bergamot dermatitis

Freund, Jules, U.S. bacteriologist, 1891-1960.
Freund complete adjuvant – water-in-oil emulsion of antigen, to which killed mycobacteria or tuberculosis bacteria are added.
Freund incomplete adjuvant – water-in-oil emulsion of antigen, without mycobacteria.

Freund, Wilhelm A., German gynecologist, 1833-1918.
Freund anomaly – a narrowing of the upper aperture of the thorax by shortening of the first rib and its cartilage.
Freund operation – (1) total abdominal hysterectomy for uterine cancer; (2) chondrotomy to relieve Freund anomaly.

Frey, Lucie, Polish neurologist, 1852-1932.
Frey syndrome – localized flushing and sweating of the ear and cheek in response to eating. *SYN:* auriculotemporal nerve syndrome

Frey, Max von, German physician, 1852-1932.
Frey hairs – short hairs of varying degrees of stiffness, set into a light wooden handle and used for assessing sensation.

Freyer, Sir Peter J., English surgeon, 1851-1921.
Freyer drain
Freyer operation – prostate enucleation.
Freyer suprapubic drain

Frias, Jaime L., 20th century Chilean pediatrician.
Opitz-Frias syndrome – see under Opitz, John M.

Fridenberg, Percy H., U.S. ophthalmologist, 1868-1960.
Fridenberg stigometric card test – an obsolete test of vision and accommodation for illiterates.

F

NOTES

Friderichsen, Carl, Danish physician, 1886-1982.
Friderichsen syndrome – *SYN:* Waterhouse-Friderichsen syndrome
Friderichsen-Waterhouse syndrome – *SYN:* Waterhouse-Friderichsen syndrome
Waterhouse-Friderichsen syndrome – see under Waterhouse

Fried, K., 20th century Israeli geneticist.
Fried syndrome – an autosomal recessive ectodermal dysplasia considered a "hair-tooth-nail syndrome." *SYN:* Fried tooth-and-nail syndrome
Fried tooth-and-nail syndrome – *SYN:* Fried syndrome

Friedlander, var. of Friedländer

Friedländer, (Friedlander), Carl, German pathologist, 1847-1887.
Friedländer bacillus – capsular types 1, 2, and 3 of this organism may be causative agents in pneumonia. *SYN: Klebsiella pneumoniae*
Friedländer disease
Friedländer pneumobacillus
Friedländer pneumonia – a form of pneumonia caused by infection with *Klebsiella pneumoniae.*
Friedländer stain for capsules – an obsolete stain employing gentian violet.

Friedman, Arnold Phineas, U.S. physician, *1909.
Friedman-Roy syndrome – familial syndrome resulting in mental deficiency, strabismus, clubfoot, and other abnormalities.

Friedman, Emanuel A., U.S. obstetrician, *1926.
Friedman curve – a graph on which hours of labor are plotted against cervical dilation in centimeters.

Friedman, M., U.S. physiologist and physician, *1903.
Friedman test – modified Aschheim-Zondek test for pregnancy.

Friedmann, Max, German physician, 1858-1925.
Friedmann syndrome – (1) juvenile epilepsy, petit mal type; (2) juvenile spastic paralysis due to congenital syphilis; (3) progressive form of encephalitis related to cerebral vasomotor disorder. *SYN:* postconcussion syndrome

Friedreich, Nikolaus, German neurologist, 1825-1882.
Friedreich ataxia – sclerosis of the posterior and lateral columns of the spinal cord, occurring in children and marked by ataxia in the lower extremities, extending to the upper, followed by paralysis and contractures. *SYN:* Biemond ataxia; hereditary spinal ataxia

Friedreich disease – an ill-defined disorder marked by rapid and widespread muscle contractions. *SYN:* Friedreich spasms; myoclonus multiplex; paramyoclonus multiplex

Friedreich phenomenon – the tympanitic percussion sound over a pulmonary cavity is slightly raised in pitch on deep inspiration.

Friedreich sign – in adherent pericardium, sudden collapse of the previously distended veins of the neck at each diastole of the heart.

Friedreich spasms – *SYN:* Friedreich disease

Friend, Charlotte, U.S. microbiologist, *1921.

Friend disease – mouse leukemia caused by the Friend virus.

Friend leukemia virus – *SYN:* Friend virus

Friend virus – a strain of the splenic group of mouse leukemia viruses, related to Moloney and Rauscher viruses. *SYN:* Friend leukemia virus; Swiss mouse leukemia virus

Fritsch, Heinrich, German gynecologist, 1844-1915.

Bozeman-Fritsch catheter – see under Bozeman

Froehde, A., 19th century German chemist.

Froehde reagent – sodium molybdate 1, in strong sulfuric acid 1000.

Froehlich, var. of Fröhlich

Fröhlich, (Froehlich), Alfred, Austrian neurologist and pharmacologist, 1871-1953.

Fröhlich dwarfism – dwarfism with Fröhlich syndrome.

Fröhlich syndrome – dystrophia adiposogenitalis, originally involving an adenohypophysial tumor. *SYN:* Launois-Cléret syndrome

Frohn, Damianus, German physician, *1843.

Frohn reagent – used to test for alkaloids and sugar.

Froin, Georges, French physician, 1874-1932.

Froin syndrome – an alteration in cerebrospinal fluid noted in loculated portions of the subarachnoid space isolated from spinal fluid circulation by an inflammatory or neoplastic obstruction. *SYN:* loculation syndrome

F

NOTES

Froment, Jules, Lyon physician, 1878-1946.
  Froment sign – flexion of the distal phalanx of the thumb when a sheet of paper is held between the thumb and index finger in ulnar nerve palsy.

Frommann, Carl, German anatomist, 1831-1892.
  Frommann lines – transverse marks on nerve fibers.

Frommel, Richard, German gynecologist, 1854-1912.
  Chiari-Frommel syndrome – see under Chiari, Johann B.
  Frommel-Chiari syndrome – *SYN:* Chiari-Frommel syndrome
  Frommel disease – prolonged lactation causing uterine involution.
  Frommel operation

Froriep, August von, German anatomist, 1849-1917.
  Froriep ganglion – a temporary collection of nerve cells on the dorsal aspect of the hypoglossal nerve in the embryo.
  Froriep induration – induration of a muscle through an interstitial growth of fibrous tissue. *SYN:* myositis fibrosa

Frost, Albert D., U.S. ophthalmologist, 1889-1945.
  Frost operation
  Frost suture – intermarginal suture between the eyelids to protect the cornea.

Frostig, Marianne B., Austrian-U.S. psychologist, *1906.
  Frostig Developmental Test of Visual Perception – designed for use with children who are learning-disabled.
  Frostig Movement Skills Test Battery – a test designed to determine learning problems by evaluating juvenile sensorimotor skills.

Frugoni, Cesare, Italian physician, *1881.
  Frugoni disease – proliferation of eosinophils causing arthralgias, respiratory and gastrointestinal problems. *SYN:* infectious eosinophilia
  Frugoni syndrome – splenomegaly due to splenic vein thrombosis.

Fryns, J.P., Belgian physician.
  Fryns syndrome – genetic disorder resulting in limb abnormalities and pulmonary defects.

Fuchs, Ernst, Austrian ophthalmologist, 1851-1930.
  angle of Fuchs – a crevice between the ciliary and pupillary zones of the iris, formed by atrophy of superficial layers of the iris in the pupillary zone.
  Dalen-Fuchs nodules – see under Dalen
  Fuchs adenoma – a benign epithelial tumor of the nonpigmented epithelium of the ciliary body, rarely exceeding 1 mm in diameter.

Fuchs atrophy – optic nerve peripheral atrophy.

Fuchs black spot – an area of pigment proliferation in the macular region in degenerative myopia.

Fuchs capsule forceps

Fuchs capsulotomy forceps

Fuchs coloboma – a congenital inferior crescent on the choroid at the edge of the optic disk. *SYN:* congenital conus

Fuchs crypt

Fuchs dystrophy – congenital degenerative eye disease.

Fuchs epithelial dystrophy – epithelial edema secondary to endothelial dystrophy of the cornea.

Fuchs heterochromic cyclitis – *SYN:* Fuchs syndrome

Fuchs keratome

Fuchs phenomenon – degeneration of third cranial nerve resulting in paradoxical retraction of lid in association with eye movements.

Fuchs spur – part of the insertion of the dilator muscle onto the iris sphincter.

Fuchs stoma – small depression on the surface of the iris near the margin of the pupil.

Fuchs syndrome – syndrome characterized by heterochromia of the iris, iridocyclitis, keratic precipitates, and cataract. *SYN:* Fuchs heterochromic cyclitis

Fuchs two-way eye syringe

Fuchs uveitis – anterior uveitis and depigmentation of the iris. *SYN:* heterochromic uveitis

Fukala, Vincenz, Austrian ophthalmologist, 1847-1911.

Fukala operation – eye lens removal.

Fukuyama, Yukio, 20th century Japanese physician.

Fukuyama dystrophy – *SYN:* Fukuyama syndrome

Fukuyama syndrome – recessive genetic trait resulting in progressive muscular dystrophy and brain disorders. *SYN:* Fukuyama dystrophy

F

Fürbringer, Paul W., German physician, 1849-1930.

Fürbringer sign – sign related to subphrenic abscess.

Furchgott, Robert F., U.S. pharmacologist, *1916, joint winner of 1998 Nobel Prize for work related to nitric oxide as a signal molecule in biological systems.

Fürmaier, A.

Fürmaier syndrome – lumbar rigidity causing difficulty in forward flexion of lumbar spine, caused by nerve root compression due to tumor or formation of posttraumatic cicatrix.

Furst, William, U.S. physician.

Ostrum-Furst syndrome – see under Ostrum

Futcher, Palmer Howard, U.S.-Canadian physician, *1910.

Futcher line – a dorsoventral line of pigmentation occurring symmetrically and bilaterally for about 10 cm along the lateral edge of the biceps muscle. *SYN:* Voigt lines

Gabler, Hedda, main character in a play by Henrik Ibsen who kills herself during pregnancy to avoid a scandal.

> **Hedda Gabler syndrome** – suicide committed while pregnant.

Gabriel, William Bashall, English surgeon, *1893.

> **Gabriel proctoscope**
>
> **Gabriel syringe** – used for injection of hemorrhoids.

Gaddum, John H., English biochemist, *1900.

> **Gaddum and Schild test** – a sensitive method for identification of epinephrine in tissue or other material.

Gaenslen, Frederick J., U.S. surgeon, 1877-1937.

> **Gaenslen fracture**
>
> **Gaenslen incision**
>
> **Gaenslen osteomyelitis**
>
> **Gaenslen sign** – pain on hyperextension of the hip with pelvis fixed by flexion of opposite hip.
>
> **Gaenslen split-heel incision**
>
> **Gaenslen technique**
>
> **Gaenslen test**

Gaertner, Hermann Treschow, Danish surgeon, 1785-1827.

> **Gaetner duct** – mesonephric duct.

Gaffky, Georg T.A., German hygienist, 1850-1918.

> **Gaffky scale** – *SYN:* Gaffky table
>
> **Gaffky table** – a numerical rating for the classification of tuberculosis. *SYN:* Gaffky scale

Gairdner, Sir William T., Scottish physician, 1824-1907.

> **Gairdner disease** – attacks of cardiac distress accompanied by apprehension. *SYN:* angor pectoris; angina pectoris sine dolore

Gaisbock, var. of Gaisböck

NOTES

Gaisböck, (Gaisbock), Felix, German physician, 1868-1955.
   Gaisböck disease – polycythemia associated with hypertension but
      without splenomegaly. *SYN:* Gaisböck syndrome; polycythemia
      hypertonica
   Gaisböck syndrome – *SYN:* Gaisböck disease

Gajdusek, D. Carleton, U.S. pediatrician, *1923, joint winner of 1976 Nobel
Prize for work related to infectious diseases.

Galant, Nikolay Fedorovich, Russian hygienist, *1893.
   Galant abdominal response
   Galant hip guide
   Galant hip prosthesis
   Galant reflex – a deep abdominal reflex in which there is a contraction of
      the abdominal muscles on tapping the anterior superior iliac spine.
      SYN: lower abdominal periosteal reflex

Galeati, Domenico, Italian physician, 1686-1775.
   Galeati glands – the tubular glands in the mucous membrane of the small
      and large intestines. *SYN:* intestinal glands

Galeazzi, Riccardo, Italian surgeon, 1886-1952.
   Galeazzi fracture – fracture of the shaft of the radius with dislocation of
      the distal radioulnar joint.
   Galeazzi patellar operation
   Galeazzi realignment
   Galeazzi sign
   Galeazzi test

Galen, Claudius, Greek physician and medical scientist in Rome, c. 130-201 A.D.
   Galen anastomosis – *SYN:* Galen nerve
   Galen bandage
   Galen dressing
   Galen foramen
   galenical – referring to medicine prepared from plants rather than
      chemicals.
   Galen nerve – communicating branch of superior laryngeal nerve with
      recurrent laryngeal nerve. *SYN:* Galen anastomosis
   Galen ventricle
   great cerebral vein of Galen – a large, unpaired vein formed by the
      junction of the two internal cerebral veins. *SYN:* great vein of Galen
   great vein of Galen – *SYN:* great cerebral vein of Galen
   veins of Galen – *SYN:* internal cerebral veins

Gall, Franz J., German-Austrian anatomist, 1758-1828.
   Gall craniology – an obsolete doctrine. *SYN:* phrenology

Gallais, Alfred, French physician.
   Gallais syndrome – *SYN:* Cushing syndrome

Gallavardin, Louis, French physician, 1875-1957.
   Gallavardin phenomenon – dissociation between the noisy and musical elements of the murmur of aortic stenosis.

Galli, surname of two brothers in whom the disease was first described.
   Galli-Galli disease – inherited disease featuring progressive reticulate hyperpigmentation of flexural areas of the skin.

Gallie, William E., Canadian surgeon, 1882-1959.
   Gallie arthrodesis
   Gallie atlantoaxial fusion technique
   Gallie fascia needle
   Gallie herniorrhaphy
   Gallie procedure
   Gallie spinal fusion
   Gallie subtalar ankle fusion
   Gallie technique
   Gallie tendon passer
   Gallie transplant – narrow strips of the femoral fascia lata used for suture material.

Galton, Sir Francis, English explorer and anthropologist, 1822-1911.
   Galton delta – a more or less well-marked triangle in a fingerprint; in dermatoglyphics, the figure at the base of each finger in the palm. *SYN:* triradius
   Galton law of regression – average parents tend to produce average offspring, but children of extreme parents inherit parental peculiarities to a lesser degree than they appear in the parents. *SYN:* law of regression to mean

G

NOTES

Galton system of classification of fingerprints – a system of classification based on the variations in the patterns of the ridges, which are grouped into arches, loops, and whorls.

Galton whistle – a cylindrical whistle attached to a compressible bulb used to test hearing.

Galvani, Luigi, Italian physician and anatomist, 1737-1798.

galvanic bath – water bath that is charged with galvanic current.

galvanic current – continuous one-direction electric current.

galvanic-faradic test – an electrodiagnostic test of muscles.

galvanic skin response – skin's response to electric stimulation.
  SYN: electrodermal response

galvanism – oral manifestations of direct current electricity occurring when dental restorations with dissimilar electric potentials (such as silver and gold) are placed in the mouth. *SYN:* voltaism

galvanometer – an instrument used to measure current.

Gambia, country in West Africa, bordering North Atlantic Ocean and Senegal.

Gambian sleeping sickness – caused by parasite *Trypanosoma brucei* and transmitted through bite of an infected tsetse fly. *SYN:* trypanosomiasis

Gamborg-Nielsen, P.

Gamborg-Nielsen keratoderma – autosomal dominant type of palmoplantar keratoderma, featuring medium-thick horny layer with a smooth surface.

Gamgee, Joseph Sampson, English surgeon, 1828-1886.

Gamgee tissue – a thick layer of absorbent cotton between two layers of absorbent gauze, used in surgical dressings.

Gammel, John A., U.S. physician.

Gammel syndrome – paraneoplastic disorder resulting in erythematous lesions associated with neoplasms of internal organs. *SYN:* erythema gyratum repens

Gamna, Carlos, Italian physician, 1896-1950.

Gamna disease – a form of chronic splenomegaly.

Gamna-Favre bodies – characteristic, relatively large, intracytoplasmic basophilic inclusion bodies observed in lymphogranuloma venereum.

Gamna-Gandy bodies – small firm spheroidal or irregular foci occurring chiefly in the spleen in such conditions as congestive splenomegaly and sickle cell disease. *SYN:* Gandy-Gamna bodies; siderotic nodules

Gandy-Gamna bodies – *SYN:* Gamna-Gandy bodies

Gamper, E., Austrian neurologist, 1887-1938.

Gamper bowing reflex – when holding the sacrum of severely brain-damaged children and, sometimes, normal but premature infants, the hips are extended and head and trunk elevate in bowlike fashion from supine position.

Gamstorp, Ingrid, Swedish pediatric neurologist, *1924.

Gamstorp disease – dominant trait resulting in periodic paralysis and usually accompanied by hyperkalemia.

Gamstorp-Wohlfart syndrome – genetic trait resulting in muscle wasting, increased muscle contractility, and increased perspiration.

Gandy, Charles, French physician, *1872.

Gamna-Gandy bodies – see under Gamna

Gandy-Gamna bodies – *SYN:* Gamna-Gandy bodies

Gandy-Nanta disease – siderotic splenomegaly.

Ganong, William F., U.S. physiologist, *1924.

Lown-Ganong-Levine syndrome – see under Lown

Ganser, Siegbert J.M., German psychiatrist, 1853-1931.

basal nucleus of Ganser – a group of large cells in the innominate substance, ventral to the lentiform nucleus. *SYN:* nucleus basalis of Ganser

Ganser commissures – the commissural fibers that lie above and behind the optic chiasm. *SYN:* commissurae supraopticae

Ganser syndrome – a psychoticlike condition, without the symptoms and signs of a traditional psychosis, occurring typically in prisoners who feign insanity. *SYN:* nonsense syndrome; syndrome of approximate relevant answers; syndrome of deviously relevant answers

nucleus basalis of Ganser – *SYN:* basal nucleus of Ganser

Gansslen, Max, German physician, 1895-1969.

Gansslen disease – autosomal dominant trait related to familial form of constitutional leukopenia.

G

NOTES

Gant, Samuel, U.S. surgeon, 1870-1944.
Gant clamp – a right-angled clamp used in hemorrhoidectomy.

Gantzer, Carol F.L., 17th century German anatomist.
Gantzer accessory bundle
Gantzer muscle – an accessory muscle extending from the superficial flexor of the digits to the deep flexor of the digits.

Ganz, William, U.S. cardiologist, *1919.
Ganz-Edwards coronary infusion catheter
Swan-Ganz balloon flotation catheter
Swan-Ganz bipolar pacing catheter
Swan-Ganz catheter – see under Swan
Swan-Ganz flow-directed catheter
Swan-Ganz pacing TD catheter

Garbe, William, Canadian dermatologist, *1908.
Sulzberger-Garbe disease – see under Sulzberger
Sulzberger-Garbe syndrome – *SYN:* Sulzberger-Garbe disease

Garceau, George J., U.S. orthopedic surgeon, 1896-1977.
Garceau approach
Garceau bougie
Garceau catheter
Garceau cheilectomy
Garceau clubfoot procedure
Garceau method – a method used to treat fractures of the surgical neck of the humerus.
Garceau tendon technique

Garcin, Raymond, French physician, 1897-1971.
Garcin syndrome – tumors of the nasopharynx involving all or most unilateral cranial nerves without involving the brain.

Garden, Robert Symon, English orthopedic surgeon.
Garden alignment index
Garden classification
Garden femoral neck fracture
Garden grades – classification system for femoral neck fractures (I-IV).
Garden procedure

Gardner, Eldon John, U.S. geneticist, 1909-1987.
Fitzgerald-Gardner syndrome – see under Fitzgerald
Gardner syndrome – multiple polyposis predisposing to carcinoma of the colon.

Gardner, Frank H., U.S. hematologist, *1919.
Gardner-Diamond syndrome – a condition usually occurring in women in which the individual bruises easily. *SYN:* autoerythrocyte sensitization syndrome

Gardner, W.J., U.S. physician.
Gardner syndrome – bilateral acoustic nerve neuromas resulting in progressive loss of hearing and neurologic complications; may result in tumors of the brain, colon, skin, pancreas, skeleton, thyroid, or mandible.

Gareis, Frank J., U.S. physician.
Gareis syndrome – mental retardation, X-linked, associated with missing extensor pollicis brevis tendons causing bilateral thumb clasping.

Gariel, Maurice, French physician, 1812-1878.
Gariel pessary – a hollow, inflatable, rubber pessary made in the form of a ring or a pear.

Garland, George M., U.S. physician, 1848-1926.
Garland triangle – a triangular area of relative resonance in the lower back, found in the same side as a pleural effusion.

Garland, Hugh G., English neurologist. 1903-1967.
Bland-White-Garland syndrome – see under Bland
Garland-Moorhouse syndrome – *SYN:* Marinesco-Sjögren syndrome
Marinesco-Sjögren-Garland syndrome – see under Marinesco

Garré, Carl, Swiss surgeon, 1857-1928.
Garré disease – fusiform thickening or increased density of bones. *SYN:* sclerosing osteitis
Garré osteomyelitis – chronic osteomyelitis with proliferative periostitis; a focal gross thickening of the periosteum with peripheral reactive bone formation resulting from mild infection.

Garrod, Sir Archibald Edward, English physician, 1857-1936.
Garrod hypothesis – one enzyme defect per gene.

NOTES

G

Garrod pads – pads on the dorsum of proximal interphalangeal joints, may be painful on flexion.

Gärtner, August, German physician, 1848-1934.

Gärtner bacillus – a widely distributed species that occurs in humans and in domestic and wild animals, especially rodents. *SYN: Salmonella enteritidis*

Gärtner method – a method of measuring venous pressure.

Gärtner tonometer – an apparatus for estimating blood pressure.

Gärtner vein phenomenon – fullness of the veins of the arm and hand held below heart level and collapsed at a certain variable distance above that level.

Gartner, Herman T., Danish anatomist and surgeon, 1785-1827.

Gartner canal – a rudimentary vestige of the mesonephric duct in the female into which the tubules of the epoöphoron open. *SYN:* Gartner duct; longitudinal duct of epoöphoron

Gartner cyst – a cyst of the principal duct in the vestigial structures of the paroöphoron in the cervix or anterolateral vaginal wall.

Gartner duct – *SYN:* Gartner canal

Gaskell, Walter H., English physiologist, 1847-1914.

Gaskell bridge – a bundle of modified cardiac muscle fibers. *SYN:* atrioventricular bundle

Gaskell clamp – an instrument for crushing the atrioventricular bundle in experimental animals and thus producing heart block.

Gass, J. Donald M., U.S. ophthalmologist, *1928.

Gass cannula

Gass cataract-aspirating cannula

Gass corneoscleral punch

Gass muscle hook

Gass scleral marker

Gass scleral punch

Irvine-Gass syndrome – see under Irvine

Gasser, Johann L., Austrian anatomist, 1723-1765.

gasserian ganglion – the large flattened sensory ganglion of the trigeminal nerve. *SYN:* trigeminal ganglion

Gasser, Konrad J., Swiss pediatrician, *1912.

Gasser cells – cytoplasmic inclusions that stain dark red-purple.

Gasser syndrome – (1) acute transient erythropoietic tissue aplasia, in children; no known cause; (2) acute renal failure, hemolytic anemia, and other disorders occurring in children under the age of 4; often associated with *Escherichia coli* infection-induced diarrhea.

Gastaut, Henri, French biologist, *1915.

Gastaut syndrome – juvenile hemiplegic epilepsy with ipsilateral signs.

Lennox-Gastaut syndrome – see under Lennox

Gatch, Willis Dew, U.S. surgeon, 1878-1961.

Gatch bed – a bed with 3 sections for independent elevation of a patient's head and knees.

Gaucher, Philippe Charles Ernest, French physician, 1854-1918.

Gaucher cells – large, finely and uniformly vacuolated cells derived from the reticuloendothelial system and found especially in the spleen, lymph nodes, liver, and bone marrow of patients with Gaucher disease.

Gaucher disease – a lysosomal storage disease. *SYN:* cerebroside lipidosis; familial splenic anemia

Gaucher type of histiocyte

pseudo-Gaucher cell – a plasma cell, microscopically resembling a Gaucher cell, found in the bone marrow in some cases of multiple myeloma.

Gauer, Otto Hans, German physiologist, 1909-1979.

Henry-Gauer response – see under Henry, James Paget

Gauss, Johann K.F., German physicist, 1777-1855.

gauss – a unit of magnetic field intensity.

gaussian curve – a specific bell-shaped frequency distribution. *SYN:* gaussian distribution; normal distribution

gaussian distribution – *SYN:* gaussian curve

Gauss, Karl J., German gynecologist, 1875-1957.

Gauss sign – marked mobility of the uterus in the early weeks of pregnancy.

Gaussel, A., French physician, 1871-1937.

Grasset-Gaussel phenomenon – *SYN:* Grasset phenomenon

G

Gavard, Hyacinthe, French anatomist, 1753-1802.
Gavard muscle – oblique fibers in the muscular coat of the stomach.

Gay, Alexander H., Russian anatomist, 1842-1907.
Gay glands – large apocrine sweat glands surrounding the anus.
SYN: circumanal glands

Gayet, Charles Jules Alphonse, French physician, 1833-1904.
Gayet disease – *SYN:* Wernicke syndrome
Gayet-Wernicke syndrome – *SYN:* Wernicke syndrome

Gay-Lussac, Joseph L., French naturalist, 1778-1850.
Gay-Lussac equation – the overall chemical equation for alcoholic
fermentation.
Gay-Lussac law – *SYN:* Charles law

Gee, Samuel J., English pediatrician and physician, 1839-1911.
Gee disease – malabsorption syndrome in infants. *SYN:* Gee-Herter
disease; Gee-Thaysen disease; Heubner-Herter disease
Gee-Herter disease – *SYN:* Gee disease
Gee-Thaysen disease – *SYN:* Gee disease

Gegenbaur, Carl, German anatomist, 1826-1903.
Gegenbaur cell – bone-producing cell.

Gehrig, Henry Louis, U.S. baseball player for the New York Yankees, 1903-
1941, victim of Lou Gehrig disease.
Lou Gehrig disease – a disease of the motor tracts of the lateral columns
and anterior horns of the spinal cord, causing progressive muscular
atrophy. *SYN:* amyotrophic lateral sclerosis; Aran-Duchenne disease;
Aran-Duchenne dystrophy; Charcot disease; Cruveilhier disease;
Cruveilhier palsy; Duchenne-Aran disease

Geigel, Richard, German physician, 1859-1930.
Geigel reflex – in the female, a contraction of the muscular fibers at the
upper edge of Poupart ligament on gently stroking the inner side of the
thigh.

Geiger, Hans, German physicist, 1882-1945.
Geiger-Müller counter – an instrument for measuring radioactivity by
counting the emission of radioactive particles.
Geiger-Müller tube

Gélineau, Jean Baptiste Edouard, French physician, 1859-1906.
Gélineau disease – *SYN:* Gélineau syndrome
Gélineau-Redlich syndrome – *SYN:* Gélineau syndrome

Gélineau syndrome – a sleep disorder that usually appears in young adulthood. *SYN:* Gélineau disease; Gélineau-Redlich syndrome; narcolepsy

Gell, Philip G., English immunologist, *1914.
   Gell and Coombs reaction – allergic reaction.

Gellé, Marie-Ernst, French otologist, 1834-1923.
   Gellé test – a test of the mobility of the ossicles using a vibrating tuning fork.

Gellerstedt, Nils, *1896.
   Ceelen-Gellerstedt syndrome – see under Ceelen

Gély, Jules A., French surgeon, 1806-1861.
   Gély suture – a cobbler's suture used in closing intestinal wounds.

Gengou, Octave, French bacteriologist, 1875-1957.
   Bordet-Gengou bacillus – see under Bordet
   Bordet-Gengou phenomenon – see under Bordet
   Bordet-Gengou potato blood agar – see under Bordet
   Bordet-Gengou reaction – *SYN:* complement fixation
   Gengou phenomenon – noncellular antigens.

Gennari, Francesco, Italian anatomist, 1750-1795.
   Gennari band – *SYN:* line of Gennari
   Gennari stria – *SYN:* line of Gennari
   line of Gennari – a prominent white line appearing in perpendicular sections of the visual cortex. *SYN:* Gennari band; Gennari stria; stripe of Gennari
   stripe of Gennari – *SYN:* line of Gennari

Georgi, Walter, German bacteriologist, 1889-1920.
   Sachs-Georgi test – see under Sachs, Hans

NOTES

G

Geraghty, John T., U.S. physician, 1876-1924.

Geraghty test – obsolete test for renal function. *SYN:* phenolsulfonphthalein test

Rowntree and Geraghty test – *SYN:* phenolsulfonphthalein test

Gerbasi, Michele, Italian physician, *1900.

Gerbasi anemia – deficiency in maternal milk leading to anemia similar to pernicious anemia in breast-fed infants.

Gerbode, Frank, U.S. cardiothoracic surgeon, 1907-1984.

Gerbode annuloplasty

Gerbode cardiovascular tissue forceps

Gerbode defect – a defect in the interventricular portion of the membranous septum, associated with a communication between the right ventricle and the right atrium through an abnormality in the tricuspid valve.

Gerbode dilator

Gerbode mitral dilator

Gerbode mitral valvulotome

Gerbode mitral valvulotomy dilator

Gerbode patent ductus clamp

Gerbode rib spreader

Gerbode sternal retractor

Gerbode valve dilator

Gerdy, Pierre N., French surgeon, 1797-1856.

Gerdy fibers – a thickening of the deep fascia in the most distal part of the base of the triangular palmar aponeurosis. *SYN:* superficial transverse metacarpal ligament

Gerdy fontanel – an occasional fontanel-like defect in the sagittal suture in the newborn. *SYN:* sagittal fontanel

Gerdy hyoid fossa – a space that contains the bifurcation of the common carotid artery. *SYN:* carotid triangle

Gerdy interatrial loop – a muscular fasciculus in the interatrial septum of the heart, passing backward from the atrioventricular groove.

Gerdy ligament – the continuation of the clavipectoral fascia downward to attach to the axillary fascia. *SYN:* suspensory ligament of axilla

Gerdy tubercle – a tubercle on the lateral side of the upper end of the tibia giving attachment to the iliotibial tract and some fibers of the tibialis anterior muscle.

Gerhardt, Carl Adolf Christian Jacob, German physician, 1833-1902.

Gerhardt disease – *SYN:* Gerhardt-Mitchell disease

Gerhardt-Mitchell disease – paroxysmal throbbing and burning pain in the skin affecting the hands and feet, accompanied by a dusky mottled redness of the parts with increased skin temperature. *SYN:* erythromelalgia; Gerhardt disease; Mitchell disease; Weir Mitchell disease

Gerhardt reaction – *SYN:* Gerhardt test for acetoacetic acid

Gerhardt-Semon law – obsolete law formerly used to account for the position of affected vocal cords after injury to the recurrent laryngeal nerve(s).

Gerhardt sign – complete bilateral paralysis of the adductor muscles of the larynx with severe inspiratory dyspnea. *SYN:* Biermer sign

Gerhardt syndrome – bilateral laryngeal abductor paralysis.

Gerhardt test for acetoacetic acid – *SYN:* Gerhardt reaction

Gerhardt, Charles F., French chemist, 1816-1856.

Gerhardt test for urobilin in the urine – the urobilin is extracted with chloroform and then treated with iodine and potassium hydrate.

Gerlach, Joseph, German anatomist, 1820-1896.

Gerlach anular tendon – the thickened portion of the circumference of the tympanic membrane that is fixed in the tympanic sulcus. *SYN:* fibrocartilaginous ring of tympanic membrane

Gerlach tonsil – a collection of lymphoid nodules near the pharyngeal opening of the auditory tube. *SYN:* tubal tonsil

Gerlach valve – a fold of mucous membrane, simulating a valve, sometimes found at the origin of the vermiform appendix. *SYN:* valve of vermiform appendix; valvula processus vermiformis

Gerlach valvula – the network of fibers at the iridocorneal angle between the anterior chamber of the eye and the venous sinus of the sclera. *SYN:* trabecular reticulum

NOTES

G

Gerlier, Felix, Swiss physician, 1840-1914.

Gerlier disease – a paroxysmal attack of severe vertigo, not accompanied by deafness or tinnitus, due to unilateral vestibular dysfunction. *SYN:* Gerlier syndrome; vestibular neuronitis

Gerlier syndrome – *SYN:* Gerlier disease

Gerold, M., German physician.

Baller-Gerold syndrome – see under Baller

Gerold-Baller syndrome – *SYN:* Baller-Gerold syndrome

Gerota, Dimitru, Romanian anatomist and surgeon, 1867-1939.

Gerota capsule – *SYN:* Gerota fascia

Gerota fascia – the condensation of the fibroareolar tissue and fat surrounding the kidney to form a sheath for the organ. *SYN:* Gerota capsule; renal fascia

Gerota method – injection of the lymphatics with a dye that is soluble in chloroform or ether but not in water.

Gersh, Isidore, U.S. histologist, *1907.

Altmann-Gersh method – see under Altmann

Gerstmann, Josef, Austrian neurologist, 1887-1969.

Gerstmann-Sträussler-Scheinker syndrome

Gerstmann-Sträussler syndrome – a more chronic cerebellar form of spongiform encephalopathy.

Gerstmann syndrome – finger agnosia, agraphia, confusion of laterality of body, and acalculia caused by lesions between the occipital area and the angular gyrus.

Geschickter, Charles F., U.S. physician.

Geschickter tumor – a bone tumor, often malignant, occurring most frequently in adults between the ages of 20 and 40; found on the femur or humerus.

Gesell, Arnold L., U.S. psychologist, 1880-1961.

Gesell Development Scales – designed to test the development of infants and preschoolers. *SYN:* Gesell test

Gesell test – *SYN:* Gesell Development Scales

Gey, George O., U.S. physician and researcher, *1899.

Gey solution – a salt solution used for culturing animal cells.

Ghilarducci, Francesco, Italian physician, 1857-1924.

Ghilarducci reaction

Ghon, Anton, Czech pathologist, 1866-1936.

Ghon complex – *SYN:* Ghon tubercle

Ghon focus – *SYN:* Ghon tubercle
Ghon lesion
Ghon node
Ghon primary lesion – *SYN:* Ghon tubercle
Ghon-Sachs bacillus – *SYN:* Sachs bacillus
Ghon tubercle – calcification seen in pulmonary parenchyma and hilar
   nodes resulting from earlier infection with tuberculosis. *SYN:* Ghon
   complex; Ghon focus; Ghon primary lesion

Giacomini, Carlo, Italian anatomist, 1841-1898.
   band of Giacomini – *SYN:* uncus band of Giacomini
   frenulum of Giacomini – *SYN:* uncus band of Giacomini
   uncus band of Giacomini – a slender whitish band crossing transversally
      the surface of the recurved part of the uncus gyri parahippocampalis.
      SYN: band of Giacomini; cauda fasciae dentatae; frenulum of Giacomini;
      tail of dentate gyrus

Gianelli, Giuseppe, Italian physician, 1799-1871.
   Gianelli sign – *SYN:* Tournay phenomenon

Giannuzzi, Giuseppe, Italian anatomist, 1839-1876.
   Giannuzzi crescents – the serous cells at the distal end of a mucous,
      tubuloalveolar secretory unit of certain salivary glands. *SYN:* Giannuzzi
      demilunes; serous demilunes
   Giannuzzi demilunes – *SYN:* Giannuzzi crescents

Gianotti, Ferdinando, Italian pediatric dermatologist, 1920-1984.
   Gianotti-Crosti syndrome – a cutaneous manifestation of hepatitis B
      infection occurring in young children. *SYN:* papular acrodermatitis of
      childhood

Giard, Alfred, French biologist, 1846-1908.
   Giardia lamblia – protozoa which causes diarrhea and abdominal
      discomfort.
   giardiasis – infection with *Giardia*.

NOTES

Gibbon, John H., U.S. surgeon, 1903-1973.
   Landis-Gibbon test – see under Landis
   Mayo-Gibbon heart-lung machine – see under Mayo, Charles Horace

Gibbon, Norman Otway Knight, English urologist.
   Gibbon catheter – urinary catheter.
   Gibbon hydrocele
   Gibbon ureteral stent

Gibbs, J. Willard, U.S. mathematician and physicist, 1839-1903.
   Gibbs-Donnan equilibrium – *SYN:* Donnan equilibrium
   Gibbs energy of activation – energy that must be added to that already
      possessed by a molecule(s) in order to initiate a reaction.
   Gibbs free energy
   Gibbs-Helmholtz equation – an equation expressing the relationship in a
      galvanic cell between the chemical energy transformed and the maximal
      electromotive force obtainable. *SYN:* Helmholtz-Gibbs theory
   Gibbs theorem – substances that lower the surface tension of the pure
      dispersion medium tend to collect in its surface, whereas substances
      that raise the surface tension tend to remain out of the surface film.
   Helmholtz-Gibbs theory – *SYN:* Gibbs-Helmholtz equation

Gibert, Camille Melchior, French dermatologist, 1797-1866.
   Gibert disease – a common inflammatory skin disorder presenting as an
      acute, self-limiting, papulosquamous eruption with a 6- to 8-week
      duration. Unknown etiology, although most probably infectious.
      SYN: Gibert pityriasis rosea
   Gibert pityriasis rosea – *SYN:* Gibert disease

Gibney, Virgil P., U.S. orthopedist, 1847-1927.
   Gibney bandage
   Gibney boot – adhesive tape treatment of a sprained ankle.
   Gibney disease
   Gibney dressing
   Gibney fixation bandage – herring bone strapping of the foot and leg for
      sprain of the ankle.
   Gibney perispondylitis
   Gibney strapping

Gibson, George A., Scottish physician, 1854-1913.
   Gibson murmur – the typical continuous murmur of patent ductus
      arteriosus.

Gibson, Kasson C., U.S. dentist, 1849-1925.
   Gibson bandage – a bandage for stabilizing a fracture of the mandible.

Gibson, Quentin Howieson, English physician.
Gibson disease – recessive trait which renders hemoglobin unable to bind with oxygen, causing dyspnea and fatigue after physical exertion.

Giedion, Andreas, Swiss pediatric cardiologist, *1925.
Giedion syndrome – genetic recessive or dominant trait causing orofacial defects and abnormalities of the phalanges. *SYN:* trichorhinophalangeal syndrome
Langer-Giedion syndrome – see under Langer, Leonard O., Jr.

Giemsa, Gustav, German bacteriologist, 1867-1948.
Giemsa chromosome banding stain – a unique chromosome staining technique used in human cytogenetics to identify individual chromosomes. *SYN:* G-banding stain
Giemsa stain – compound used for demonstrating Negri bodies, *Tunga* species, spirochetes and protozoans, and differential staining of blood smears.

Gierke, Edgar von, German pathologist, 1877-1945.
Fibiger-Debré-von Gierke syndrome – *SYN:* Debré-Fibiger syndrome
Gierke disease – glycogenosis due to glucose 6-phosphatase deficiency, resulting in accumulation of excessive amounts of glycogen of normal chemical structure, particularly in liver and kidney. *SYN:* type 1 glycogenosis; von Gierke disease; von Gierke syndrome
von Gierke disease – *SYN:* Gierke disease
von Gierke syndrome – *SYN:* Gierke disease

Gierke, Hans P.B., German anatomist, 1847-1886.
Gierke corpuscles – *SYN:* thymic corpuscles
Gierke respiratory bundle – primary sensory fibers that enter with the vagus, glossopharyngeal, and facial nerves, and in part convey information from stretch receptors and chemoreceptors in the walls of the cardiovascular, respiratory, and intestinal tracts. *SYN:* solitary tract

Gieson, Ira van, see under van Gieson

G

NOTES

Gifford, Harold, U.S. ophthalmologist, 1858-1929.
    Gifford applicator
    Gifford corneal applicator
    Gifford corneal curette
    Gifford fixation forceps
    Gifford holder
    Gifford iris forceps
    Gifford keratotomy
    Gifford needle holder
    Gifford reflex – constriction of both pupils when an effort is made to close eyelids forcibly held apart. *SYN:* eye-closure pupil reaction
    Gifford sign – difficulty in everting the upper eyelid in Graves disease.

Gigli, Leonardo, Italian gynecologist, 1863-1908.
    Gigli operation – severance of the pubic bone a few centimeters lateral to the symphysis to permit the passage of a living child. *SYN:* pubiotomy
    Gigli pubiotomy
    Gigli saw – a hand-held wire saw for use in craniotomy or pubiotomy.
    Gigli-saw blade
    Gigli-saw conductor
    Gigli-saw guide
    Gigli-saw handle
    Gigli-saw wire

Gilbert, Nicholas A., French physician, 1858-1927.
    Gilbert disease – *SYN:* familial nonhemolytic jaundice
    Gilbert syndrome – *SYN:* familial nonhemolytic jaundice

Gilbert, Walter, U.S. microbiologist and Nobel laureate, *1932.
    Maxim-Gilbert sequencing – see under Maxim

Gilbert-Dreyfus, Savoie, French physician.
    Gilbert-Dreyfus syndrome – *SYN:* androgen insensitivity syndrome, partial; incomplete testicular feminization

Gilchrist, Thomas Casper, U.S. physician, 1862-1927.
    Gilchrist disease – a chronic granulomatous and suppurative disease caused by *Blastomyces dermatitidis*. *SYN:* blastomycosis
    Gilchrist mycosis – obsolete term for blastomycosis.

Gilford, Hastings, English physician, 1861-1941.
    Hutchinson-Gilford disease – see under Hutchinson, Sir Jonathan
    Hutchinson-Gilford syndrome – *SYN:* Hutchinson-Gilford disease

Gilles de la Tourette, Georges, French physician, 1857-1904.
   Gilles de la Tourette disease – *SYN:* Tourette syndrome
   Gilles de la Tourette syndrome – *SYN:* Tourette syndrome
   Tourette disease – *SYN:* Tourette syndrome
   Tourette syndrome – a disorder characterized by multiple motor and vocal
      tics. *SYN:* Gilles de la Tourette disease; Gilles de la Tourette syndrome;
      Tourette disease

Gillespie, Frank D., U.S. ophthalmologist, *1927.
   Gillespie syndrome – hereditary syndrome resulting in absence of the iris
      and other abnormalities.

Gillette, Eugène P., French surgeon, 1836-1886.
   Gillette suspensory ligament – longitudinal fiber of the esophagus that
      attaches to the posterior aspect of the cricoid cartilage of the larynx.
      SYN: cricoesophageal tendon

Gilliam, David Tod, U.S. gynecologist, 1844-1923.
   Gilliam operation – an operation for retroversion of the uterus by suturing
      round ligaments to abdominal wall fascia.
   Gilliam suspension of uterus

Gillies, Sir Harold D., English plastic surgeon, 1882-1960.
   Filatov-Gillies flap – *SYN:* Filatov flap
   Filatov-Gillies tubed pedicle – *SYN:* Filatov flap
   Gillies approach
   Gillies construction of replacement thumb
   Gillies ectropion graft
   Gillies elevation procedure
   Gillies flap
   Gillies graft
   Gillies hook
   Gillies horizontal dermal suture
   Gillies implant
   Gillies incision

G

NOTES

Gillies needle holder
Gillies operation – a technique for reducing fractures of the zygoma and the zygomatic arch through an incision in the temporal region above the hairline.
Gillies prosthesis
Gillies scissors
Gillies skin hook
Gillies tissue forceps
Gillies up-and-down flap
Gillies zygomatic hook

Gilman, Alfred G., joint winner of 1994 Nobel Prize for work related to G-proteins.

Gilmer, Thomas L., U.S. oral surgeon, 1849-1931.
Gilmer intermaxillary fixation – *SYN:* Gilmer wiring
Gilmer tooth splint
Gilmer wiring – a method of intermaxillary fixation in which single opposing teeth are wired circumferentially, and the wires are twisted together. *SYN:* Gilmer intermaxillary fixation

Gil-Vernet, Jose Maria Vila, Spanish urologist, *1922.
Gil-Vernet dissection
Gil-Vernet operation – extension of a standard pyelotomy into the lower pole infundibulum through the avascular plane between the posterior and basilar segmental renal arteries. *SYN:* extended pyelotomy
Gil-Vernet pyelolithotomy
Gil-Vernet renal sinus retractor
Gil-Vernet retractor

Gimard, see under Martin de Gimard

Gimbel, Howard V., Canadian ophthalmologist, *1934, invented continuous-tear capsulotomy technique and divide-and-conquer phacoemulsification technique.

Gimbernat, Don Manuel L.A. de, Spanish anatomist and surgeon, 1734-1816.
Gimbernat ligament – a curved fibrous band that forms the medial boundary of the femoral ring. *SYN:* lacunar ligament

Giovannini, Sebastiano, Italian physician, 1851-1920.
Giovannini disease – fungal infection of the hair.

Girard, A., Swiss-born U.S. surgeon, 1841-1914.
Girard reagent – the hydrazine of betaine chloride, used to extract ketonic steroids by forming water-soluble hydrazones with them.

Girdlestone, Gathorne Robert, English orthopaedist, 1881-1950.
Girdlestone procedure – complete resection or excision of the head and neck of the femur.
Girdlestone resection
Girdlestone resection arthroplasty

Giroux, Jean Marie, Canadian physician.
Giroux-Barbeau syndrome – dominant trait causing plaques in the neonate with development of neurologic disorders in adulthood.

Givens, Maurice H., U.S. biochemist, *1888.
Givens method – measurement of digestion.

Gjessing, Leiv Rolvssoen, Norwegian physician, *1918.
Gjessing syndrome – nitrogen retention resulting in periodic catatonia which responds to thyroid therapy.

Glanzmann, Eduard, Swiss clinician, 1887-1959.
Glanzmann disease – *SYN:* Glanzmann thrombasthenia
Glanzmann-Naegeli syndrome– *SYN:* Glanzmann thrombasthenia
Glanzmann and Riniker lymphocytophthisis – agammaglobulinemia, absent thymus, severe cytopenia, recurring infections, and inability to form antibodies.
Glanzmann thrombasthenia – a hemorrhagic diathesis due to defect in platelet membrane glycoprotein IIb-IIIa complex. *SYN:* constitutional thrombopathy; Glanzmann disease; Glanzmann-Naegeli syndrome; hereditary hemorrhagic thrombasthenia

Glaser, Johann H., Swiss anatomist, 1629-1675.
glaserian artery – *SYN:* anterior tympanic artery
glaserian fissure – *SYN:* petrotympanic fissure

G

NOTES

Glasgow, William C., U.S. physician, 1845-1907.
Glasgow sign – a systolic murmur heard over the brachial artery in aortic aneurysm.

Glauber, Johann R., German chemist, 1604-1668.
Glauber salt – an ingredient of many of the natural laxative waters, and also used as a hydragogue cathartic. *SYN:* sodium sulfate

Gleason, Donald F., U.S. pathologist, *1920.
Gleason score
Gleason tumor grade – a classification of adenocarcinoma of the prostate.

Glénard, F., French physician, 1848-1920.
Glénard disease – intraabdominal organ ptosis.

Glenn, William Wallace Lumpkin, U.S. cardiovascular surgeon, 1914-2003.
Glenn operation – superior vena cava to pulmonary artery shunt to bypass right side of heart.

Glenner, George B., U.S. pathologist and histologist, *1927.
Glenner-Lillie stain for pituitary – a modification of Mann methyl blue-eosin stain.

Gley, Marcel E.E., French physiologist, 1857-1930.
Gley cells – testicular interstitial cells.
Gley glands

Glisson, Francis, English physician, anatomist, physiologist and pathologist, 1597-1677.
Glisson capsule – a layer of connective tissue ensheathing the liver, hepatic artery, portal vein, and bile ducts. *SYN:* fibrous capsule of liver
Glisson cirrhosis – chronic perihepatitis with thickening and subsequent contraction, resulting in atrophy and deformity of the liver. *SYN:* capsular cirrhosis of liver
Glisson disease
Glisson sling – used in cervical traction to support the head.
Glisson sphincter – the smooth muscle sphincter of the hepatopancreatic ampulla within the duodenal papilla. *SYN:* sphincter of hepatopancreatic ampulla

Glogau, Richard G., U.S. dermatologist.
Glogau classification – used to document the level of actinic damage present prior to chemical peeling procedures.

Gluge, Gottlieb, German histologist, 1812-1898.
Gluge corpuscles – large pus cells containing fat droplets.

Gmelin, Leopold, German physiologist and chemist, 1788-1853.
   Gmelin test – a test for bile in body fluid. *SYN:* Rosenbach-Gmelin test
   Rosenbach-Gmelin test – *SYN:* Gmelin test

Godélier, Charles P., French physician, 1813-1877.
   Godélier law – tuberculosis of the peritoneum is always associated with tuberculosis of the pleura on one or both sides.

Godman, John D., U.S. anatomist, 1794-1830.
   Godman fascia – an extension of the pretracheal fascia into the thorax and onto the pericardium.

Godtfredsen, Erik, English ophthalmologist, *1913.
   Godtfredsen syndrome – invasive tumor of the cavernous sinus causing ipsilateral blindness, trigeminal neuralgia, paralysis of 12th cranial nerve, and ophthalmoplegia.

Godwin, John T., U.S. pathologist, *1917.
   Godwin tumor – benign tumorlike masses of lymphoid tissue in the parotid gland, containing scattered small islands of epithelial cells. *SYN:* benign lymphoepithelial lesion

Goeckerman, William H., U.S. dermatologist, 1884-1954.
   Goeckerman light therapy
   Goeckerman treatment – a treatment for psoriasis.

Goedel, A., German physician.
   Epstein-Goedel syndrome – see under Epstein, E.

Goeminne, Luc, Belgian physician.
   Goeminne syndrome – congenital disorder resulting in torticollis, facial asymmetry, renal problems, pigmented nevi, varicose veins of lower extremities, hyperpigmentation.

Gofman, Moses, German physician, *1887.
   Gofman test – a test for various serum lipoproteins that contain cholesterol, as an index of the tendency to the development of atheromatous lesions and arteriosclerosis.

G

NOTES

Goggia, Carlo P., Italian physician, 1871-1948.
Goggia sign – fibrillation of the biceps muscle, when pinched and tapped, is confined to a limited area in cases of debilitating disease, whereas in health it is general.

Goldberg, Morton F., U.S. physician, *1937.
Goldberg syndrome – galactosialidosis.

Goldblatt, Harry, U.S. pathologist, 1891-1977.
Goldblatt clamp
Goldblatt hypertension – increased blood pressure following obstruction of blood flow to one kidney. *SYN:* Goldblatt phenomenon
Goldblatt kidney – a kidney whose arterial blood supply has been compromised, as a consequence of which arterial hypertension develops.
Goldblatt phenomenon – *SYN:* Goldblatt hypertension

Goldenhar, Maurice, French physician, 1924-2001.
Goldenhar syndrome – a syndrome characterized by epibulbar dermoids, preauricular appendages, micrognathia, and vertebral and other anomalies. *SYN:* oculoauriculovertebral dysplasia

Goldflam, Samuel V., Polish neurologist, 1852-1932.
Erb-Goldflam disease – *SYN:* Goldflam disease
Goldflam disease – disorder of neuromuscular transmission, marked by fluctuating weakness, of oculofacial and proximal limb muscles. *SYN:* Erb-Goldflam disease; Goldflam symptom complex; Hoppe-Goldflam disease; myasthenia gravis
Goldflam symptom complex – *SYN:* Goldflam disease
Hoppe-Goldflam disease – *SYN:* Goldflam disease

Goldman, David E., U.S. physiologist, *1911.
Goldman equation – an equation derived to predict membrane potentials in terms of the membrane's permeability to ions and their concentrations on either side. *SYN:* constant field equation; Goldman-Hodgkin-Katz equation
Goldman-Hodgkin-Katz equation – *SYN:* Goldman equation

Goldman, Henry M., U.S. periodontist, *1911.
Goldman-Fox knives – a set of knives used in periodontal surgery.

Goldmann, Hans, Swiss ophthalmologist, 1899-1991.
Goldmann applanation tonometer – an applanation tonometer that flattens only 3 sq mm of cornea, used with a slit-lamp.
Goldmann contact lens

Goldmann contact lens prism
Goldmann expressor
Goldmann goniolens
Goldmann implant
Goldmann lens
Goldmann macular contact lens
Goldmann multimirror lens implant
Goldmann perimeter – a projection perimeter that adds further precision by controlling the surrounding illumination.
Goldmann serrated knife
Goldmann tonometer

Goldscheider, Johannes Karl August Eugen Alfred, German neurologist, 1858-1935.
Goldscheider disease – loosening of the epidermis with formation of bullae. *SYN:* epidermolysis bullosa
Goldscheider test – determination of the temperature sense by touching the skin with a sharp-pointed metallic rod, heated to varying degrees.

Goldstein, Hyman Isaac, U.S. physician, 1887-1954.
Goldstein toe sign – increased space between the great toe and the second toe, seen in mongolism and occasionally in cretinism.

Goldstein, Joseph L., U.S. physician, *1940, joint winner of 1985 Nobel Prize for work related to cholesterol.

Goldstein, K., U.S. neurologist, 1878-1965.
Goldstein catastrophic reaction – when trying to perform a cognitive skill which has been lost, patients are seen to exhibit extreme agitation and anger.

Goldthwait, Joel E., U.S. surgeon, 1866-1961.
Goldthwait sign – in sprain of sacroiliac ligaments, flexion of the hip with extended knee elicits pain in the sacroiliac region.

G

NOTES

Golé, L., 20th century French physician.
Touraine-Solente-Golé syndrome – see under Touraine

Golgi, Camillo, Italian histologist and Nobel laureate, 1844-1926.
Golgi apparatus – a membranous system of cisternae and vesicles concerned with intracellular transport of membrane-bounded secretory proteins. *SYN:* dictyosome; Golgi body; Golgi complex; Golgi internal reticulum; Holmgrén-Golgi canals
Golgi body – *SYN:* Golgi apparatus
Golgi cells
Golgi complex – *SYN:* Golgi apparatus
Golgi corpuscle
Golgi internal reticulum – *SYN:* Golgi apparatus
Golgi-Mazzoni corpuscle – an encapsulated sensory nerve ending.
Golgi osmiobichromate fixative – an osmic-bichromate mixture used to demonstrate nerve cells and their processes.
Golgi stain – any of several methods for staining nerve cells, nerve fibers, and neuroglia.
Golgi tendon organ – a proprioceptive sensory nerve ending embedded among the fibers of a tendon. *SYN:* neurotendinous organ; neurotendinous spindle
Golgi zone – part of the cytoplasm occupied by the Golgi apparatus.
Holmgrén-Golgi canals – *SYN:* Golgi apparatus

Goll, Friedrich, Swiss anatomist, 1829-1903.
Goll column – *SYN:* fasciculus gracilis
nucleus of Goll – the medial one of the three nuclei of the dorsal column. *SYN:* gracile nucleus
tract of Goll – *SYN:* fasciculus gracilis

Goltz, Robert William, U.S. dermatologist, *1923.
Goltz syndrome – *SYN:* focal dermal hypoplasia

Gombault, François A.A., French neurologist and pathologist, 1844-1904.
Gombault triangle

Gomori, George, Hungarian histochemist in the U.S., 1904-1957.
Gomori chrome alum hematoxylin-phloxine stain – a technique used to demonstrate cytoplasmic granules.
Gomori method for chromaffin
Gomori nonspecific alkaline phosphatase stain – for histological demonstration of enzymes.
Gomori one-step trichrome stain – a connective tissue stain.

Gomori silver impregnation stain – a reliable method for reticulin, as an aid in the diagnosis of neoplasm and early cirrhosis of the liver.

Grocott-Gomori methenamine-silver stain – a modification of Gomori methenamine-silver stain for fungi.

Gompertz, Benjamin, English actuary, 1779-1865.

Gompertz hypothesis – a theory that the force of mortality increases in geometrical progression.

Gompertz law – after age 35-40, the increase in mortality with age tends to be logarithmic.

Gonin, Jules, Swiss ophthalmic surgeon, 1870-1935.

Gonin cautery

Gonin marker

Gonin operation – retinal detachment repair.

Good, Robert A., U.S. pediatrician, *1922.

Good syndrome – agammaglobulinemia resulting in recurrent infections.

Goodell, William, U.S. gynecologist, 1829-1894.

Goodell dilator – obsolete term for a uterine dilator.

Goodell sign – softening of the cervix and vagina as being usually indicative of pregnancy.

Goodenough, Florence L., U.S. psychologist, *1886.

Goodenough Draw-a-Man Test – an intelligence test.

Goodman, Richard M., Israeli geneticist, 1932-1987.

Goodman syndrome – a hereditary syndrome of congenital deafness and onychodystrophy.

Goodpasture, Ernest W., U.S. pathologist, 1886-1960.

Goodpasture disease

Goodpasture epitope

Goodpasture reactivity

Goodpasture stain – a stain for gram-negative bacteria, using aniline fuchsin.

NOTES

G

Goodpasture syndrome – glomerulonephritis that usually progresses rapidly to produce death from renal failure, and the lungs at autopsy show extensive hemosiderosis or recent hemorrhage.

Goodsall, David H., English surgeon, 1843-1906.
Goodsall rule – a guide for classifying anal fistulas.

Goormaghtigh, Norbert, Belgian physician, 1890-1960.
Goormaghtigh cells – modified smooth muscle cells primarily of the afferent arteriole of the renal glomerulus. *SYN:* juxtaglomerular cells

Gopalan, C., Indian biochemist, *1918.
Gopalan syndrome – severe discomfort of the feet associated with elevated skin temperature and excessive sweating.

Gordius, in Greek mythology, a peasant in a cart who became the king of Phrygia after an oracle's prediction; he tied his cart to a pole with a complicated knot which was later severed, legend has it, by Alexander the Great.
Gordius worm – long, thin parasites resembling horse hairs, often existing in an intricately tangled mass. *SYN:* horse hair worm

Gordon, Alfred, U.S. neurologist, 1874-1953.
Gordon reflex – dorsal flexion of the great toe produced by firm lateral pressure on the calf muscles. *SYN:* paradoxical flexor reflex
Gordon sign – a sign of organic hemiplegia. *SYN:* finger phenomenon
Gordon symptom – the occurrence of an appreciable interval after the production of a reflex before relaxation. *SYN:* tonic reflex

Gordon, Hymie, South African physician.
Gordon syndrome – condition characterized by cleft palate and club foot along with spinal stenosis, narrow intervertebral spaces, and other abnormalities.

Gordon, Mervyn H., English physician, 1872-1953.
Gordon test – a spinal fluid test for proteins.

Gordon, Richard D., Australian endocrinologist, *1934.
Gordon test – a test formerly used for Hodgkin disease.

Gorham, Lemuel W., U.S. physician, 1885-1968.
Gorham disease – extensive decalcification of a single bone. *SYN:* disappearing bone disease

Gorlin, Richard, U.S. physiologist and cardiologist, *1926.
Gorlin formula – a formula for calculating the area of the orifice of a cardiac valve.

Gorlin, Robert James, U.S. oral pathologist, *1923.
Gorlin-Chaudhry-Moss syndrome – craniofacial dysostosis, patent ductus arteriosus, hypertrichosis, hypoplasia of the labia majora, and dental and ocular abnormalities.
Gorlin sign – unusual ease in touching the tip of the nose with the tongue.
Gorlin syndrome – a syndrome of myriad basal cell nevi with development of basal cell carcinomas in adult life. *SYN:* basal cell nevus syndrome

Gorman, P.
Paget-Gorman sign language – *SYN:* Paget sign language

Goslee, Hart J., U.S. dentist, 1871-1930.
Goslee tooth – metal-based artificial tooth.

Gosselin, Léon Athanese, French surgeon, 1815-1887.
Gosselin fracture – V-shaped fracture of distal end of tibia.

Göthlin, Gustaf F., Swedish physiologist, 1874-1949.
Göthlin test – a capillary fragility test to determine the presence or absence of scurvy.

Gottlieb, Bernhard, Viennese dentist, 1885-1950.
Gottlieb epithelial attachment – a band of epithelium that forms a protective barrier between periodontal tissue and materials in the oral cavity.

Gottron, Heinrich Adolf, German physician, 1890-1974.
Arndt-Gottron syndrome – see under Arndt, Georg

Gottschaldt, Kurt, German psychologist, *1902.
Gottschaldt figures – geometric figures used to test perception of forms.

Gottstein, Jacob, German otologist, 1832-1895.
Gottstein fibers – fibers related to auditory nerve.

Gougerot, Claude, French physician.
Beuermann-Gougerot disease – *SYN:* Schenck disease

NOTES

G

Gougerot, Henri, French physician, 1881-1955.
    Gougerot and Blum disease – an eruption of lichenoid papules on the legs. *SYN:* pigmented purpuric lichenoid dermatosis
    Gougerot-Carteaud syndrome – discrete and confluent gray-brown papules of the anterior and posterior midchest. *SYN:* confluent and reticulate papillomatosis
    Gougerot disease – dermatologic disorder resulting in papular lesions, macules and dermal/dermohypodermal nodularity. *SYN:* Gougerot trilogy
    Gougerot-Sjögren disease – *SYN:* Sjögren syndrome
    Gougerot trilogy – *SYN:* Gougerot disease

Gould, Sir Alfred P., English surgeon, 1852-1922.
    Gould electromagnetic flowmeter
    Gould suture – an intestinal mattress suture.

Gouley, John W.S., U.S. urologist, 1832-1920.
    Gouley catheter
    Gouley dilator
    Gouley guide
    Gouley tunneled urethral sound
    Gouley urethral sound

Gouverneur, R., French physician.
    Gouverneur syndrome – fistula of vesicointestinal region with associated suprapubic pain, urinary frequency, pain on urination, and tenesmus.

Gowers, Sir William Richard, English neurologist, 1845-1915.
    Gowers column – a bundle of fibers that conveys proprioceptive and exteroceptive information largely from the opposite lower extremity. *SYN:* anterior spinocerebellar tract; Gowers tract
    Gowers contraction – contraction of the calf muscles when the anterior surface of the leg is struck. *SYN:* front-tap contraction
    Gowers disease – a distal type of progressive muscular dystrophy. *SYN:* saltatory spasm
    Gowers solution – solution used to count red blood cells.
    Gowers syndrome – syndrome consisting of palpitation, chest pain, respiratory difficulties, and disturbances in gastric motility, now considered psychogenic. *SYN:* vagal attack; vasovagal attack
    Gowers tract – *SYN:* Gowers column

Goyer, R.A.
    Goyer syndrome – autosomal dominant condition featuring hearing loss, ichthyosis, and renal disease.

Graaf, Reijnier de, Dutch physiologist and histologist, 1641-1673.
  graafian follicle – a follicle in which the oocyte attains its full size.
    SYN: vesicular ovarian follicle

Gradenigo, Giuseppe, Italian physician, 1859-1926.
  Gradenigo syndrome – petrositis with abducens paralysis and pain in the temporal region, due to localized meningitis involving the fifth and sixth nerves.

Graefe, (Gräfe, Graffe), Albrecht von, German ophthalmologist, 1828-1870.
  Graefe cataract knife
  Graefe disease – chronic progressive ophthalmoplegia.
  Graefe eye speculum
  Graefe forceps – a small thumb forceps with one horizontal row of six or eight delicate teeth across each tip.
  Graefe iris forceps
  Graefe knife – a narrow-bladed knife used in making a section of the cornea.
  Graefe operation – (1) cataract removal by a limbal incision with capsulotomy and iridectomy; (2) iridectomy for glaucoma.
  Graefe sign – in Graves disease, lag of the upper eyelid as it follows the rotation of the eyeball downward. *SYN:* von Graefe sign
  Graefe spots – small areas over the vertebrae or near the supraorbital foramen, pressure upon which causes relaxation of blepharofacial spasm.
  pseudo-Graefe phenomenon – retraction of the upper eyelid on downward movement of the eyes.
  von Graefe cautery
  von Graefe cystotome
  von Graefe electrocautery
  von Graefe knife needle
  von Graefe sign – *SYN:* Graefe sign
  von Graefe strabismus hook

NOTES

Graefenberg, (Gräfenberg), Ernst, German gynecologist in U.S., 1881-1957.
 Graefenberg ring – obsolete term for a silver or silkworm gut ring designed for insertion into the uterine cavity as a means of contraception.

Gräfe, var. of Graefe

Gräfenberg, var. of Graefenberg

Graffe, var. of Graefe

Graffi, Arnold, German pathologist, *1910.
 Graffi virus – a mouse myeloleukemia virus from filtrates of transplantable tumors.

Graham, Evarts Ambrose, U.S. surgeon, 1883-1957.
 Graham-Cole test – a radiographic study of the gallbladder.
   SYN: cholecystography

Graham, Thomas, English chemist, 1805-1869.
 Graham law – the relative rapidity of diffusion of two gases varies inversely as the square root of their densities, i.e., their molecular weights.

Graham Little, see under Little, Sir Ernest Gordon Graham

Graham Steell, see under Steell

Gram, Hans Christian Joachim, Danish bacteriologist, 1853-1938.
 Gram iodine – a solution containing iodine and potassium iodide, used in Gram stain.
 Gram stain – a method for differential staining of bacteria.
 Weigert-Gram stain – see under Weigert

Grancher, Jacques Joseph, French physician, 1843-1907.
 Grancher disease – pneumonia with lung splenization.

Grandry, M., 19th century French anatomist.
 Grandry corpuscles – general sensory endings in the beak, mouth, and tongue of birds.

Granger, Amedee, U.S. radiologist, 1879-1939.
 Granger line – on lateral skull x-ray, the line produced by the groove of the optic chiasm or sulcus prechiasmatis.

Granit, Ragnar A., Finnish-Swedish neurophysiologist and Nobel laureate, 1900-1991.
 Granit loop – the reflex arc consisting of small anterior horn cells and neuroma which initiates the afferent impulses that pass through the posterior root to the anterior horn cells. *SYN:* gamma loop

Grant, R.T.

    Grant syndrome – type of physical urticaria, characterized by multiple small, pruritic wheals surrounded by large areas of erythema, often precipitated by a rise in body core temperature, as in warm bath, exercise, pyrexia.

Grasbeck, Ralph, Finnish physician, *1930.

    Grasbeck-Imerslund syndrome – *SYN:* Imerslund-Grasbeck syndrome
    Imerslund-Grasbeck syndrome – see under Imerslund

Graser, Ernst, German physician, 1860-1929.

    Graser diverticulum – *SYN:* sigmoid diverticulum

Grashey, Hubert, German neurologist.
    Grashey aphasia

Grasset, Joseph, French physician, 1849-1918.

    Grasset-Gaussel phenomenon – *SYN:* Grasset phenomenon
    Grasset law – *SYN:* Landouzy-Grasset law
    Grasset phenomenon – in organic paralysis of the lower extremity, the patient, lying on his back, can raise either limb separately but not both together. *SYN:* Grasset-Gaussel phenomenon
    Grasset sign – normal contraction of the sternocleidomastoid muscle on the paralyzed side in cases of hemiplegia.
    Landouzy-Grasset law – see under Landouzy

Gratiolet, Louis P., French anatomist, physiologist, and physician, 1815-1865.

    Gratiolet fibers – the massive fanlike fiber system passing from the lateral geniculate body of the thalamus to the visual cortex. *SYN:* Gratiolet radiation; optic radiation
    Gratiolet radiation – *SYN:* Gratiolet fibers

Gräupner, Sigurd C., German physician, 1861-1916.

    Gräupner method – obsolete term for a test of the sufficiency of the heart muscle.

NOTES

G

Graves, Robert James, Irish physician, 1796-1853.
   Graves disease – thyroid dysfunction and all or any of its clinical associations. *SYN:* Basedow disease; Marsh disease; ophthalmic hyperthyroidism; Parry disease
   Graves ophthalmopathy – exophthalmos associated with thyroid disease. *SYN:* endocrine ophthalmopathy; Graves orbitopathy
   Graves orbitopathy – *SYN:* Graves ophthalmopathy

Grawitz, Paul, German pathologist, 1850-1932.
   Grawitz basophilia – a condition in which basophilic erythrocytes are found in circulating blood, as in certain instances of leukemia, advanced anemia, malaria, and plumbism. *SYN:* basophilia
   Grawitz tumor – obsolete term for renal adenocarcinoma.

Grebe, Hans, German physician *1913.
   Grebe syndrome – genetic trait resulting in dwarfism with extremely short limbs, legs being more severely affected than arms.

Greeff, C. Richard, German ophthalmologist, 1862-1938.
   Prowazek-Greeff bodies – see under Prowazek

Greene, Charles L., U.S. physician, 1862-1929.
   Greene sign – cardiac border displacement due to pleural effusion.

Greenfield, Joseph G., English neuropathologist, 1884-1958.
   Greenfield disease – metabolic disorder.

Greengard, Paul, U.S. biochemist, *1925, joint winner of 2000 Nobel Prize for work related to nervous system signal transduction.

Greenhow, Edward Headlam, English physician, 1814-1888.
   Greenhow disease – excoriations and melanoderma caused by scratching the bites of the body louse, *Pediculus corporis*. *SYN:* parasitic melanoderma

Gregg, Sir Norman, Australian ophthalmologist, 1902-1966.
   Gregg triad – deafness, cataracts, and heart defects found in children whose mothers contracted rubella while pregnant.

Greig, David M., Scottish physician, 1864-1936.
   Greig syndrome – increased width between the eyes due to an enlarged sphenoid bone. *SYN:* ocular hypertelorism

Greissinger, Georg, German prosthetist, 1903-1972.
   Greissinger foot – prosthetic foot that has ankle motion in all directions.

Greither, Aloys, German dermatologist, 1914-1986.

    Greither keratosis – an autosomal dominant palmoplantar keratoderma that extends onto the dorsa of the hands and feet, with onset in infancy and increasing severity with increasing age. *SYN:* Greither palmoplantar progressive keratoderma; Greither syndrome

    Greither palmoplantar progressive keratoderma – *SYN:* Greither keratosis

    Greither syndrome – *SYN:* Greither keratosis

Greulich, William Walter, radiologist.

    Greulich and Pyle atlas – collection of plates, illustrations, text, and x-rays providing data on bone age.

Grey Turner, see under Turner, George Grey

Gridley, Mary F., U.S. medical technologist, 1908-1954.

    Gridley stain – a silver staining method for reticulum.

    Gridley stain for fungi – a method for fixed tissue sections.

Griesinger, Wilhelm, German neurologist, 1817-1868.

    bilious typhoid of Griesinger – *SYN:* Griesinger disease

    Duchenne-Griesinger disease – *SYN:* Duchenne dystrophy

    Griesinger disease – a severe form of louse-borne relapsing fever caused by *Borrelia recurrentis*. *SYN:* bilious typhoid of Griesinger

    Griesinger symptom – edema of the superficial tissues at the tip of the mastoid process in cases of thrombosis of the sigmoid sinus.

Griffiths, Ruth, English psychologist, *1909.

    Griffiths Mental Development Scale – designed to determine developmental level of infants and children up to age two.

Grignolo, Antonio, Italian ophthalmologist.

    Grignolo syndrome – anterior chamber pus accumulation, inflammation of the iris, uveal inflammation, exudative erythema, frequently exacerbated.

G

NOTES

Grindon, Joseph, U.S. physician.
   Grindon disease – inflammation of hair follicles resulting in reversible baldness.

Grinspan, D., Argentinian physician.
   Grinspan syndrome – lichen planus, hypertension, and diabetes mellitus.

Griscelli, Claude, French physician.
   Griscelli syndrome – genetic trait causing partial albinism and frequent episodes of fever, decrease in blood platelets, and neutropenia.

Grisel, P., French physician.
   Grisel syndrome – torticollis resulting from subluxation of atlantoaxial joint.

Gritti, Rocco, Italian surgeon, 1828-1920.
   Gritti operation – *SYN:* Gritti-Stokes amputation
   Gritti-Stokes amputation – supracondylar amputation of the femur.
   SYN: Gritti operation

Grob, Max, Swiss physician, 1901-1976.
   Grob syndrome – syndrome characterized by craniofacial and digit abnormalities as well as mental deficiency.

Grocco, Pietro, Italian physician, 1857-1916.
   Grocco sign – acute dilation of the heart following a muscular effort.
   Grocco triangle – a triangular patch of dullness at the base of the chest near the spinal column, on the side opposite a pleural effusion.
   SYN: paravertebral triangle
   Orsi-Grocco method – see under Orsi

Groenouw, Arthur, German ophthalmologist, 1862-1945.
   Groenouw corneal dystrophy – a granular type of corneal dystrophy.

Groffith, Joseph, English physician.
   Groffith degeneration – degeneration of undescended testicles.

Grönblad, Ester Elisabeth, Swedish ophthalmologist, 1898-1942.
   Grönblad-Strandberg syndrome – angioid streaks of the retina together with pseudoxanthoma elasticum of the skin.

Gross, Ludwik, 20th century U.S. oncologist.
   Gross leukemia virus – *SYN:* Gross virus
   Gross virus – a strain of mouse leukemia virus. *SYN:* Gross leukemia virus

Gross, Samuel David, U.S. physician, 1805-1884.
   Gross disease – disease in which the walls of the anus develop large pouches which may contain hardened feces.

Grover, Ralph W., U.S. dermatologist, *1920.
Grover disease – a pruritic papular eruption. *SYN:* transient acantholytic dermatosis

Groves, Ernest William Hey, English surgeon, 1872-1944.
Hey Groves clamp – orthopedic clamp.

Grubben, C., Belgian human geneticist.
Grubben syndrome – autosomal recessive syndrome featuring postnatal growth deficiency, hypotonia, psychomotor retardation, partial agenesis of the corpus callosum, abnormal speech development, small hands and feet, eczema, and skin hyperlaxity.

Gruber, George B., German physician, 1884-1977.
Martin-Gruber anastomosis – see under Martin, August E.
Meckel-Gruber syndrome – see under Meckel, Johann Friedrich, the younger

Gruber, Josef, Austrian otologist, 1827-1900.
Gruber method – a modification of the Politzer method (related to permeability of eustachian tube) in which the patient does not swallow, but says "hoc" at the instant of compression of the bag.

Gruber, Max von, German hygienist, 1853-1927.
Gruber reaction – *SYN:* Widal reaction
Gruber-Widal reaction – *SYN:* Widal reaction

Gruber, Wenzel (Wenaslaus) L., Russian anatomist, 1814-1890.
Gruber cul-de-sac – a lateral diverticulum in the suprasternal space.
Gruber-Landzert fossa – the variable peritoneal recess which lies behind the inferior duodenal fold and along the ascending part of the duodenum. *SYN:* inferior duodenal recess

Gruby, David, French physician, 1810-1898.
Gruby disease – *SYN:* tinea tonsurans

Grutz, var. of Grütz

NOTES

Grütz, (Grutz), Otto, German dermatologist, *1886.
  Bürger-Grütz disease – see under Bürger
  Bürger-Grütz syndrome – see under Bürger

Grynfeltt, Joseph C., French surgeon, 1840-1913.
  Grynfeltt triangle – lumbar hernia occurs in this space. *SYN:* Lesshaft
    triangle

Grzybowski, M., Polish dermatologist, 1895-1949.
  Grzybowski disease – sporadic condition in which numerous tiny
    keratoacanthomas develop in an eruptive pattern, often in middle age.

Guarnieri, Giuseppi, Italian physician, 1856-1918.
  Guarnieri bodies – intracytoplasmic acidophilic inclusion bodies observed
    in epithelial cells in smallpox and vaccinia infections, and which include
    aggregations of Paschen bodies or virus particles.
  Guarnieri gelatin agar – a type of agar used for the cultivation of
    Streptococcus pneumoniae.

Gubler, Adolphe, French physician, 1821-1879.
  Gubler line – the level of the superficial origin of the trigeminus on the
    pons, a lesion below which causes Gubler paralysis.
  Gubler paralysis – *SYN:* Gubler syndrome
  Gubler syndrome – a form of alternating hemiplegia characterized by
    contralateral hemiplegia and ipsilateral facial paralysis. *SYN:* Gubler
    paralysis; Millard-Gubler syndrome
  Gubler tumor – a fusiform swelling on the wrist in lead palsy.
  Millard-Gubler syndrome – *SYN:* Gubler paralysis

Gudden, Bernhard A. von, German neurologist, 1824-1886.
  Gudden commissures – the commissural fibers that lie above and behind
    the optic chiasm. *SYN:* commissurae supraopticae
  Gudden ganglion – a median, unpaired, ovoid cell group at the base of
    the midbrain tegmentum between the cerebral peduncles. *SYN:*
    interpeduncular nucleus
  Gudden tegmental nuclei – collective term for two small round cell groups
    in the caudal part of the midbrain associated with the mamillary body by
    way of the mamillary peduncle and mamillotegmental tract. *SYN:*
    tegmental nuclei

Guedel, Arthur Ernest, U.S. anesthetist, *1883.
  Guedel airway – rubber oropharyngeal airway.

Guéneau de Mussy, Noël F.O., French physician, 1813-1885.
   de Mussy point – in the presence of diaphragmatic pleurisy, a point on the left sternal border at the end of the tenth rib which is exceedingly painful when pressure is applied. *SYN:* Guéneau de Mussy point
   Guéneau de Mussy point – *SYN:* de Mussy point

Guérin, Alphonse F.M., French surgeon, 1816-1895.
   Guérin fold – *SYN:* Guérin valve
   Guérin fracture – a fracture of the facial bones. *SYN:* horizontal fracture; Le Fort I fracture
   Guérin glands – *SYN:* glands of the female urethra
   Guérin sinus – a cul-de-sac or diverticulum behind the valve of the navicular fossa.
   Guérin valve – a fold of mucous membrane sometimes found in the root of the navicular fossa of the urethra. *SYN:* Guérin fold; valve of navicular fossa

Guérin, Camille, French bacteriologist, 1872-1961.
   Bacille bilié de Calmette-Guérin – see under Calmette
   Bacille Calmette-Guérin – *SYN:* Bacille bilié de Calmette-Guérin
   bacillus Calmette-Guérin – *SYN:* Bacille bilié de Calmette-Guérin
   bacillus Calmette-Guérin vaccine – see under Calmette
   Calmette-Guérin bacillus – *SYN:* Bacille bilié de Calmette-Guérin
   Calmette-Guérin vaccine – *SYN:* bacillus Calmette-Guérin vaccine

Guidi, Guido, Italian physician, 1508-1569.
   Guidi canal – *SYN:* pterygoid canal

Guillain, Georges, French neurologist, 1876-1961.
   Guillain-Barré reflex – plantar flexion of the foot and toes elicited by tapping the sole near its outer edge. *SYN:* aponeurotic reflex
   Guillain-Barré syndrome – a syndrome marked by paresthesia of the limbs, muscular weakness or a flaccid paralysis, and increased protein in the cerebrospinal fluid without increase in cell count. *SYN:* acute idiopathic polyneuritis

G

NOTES

Landry-Guillain-Barré syndrome – *SYN:* Landry syndrome

Guillemin, Roger, French-U.S. physician, *1924, joint winner of 1977 Nobel Prize for work related to production of peptide hormone.

Guillotin, Joseph I., French physician, 1738-1814.
> **guillotine** – instrument for decapitation; the term is also applied to some surgical instruments that work in a similar fashion.

Guldberg, C., Norwegian chemist, 1862-1902.
> **Guldberg-Waage law** – the rate of a chemical reaction is proportional to the concentrations of the reacting substances. *SYN:* law of mass action

Gull, Sir William Whitey, English physician, 1816-1890.
> **Gull disease** – hypothyroidism.

Gullstrand, Allvar, Swedish ophthalmologist and Nobel laureate, 1862-1930.
> **Gullstrand slitlamp** – in ophthalmology, an instrument consisting of a microscope combined with a rectangular light source that can be narrowed into a slit. *SYN:* slitlamp

Gumprecht, Ferdinand, German physician, *1864.
> **Gumprecht shadows** – immature leukocytes that have undergone partial breakdown. *SYN:* smudge cells
> **Klein-Gumprecht shadow nuclei** – see under Klein, Edward E.

Gunn, Robert Marcus, English ophthalmologist, 1850-1909.
> **Gunn dots** – minute, highly glistening, white or yellowish specks usually seen in the posterior part of the fundus.
> **Gunn phenomenon** – an increase in the width of the eyelids during chewing. *SYN:* Gunn syndrome; jaw-winking syndrome; Marcus Gunn syndrome
> **Gunn pupil** – *SYN:* Marcus Gunn pupil
> **Gunn sign** – compression of the underlying vein at arteriovenous crossings seen ophthalmoscopically in arteriolar sclerosis. *SYN:* Marcus Gunn sign
> **Gunn syndrome** – *SYN:* Gunn phenomenon
> **Marcus Gunn pupil** – relative afferent pupillary defect. *SYN:* Gunn pupil
> **Marcus Gunn sign** – *SYN:* Gunn sign
> **Marcus Gunn syndrome** – *SYN:* Gunn phenomenon

Gunning, var. of Günning

Günning, (Gunning), Jan W., Dutch chemist, 1827-1901.
> **Günning reaction** – the formation of iodoform from acetone by iodine and ammonia in alcohol.
> **Günning test** – test for urine acetone.

Gunning, Thomas B., U.S. dentist, 1813-1889.
   Gunning splint – a prosthesis fabricated from models of edentulous maxillary and mandibular arches in order to aid in reduction and fixation of a fracture.

Günther, Hans, German physician, 1884-1956.
   Günther disease – autosomal recessive type of erythropoietic porphyria.

Günz, Justus, German anatomist, 1714-1751.
   Günz ligament – a portion of the superficial layer of the obturator membrane.

Günzberg, Alfred, German physician, 1861-1937.
   Günzberg reagent – phloroglucin and vanillin used as a reagent in Günzberg test.
   Günzberg test – a test for hydrochloric acid utilizing phloroglucin vanillin (Günzberg reagent), with which a bright red color is produced in the presence of the acid.

Gurdjieff, Georg Ivanovich, Armenian philosopher, 1877-1949.
   Gurdjieff exercises – rhythmic exercises used for self-development.

Gussenbauer, Carl, German surgeon, 1842-1903.
   Gussenbauer suture – a figure-of-eight suture for the intestine, resembling the Czerny-Lembert suture but not including the mucous membrane.

Guthrie, George J., English ophthalmologist, 1785-1856.
   Guthrie muscle – constricts membranous urethra. *SYN:* sphincter urethrae

Guthrie, Robert, U.S. pediatrician, *1916.
   Guthrie test – bacterial inhibition assay for detection of phenylketonuria in the newborn.

Guthrie-Smith, Olive F., English physical therapist, 1883-1956.
   Guthrie-Smith apparatus – *SYN:* Guthrie-Smith bed
   Guthrie-Smith bed – *SYN:* Guthrie-Smith apparatus
   Guthrie-Smith suspension exercises – *SYN:* weightless exercises

NOTES

G

Gutierrez, Robert, U.S. physician, *1895.
    Gutierrez syndrome – *SYN:* horseshoe kidney

Gutmann, Carl, German physician, *1872.
    Michaelis-Gutmann body – see under Michaelis

Guttman, Louis, Israeli psychologist, *1906.
    Guttman scale – attitude scale. *SYN:* cumulative scale

Guttmann, Paul, German physician, 1834-1893.
    Guttmann sign – thyroid gland bruit heard in patients with thyrotoxicosis.

Gutzeit, Max A.G., German chemist, 1847-1915.
    Gutzeit test – a test for arsenic.

Guyon, Felix J.C., French surgeon, 1831-1920.
    Guyon amputation – amputation above the malleoli, a modification of Syme amputation.
    Guyon bougie
    Guyon canal
    Guyon catheter guide
    Guyon clamp
    Guyon curettage
    Guyon dilator
    Guyon exploratory bougie
    Guyon isthmus – an elongated constriction at the junction of the body and cervix of the uterus. *SYN:* isthmus of uterus
    Guyon sign – ballottement of the kidney in cases of nephroptosis, especially when there is also a renal tumor.
    Guyon sound
    Guyon ureteral sound
    Guyon vessel clamp

Haab, Otto, Swiss ophthalmologist, 1850-1931.
    Haab degeneration
    Haab eye knife
    Haab magnet – a magnet that is used to extract metallic foreign bodies
       from the eye.
    Haab needle
    Haab reflex – a pupillary reflex. *SYN:* cerebral cortex reflex
    Haab scleral resection knife

Haber, Henry, Czech-born English dermatopathologist, 1900-1962.
    Haber syndrome – a permanent flushing and telangiectasia of the face
       with prominent follicular openings, small papules with scaling, and
       minute pitted areas.

Habermann, Rudolf, German dermatologist, 1884-1941.
    Habermann disease
    Mucha-Habermann disease – see under Mucha
    Mucha-Habermann syndrome – *SYN:* Mucha-Habermann disease

Hadfield, Geoffrey, English physician, 1889-1968.
    Clarke-Hadfield syndrome – see under Clarke, Cecil

Hadorn, W., Swiss physician.
    Albright-Hadorn syndrome – see under Albright

Haeckel, Ernst, German naturalist, 1834-1919.
    Haeckel gastrea theory – that the two-layered gastrula is the ancestral
       form of all multicellular animals. *SYN:* gastrea theory
    Haeckel law – the theory that ontogeny is an abbreviated recapitulation of
       phylogeny. *SYN:* recapitulation theory

Haenel, Hans G., German neurologist, 1874-1942.
    Haenel symptom – absence of sensation on pressure of the eyeball in the
       tabes.

NOTES

Haenszel, William, U.S. epidemiologist and statistician, *1910.
  Mantel-Haenszel test – see under Mantel

Haferkamp, Otto, German physician, *1929.
  Haferkamp syndrome – syndrome resulting in anemia, arteriosclerosis of renal arteries, fat metabolism disorders.

Haffkine, Waldemar M.W., Russian physician, 1860-1930.
  Haffkine vaccine – a killed culture of *Vibrio cholerae*; a killed plague bacillus (*Yersinia pestis*) vaccine.

Hagedorn, Werner, German surgeon, 1831-1894.
  Hagedorn cheiloplasty
  Hagedorn needle – a curved surgical needle that is flattened on the sides.
  Hagedorn needle holder
  Hagedorn operation
  Hagedorn suture needle

Haglund, S.E. Patrick, Swedish orthopedist, 1870-1937.
  Haglund deformity – *SYN:* Haglund disease
  Haglund disease – an abnormal prominence of the posterior superior lateral aspect of the os calcis, caused by a gait disorder. *SYN:* Haglund deformity

Hagner, Francis R., U.S. surgeon, 1873-1940.
  Hagner bag – bag used to prevent postprostatectomy hemorrhage.
  Hagner bag catheter
  Hagner hemostatic bag
  Hagner operation
  Hagner urethral bag

Hahn, Eugen H., German physician, 1841-1902.
  Hahn sign – side-to-side head rotation seen in childhood cerebellar disease.

Haidinger, Wilhelm von, Austrian mineralogist, 1795-1871.
  Haidinger brushes – the perception of two dark yellowish brushes when an evenly illuminated surface is viewed through a polarizing lens.

Hailey, Hugh Edward, U.S. dermatologist, *1909.
  Hailey-Hailey disease – recurrent eruption of vesicles and bullae. *SYN:* benign familial chronic pemphigus

Hailey, William Howard, U.S. dermatologist, 1898-1967.
  Hailey-Hailey disease – recurrent eruption of vesicles and bullae. *SYN:* benign familial chronic pemphigus

Hajdu, Nicholas, Czech physician, *1908.
  Cheney-Hajdu syndrome – *SYN:* Hajdu-Cheney syndrome
  Hajdu-Cheney syndrome – missing terminal phalanges on extremities
    giving appearance of clubbing; may be accompanied by scoliosis, tooth
    loss, and other defects. *SYN:* Cheney-Hajdu syndrome

Hakim, S., 20th century U.S. neurologist.
  Hakim-Adams syndrome – *SYN:* Hakim syndrome
  Hakim catheter
  Hakim reservoir
  Hakim shunt
  Hakim syndrome – in the presence of normal pressure hydrocephalus,
    the patient experiences urinary incontinence, dementia, gait apraxia.
    SYN: Hakim-Adams syndrome; HA syndrome
  Hakim tube
  Hakim valve

Hakola, H.P.A., Finnish physician.
  Hakola syndrome – genetic trait resulting in progressive dementia and
    cystic changes in bones.

Halbeisen, William A., U.S. physician, *1915.
  Stryker-Halbeisen syndrome – see under Stryker, Garold V.

Halberstaedter, Ludwig, German physician, 1876-1949.
  Halberstaedter-Prowazek bodies – *SYN:* Prowazek-Greeff bodies

Halbrecht, J., U.S. physician.
  Halbrecht syndrome – jaundice appearing in newborns within 24 hours of
    birth and related to ABO blood type incompatibility between mother and
    infant.

Haldane, John S., Scottish physiologist at Oxford, 1860-1936.
  Haldane apparatus – a device used for analyzing respiratory gases.
  Haldane chamber – an obsolete chamber for metabolic studies on
    animals.

NOTES

Haldane effect – the promotion of carbon dioxide dissociation by oxygenation of hemoglobin.

Haldane-Priestley sample – an approximation of alveolar gas obtained from the end of a sudden maximal expiration into a Haldane tube.

Haldane relationship – a mathematical relationship between the equilibrium constant of an enzyme-catalyzed reaction and all of that enzyme's kinetic parameters.

Haldane transformation – multiplication of inspired oxygen concentration by the ratio of expired to inspired nitrogen concentration in the calculation of oxygen consumption or respiratory quotient by the open circuit method.

Haldane tube – a tube for securing human alveolar air samples.

Hales, Stephen, English physiologist, 1677-1761.

Hales piesimeter – a glass tube inserted into an artery at right angles to its axis to measure pressure.

Hallauer, Otto, 19th century Swiss ophthalmologist.

Hallauer glasses – glasses which prohibit blue and ultraviolet rays from passing through them.

Hallberg, Josef H., 20th century U.S. electrician.

Hallberg effect – peaks and troughs in wave fields have opposite electrical signs.

Hallé, Adrien J.M.N., French physician, 1859-1947.

Hallé point – a point where the ureter can be most readily palpated.

Haller, Albrecht von, Swiss physiologist, 1708-1777.

Haller annulus – *SYN:* Haller insula

Haller ansa – *SYN:* communicating branch of facial nerve with glossopharyngeal nerve

Haller arches

Haller circle – (1) a network of branches of the short ciliary arteries on the sclera around the point of entrance of the optic nerve. *SYN:* vascular circle of optic nerve; (2) a venous plexus in the areola surrounding the nipple. *SYN:* areolar venous plexus

Haller cones – the coiled portion of the efferent ductules that constitute the head of the epididymis. *SYN:* lobules of epididymis

Haller habenula – rarely used term for the cordlike remains of the vaginal process of the peritoneum. *SYN:* Scarpa habenula

Haller insula – a doubling of the thoracic duct for part of its course through the thorax. *SYN:* Haller annulus

Haller line – a thickened band of pia mater along the midline of the anterior surface of the spinal cord. *SYN:* linea splendens

Haller plexus – a nervous plexus of sympathetic filaments and branches of the external laryngeal nerve on the surface of the inferior constrictor muscle of the pharynx.

Haller rete – the network of canals at the termination of the straight tubules in the mediastinum testis. *SYN:* rete testis

Haller tripod – abdominal artery. *SYN:* celiac trunk

Haller tunica vasculosa – the vascular, pigmentary, or middle coat of the eye, comprising the choroid, ciliary body, and iris. *SYN:* vascular tunic of eye

Haller unguis – the lower of two elevations on the medial wall of the posterior horn of the lateral ventricle of the brain. *SYN:* calcar avis

Haller vas aberrans – a narrow, coiled tubule frequently connected to the first part of the ductus deferens or to the lower part of the ductus epididymitis. *SYN:* inferior aberrant ductule

Haller vascular tissue – the outer portion of the choroid of the eye containing the largest blood vessels. *SYN:* vascular lamina of choroid

Hallermann, Wilhelm, German ophthalmologist, 1901-1975.

Hallermann-Streiff-François syndrome – *SYN:* Hallermann-Streiff syndrome

Hallermann-Streiff syndrome – a syndrome of bony anomalies of the calvaria, face, and jaw, with curved nose and multiple ocular defects. *SYN:* dyscephalia mandibulo-oculofacialis; François syndrome; Hallermann-Streiff-François syndrome

Hallervorden, Julius, German neurologist, 1882-1965.

Hallervorden-Spatz disease – *SYN:* Hallervorden-Spatz syndrome

Hallervorden-Spatz syndrome – a disorder characterized by dystonia with other extrapyramidal dysfunctions. *SYN:* Hallervorden-Spatz disease; Hallervorden syndrome; status dysmyelinisatus

Hallervorden syndrome – *SYN:* Hallervorden-Spatz syndrome

NOTES

Hallgren, Bertil, 20th century Swedish geneticist.
  Hallgren syndrome – vestibulocerebellar ataxia, pigmentary retinal dystrophy, congenital deafness, and cataract.

Halliday, John, Australian physician.
  Halliday hyperostosis – excessive bone growth in skull, ribs, and clavicles accompanied by osteoblastic activity in other bones.

Hallion, Louis, French physiologist, 1862-1940.
  Hallion test – a test of collateral circulation. *SYN:* Tuffier test

Hallopeau, François Henri, French dermatologist, 1842-1919.
  Hallopeau disease – a sterile pustular eruption of the fingers and toes. *SYN:* pemphigus vegetans; pustulosis palmaris et plantaris
  Hallopeau-Siemens syndrome

Hallwachs, Wilhelm L.F., German physiologist, 1859-1922.
  Hallwachs effect – electronic or electric effects produced by action of light.

Halstead, Ward C., U.S. psychologist, 1908-1968.
  Halstead-Reitan battery – a battery of neuropsychological tests used to study brain-behavior functions. *SYN:* Tactual Performance Test

Halsted, William Stewart, U.S. surgeon, 1852-1922.
  Halsted clamp
  Halsted curved mosquito forceps
  Halsted hemostat
  Halsted incision
  Halsted law – transplanted tissue will grow only if there is a lack of that tissue in the host.
  Halsted mattress sutures
  Halsted operation – excision of the breast as well as the pectoral muscles, lymphatic-bearing tissue in the axilla, and various other tissues. *SYN:* radical mastectomy
  Halsted suture – a suture used for exact skin approximation.

Haltia, M., Finnish physician.
  Haltia-Santavuori syndrome – autosomal recessive trait described as an inborn error of metabolism, with onset in the second year of life. *SYN:* neuronal ceroid lipofuscinosis

Ham, Thomas Hale, U.S. physician, *1905.
  Ham test – lysis of the patient's red cells in acidified fresh serum. *SYN:* acidified serum test

Hamburger, Hartog J., Dutch physiologist, 1859-1924.
   Hamburger law – albumins and phosphates pass from red corpuscles to serum, and chlorides pass from serum to cells when blood is acid; the reverse occurs when blood is alkaline.
   Hamburger phenomenon – movement of chloride from plasma to erythrocyte interior, or vice versa. *SYN:* chloride shift

Hamilton, Frank Hastings, U.S. surgeon, 1813-1886.
   Hamilton pseudophlegmon – a trophic affection of the subcutaneous connective tissue, marked by a circumscribed swelling which may become indurated and red, but never suppurates.

Hamilton, James B., U.S. physician.
   Hamilton classification – *SYN:* Norwood classification
   Hamilton-Norwood classification – *SYN:* Norwood classification

Hamilton, J.B., U.S. endocrinologist.
   Hamilton sign – normal androgenic function in males over 30 years of age, characterized by hairs growing on the antitragus.

Hamman, Louis, U.S. physician, 1877-1946.
   Hamman crunch
   Hamman disease – *SYN:* Hamman syndrome
   Hamman murmur – *SYN:* Hamman sign
   Hamman-Rich syndrome – *SYN:* usual interstitial pneumonia of Liebow
   Hamman sign – a crunching, rasping sound, synchronous with heartbeat, heard over the precordium and sometimes at a distance from the chest in mediastinal emphysema. *SYN:* Hamman murmur
   Hamman syndrome – spontaneous mediastinal emphysema, resulting from rupture of alveoli. *SYN:* Hamman disease

Hammarsten, Olof, Swedish physiological chemist, 1841-1932.
   Hammarsten reagent – a mixture of hydrochloric acid and alcohol to test for bile.

NOTES

Hammerschlag, Albert, Austrian physician, 1863-1935.
Hammerschlag method – a hydrometric method of determining the specific gravity of the blood.

Hammond, William A., U.S. neurologist, 1828-1900.
Hammond disease – a condition in which there is a constant succession of involuntary movements of the fingers and hands, and sometimes of the toes and feet. *SYN:* athetosis

Hampton, Aubrey Otis, U.S. radiologist, 1900-1955.
Hampton hump – a juxtapleural pulmonary soft tissue density on a chest x-ray, described as a manifestation of pulmonary infarction.
Hampton line – a thin radiolucent band across the neck of a contrast-filled benign gastric ulcer, indicating mucosal edema.
Hampton maneuver – rolling a supine patient to the right and then left side to obtain an air contrast x-ray in gastrointestinal fluoroscopy.
Hampton technique – obsolete term for atraumatic, nonpalpation, fluoroscopic examination of the upper gastrointestinal tract in peptic ulcer disease with acute hemorrhage.

Hancock, Henry, English surgeon, 1809-1880.
Hancock amputation – amputation of the foot through the astragalus.

Hand, Alfred, Jr., U.S. pediatrician, 1868-1949.
Hand-Schüller-Christian disease – the chronic disseminated form of Langerhans cell histiocytosis. *SYN:* Christian disease (1); Christian syndrome; normal cholesteremic xanthomatosis; Schüller disease; Schüller syndrome

Hanflig, Samuel S., U.S. orthopedic surgeon, 1901-1966.
Hanflig technique of neck traction – a method of cervical traction.

Hanfmann, Eugenia, Russian-U.S. psychologist, *1905.
Hanfmann-Kasanin Concept Formation Test – a test to assess conceptual thinking.

Hanhart, Ernst, Swiss internist and geneticist, 1891-1973.
Hanhart syndrome – hypoplasia of the mandible with malformed and missing teeth, birdlike face, and severe deformities of the hands and forearms and sometimes of feet and legs. *SYN:* micrognathia with peromelia
Richner-Hanhart syndrome– see under Richner

Hanks, Horace Tracy, U.S. surgeon, 1837-1900.
Hanks dilator – uterine dilator of solid metal construction.

Hanlon, C. Rollins, U.S. cardiovascular and thoracic surgeon, *1915.
  Blalock-Hanlon operation – see under Blalock

Hannover, Adolph, Danish anatomist, 1814-1894.
  Hannover canal – the potential space between the ciliary zonule and the vitreous body.

Hanot, Victor C., French physician, 1844-1896.
  Hanot cirrhosis – a condition characterized by obstructive jaundice with hyperlipemia, pruritus, and hyperpigmentation of the skin. *SYN:* primary biliary cirrhosis

Hansemann, D.P. von, see under von Hansemann

Hansen, Gerhard Henrik Armauer, Norwegian physician, 1841-1912.
  Fosdick-Hansen-Epple test – see under Fosdick
  Hansen bacillus – a species that causes Hansen disease. *SYN:* *Mycobacterium leprae*
  Hansen disease – *SYN:* leprosy

Hantaan, river in South Korea.
  Hantaan virus – member of Hantavirus family, named for area of South Korea where it first occurred, characterized by fever and renal failure.

Happle, Rudolph.
  Happle syndrome – X-linked dominant ichthyosis.

Hapsburg, Austrian royal family who ruled most of central and part of western Europe for centuries.
  disease of the Hapsburgs – factor VIII deficiency causing blood coagulation disorder. *SYN:* classic hemophilia; hemophilia A

Harada, Einosuke, Japanese ophthalmologist, 1892-1947.
  Harada disease – *SYN:* Harada syndrome
  Harada syndrome – bilateral retinal edema, uveitis, choroiditis, and retinal detachment, with deafness, graying of the hair, and alopecia. *SYN:* Harada disease; uveoencephalitis; uveomeningitis syndrome
  Vogt-Koyanagi-Harada syndrome– see under Vogt, Alfred

NOTES

Harden, Sir Arthur, English biochemist and Nobel laureate, 1865-1940.
Harden-Young ester – important intermediate in sugar metabolism.

Harder, Johann J., Swiss anatomist, 1656-1711.
Harder gland – the deep gland of the semilunar conjunctival fold found in animals such as pig and deer.

Harding, Harold E., 20th century English pathologist.
Harding-Passey melanoma – a melanin-forming tumor that is transplantable to mice of many strains.

Hardy, Godfrey H., English mathematician, 1877-1947.
Hardy-Weinberg equilibrium – the state in which the genetic structure of the population conforms to the prediction of the Hardy-Weinberg law. SYN: random mating equilibrium
Hardy-Weinberg law – if mating occurs at random with respect to any one autosomal locus in a population in which the gene frequencies are equal in the two sexes, and the factors tending to change gene frequencies are absent or negligible, then in one generation the probabilities of all possible genotypes will on average equal the same proportions as if the genes were assembled at random.

Hardy, LeGrand, U.S. ophthalmologist, 1895-1954.
Hardy enucleator
Hardy-Rand-Ritter test – a test for color vision deficiency.

Hare, Edward S., English surgeon, 1812-1838.
Hare syndrome – SYN: Pancoast syndrome

Harkavy, Joseph, U.S. physician, *1890.
Harkavy syndrome – probable allergic reaction causing pleurisy, pericarditis, and neurologic symptoms.

Harken, Dwight, U.S. Army surgeon.
Harken cardiovascular forceps
Harken clamp
Harken-Cooley forceps
Harken needle
Harken prosthetic valve
Harken retractor
Harken rib spreader
Harken valve

Harley, George, Scottish physician, 1829-1896.
Harley disease – hemoglobin in the urine.

Harnasch, Hans M.E., German physician, *1907.
   Harnasch disease – loss of bone tissue in hands and feet.

Harrington, David O., U.S. ophthalmologist, *1904.
   Harrington-Flocks test – an obsolete rapid screening test for visual field defects.

Harrington, Paul R., U.S. orthopedic surgeon, *1911.
   Harrington clamp
   Harrington deep surgical scissors
   Harrington flat wrench
   Harrington hook driver
   Harrington instrumention
   Harrington operation
   Harrington retractor
   Harrington rod instrumentation
   Harrington scissors
   Harrington spinal elevator
   Harrington spinal fusion
   Harrington spinal instrumentation
   Harrington strut
   Harrington thoracic forceps
   Harrington tonometer

Harris, Henry A., English anatomist, 1886-1968.
   Harris lines – dense lines parallel to the growth plates of long bones on x-rays. *SYN:* growth arrest lines

Harris, Henry F., U.S. physician, 1867-1926.
   Harris hematoxylin – an alum type of hematoxylin.

Harris, R.I., 20th century Canadian orthopedist.
   Harris anterolateral approach
   Harris brace-type reamer
   Harris broach
   Harris cemented hip prosthesis

NOTES

Harris cement gun
Harris center-cutting acetabular reamer
Harris condylocephalic nailing
Harris condylocephalic rod
Harris femoral component removal
Harris growth arrest line
Harris hip scale
Harris hip status system
Harris lateral approach
Harris medullary nail
Harris plate
Harris prosthesis
Harris splint sling
Harris superior acetabular graft
Harris view
Harris wire tier
Salter-Harris classification of epiphysial plate injuries – see under
    Salter, Robert

Harris, Robert L., Canadian surgeon.
    Harris footprint mat – a rubber mat that is used for taking footprints.

Harris, Seale, U.S. physician, 1870-1957.
    Harris syndrome – hypoglycemia due to pancreatic disorders.

Harris, Wilfred, English physician, 1869-1960.
    Harris migraine – recurrent facial pain and headache, more common in
        men than in women. *SYN:* periodic migrainous neuralgia

Harrison, Edward, English physician, 1766-1838.
    Harrison groove – a deformity of the ribs.

Hartel, Fritz, 20th century German surgeon.
    Hartel technique – a method of reaching the gasserian ganglion for the
        relief of trigeminal neuralgia.

Hartline, Haldan Keffer, U.S. physician and physiologist, joint winner of 1967
Nobel Prize for work related to the eye.

Hartman, LeRoy L., U.S. dentist, 1893-1951.
    Hartman solution – a solution used to desensitize dentin in dental
        operations.

Hartmann, Alexis F., U.S. pediatrician, 1898-1964.
    Hartmann solution – *SYN:* lactated Ringer solution
    Shaffer-Hartmann method – see under Shaffer

Hartmann, Arthur, German laryngologist, 1849-1931.
   Hartmann adenoidal curette
   Hartmann curette – a curette for the removal of adenoids.
   Hartmann ear forceps
   Hartmann ear rongeur
   Hartmann eustachian catheter
   Hartmann mastoid rongeur
   Hartmann nasal dressing forceps
   Hartmann nasal speculum
   Hartmann punch
   Hartmann tonsillar punch
   Hartmann tuning fork

Hartmann, Henri A.C.A., French surgeon, 1860-1952.
   Hartmann colostomy
   Hartmann knife
   Hartmann mosquito forceps
   Hartmann operation – resection of the rectosigmoid colon beginning at or just above the peritoneal reflexion and extending proximally, with closure of the rectal stump and end-colostomy.
   Hartmann pouch – a spheroid or conical pouch at the junction of the neck of the gallbladder and the cystic duct. *SYN:* ampulla of gallbladder; fossa provesicalis; pelvis of gallbladder
   Hartmann resection
   Hartmann speculum

Hartnup, surname of the English family first described with this condition.
   Hartnup disease – autosomal recessive metabolic disease characterized by skin rash, emotional lability, unsteady gait, and various neurological symptoms. *SYN:* Hartnup syndrome
   Hartnup syndrome – *SYN:* Hartnup disease

Hartwell, Leland H., U.S. scientist, *1939, joint winner of 2001 Nobel Prize for work related to key regulators of cell cycles.

NOTES

Harvey, William, English physician, 1578-1657.
   Harvey sign – related to venous refill.

Häser, Heinrich, German physician, 1811-1884.
   Häser formula – a formula to determine the number of grams of urinary
      solids per liter. *SYN:* Christison formula; Trapp formula; Trapp-Häser
      formula
   Trapp-Häser formula – *SYN:* Häser formula

Hashimoto, Hakaru, Japanese surgeon, 1881-1934.
   Hashimoto disease – *SYN:* Hashimoto thyroiditis
   Hashimoto struma – *SYN:* Hashimoto thyroiditis
   Hashimoto thyroiditis – diffuse infiltration of the thyroid gland with
      lymphocytes. *SYN:* autoimmune thyroiditis; Hashimoto disease;
      Hashimoto struma; lymphadenoid goiter; struma lymphomatosa;

Haslam, John, English physician, 1764-1844.
   Haslam-Pinel syndrome – a type of schizophrenia. *SYN:* Pinel-Haslam
      syndrome
   Pinel-Haslam syndrome – *SYN:* Haslam-Pinel syndrome

Hasner, Joseph Ritter von, Czech ophthalmologist, 1819-1892.
   Hasner fold – a fold of mucous membrane guarding the lower opening of
      the nasolacrimal duct. *SYN:* Hasner valve; lacrimal fold
   Hasner lid
   Hasner operation
   Hasner valve – *SYN:* Hasner fold

Hassall, Arthur, English physician, 1817-1894.
   Hassall bodies – small spherical bodies of keratinized and usually
      squamous epithelial cells found in the medulla of the lobules of the
      thymus. *SYN:* Hassall concentric corpuscle; thymic corpuscle; Virchow-
      Hassall bodies
   Hassall concentric corpuscle – *SYN:* Hassall bodies
   Hassall-Henle bodies – hyaline bodies on the posterior surface of
      Descemet membrane at the periphery of the cornea. *SYN:* Henle warts
   Virchow-Hassall bodies – *SYN:* Hassall bodies

Hasselbalch, Karl, Danish biochemist and physician, 1874-1962.
   Henderson-Hasselbalch equation – see under Henderson

Haudek, Martin, Austrian radiologist, 1880-1931.
   Haudek niche – an obsolete term for the radiographic appearance in
      profile of contrast material filling a gastric ulcer in the wall of the
      stomach.

Hauptmann, Alfred, German physician, 1881-1948.
   Hauptmann-Thannhauser syndrome – muscular dystrophy
   accompanied by cardiomyopathy and early contractures.

Hauser, G.A., 20th century German gynecologist.
   Mayer-Rokitansky-Küster-Hauser syndrome – see under Mayer, Paul
   Rokitansky-Küster-Hauser syndrome – *SYN:* Mayer-Rokitansky-Küster-
   Hauser syndrome

Havers, Clopton, English anatomist, 1650-1702.
   Havers glands – collections of adipose tissue in the hip, knee, and other
   joints, covered by synovial membrane. *SYN:* synovial glands
   haversian canals – vascular canals that run longitudinally in the center of
   haversian systems of compact osseous tissue. *SYN:* Leeuwenhoek
   canals
   haversian lamella – one of the concentric tubular layers of bone
   surrounding the central canal in an osteon. *SYN:* concentric lamella
   haversian spaces – spaces in bone formed by the enlargement of
   haversian canals.
   haversian system – a central canal containing capillaries and the
   concentric osseous lamellae around it occurring in compact bone.
   SYN: osteon

Hawley, C.A., 20th century U.S. orthodontist.
   Hawley appliance – *SYN:* Hawley retainer
   Hawley bite plate
   Hawley chart
   Hawley retainer – a removable wire and acrylic palatal appliance used to
   stabilize teeth following orthodontic tooth movement. *SYN:* Hawley
   appliance

Hawley, George Waller, U.S. surgeon, 1875-1940.
   Hawley table – operating table for orthopedic procedures.

NOTES

Haworth, Sir Walter Norman, English chemist and Nobel laureate, 1883-1950.

> **Haworth conformational formulas of cyclic sugars** – for the pyranoses, these depict those shapes on which 0 to 2 ring-atoms lie outside the plane of the ring.
>
> **Haworth perspective formulas of cyclic sugars** – these formulas depict the planar conformation, a situation not usually met.

Haw River, river running through Chatham County, North Carolina, and into Jordan Lake.

> **Haw River syndrome** – a dominant neurodegenerative disease that has affected five generations of a rural African American family; symptoms resemble those of Huntington disease.

Haxthausen, Holger, Danish dermatologist, 1892-1958.

> **Blegvad-Haxthausen syndrome** – see under Blegvad
>
> **Haxthausen disease** – *SYN:* Haxthausen panniculitis
>
> **Haxthausen hyperkeratosis** – *SYN:* Haxthausen syndrome
>
> **Haxthausen panniculitis** – a form of localized panniculitis caused by cold injury to subcutaneous fat. *SYN:* Haxthausen disease
>
> **Haxthausen syndrome** – hyperkeratosis of the soles, and later the palms, in women older than 45 years of age; association with obesity has been reported. *SYN:* Haxthausen hyperkeratosis

Hayem, Georges, French physician, 1841-1933.

> **Hayem hematoblast** – an irregularly shaped, disklike cytoplasmic fragment of a megakaryocyte found in the peripheral blood where it functions in clotting. *SYN:* platelet
>
> **Hayem solution** – a blood diluent used prior to counting red blood cells.
>
> **Hayem-Widal syndrome** – obsolete term for acquired hemolytic icterus. *SYN:* Widal syndrome

Hayflick, Leonard, U.S. microbiologist, *1928.

> **Hayflick limit** – the limit of human cell division in subcultures.

Haygarth, John, English physician, 1740-1827.

> **Haygarth nodes** – exostoses associated with lateral deflection of the fingers toward the ulnar side, occurring in rheumatoid arthritis. *SYN:* Haygarth nodosities
>
> **Haygarth nodosities** – *SYN:* Haygarth nodes

Head, Sir Henry, English neurologist, 1861-1940.

> **Head areas** – areas of skin exhibiting reflex hyperesthesia and hyperalgesia due to visceral disease.

Head lines – bands of cutaneous hyperesthesia associated with acute or chronic inflammation of the viscera. *SYN:* Head zones; tender lines; tender zones

Head zones – *SYN:* Head lines

Heaf, Frederick R.G., English physician, 1894-1973.
Heaf gun – inoculation gun.

Heaney, Noble Sproat, U.S. gynecological surgeon and obstetrician, 1880-1955.

Heaney clamp
Heaney curette
Heaney hysterectomy forceps
Heaney needle holder
Heaney operation – technique for vaginal hysterectomy.
Heaney retractor
Heaney suture
Heaney uterine curette
Heaney vaginal hysterectomy

Heath, Christopher, English surgeon, 1835-1905.
Heath clip
Heath curette
Heath dilator
Heath dissector
Heath forceps
Heath operation – division of mandibular ascending rami.
Heath scissors
Heath trephine flap dissector
Parker-Heath anterior chamber syringe
Parker-Heath cautery
Parker-Heath electrocautery
Parker-Heath piggyback probe

NOTES

Hebb, Donald O., Canadian psychologist, *1904.
Hebb learning theory

Heberden, William, Sr., English physician, 1710-1801.
Heberden angina – severe constricting pain in the chest. *SYN:* angina pectoris; Rougnon-Heberden disease
Heberden anomaly
Heberden asthma
Heberden disease – small-joint rheumatism, with distal interphalangeal joint nodules and angina.
Heberden nodes – small exostoses found on the terminal phalanges of the fingers in osteoarthritis. *SYN:* Heberden nodosities; Rosenbach disease (1); tuberculum arthriticum
Heberden nodosities – *SYN:* Heberden nodes
Heberden rheumatism
Rougnon-Heberden disease – *SYN:* Heberden angina

Hebra, Ferdinand von, Austrian dermatologist, 1816-1880.
Hebra disease – an acute eruption of macules, papules, or subdermal vesicles presenting a multiform appearance. *SYN:* erythema multiforme; familial nonhemolytic jaundice
Hebra prurigo – a severe form of chronic dermatitis with secondary infection. *SYN:* prurigo agria; prurigo ferox

Hecht, Victor, early 20th century Austrian pathologist.
Hecht pneumonia – a rare complication of measles, with the postmortem finding of multinucleated giant cells lining the alveoli. *SYN:* giant cell pneumonia

Heck, John W., U.S. dentist, *1923.
Heck disease – multiple soft nodular lesions of the lips, buccal mucosa, tongue, and other oral sites in children and adolescents. *SYN:* focal epithelial hyperplasia

Hedblom, Carl Arthur, U.S. physician, 1879-1934.
Hedblom syndrome – inflammation of the diaphragm.

Hedda Gabler, see under Gabler, Hedda

Hedström, Gustav, Swedish endodontist.
Hedström file – a coarse root canal file similar to a rasp.

Heerfordt, Christian Frederick, Danish ophthalmologist, 1871-1953.
Heerfordt disease – chronic enlargement of the parotid glands and inflammation of the uveal tract accompanied by a long-continued fever of low degree. *SYN:* uveoparotid fever

Heerfordt syndrome

Hefke, Hans William, U.S. radiologist, *1871.
Hefke-Turner sign – inflammatory hip disease found in children.
SYN: Turner-Hefke sign
Turner-Hefke sign – SYN: Hefke-Turner sign

Hegar, Alfred, German gynecologist, 1830-1914.
Hegar bougie
Hegar dilators – a series of cylindrical bougies of graduated sizes used to dilate the cervical canal.
Hegar needle holder
Hegar operation
Hegar sign – softening and compressibility of the lower segment of the uterus in early pregnancy.
Mayo-Hegar needle holder

Hegglin, Robert M.P., Swiss internist, 1907-1970.
Hegglin anomaly – a disorder in which neutrophils and eosinophils contain Döhle bodies and in which there is faulty maturation of platelets, with thrombocytopenia. SYN: May-Hegglin anomaly
Hegglin syndrome – an energy-dynamic cardiac insufficiency during diabetic coma and other metabolic disorders. SYN: May-Hegglin syndrome
May-Hegglin anomaly – SYN: Hegglin anomaly
May-Hegglin syndrome – SYN: Hegglin syndrome

Hehner, Otto, English chemist, 1853-1924.
Hehner number – the weight or percentage of the nonvolatile fatty acids yielded by 5 g of a saponified fat or oil. SYN: Hehner value
Hehner value – SYN: Hehner number

Heidbreder, Edna, U.S. psychologist, *1890.
Heidbreder test – SYN: Minnesota Mechanical Ability Test

NOTES

Heidelberg, city in Germany.
  Heidelberg arm – a pneumatic prosthesis with a hand, created at the University Clinic in Heidelberg, Germany.

Heidenhain, Adolf, German neurologist, *1893.
  Heidenhain syndrome – dementia of presenile type, associated with limb rigidity, ataxia, and blindness due to lesions of neurons.

Heidenhain, Rudolph P., German histologist and physiologist, 1834-1897.
  Biondi-Heidenhain stain – see under Biondi
  Heidenhain azan stain – a technique to stain nuclei and erythrocytes red, muscle orange, glia fibrils reddish, mucin blue, and collagen and reticulum dark blue.
  Heidenhain crescents – the serous cells at the distal end of a mucous, tubuloalveolar secretory unit of certain salivary glands. *SYN:* Heidenhain demilunes; serous demilunes
  Heidenhain demilunes – *SYN:* Heidenhain crescents
  Heidenhain iron hematoxylin stain – an iron alum hematoxylin stain used for staining muscle striations and mitotic structures blue-black.
  Heidenhain law – glandular secretion is always accompanied by an alteration in the structure of the gland.
  Heidenhain pouch – a small sac or pouch of the stomach fashioned for the purpose of obtaining gastric juice and for studying gastric secretion in physiologic experiments.

Heilbronner, Karl, Dutch physician, 1869-1914.
  Heilbronner thigh – in cases of organic paralysis, flattening and broadening of the thigh, when the patient lies supine on a hard mattress.

Heim, Ernst L., German physician, 1747-1834.
  Heim-Kreysig sign – in adherent pericardium, an indrawing of the intercostal spaces, synchronous with cardiac systole. *SYN:* Kreysig sign

Heimlich, Harry J., U.S. thoracic surgeon, *1920.
  Heimlich maneuver – a method used to expel an obstructing bolus of food from the throat.
  Heimlich operation
  Heimlich tube
  Heimlich valve

Heine, Jacob von, see under von Heine

Heine, Leopold, German ophthalmologist, 1870-1940.
  Heine operation – cyclodialysis.

Heineke, Walter, German surgeon, 1834-1901.
Heineke colon resection
Heineke gastroenterostomy
Heineke hypospadias operation
Heineke-Mikulicz herniorrhaphy
Heineke-Mikulicz pyloroplasty – procedure in which a short longitudinal
incision is made over the pylorus and closed transversely.

Heiner, Douglas C., U.S. pediatrician, *1925.
Heiner syndrome – an infant's failure to thrive due to serum antibodies in
cow's milk.

Heinz, Robert, German pathologist, 1865-1924.
Heinz bodies – intracellular inclusions composed of denatured
hemoglobin.
Heinz body anemia
Heinz body test – a test for glucose 6-phosphate dehydrogenase-deficient
red blood cells.
Heinz-Ehrlich body – *SYN:* Ehrlich inner body

Heister, Lorenz, German anatomist, 1683-1758.
Heister diverticulum
Heister valve – a series of crescentic folds of mucous membrane in the
upper part of the cystic duct, arranged in a somewhat spiral manner.
SYN: spiral fold of cystic duct

Hejna, Robert F., U.S. speech pathologist.
Hejna test – measure of speech articulation.

Held, Hans, German anatomist, 1866-1942.
Held bundle – a bundle of thick, heavily myelinated fibers that ends in the
medial region of the anterior horn of the cervical spinal cord and
appears to be involved in head movements during visual and auditory
tracking. *SYN:* tectospinal tract
Held decussation – the crossing of some of the fibers arising from the
cochlear nuclei to form the lateral lemniscus.

NOTES

Helie, Louis T., French gynecologist, 1804-1867.

Helie bundle – a vertically arched bundle of fibers in the superficial layer of the myometrium.

Heller, Arnold Ludwig Gotthilf, German pathologist, 1840-1913.

Döhle-Heller aortitis – see under Döhle

Heller plexus – plexus of small arteries in the wall of the intestine.

Heller, Ernst, German surgeon, 1877-1964.

Heller operation – esophagomyotomy at the gastroesophageal region.

Heller, Julius, German dermatologist, 1864-1931.

median canaliform dystrophy of Heller – longitudinal groove of the nail plate, usually in midline, with fir tree-like pattern of ridges. It most often affects the thumb nails, and some patients give a definite history of trauma.

Hellerström, Sven Curt Alfred, Swedish dermatologist, *1901.

Hellerström disease – encephalitis associated with erythema chronicum migrans (Afzelius), as manifestation of Lyme disease.

Hellin, Dyonizy, Polish pathologist, 1867-1935.

Hellin law – law expressing the frequencies of twins and triplets.

Helly, Konrad, Swiss pathologist, *1875.

Helly fixative – a microanatomic fixative for cytoplasmic granules and nuclear staining.

Helly fluid

Helmholtz, Hermann L.F. von, German physician, physicist, and physiologist, 1821-1894.

Gibbs-Helmholtz equation – see under Gibbs

Helmholtz axis ligament – a ligament forming the axis about which the malleus rotates. *SYN:* axis ligament of malleus

Helmholtz coil

Helmholtz energy – energy equivalent to the internal energy minus the entropy contribution.

Helmholtz-Gibbs theory – *SYN:* Gibbs-Helmholtz equation

Helmholtz keratometer

Helmholtz ophthalmoscope

Helmholtz theory of accommodation – the ciliary muscle relaxes for near vision and allows the anterior aspect of the lens to become more convex.

Helmholtz theory of color vision – *SYN:* Young-Helmholtz theory of color vision

Helmholtz theory of hearing – that the basilar membrane of the cochlea acts as a resonating structure, recording low tones from its apical turns and high tones from its basal turns. *SYN:* resonance theory of hearing
Young-Helmholtz theory of color vision – see under Young, Thomas

Helmont, Jean B. van, see under van Helmont

Helweg, Hans K.S., Danish physician, 1847-1901.
Helweg bundle – a slender bundle of nerve fibers in the peripheral zone of the lateral funiculus of the spinal cord. *SYN:* olivospinal tract

Helweg-Larssen, Hans F., Danish dermatologist 1917-1969.
Helweg-Larssen syndrome – familial anhidrosis present from birth, with neurolabyrinthitis developing in the fourth or fifth decade.

Helwig, Elson Bowman, U.S. physician, *1907.
Helwig disease – an epithelial tumor commonly presenting as a papule on the face of an adult.

Hench, Philip S., U.S. physician, 1896-1965.
Hench-Rosenberg syndrome – the sudden onset of arthritis, usually affecting a single joint, with no appearance on x-ray examination. *SYN:* Rosenberg-Hench syndrome
Rosenberg-Hench syndrome – *SYN:* Hench-Rosenberg syndrome

Henderson, Lawrence J., U.S. biochemist, 1879-1942.
Henderson-Hasselbalch equation – a formula relating the pH value of a solution to the value of the acid in the solution and the ratio of the acid and the conjugate base concentrations.

Hendon, West Hendon Hospital, England.
Hendon arm – children's upper limb prosthesis, created at England's West Hendon Hospital.

Henke, Wilhelm, German anatomist, 1834-1896.
Henke space – retropharyngeal space.
Henke triangle

NOTES

Henkin, R.I., U.S. physician.
  Henkin syndrome – syndrome of unknown etiology that affects the senses of taste and smell.

Henle, Friedrich Gustar Jacob, German anatomist, pathologist, and histologist, 1809-1885.
  crypts of Henle – infoldings of conjunctiva.
  Hassall-Henle bodies – see under Hassall
  Henle ampulla – the dilation of the ductus deferens where it approaches its contralateral partner before it is joined by the duct of the seminal vesicle. *SYN:* ampulla of ductus deferens
  Henle ansa – *SYN:* nephronic loop
  Henle fenestrated elastic membrane – *SYN:* elastic laminae of arteries
  Henle fiber layer – the layer of inner cone fibers in the central area of the retina.
  Henle fissures – minute spaces filled with connective tissue between the muscular fasciculi of the heart.
  Henle glands – accessory lacrimal glands. *SYN:* Baumgarten glands
  Henle layer – the outer layer cells of the inner root sheath of the hair follicle.
  Henle ligament
  Henle loop – *SYN:* nephronic loop
  Henle membrane – the transparent inner layer of the choroid in contact with the pigmented layer of the retina. *SYN:* lamina basalis choroideae
  Henle nervous layer – the layer of the retina from the outer plexiform to the nerve fiber layer inclusive. *SYN:* entoretina
  Henle reaction – dark brown staining of the medullary cells of the adrenal bodies when treated with the salts of chromium, the cortical cells remaining unstained.
  Henle sheath – the delicate connective tissue enveloping individual nerve fibers within a peripheral nerve. *SYN:* endoneurium
  Henle sphincter
  Henle spine – small bony prominence anterior to the supramastoid pit at the posterosuperior margin of the bony external acoustic meatus. *SYN:* suprameatal spine
  Henle tubules – the straight portions of the uriniferous tubules that form Henle loop, distinguished as the descending and ascending tubules of Henle.
  Henle warts – *SYN:* Hassall-Henle bodies

Henneberg, Richard, German neurologist, 1868-1962.
  Henneberg reflex – reflex of the hard palate. *SYN:* Laehr-Henneberg reflex

Laehr-Henneberg reflex – *SYN:* Henneberg reflex

Henning, Wilhelm, German physician, 1716-1794.
    Henning sign – stomach angle takes on a Gothic arch shape in the presence of chronic gastric ulcer.

Henoch, Eduard Heinrich, German pediatrician, 1820-1910.
    Henoch chorea – a disorder in which sudden spasmodic coordinated movements of certain muscles or groups of physiologically related muscles occur at irregular intervals. *SYN:* spasmodic tic
    Henoch purpura – *SYN:* Henoch-Schönlein purpura
    Henoch-Schönlein purpura – an eruption of nonthrombocytopenic purpuric lesions due to dermal leukocytoclastic vasculitis. *SYN:* acute vascular purpura; anaphylactoid purpura; Henoch purpura; Henoch-Schönlein syndrome; purpura nervosa; purpura rheumatica; Schönlein disease; Schönlein-Henoch purpura; Schönlein purpura
    Henoch-Schönlein syndrome – *SYN:* Henoch-Schönlein purpura
    Schönlein-Henoch syndrome – *SYN:* Henoch-Schönlein purpura

Henry, James Paget, U.S. physiologist, *1914.
    Henry-Gauer response – inhibition of antidiuretic hormone secretion due to a rise in atrial pressure that stimulates atrial stretch receptors.

Henry, Joseph, U.S. physicist, 1797-1878.
    Dalton-Henry law – see under Dalton

Henry, William, English chemist, 1775-1837.
    Henry law – at equilibrium, at a given temperature, the amount of gas dissolved in a given volume of liquid is directly proportional to the partial pressure of that gas in the gas phase.

Henseleit, K., German internist, *1907.
    Krebs-Henseleit cycle – see under Krebs, Sir Hans Adolph

NOTES

Hensen, Victor, German anatomist and physiologist, 1835-1924.

Hensen canal – a short membranous tube passing from the lower end of a saccule to the cochlear duct of the membranous labyrinth. *SYN:* Hensen duct; uniting duct

Hensen cell – one of the supporting cells in the organ of Corti.

Hensen disk – *SYN:* Hensen line

Hensen duct – *SYN:* Hensen canal

Hensen knot – a local thickening of the blastoderm at the cephalic end of the primitive streak of the embryo. *SYN:* Hensen node; primitive node

Hensen line – the paler area in the center of the A band of a striated muscle fiber, comprising the central portion of thick filaments that are not overlapped by thin filaments. *SYN:* H band; Hensen disk

Hensen node – *SYN:* Hensen knot

Hensen stripe – a band on the undersurface of the membrana tectoria of the cochlear duct.

Hensing, Friedrich W., German anatomist, 1719-1745.

Hensing ligament – the left superior colic ligament.

Herbert, Herbert, English ophthalmic surgeon, 1865-1942.

Herbert pits – corneal cavities.

Herbst, Ernst F.G., German anatomist, 1803-1893.

Herbst corpuscles – tactile corpuscles found in birds.

Herelle, var. of d'Herelle

Hering, Heinrich Ewald, German physiologist, 1866-1948.

Hering-Breuer reflex – inflation of the lungs arrests inspiration with expiration then ensuing; deflation of the lungs brings on inspiration.

sinus nerve of Hering – a branch of the glossopharyngeal nerve that innervates the baroreceptors in the wall of the carotid sinus and the chemoreceptors in the carotid body. *SYN:* carotid sinus nerve

Hering, Karl E.K., German physiologist, 1834-1918.

canal of Hering – a ductule occurring between a bile canaliculus and an interlobular bile duct. *SYN:* cholangiole

Hering test – a test of binocular vision.

Hering theory of color vision – that there are three opponent visual processes: blue-yellow, red-green, and white-black.

Semon-Hering theory – see under Semon, Richard W.

Traube-Hering curves – see under Traube

Traube-Hering waves – *SYN:* Traube-Hering curves

Herlitz, Gillis, Swedish pediatrician, *1902.
Herlitz syndrome – epidermolysis bullosa in which the bullae are persistent, nonhealing, and often present in the oral mucosa and trachea. *SYN:* epidermolysis bullosa lethalis

Herman, Eufemius, Polish physician.
Herman syndrome – a syndrome characterized by pyramidal, extrapyramidal, and mental disorders, and livedo racemosa universalis.

Hermann, Friedrich, German anatomist, 1859-1920.
Hermann fixative – a hardening fixative of glacial acetic acid, osmic acid, and platinum chloride.

Hermans, P.E., U.S. physician.
Hermans syndrome – hyperplasia of the ileum caused by globulin deficiency and resulting in recurrent diarrhea and infections.

Hermansky, F., Czech physician.
Hermansky-Pudlak syndrome – autosomal recessive trait characterized by early fibromatosis and related abnormalities.

Herrenschwand, Friedrich von, German ophthalmologist, *1881.
Herrenschwand syndrome – sympathetic lesions causing differences in color of the iris.

Herring, Percy T., English physiologist, 1872-1967.
Herring bodies – accumulations of neurosecretory granules in dilated terminal endings of axons in the neurohypophysis.

Herrmann, Christian, Jr., U.S. physician, *1921.
Herrmann syndrome – a nervous system disorder with photomyoclonus and hearing loss followed by diabetes mellitus, progressive dementia, pyelonephritis, and glomerulonephritis.

Hers, Henri-Géry, 20th century Belgian physiologist and biochemist.
Hers disease – *SYN:* type 6 glycogenosis

NOTES

Hershey, Alfred D., U.S. biologist, *1908, joint winner of the 1969 Nobel Prize for research on mechanisms and materials of virus inheritance.

Hersman, C.F., U.S. physician.
    Hersman disease – progressive enlargement of the hands, of unknown etiology.

Herter, Christian A., U.S. physician, 1865-1910.
    Gee-Herter disease – *SYN:* Gee disease
    Herter disease – gluten sensitivity, manifested by diarrhea, malabsorption, steatorrhea, nutritional and vitamin deficiencies. *SYN:* celiac disease
    Heubner-Herter disease – *SYN:* Gee disease

Hertwig, Richard, German zoologist, 1850-1937.
    Magendie-Hertwig sign – see under Magendie
    Magendie-Hertwig syndrome – *SYN:* Magendie-Hertwig sign

Hertwig, Wilhelm A.O., German embryologist, 1849-1922.
    Hertwig sheath – the merged outer and inner epithelial layers of the enamel organ, which extends beyond the anatomical crown and initiates formation of dentin in the root of a developing tooth.

Hertz, Heinrich R., German physicist, 1857-1894.
    hertz – a unit of frequency equivalent to 1 cycle per second.
    hertzian experiments – experiments demonstrating that electromagnetic induction is propagated in waves analogous to waves of light but not affecting the retina.

Herxheimer, Karl, German dermatologist, 1861-1944.
    Herxheimer reaction – an inflammatory reaction in syphilitic tissues induced by specific treatment with Salvarsan, mercury, or antibiotics. *SYN:* Jarisch-Herxheimer reaction
    Herxheimer spiral
    Jarisch-Herxheimer reaction – *SYN:* Herxheimer reaction

Herying, Théodor, Polish otolaryngologist, 1847-1925.
    Herying sign – pus in a maxillary sinus causing a shadow under the eyes when tested with a flashlight in the mouth.

Heryng, Richard L., Austrian pathologist, 1824-1881.
    Heryng sign – infraorbital shadow related to diseases affecting the maxillary sinuses.

Herz, Max, Austrian physician, 1865-1936.
    Herz method – *SYN:* Herz system
    Herz system – a system of therapy consisting of baths, walks, and exercises. *SYN:* Herz method

Heschl, Richard L., Austrian pathologist, 1824-1881.

    Heschl gyri – two or three convolutions running transversely on the upper surface of the temporal lobe bordering on the sylvian fissure, separated from each other by the transverse temporal sulci. *SYN:* transverse temporal gyri

Hess, Alfred F., U.S. physician, 1875-1933.

    Hess test – *SYN:* Rumpel-Leede test

Hess, Carl von, German ophthalmologist, 1863-1923.

    Hess capsule iris forceps
    Hess expressor
    Hess eyelid operation
    Hess lens scoop
    Hess lens spoon
    Hess ptosis operation
    Hess screen – a screen used in the measurement of ocular deviation.
    Hess tonsil expressor

Hess, Walter R., Swiss physiologist and Nobel laureate, 1881-1973.

    trophotropic zone of Hess – an area in the hypothalamus concerned with positive rewarding bodily sensations.

Hesselbach, Franz K., German anatomist and surgeon, 1759-1816.

    Hesselbach fascia – the part of the superficial fascia of the thigh that covers the saphenous opening. *SYN:* cribriform fascia

    Hesselbach hernia – hernia with diverticula through the cribriform fascia, presenting a lobular outline.

    Hesselbach ligament – fibrous or muscular strands extending from the lower border of the transversus muscle to the lacunar ligament and pectineal fascia. *SYN:* interfoveolar ligament

    Hesselbach triangle – the triangular area in the lower abdominal wall bounded by the inguinal ligament, the border of the rectus abdominis, and the inferior epigastric vessels. *SYN:* inguinal triangle

---

NOTES

Hessing, Friedrich von, German orthopedic surgeon, 1838-1918.
Hessing brace – a brace of steel and molded leather designed to encase the body.

Heublein, Arthur C., U.S. radiologist, 1879-1932.
Heublein method – use of low-dose ionizing irradiation over the whole body.

Heubner, Johann O.L., German pediatrician, 1843-1926.
artery of Heubner – a cerebral artery. *SYN:* medial striate artery
Heubner arteritis – inflammation of arteries within the circle of Willis secondary to chronic basal meningitis from tubercle bacillus or particular fungi.
Heubner-Herter disease – *SYN:* Gee disease

Heuser, Chester, U.S. embryologist, 1885-1965.
Heuser membrane – a layer of cells delaminated from the inner surface of the blastocystic cytotrophoblast and from the envelope of the primary yolk sac during the second week of embryonic life. *SYN:* exocelomic membrane

Hey, William, English surgeon, 1736-1819.
Hey amputation – amputation of the foot in front of the tarsometatarsal joint.
Hey hernia – *SYN:* Cooper hernia
Hey internal derangement – dislocation of the semilunar cartilages of the knee joint.
Hey ligament – the upper part of the falciform margin of the opening in the fascia lata through which the greater saphenous vein passes. *SYN:* superior horn of falciform margin of saphenous opening
Hey skull saw

Heyde, Edward C., U.S. physician.
Heyde syndrome – occurrence of gastrointestinal bleeding and aortic stenosis after replacement of aortic valve.

Heyer, W.T., U.S. scientist, *1902.
Heyer-Pudenz valve – a valve used in the shunting procedure for hydrocephalus. *SYN:* Pudenz valve

Hey Groves, see under Groves, Ernest William Hey

Heymann, Walter, Belgian-U.S. physician, 1901-1985.
Heymann nephritis – experimental membranous glomerulonephritis created in laboratory rats.

Heymans, Corneille J.F., Belgian physiologist, 1892-1968.
　　Heymans law – theory regarding stimuli.

Heyns, O.S., 20th century South African obstetrician.
　　Heyns abdominal decompression apparatus – a vacuum chamber
　　　enclosing the abdomen of the pregnant woman, creating pressure
　　　during the first stage of labor.

Hibbs, Russell A., U.S. surgeon, 1869-1932.
　　Hibbs approach
　　Hibbs arthrodesis
　　Hibbs biting forceps
　　Hibbs blade
　　Hibbs bone chisel
　　Hibbs bone gouge
　　Hibbs chisel elevator
　　Hibbs costal elevator
　　Hibbs foot procedure
　　Hibbs fracture appliance
　　Hibbs fracture frame
　　Hibbs hammer
　　Hibbs hip arthrodesis
　　Hibbs laminectomy retractor
　　Hibbs mallet
　　Hibbs onlay graft fusion of the lumbar spine
　　Hibbs operation – a type of spinal fusion.
　　Hibbs osteotome
　　Hibbs periosteal elevator
　　Hibbs retractor
　　Hibbs retractor blade
　　Hibbs self-retracting retractor
　　Hibbs spinal fusion
　　Hibbs sponge

NOTES

Hibbs technique

Hicks, see under Braxton Hicks

Higashi, Ototaka, Japanese physician. *1924.
  Chédiak-Higashi anomaly – *SYN:* Chédiak-Steinbrinck-Higashi syndrome
  Chédiak-Higashi disease – *SYN:* Chédiak-Steinbrinck-Higashi syndrome
  Chédiak-Steinbrinck-Higashi anomaly – *SYN:* Chédiak-Steinbrinck-
    Higashi syndrome
  Chédiak-Steinbrinck-Higashi syndrome – see under Chédiak

Highmore, Nathaniel, English anatomist, 1613-1685.
  antrum of Highmore – the largest of the paranasal sinuses occupying the
    body of the maxilla, communicating with the middle meatus of the nose.
    SYN: maxillary sinus
  corpus highmori – *SYN:* Highmore body
  corpus highmorianum – *SYN:* Highmore body
  Highmore body – a mass of fibrous tissue continuous with the tunica
    albuginea, projecting into the testis from its posterior border. *SYN:* corpus
    highmori; corpus highmorianum; mediastinum testis

Hildenbrand, Johann Valentin Edler von, Austrian physician, 1763-1818.
  Hildenbrand disease – disease caused by *Rickettsia*, transmitted by body
    lice. *SYN:* camp fever; jail fever; ship fever

Hilgenreiner, Heinrich, German orthopedist and surgeon, *1870.
  Hilgenreiner line – a line drawn on pelvic radiographs to evaluate the
    acetabular angle and iliac index.

Hill, Archibald V., English biophysicist and Nobel laureate, 1886-1977.
  Hill equation – used to express the fractional saturation of a molecule with
    a ligand as a function of ligand concentration.
  Hill plot – a graphical representation of enzyme kinetic data or of binding
    phenomena to assess the degree of cooperativity of a system.

Hill, Harold A., U.S. radiologist, *1901.
  Hill-Sachs lesion – an irregularity seen in the head of the humerus
    following dislocation of the shoulder.

Hill, Lucius, U.S. thoracic surgeon, *1921.
  Hill operation – repair of hiatus hernia.

Hill, Robert, English plant physiologist, *1899.
  Hill reaction – that portion of the photosynthesis reaction that involves the
    photolysis of water and the liberation of oxygen and does not include
    carbon dioxide fixation.

Hill, Sir Leonard Erskine, English physiologist, 1866-1952.
    Hill phenomenon – *SYN:* Hill sign
    Hill sign – in aortic insufficiency, greater systolic blood pressure in the legs than in the arms. *SYN:* Hill phenomenon

Hillis, David S., U.S. obstetrician and gynecologist, 1873-1942.
    DeLee-Hillis stethoscope
    Hillis-Müller maneuver – manual pressure on the term fundus while a finger in the vagina determines the descent of the fetal head into the pelvis.

Hilton, John, English surgeon, 1804-1878.
    Hilton law – the nerve supplying a joint also supplies the muscles that move the joint and the skin covering the articular insertion of those muscles.
    Hilton method – division of the nerves supplying a part, for the relief of pain in ulcers.
    Hilton sac – a small diverticulum provided with mucous glands.
        SYN: saccule of larynx
    Hilton white line – a zone in the mucosa of the anal canal said to be palpable. *SYN:* white line of anal canal

Hines, Edgar A., U.S. physician, 1906-1978.
    Hines and Brown test – test for a lesion of central or sympathetic nervous system.

Hinman, Frank, Jr., U.S. urologist, *1915.
    Hinman syndrome – detrusor-sphincter incoordination.
        SYN: nonneurogenic neurogenic bladder

Hinton, William A., U.S. physician, 1883-1959.
    Hinton test – a formerly widely used precipitin test for syphilis.
    Muller-Hinton agar – see under Muller, Hermann Joseph

Hippel, Eugen von, see under von Hippel

NOTES

Hippocrates, Greek physician, 460-370 B.C.
  Hippocrates bandage
  hippocratic – relating to, described by, or attributed to Hippocrates.
  hippocratic facies – sunken appearance of facial features seen in dehydration.
  hippocratic fingers – clubbing of the fingers.
  Hippocratic Oath – an oath demanded of physicians about to enter the practice of their profession.
  hippocratic splash – *SYN:* hippocratic succussion
  hippocratic succussion – a diagnostic procedure to test for obstruction of the pylorus of stomach. *SYN:* hippocratic splash
  hippocratism – a system of medicine attributed to Hippocrates and his disciples that is based on the imitation of nature's processes in the therapeutic management of disease.

Hirsch, (origin unknown).
  Hirsch-Peiffer stain – see under Peiffer

Hirschberg, Julius, German ophthalmologist, 1843-1925.
  Hirschberg method – a method of measuring the amount of deviation of a strabismic eye.

Hirschfeld, Isador, U.S. dentist, 1881-1965.
  Hirschfeld canals – canals that extend vertically through alveolar bone between the roots of mandibular and maxillary incisor and maxillary bicuspid teeth. *SYN:* interdental canals
  Hirschfeld file
  Hirschfeld method
  Hirschfeld silver point

Hirschsprung, Harald, Danish physician, 1830-1916.
  Hirschsprung disease – congenital dilation and hypertrophy of the colon. *SYN:* congenital megacolon

His, Wilhelm, Jr., German physician, 1863-1934.
  His band – *SYN:* His bundle
  His bundle – modified cardiac muscle fibers. *SYN:* atrioventricular bundle; His band; Kent bundle; Kent-His bundle
  His bundle electrogram – an electrogram recorded from the His bundle.
  His bundle heart block
  His bundle recording
  His spindle – a fusiform dilation of the aorta immediately beyond the isthmus. *SYN:* aortic spindle

His-Tawara system – the complex system of interlacing Purkinje fibers within the ventricular myocardium.
Kent-His bundle – *SYN:* His bundle

His, Wilhelm, Sr., Swiss anatomist and embryologist in Germany, 1831-1904.
duct of His – *SYN:* Bochdalek duct
His copula – a median elevation in the floor of the embryonic pharynx that is incorporated in the root of the tongue. *SYN:* hypobranchial eminence
His line – a line dividing the face into an upper and a lower, or dental part.
His perivascular space – *SYN:* Virchow-Robin space
His rule – an obsolete calculation for the duration of pregnancy.
isthmus of His – the anterior portion of the rhombencephalon connecting with the mesencephalon. *SYN:* rhombencephalic isthmus

Hiskey, Marshall S., U.S. psychologist.
Hiskey-Nebraska Test of Learning Aptitude

Hiss, Philip, U.S. bacteriologist, 1868-1913.
Hiss stain – a stain for demonstrating the capsules of microorganisms, using gentian violet or basic fuchsin followed by a copper sulphate wash.

Hitchings, George H., joint winner of 1988 Nobel Prize for work related to drug treatment.

Hitzig, Edward, German neurologist, 1838-1907.
Hitzig girdle – breast-level analgesia caused by tabes dorsalis.
Hitzig test – test of vestibular apparatus in the ear.

Hitzig, Julius Eduard, German physician, 1838-1907.
Hitzig syndrome – involuntary movement of muscles innervated by cranial nerve 7.

Hjärre, A., German pathologist, 1897-1958.
Hjärre disease – a granulomatous disease of the intestines and liver of chickens. *SYN:* coli granuloma

Hoboken, Nicholas van, Dutch anatomist and physician, 1632-1678.
Hoboken gemmules – *SYN:* Hoboken nodules

NOTES

Hoboken nodules – gross dilations on the outer surface of the umbilical arteries. *SYN:* Hoboken gemmules

Hoboken valves – the flangelike protrusions into the lumen of the umbilical arteries where they are twisted or kinked in their course through the umbilical cord.

Hoche, Alfred E., German psychiatrist, 1865-1943.
Hoche bundle
Hoche tract

Hochenegg, Julius von, Austrian surgeon, 1859-1940.
Hochenegg operation – excision of the rectum, preserving the anal sphincter.
Hochenegg ulcer – hard tumor of the rectum resulting in defecation difficulty, fecal blood, colic, and mucus.

Hockey, Athel, Australian physician.
Hockey syndrome – genetic trait linked to mental retardation, precocious puberty, and obesity.

Hodara, Manehem, Turkish physician, d. 1926.
Hodara disease – condition of the scalp causing hair breakage.

Hodge, Harold Carpenter, U.S. dentist, *1904.
Capdepont-Hodge syndrome – *SYN:* Capdepont syndrome

Hodge, Hugh L., U.S. gynecologist, 1796-1873.
Hodge maneuver
Hodge obstetrical forceps
Hodge pessary – a double-curve oblong pessary employed for the correction of retrodeviations of the uterus.

Hodgen, John T., U.S. surgeon, 1826-1882.
Hodgen apparatus
Hodgen splint – a suspension leg splint for fractures of the middle or lower end of the femur.

Hodgkin, Alan L., English physiologist and Nobel laureate, *1914.
Goldman-Hodgkin-Katz equation – *SYN:* Goldman equation

Hodgkin, Thomas, English physician, 1798-1866.
Hodgkin disease – malignant neoplasm of lymphoid cells of uncertain origin, associated with inflammatory infiltration of lymphocytes and eosinophilic leukocytes and fibrosis. *SYN:* lymphadenoma
Hodgkin-Key murmur – a musical diastolic murmur.
Hodgkin sarcoma
non-Hodgkin lymphoma – a lymphoma other than Hodgkin disease.

Hodgkin, W.E., 20th century U.S. pediatrician.
Rapp-Hodgkin syndrome – see under Rapp

Hodgson, Joseph, English physician, 1788-1869.
Hodgson disease – dilation of the arch of the aorta associated with insufficiency of the aortic valve.

Hoeppli, Reinhard J.C., German parasitologist, 1893-1973.
Splendore-Hoeppli phenomenon – see under Splendore

Hoet, Joseph Jules, Belgian physician, *1925.
Hoet-Abaza syndrome – syndrome characterized by postpartum obesity and diabetes mellitus.

Hofbauer, J. Isfred I., U.S. gynecologist, 1878-1961.
Hofbauer cell – a large cell in the connective tissue of the chorionic villi.

Hoff, Jacobus H. van't, see under van't Hoff

Hoffa, Albert, German surgeon, 1859-1908.
Hoffa fat
Hoffa operation – to relieve congenital dislocation of the hip.
Hoffa tendon shortening

Hoffmann, August, German chemist, 1818-1892.
Frei-Hoffmann reaction – *SYN:* Frei test

Hoffmann, Johann, German neurologist, 1857-1919.
Hoffmann muscular atrophy – progressive dysfunction of the anterior horn cells in the spinal cord and brainstem cranial nerves. *SYN:* infantile spinal muscular atrophy
Hoffmann phenomenon – excessive irritability of the sensory nerves to electrical or mechanical stimuli in tetany.
Hoffmann reflex – *SYN:* Hoffmann sign
Hoffmann sign – in latent tetany, mild mechanical stimulation of the trigeminal nerve causes severe pain. *SYN:* Hoffmann reflex
Werdnig-Hoffmann disease – *SYN:* Werdnig-Hoffmann muscular atrophy
Werdnig-Hoffmann muscular atrophy – see under Werdnig

NOTES

Hoffmann, Moritz, German anatomist, 1622-1698.
   Hoffmann duct – the excretory duct of the pancreas. *SYN:* pancreatic duct

Hofmann, Georg von, Austrian bacteriologist, 1843-1890.
   Hofmann bacillus – a nonpathogenic species found in normal throats. *SYN:* *Corynebacterium pseudodiphtheriticum*

Hofmeister, Franz, German biochemist, 1850-1922.
   Hofmeister series – a series of cations and of anions. *SYN:* lyotropic series

Hofmeister, Franz von, German surgeon, 1867-1926.
   Hofmeister anastomosis
   Hofmeister antecolic gastrojejunostomy
   Hofmeister drainage bag
   Hofmeister endometrial biopsy curette
   Hofmeister gastrectomy – operation in which a portion of the stomach is removed and a retrocolic gastrojejunostomy is constructed.
   Hofmeister gastroenterostomy
   Hofmeister operation – partial gastrectomy with closure of a portion of the lesser curvature and retrocolic anastomosis of the remainder to jejunum.
   Hofmeister-Pólya anastomosis
   Hofmeister technique

Hogness, D.S., U.S. molecular biologist, *1925.
   Grunstein-Hogness assay – a procedure for identifying plasmid clones by colony hybridization.
   Hogness box

Hohmann, Georg, German surgeon, *1880.
   Hohmann bunionectomy
   Hohmann clamp
   Hohmann osteotome
   Hohmann osteotomy
   Hohmann retractor
   Hohmann tennis elbow procedure

Hoigne, Rolf V., Swiss physician, *1923.
   Hoigne syndrome – neurologic disorders caused by injecting penicillin into the bloodstream.

Holden, Luther, English anatomist, 1815-1905.
   Holden line – the crease or furrow of the skin of the groin caused by flexion of the thigh.

Holl, Mortiz, Austrian surgeon, 1852-1920.

Holl ligament – ligament joining the corpora cavernosa clitoridis in front of the urinary meatus.

Hollander, Franklin, U.S. physiologist, 1899-1966.

Hollander test – a test to determine the completeness of vagotomy for peptic ulcer. *SYN:* insulin hypoglycemia test

Hollenhorst, Robert W., U.S. ophthalmologist, *1913.

Hollenhorst plaques – glittering, orange-yellow, atheromatous emboli in the retinal arterioles that contain cholesterin crystals and originate in the carotid artery or great vessels.

Holley, Robert W., U.S. biochemist, *1928, joint winner of 1968 Nobel Prize for work related to genetic code.

Holliday, R.

Holliday junction – the cross-strand structure formed when two DNA duplexes cross in a recombination event. *SYN:* Holliday structure

Holliday structure – *SYN:* Holliday junction

Holly, F., U.S. obstetrician.

Holly anemia – anemia due to greatly depressed and inadequately functioning bone marrow, sometimes occurring during pregnancy.

Holmes, Sir Gordon M., English neurologist, 1876-1965.

Holmes-Adie pupil – *SYN:* Adie syndrome

Holmes-Adie syndrome – *SYN:* Adie syndrome

Stewart-Holmes sign – see under Stewart, Thomas Grainger

Holmes, Thomas, U.S. psychiatrist, *1918.

Holmes-Rahe questionnaire – *SYN:* Rahe-Holmes questionnaire

Rahe-Holmes questionnaire – see under Rahe

Holmes, W.

Holmes stain – a silver nitrate staining method for nerve fibers.

NOTES

Holmgren, Alarik F., Swedish physiologist, 1831-1897.
Holmgren wool test – a test for color blindness in which the subject matches variously colored skeins of wool.

Holmgrén, Emil A., Swedish histologist, 1866-1922.
Holmgrén-Golgi canals – *SYN:* Golgi apparatus

Holt, Mary, 20th century English cardiologist.
Holt-Oram syndrome – atrial septal defect in association with fingerlike or absent thumb and other deformities of the forearm.

Holt, Sarah B., English physician.
Holt syndrome – genetic trait resulting in supernumerary digits on hands and feet as well as abnormal shortness of metacarpal/metatarsal bones.

Holter, Norman, U.S. biophysicist, 1914-1983.
Holter monitor – ambulatory monitoring technique used to obtain uninterrupted electrocardiographic signal readings.
Holter pump
Holter shunt
Holter tube
Holter valve

Holth, Sören, Norwegian ophthalmologist, 1863-1937.
Holth corneoscleral punch
Holth forceps
Holth iridencleisis
Holth operation – punch procedure done to remove sclera.
Holth punch forceps
Holth sclerectomy
Holth sclerectomy punch

Holthouse, Carsten, English surgeon, 1810-1901.
Holthouse hernia – inguinal hernia with extension of the loop of intestine along Poupart ligament.

Holzknecht, Guido, Austrian radiologist, 1872-1931.
Holzknecht unit – an obsolete unit of x-ray dosage equal to one-fifth of the erythema dose.

Homans, John, U.S. surgeon, 1877-1954.
Homans sign – slight pain at the back of the knee indicative of incipient or established thrombosis in the veins of the leg.

Home, Sir Everard, English surgeon, 1756-1832.
Home lobe – the enlarged middle lobe of the prostate gland.

Hooke, Robert, English experimental physicist, 1635-1703.
  hookean behavior – the behavior of a perfectly elastic body.
  Hooke law – the stress applied to stretch or compress a body is
    proportional to the strain, or change in length thus produced.

Hooker, Charles W.
  Hooker-Forbes test – a test for compounds with progestational activity.

Hoover, Charles F., U.S. physician, 1865-1927.
  Hoover signs – in organic hemiplegia the patient attempts to lift a
    paralyzed leg, counterpressure will be made with the other heel,
    whether any movement occurs in the paralyzed limb or not.

Hope, James, English physician, 1801-1841.
  Hope murmur
  Hope resuscitator
  Hope sign – double heartbeat heard in presence of aortic aneurysm.

Hopf, Gustav, German dermatologist, 1900-1979.
  Hopf disease – *SYN:* Hopf keratosis
  Hopf keratosis – genetic trait resulting in wartlike nevi on the dorsum of
    hands and feet. *SYN:* Hopf disease

Hopkins, Sir Frederick G., English biochemist and Nobel laureate,
1861-1947.
  Benedict-Hopkins-Cole reagent – see under Benedict, Stanley R.

Hopmann, Carl M., German rhinologist, 1849-1925.
  Hopmann papilloma – a papillomatous overgrowth of the nasal mucous
    membrane. *SYN:* Hopmann polyp
  Hopmann polyp – *SYN:* Hopmann papilloma

Hoppe, Herman H., U.S. neurologist, 1867-1919.
  Hoppe-Goldflam disease – *SYN:* Goldflam disease

Horan, M.B.
  Nance-Horan syndrome – see under Nance

NOTES

Horecker, Bernard L., U.S. biochemist, *1914.
Warburg-Lipman-Dickens-Horecker shunt – *SYN:* Dickens shunt

Horne, Jan (Johannes) van, see under van Horne

Horner, Johann Friedrich, Swiss ophthalmologist, 1831-1886.
Bernard-Horner syndrome – *SYN:* Horner syndrome
Horner pupil – constricted pupil due to impairment of sympathetic nerve innervation of the dilator muscle of the pupil.
Horner syndrome – ptosis, miosis, and anhidrosis on the side of the sympathetic palsy. *SYN:* Bernard-Horner syndrome; Bernard syndrome; ptosis sympathetica
Horner-Trantas dots – evanescent white cellular infiltrates occurring in the bulbar form of vernal keratoconjunctivitis.

Horner, William E., U.S. anatomist, 1793-1853.
Horner muscle – *SYN:* lacrimal part of orbicularis oculi muscle
Horner teeth – incisor teeth having a horizontal hypoplastic groove.

Horsfall, Frank L., Jr., U.S. physician, 1906-1971.
Tamm-Horsfall mucoprotein – see under Tamm
Tamm-Horsfall protein

Horsley, Sir Victor A.H., English surgeon, 1857-1916.
Horsley anastomosis
Horsley bone cutter
Horsley bone-cutting forceps
Horsley bone rongeur
Horsley bone wax – a mixture of antiseptic agents, oil, and wax used to stop bleeding by plugging bone cavities or haversian canals. *SYN:* bone wax
Horsley cranial rongeur
Horsley dural separator
Horsley elevator
Horsley forceps
Horsley suture
Horsley trephine

Hortega, Pio del Rio, Spanish neurohistologist in South America, 1882-1945.
Hortega cells – small neuroglial cells that may become phagocytic in areas of neural damage or inflammation. *SYN:* microglia
Hortega neuroglia stain – one of several silver carbonate methods to demonstrate astrocytes, oligodendroglia, and microglia.

Horton, Bayard T., U.S. physician, 1895-1980.
    Horton arteritis – a subacute, granulomatous arteritis involving the external carotid arteries, especially the temporal artery. *SYN:* temporal arteritis
    Horton cephalalgia – unilateral orbitotemporal headaches associated with ipsilateral photophobia, lacrimation, and nasal congestion. *SYN:* cluster headache; Horton headache
    Horton headache – *SYN:* Horton cephalalgia

Horvitz, H. Robert, U.S. biologist, *1947, joint winner of 2002 Nobel Prize for work related to genetic regulation of organ development and cell death.

Hounsfield, Godfrey N., English electronics engineer and Nobel laureate, *1919.
    Hounsfield number – a normalized value of the calculated x-ray absorption coefficient of a pixel in a computed tomogram. *SYN:* CT number
    Hounsfield unit – a normalized index of x-ray attenuation used in CT imaging.

Housepian, Edgar M., U.S. neurosurgeon.
    Housepian aneurysm clip
    Housepian forceps

Houssay, Bernardo A., Argentinian physiologist and Nobel laureate, 1887-1971.
    Houssay animal – an animal that has had its pancreas and hypophysis excised.
    Houssay phenomenon
    Houssay syndrome – the amelioration of diabetes mellitus by a destructive lesion in, or surgical removal of, the pituitary gland.

Houston, John, Irish physician, 1802-1845.
    Houston folds – *SYN:* transverse rectal folds
    Houston muscle – a variation of the bulbospongiosus muscle in the penis. *SYN:* compressor venae dorsalis penis

NOTES

Houston valves – *SYN:* transverse rectal folds

Hovius, Jacob, Dutch ophthalmologist, 1710-1786.
canal of Hovius – an anastomotic circle between the anterior twigs of the venae vorticosae in the eyes of some animals, but not in normal human eyes.

Howard, John Eager, U.S. internist and endocrinologist, 1902-1985.
Ellsworth-Howard test – see under Ellsworth
Howard test – a differential ureteral catheterization test.

Howell, William, U.S. physiologist, 1860-1945.
Howell-Jolly bodies – spherical or ovoid eccentrically located granules occasionally observed in the stroma of circulating erythrocytes that occur most frequently after splenectomy or in megaloblastic or severe hemolytic anemia. *SYN:* Jolly bodies
Howell unit – equivalent approximately to 0.002 mg of pure heparin. *SYN:* heparin unit

Howship, John, English surgeon, 1781-1841.
Howship lacunae – tiny depressions, pits, or irregular grooves in bone that are being resorbed by osteoclasts. *SYN:* resorption lacunae
Romberg-Howship symptom – see under Romberg, Moritz Heinrich von

Hoyer, Heinrich F., Polish anatomist and histologist, 1834-1907.
Hoyer anastomoses – *SYN:* Sucquet-Hoyer canals
Hoyer canals – *SYN:* Sucquet-Hoyer canals
Sucquet-Hoyer anastomoses – *SYN:* Sucquet-Hoyer canals
Sucquet-Hoyer canals – see under Sucquet

Hubbard, Carl P., 20th century U.S. engineer.
Hubbard tank – a tank designed for full-body immersion. *SYN:* full-body tank

Hubel, David H., Canadian-U.S. neurobiologist, *1926, joint winner of 1981 Nobel Prize for work related to vision.

Hubrecht, Ambrosius A.W., Dutch zoologist and comparative anatomist, 1853-1915.
Hubrecht protochordal knot – a local thickening of the blastoderm at the cephalic end of the primitive streak of the embryo. *SYN:* primitive node

Huchard, Henri, French physician, 1844-1910.
Huchard disease – hypertension that occurs without preexisting renal disease or known cause. *SYN:* essential hypertension

Huchard sign – when patients with hypertension change from standing to supine position, the heart rate drop is less than that for normotensive patients.

Huckleberry Finn, see under Finn, Huckleberry

Hudson, Arthur Cyril, English ophthalmologist, 1875-1962.
Hudson-Stähli line – a brown, horizontal line across the lower third of the cornea.

Huebner, O.
Nierhoff-Huebner syndrome – see under Nierhoff

Hueck, Alexander F., German anatomist, 1802-1842.
Hueck ligament – the network of fibers at the iridocorneal angle between the anterior chamber of the eye and the venous sinus of the sclera. *SYN:* trabecular reticulum

Huet, var. of Huët

Huët, (Huet), G.J., Dutch physician, *1879.
Huët-Pelger anomaly – *SYN:* Pelger-Huët nuclear anomaly
Pelger-Huët nuclear anomaly – see under Pelger

Hueter, Karl, German surgeon, 1838-1882.
Hueter maneuver – pressing the patient's tongue downward and forward with the left forefinger in passing a stomach tube.
Hueter sign – in case of fracture, the vibration expected on tapping the bone is not transmitted when tissue intervenes between the fractured parts of bone.

Hüfner, Carl Gustav von, German physician, 1840-1908.
Hüfner equation – an equation expressing the relationship between myoglobin dissociation and oxygen partial pressure.

Huggins, Charles B., Canadian-U.S. surgeon and Nobel laureate, 1901-1994.
Huggins operation – orchidectomy performed for palliation or cure of cancer of the prostate. *SYN:* castration

NOTES

Huguier, Pierre C., French surgeon, 1804-1873.

Huguier canal – a canal in the petrotympanic or glaserian fissure, near its posterior edge, through which the chorda tympani nerve issues from the skull. *SYN:* anterior canaliculus of chorda tympani

Huguier circle – anastomosis around the isthmus of the uterus between the right and left uterine arteries.

Huguier sinus – a depression on the medial wall of the middle ear which has the oval window in its lower portion. *SYN:* fossula fenestrae vestibuli

Huhner, Max, U.S. urologist, 1873-1947.

Huhner test – determination of sperm quantity and motility in specimens obtained from the cervical canal following coitus, performed around the time of ovulation.

Humm, Doncaster George, U.S. psychologist, 1887-1959.

Humm-Wadsworth Temperament Scale – personality inventory.

Hummelsheim, Eduard K.M.J., German ophthalmologist, 1868-1952.

Hummelsheim operation – transplantation of a normal ocular rectus muscle, to substitute for a paralyzed muscle.

Humphry, Sir George M., English surgeon, 1820-1896.

Humphry ligament – the ligamentous band that passes anterior to the posterior cruciate ligament, extending between the posterior portion of the lateral meniscus and the upper end of the anterior cruciate ligament. *SYN:* anterior meniscofemoral ligament

Hunermann, Carl, German pediatrician, 1900-1943.

Conradi-Hunermann disease – *SYN:* Conradi disease

Hunner, Guy L., U.S. surgeon, 1868-1957.

Fenwick-Hunner ulcer – *SYN:* Hunner ulcer

Hunner stricture – bladder stricture produced by interstitial cystitis (Hunner ulcer).

Hunner ulcer – a focal and often multiple lesion involving all layers of the bladder wall in chronic interstitial cystitis. *SYN:* elusive ulcer; Fenwick-Hunner ulcer

Hunt, James Ramsay, U.S. neurologist, 1872-1937.

Hunt atrophy – obsolete term for atrophy of the small muscles of the hand, without sensory disturbances.

Hunt neuralgia – a severe paroxysmal lancinating pain deep in the ear. *SYN:* geniculate neuralgia

Hunt paradoxical phenomenon – in torsion dystonia, extension of the foot in response to passive flexion and flexion in response to attempted passive extension.

Hunt syndrome – (1) an intention tremor beginning in one extremity and subsequently involving other parts of the body. *SYN:* progressive cerebellar tremor; (2) facial paralysis, otalgia, and herpes zoster resulting from viral infection of the seventh cranial nerve and geniculate ganglion. *SYN:* herpes zoster oticus; (3) a form of juvenile paralysis agitans associated with primary atrophy of the pallidal system. *SYN:* paleostriatal syndrome pallidal syndrome; Ramsay Hunt syndrome

Ramsay Hunt syndrome – *SYN:* Hunt syndrome

Hunt, R. Timothy, English scientist, *1943, joint winner of 2001 Nobel Prize for work related to key regulators of cell cycles.

Hunt, William E., U.S. neurosurgeon, *1921.

Hunt angled serrated ring forceps
Hunt angled-tip forceps
Hunt grasping forceps
Tolosa-Hunt syndrome – see under Tolosa

Hunter, Charles H., Canadian physician, 1872-1955.

Hunter syndrome – an error of mucopolysaccharide metabolism. *SYN:* type II mucopolysaccharidosis

Hunter, John, Scottish surgeon, anatomist, physiologist, and pathologist, 1728-1793.

Hunter canal – the space in the middle third of the thigh that gives passage to the femoral vessels and saphenous nerve. *SYN:* adductor canal

Hunter gubernaculum – an obsolete term for gubernaculum testis.
hunterian chancre – chancre resulting from syphilis.
hunterian perforator
Hunter operation – ligation of the artery proximal and distal to an aneurysm.

NOTES

Hunter-Schreger bands – alternating light and dark lines seen in dental enamel. *SYN:* Hunter-Schreger lines; Schreger lines
Hunter-Schreger lines – *SYN:* Hunter-Schreger bands

Hunter, William, English pathologist, 1861-1937.
Hunter glossitis – *SYN:* Moeller-Hunter syndrome
Moeller-Hunter syndrome – see under Moeller, Julius Otto Ludwig

Hunter, William, Scottish anatomist and obstetrician, 1718-1783.
Hunter ligament – *SYN:* round ligament of the uterus
Hunter line – a fibrous band running vertically the entire length of the center of the anterior abdominal wall, receiving the attachments of the oblique and transverse abdominal muscles. *SYN:* linea alba
Hunter membrane – the mucous membrane of the pregnant uterus. *SYN:* deciduous membrane

Huntington, George, U.S. physician, 1850-1916.
Huntington chorea – an inherited degenerative disorder of the cerebral cortex and corpus striatum. *SYN:* chronic progressive chorea; degenerative chorea; hereditary chorea; Huntington disease
Huntington disease – *SYN:* Huntington chorea

Huriez, C., French dermatologist, 1907-1984.
Huriez syndrome – an autosomal dominant syndrome presenting in infancy with sclerodactyly, diffuse keratoderma more marked on the soles than palms, nail abnormalities and hypohidrosis. Some patients developed cutaneous squamous cell carcinoma.

Hurler, Gertrud, German pediatrician, 1889-1965.
Hurler disease – *SYN:* Hurler syndrome
Hurler syndrome – mucopolysaccharidosis with severe abnormality in development of skeletal cartilage and bone, corneal clouding, hepatosplenomegaly, mental retardation, and gargoyle-like facies. *SYN:* dysostosis multiplex; Hurler disease; lipochondrodystrophy; Pfaundler-Hurler syndrome; type IH mucopolysaccharidosis
Pfaundler-Hurler syndrome – *SYN:* Hurler syndrome

Hurst, Edward Weston, Australian bacteriologist, 1900-1980.
Hurst disease – *SYN:* acute hemorrhagic leukoencephalitis

Hürthle, Karl W., German histologist, 1860-1945.

Hürthle cell – a large, granular eosinophilic cell derived from thyroid follicular epithelium by accumulation of mitochondria, e.g., in Hashimoto disease. *SYN:* Askanazy cell

Hürthle cell adenoma – a follicular adenoma of the thyroid in which the epithelium has undergone metaplasia into Hürthle cells.

Hürthle cell carcinoma – *SYN:* Hürthle cell tumor

Hürthle cell tumor – neoplasm of the thyroid gland. *SYN:* Hürthle cell carcinoma

Huschke, Emil, German anatomist, 1797-1858.

Huschke auditory teeth – tooth-shaped formations or ridges occurring on the vestibular lip of the limbus lamina spiralis of the cochlear duct. *SYN:* auditory teeth

Huschke canal

Huschke cartilages – two horizontal cartilaginous rods at the edge of the cartilaginous septum of the nose.

Huschke foramen – an opening in the floor of the bony part of the external acoustic meatus near the tympanic membrane.

Huschke ligament

Huschke valve – a fold of mucous membrane guarding the lower opening of the nasolacrimal duct. *SYN:* lacrimal fold

Hutchinson, Sir Jonathan, English surgeon and pathologist, 1828-1913.

Hutchinson crescentic notch – the semilunar notch on the incisal edge of Hutchinson teeth, encountered in congenital syphilis.

Hutchinson disease – age-related guttate choroiditis.

Hutchinson facies – the peculiar facial expression produced by drooping eyelids and motionless eyes in external ophthalmoplegia.

Hutchinson freckle – a brown or black mottled, irregularly outlined, slowly enlarging lesion. *SYN:* lentigo maligna

Hutchinson-Gilford disease – a condition in which normal development in the first year is followed by gross retardation of growth, with dry wrinkled

NOTES

skin, total alopecia, and birdlike facies. *SYN:* Hutchinson-Gilford syndrome; progeria

Hutchinson-Gilford syndrome – *SYN:* Hutchinson-Gilford disease

Hutchinson mask – the sensation experienced in tabetic neurosyphilis as if the face were covered with a mask or with cobwebs.

Hutchinson patch – interstitial or parenchymatous keratitis giving rise to neovascularization of the cornea. *SYN:* salmon patch

Hutchinson pupil – dilation of the pupil on the side of the lesion as part of a third nerve palsy.

Hutchinson teeth – the teeth of congenital syphilis in which the incisal edge is notched and narrower than the cervical area. *SYN:* notched teeth; screwdriver teeth; syphilitic teeth

Hutchinson triad – parenchymatous keratitis, labyrinthine disease, and Hutchinson teeth, significant of congenital syphilis.

Hutchison, Sir Robert, English pediatrician, 1871-1960.
Hutchison syndrome – adrenal neuroblastoma of infants with metastasis to the orbit.

Hutinel, Victor H., French pediatrician, 1849-1933.
Hutinel disease – juvenile tuberculous pericarditis.

Hutton, Lauren, 20th century U.S. model and film actress.
Lauren Hutton sign – *SYN:* David Letterman sign

Huxley, Sir Andrew Fielding, English physiologist, *1917, joint winner of 1963 Nobel Prize for work related to nerve cell membrane.

Huxley, Thomas Henry, English biologist, physiologist, and comparative anatomist, 1825-1895.
Huxley layer – the layer of cells interposed between Henle layer and the cuticle of the inner root sheath of the hair follicle. *SYN:* Huxley membrane; Huxley sheath
Huxley membrane – *SYN:* Huxley layer
Huxley sheath – *SYN:* Huxley layer

Huygens, Christian, Dutch physicist, 1629-1695.
Huygens ocular – the compound ocular of a microscope, composed of two planoconvex lenses so arranged that the plane side of each is directed toward the observer.
Huygens principle – used in ultrasound technology.

Hyde, James N., U.S. dermatologist, 1840-1910.

Hyde disease – an eruption of hard nodules in the skin caused by rubbing and accompanied by intense itching. *SYN:* picker's nodules; prurigo nodularis

Hynes, Wilfred, English plastic surgeon, *1903.

Anderson-Hynes pyeloplasty – see under Anderson, James C.

Hynes pharyngoplasty – an operation to narrow the pharynx in order to improve speech.

Hyrtl, Joseph, Austrian anatomist, 1810-1894.

Hyrtl anastomosis – *SYN:* Hyrtl loop

Hyrtl canal

Hyrtl epitympanic recess – the upper portion of the tympanic cavity above the tympanic membrane. *SYN:* epitympanic recess; Hyrtl recess

Hyrtl foramen – an occasional foramen in the sphenoid bone through which passes the motor portion of the trigeminal nerve. *SYN:* porus crotaphytico-buccinatorius

Hyrtl loop – a communicating loop between the right and left hypoglossal nerves. *SYN:* Hyrtl anastomosis

Hyrtl nerve

Hyrtl recess – *SYN:* Hyrtl epitympanic recess

Hyrtl sphincter – a band, generally incomplete, of circular muscular fibers in the rectum about 10 cm above the anus (upper rectal ampulla).

Ibrahim, Murad Jussuf Bey, Egyptian pediatrician, 1877-1953.
  Beck-Ibrahim syndrome – see under Beck, Soma Cornelius
  Ibrahim disease – *SYN:* Beck-Ibrahim syndrome

Iceland, an island in the North Atlantic where the disease is prevalent.
  Iceland disease – chronic fatigue syndrome. *SYN:* epidemic
  neuromyasthenia

Ieshima, Atsushi, Japanese physician.
  Ieshima syndrome – genetic trait resulting in psychomotor retardation and
  multiple abnormalities.

Ignarro, Louis J., U.S. pharmacologist, *1941, joint winner of 1998 Nobel
Prize for work related to nitric oxide as a signal molecule in biological systems.

Ilosvay, Lajos de, Hungarian chemist, *1851.
  Ilosvay reagent – test for nitrites.

Imerslund, Olga, Norwegian physician.
  Grasbeck-Imerslund syndrome – *SYN:* Imerslund-Grasbeck syndrome
  Imerslund-Grasbeck syndrome – familial enterocyte cobalamin
  malabsorption. *SYN:* Grasbeck-Imerslund syndrome; malabsorption
  syndrome

Imhoff, Karl, German engineer, 1876-1965.
  Imhoff tank – tank for digestion.

Imlach, Francis, Scottish anatomist and surgeon, 1819-1891.
  Imlach fat-pad – fat surrounding the round ligament of the uterus in the
  inguinal canal.
  Imlach ring – that part of the inguinal canal which lodges the round
  ligament of the uterus.

Imrie, C.W., Scottish surgeon.
Imrie sign – flushing of the face during initial phase of acute pancreatitis; may be accompanied by gastrointestinal symptoms.

Ingrassia, Giovanni F., Italian anatomist, 1510-1580.
Ingrassia apophysis – *SYN:* Ingrassia wing
Ingrassia wing – one of a bilateral pair of triangular, pointed plates extending laterally from the anterolateral body of the sphenoid bone. *SYN:* Ingrassia apophysis; lesser wing of sphenoid bone

Iru Kandji, Australian aboriginal tribe.
Iru Kandji syndrome – syndrome resulting from a jellyfish sting; produces shock and muscle pain as well as gastrointestinal symptoms.

Irvine, A. Ray, Jr., U.S. ophthalmologist, *1917.
Irvine corneal scissors
Irvine-Gass syndrome – macular edema, aphakia, and vitreous humor adherent to incision for cataract extraction.
Irvine operation
Irvine probe-pointed scissors

Isaacs, Hyam, South African neurophysiologist, *1927.
Isaacs syndrome – peripheral nerve disease resulting in rigidity of the muscles. *SYN:* stiff man syndrome

Isaacs, R., U.S. physician, *1891.
Isaacs granules – refractile granules seen in normal unstained erythrocytes.

Isambert, Emile, French physician, 1828-1876.
Isambert disease – miliary tuberculosis.

Ishak, K.G.
Luna-Ishak stain – see under Luna

Ishihara, Shinobu, Japanese ophthalmologist, 1879-1963.
Ishihara I-Temp cautery
Ishihara IV slit lamp
Ishihara plate
Ishihara test – a test for color vision deficiency.
Ishihara test chart book

Iso, Ryosuke, 20th century Japanese physician.
Iso-Kikuchi syndrome – syndrome featuring abnormal nail of the index finger (nail is absent, small, or consists of two nails of different size) and bifurcation of the distal phalanx of the index finger.

Israel, James Adolf, German urologist, 1848-1926.
Actinomyces israelii

Itard, Jean M.G., French otologist, 1774-1838.
Cholewa-Itard sign – *SYN:* Itard-Cholewa sign
Itard-Cholewa sign – tympanic membrane anesthesia due to otosclerosis.
SYN: Cholewa-Itard sign

Ito, Hayozo, Japanese physician, *1865.
Ito-Reenstierna test – *SYN:* Ducrey test

Ito, Minor, Japanese dermatologist, 1884-1982.
hypomelanosis of Ito – inherited hypopigmented macules variably
associated with epidermal nevi, alopecia, and ocular, skeletal, and
neural abnormalities. *SYN:* incontinentia pigmenti achromians
Ito nevus – pigmentation of skin innervated by lateral branches of the
supraclavicular nerve and the lateral cutaneous nerve of the arm.

Ito, T., 20th century Japanese physician.
Ito cells – fat-containing cells lining hepatic sinusoids.

Itsenko, N.M., Russian physician, 1889-1954.
Itsenko-Cushing syndrome – *SYN:* Cushing syndrome

Ivemark, Björn, Swedish pathologist, *1925.
Ivemark syndrome – a possibly heritable disorder in which organs of the
left side of the body are a mirror image of their counterpart on the right
side, with associated splenic agenesis and cardiac malformations.

Ivy, Andrew Conway, U.S. physiologist, 1893-1978.
Ivy bleeding time test

Ivy, Robert H., U.S. oral and plastic surgeon, 1881-1974.
Ivy loop wiring – placement of a wire around two adjacent teeth to provide
an attachment for intermaxillary elastics.

Izar, Guido, 20th century Italian pathologist.
Izar reagent

NOTES

Jabon, Marcel M.J., French physician, *1898.

Jabon syndrome – gastrointestinal syndrome produced when antibiotic therapy destroys normal flora and allows specific strains of staphylococci to flourish.

Jaboulay, Mathieu, French surgeon, 1860-1913.

Jaboulay amputation – amputation of an entire leg together with the os coxae. *SYN:* hemipelvectomy

Jaboulay button

Jaboulay method – anastomosis of arteries by splitting the cut ends a short distance, suturing the flaps together, and applying intima to intima. *SYN:* broad marginal confrontation method

Jaboulay pyloroplasty – a side-to-side gastroduodenostomy.

Jaccoud, François Sigismond, French physician, 1830-1913.

Jaccoud arthritis – a rare form of chronic arthritis, reported to occur after attacks of acute rheumatic fever. *SYN:* Jaccoud arthropathy

Jaccoud arthropathy – *SYN:* Jaccoud arthritis

Jaccoud syndrome

Jackson, Jabez N., U.S. surgeon, 1868-1935.

Jackson anterior commissure laryngoscope

Jackson approximation forceps

Jackson broad staple forceps

Jackson button forceps

Jackson conventional foreign body forceps

Jackson cross-action forceps

Jackson double-prong forceps

Jackson dull rotation forceps

Jackson esophagoscope

Jackson flexible upper lobe bronchus forceps

Jackson globular object forceps

NOTES

Jackson membrane – a thin vascular membrane or veil-like adhesion covering the anterior surface of the ascending colon from the cecum to the right flexure. *SYN:* Jackson veil

Jackson papilloma forceps

Jackson pin-bending costophrenic forceps

Jackson sharp-pointed rotation forceps

Jackson spinal surgery and imaging table

Jackson steel-stem woven filiform bougie

Jackson triangular brass dilator

Jackson veil – *SYN:* Jackson membrane

Jackson, John Hughlings, English neurologist, 1835-1911.

jacksonian epilepsy – *SYN:* jacksonian seizure

jacksonian seizure – a seizure originating in or near the rolandic neocortex which clinically involves one part of the body. *SYN:* jacksonian epilepsy

Jackson law – loss of mental functions due to disease retraces in reverse order its evolutionary development.

Jackson rule – after an epileptic attack, simple and quasiautomatic functions are less affected and more rapidly recovered than the more complex ones.

Jackson sign – during quiet respiration the movement of the paralyzed side of the chest may be greater than that of the opposite side, while in forced respiration the paralyzed side moves less than the other.

Jacob, Arthur, Irish physician, 1790-1874.

Jacob membrane

Jacob ulcer

Jacob, François, French biologist, *1920, joint winner of 1965 Nobel Prize for work related to synthesis of viruses and enzymes.

Jacob, Octave, French physician.

Jacob disease – inability to open the mouth secondary to mandibular constriction.

Jacobaeus, Hans C., Swedish surgeon, 1879-1937.

Jacobaeus operation – obsolete term for pleurolysis.

Jacobaeus thoracoscope

Jacobi, Eduard, German dermatologist, 1862-1915.

Jacobi poikiloderma – an unusual type of mycosis fungoides in which the skin shows areas of atrophy, pigmentary change, and telangiectasia.

Jacobs, Eugene C., U.S. physician, *1905.

    Jacobs syndrome – scrotal dermatitis, conjunctivitis, and stomatitis observed in American prisoners of war who were fed a diet of rice.

Jacobson, Julius, German ophthalmologist, 1828-1889.

    Jacobson neuralgia – *SYN:* Reichert syndrome

    Jacobson retinitis – *SYN:* syphilitic retinitis

Jacobson, Ludwig L., Danish anatomist, 1783-1843.

    Jacobson anastomosis – a portion of the tympanic plexus.

    Jacobson canal – a minute canal in the wedge of bone separating the jugular canal and carotid canal. *SYN:* tympanic canaliculus

    Jacobson cartilage – a narrow strip of cartilage located between the lower edge of the cartilage of the nasal septum and the vomer. *SYN:* cartilago vomeronasalis

    Jacobson nerve – *SYN:* tympanic nerve

    Jacobson organ – a fine vestigial horizontal canal ending in a blind pouch in the mucous membrane of the nasal septum. *SYN:* vomeronasal organ

    Jacobson plexus – a plexus on the promontory of the labyrinthine wall of the tympanic cavity, formed by the tympanic nerve, an anastomotic branch of the facial nerve, and sympathetic branches from the internal carotid plexus. *SYN:* tympanic plexus

    Jacobson reflex – flexion of the fingers elicited by tapping the flexor tendons over the wrist joint or the lower end of the radius.

Jacod, Maurice, French neurologist, *1880.

    Jacod syndrome – total ophthalmoplegia, blindness, and trigeminal neuralgia. *SYN:* Jacod triad

    Jacod triad – *SYN:* Jacod syndrome

Jacquart, Henri, 19th century French physician.

    Jacquart facial angle – a facial angle with the intersection always at the nasal spine point.

NOTES

Jacquemet, Marcel, French anatomist, 1872-1908.
Jacquemet recess – a pouch of peritoneum between the gallbladder and the liver.

Jacquemin, Emile, 19th century French chemist.
Jacquemin test – a test for phenol.

Jacques, James Archibald, manager of an English rubber company, 1815-1878.
Jacques catheter – urethral catheter.

Jacques, Paul, 19th century French physician.
Jacques plexus – a nerve plexus within the muscular coat of the fallopian tube.

Jacquet, Leonard Marie Lucien, French dermatologist, 1860-1914.
Jacquet erythema – diaper rash. *SYN:* diaper dermatitis

Jadassohn, Josef, German dermatologist in Switzerland, 1863-1936.
Borst-Jadassohn type intraepidermal epithelioma – see under Borst
Franceschetti-Jadassohn syndrome – *SYN:* Naegeli syndrome
Jadassohn-Lewandowski syndrome – ectodermal dysplasia of abnormal thickness and elevation of nail plates with palmar and plantar hyperkeratosis. *SYN:* pachyonychia congenita
Jadassohn nevus – congenital papillary acanthosis of the epidermis, with hyperplasia of sebaceous glands developing at puberty and presence of apocrine glands in nonapocrine areas of the skin. *SYN:* nevus sebaceus
Jadassohn-Pellizzari anetoderma – cutaneous atrophy preceded by erythematous or urticarial lesions of the trunk and upper portions of the extremities.
Jadassohn-Tièche nevus – a dark blue or blue-black nevus covered by smooth skin and formed by heavily pigmented spindle-shaped or dendritic melanocytes in the reticular dermis. *SYN:* blue nevus

Jadelot, Jean F.N., French physician, 1791-1830.
Jadelot furrows – *SYN:* Jadelot lines
Jadelot lines – facial lines in children. *SYN:* Jadelot furrows

Jaeger, Eduard, Ritter von Jaxtthal, Austrian ophthalmologist, 1818-1884.
Jaeger hook
Jaeger keratome knife
Jaeger lid plate
Jaeger lid retractor
Jaeger reading chart

Jaeger strabismus hook

Jaeger test types – type of different sizes used for testing the acuity of near vision.

Jaffe, Henry Lewis, U.S. pathologist, 1896-1979.
Jaffe-Campanacci syndrome – *SYN:* Campanacci syndrome
Jaffe-Lichtenstein disease – obsolete term for fibrous dysplasia of bone.

Jaffe, Max, German biochemist, 1841-1911.
Jaffe reaction – the basis of most routine creatinine tests.
Jaffe test – a qualitative test for the presence of indicanuria.

Jakob, Alfons M., German neuropsychiatrist, 1884-1931.
Creutzfeldt-Jakob disease – see under Creutzfeldt
Jakob-Creutzfeldt disease – *SYN:* Creutzfeldt-Jakob disease

Jaksch, Rudolf Ritter Von Wartenhorst, Austrian physician, 1855-1940.
Jaksch anemia – *SYN:* Jaksch syndrome
Jaksch syndrome – a form of chronic anemia in infants and children under 3 years of age. *SYN:* Jaksch anemia

James, George C.W., 20th century U.S. radiologist.
Swyer-James-Macleod syndrome – *SYN:* Swyer-James syndrome (2)
Swyer-James syndrome – see under Swyer

James, Thomas N., U.S. cardiologist and physiologist, *1925.
James fibers – atrio-His bundle connections thought to be the basis for the short P-R interval syndrome. *SYN:* James tracts
James tracts – *SYN:* James fibers

James, William, U.S. psychologist, 1842-1910.
James-Lange theory – that bodily changes, such as tachycardia or sweating, precede rather than follow the conscious perception of an emotion and by themselves evoke the emotional feeling.

Jampel, Robert Steven, U.S. ophthalmologist, *1926.
Schwartz-Jampel-Aberfeld syndrome – *SYN:* Schwartz-Jampel syndrome

NOTES

Schwartz-Jampel syndrome – myotonic chondrodystrophy.
   SYN: Schwartz-Jampel-Aberfeld syndrome

Janet, Pierre M.F., French neurologist, 1859-1947.
   Janet disease – psychasthenia.
   Janet test – a test for functional or organic anesthesia.

Janeway, Edward G., U.S. physician, 1841-1911.
   Janeway lesion – a small erythematous or hemorrhagic lesion seen in some cases of bacterial endocarditis.

Janeway, Theodore Caldwell, U.S. physician, 1872-1917.
   Janeway sphygmomanometer

Jannetta, Peter J., U.S. neurosurgeon, *1932.
   Jannetta aneurysm neck dissector
   Jannetta bayonet forceps
   Jannetta bayonet needle holder
   Jannetta bayonet scissors
   Jannetta dissector
   Jannetta elevator
   Jannetta microbayonet forceps
   Jannetta needle holder
   Jannetta posterior fossa retractor
   Jannetta procedure – decompression of microvascular structures.
   Jannetta sterilizing rack

Jansen, Albert, German otologist, 1859-1933.
   Jansen bayonet nasal forceps
   Jansen ear forceps
   Jansen ear rongeur
   Jansen mastoid raspatory
   Jansen-Middleton punch forceps
   Jansen mouth gag
   Jansen operation – an operation for frontal sinus disease, the lower wall and lower portion of the anterior wall being removed and the mucous membrane curetted away.
   Jansen scalp retractor

Jansen, Murk, Dutch orthopedic surgeon, 1867-1935.
   Jansen syndrome – rare congenital disease that causes anatomical abnormalities.

Jansky, Jan, Czech physician, 1873-1921.
   Bielschowsky-Jansky disease – *SYN:* Jansky-Bielschowsky disease

Jansky-Bielschowsky disease – cerebral sphingolipidosis, early juvenile
   type. *SYN:* Bielschowsky-Jansky disease
Jansky classification – the classification of human blood groups now
   designated O, A, B, and AB.

Janus, in Roman mythology, the two-faced god of gates; one face looks
forward and the other face looks backward.
   Janus-faced – marked by deliberate deceitfulness. *SYN:* double-faced;
      duplicitous; two-faced

Jaquet, Alfred, Swiss pharmacologist, 1865-1937.
   Jaquet apparatus – apparatus for recording cardiac and venous impulses.

Jarcho, Julius, Russian-U.S. obstetrician, 1882-1963.
   Jarcho pressometer – instrument used in hysterosalpingography.
   Jarcho self-retaining uterine cannula
   Jarcho uterine tenaculum

Jarcho, Saul, U.S. physician, *1906.
   Jarcho syndrome – bone marrow metastatic carcinoma.

Jarisch, Adolf, Austrian dermatologist, 1850-1902.
   Bezold-Jarisch reflex – see under Bezold, Albert von
   Jarisch-Herxheimer reaction – *SYN:* Herxheimer reaction

Jarjavay, Jean F., French anatomist and surgeon, 1815-1868.
   Jarjavay ligament – a fold of peritoneum containing the rectouterine
      muscle. *SYN:* sacrouterine fold

Jaworski, Walery, Polish physician, 1849-1924.
   Jaworski bodies – mucous shreds in the gastric contents in
      hyperchlorhydria.

Jeanselme, A. Edouard, French dermatologist, 1858-1935.
   Jeanselme nodules – a form of tertiary yaws that is characterized by the
      occurrence of nodules on the arms and legs, situated usually near the
      joints. *SYN:* juxtaarticular nodules

NOTES

Jefferson, Sir Geoffrey, English neurologist, 1886-1961.
    Jefferson syndrome – *SYN:* internal carotid artery aneurysm

Jeghers, Harold Joseph, U.S. physician, 1904-1990.
    Jeghers-Peutz syndrome – *SYN:* Peutz-Jeghers syndrome
    Peutz-Jeghers syndrome – see under Peutz

Jekyll and Hyde, main characters in Robert Louis Stevenson's classic novel about a doctor who turns into a murderous madman and back again during experimentation with an elixir.
    Jekyll and Hyde personality – one who is vile, cruel, and aggressive in private but who is charming, deceptive, and verbally facile in public.

Jellinek, Edward J., English physician, 1890-1963.
    Jellinek formula – a method of estimating the prevalence of alcoholism in a nation's population.

Jellinek, Stefan, Austrian physician, *1871.
    Jellinek sign – in Graves disease, a brownish pigmentation of the eyelids, especially the upper ones.

Jendrassik, Ernö, Hungarian physician, 1858-1921.
    Jendrassik maneuver – a method of emphasizing the patellar reflex: the subject hooks his hands together by the flexed fingers and pulls against them with all his strength.

Jenner, Harley D., Canadian physician, *1907.
    Jenner-Kay unit – that amount of phosphatase that liberates 1 mg of phosphorus.

Jenner, Louis, English physician, 1866-1904.
    Jenner stain – used for staining of blood smears.

Jenner, Sir Edward, English physician, 1749-1823.
    jennerian vaccination – vaccination to prevent smallpox.

Jensen, Carl O., Danish veterinary surgeon and pathologist, 1864-1934.
    Jensen sarcoma – a mouse tumor transmissible by inoculation.

Jensen, Edmund Z., Danish ophthalmologist, 1861-1950.
    Jensen disease – retinochoroiditis close to the optic disk.
        SYN: retinochoroiditis juxtapapillaris
    Jensen intraocular lens forceps
    Jensen lens forceps
    Jensen polisher
    Jensen scratcher
    Jensen ties

Jerne, Niels K., Danish immunologist, *1911, joint winner of the 1984 Nobel Prize for medicine and physiology.

Jervell, Anton, Norwegian cardiologist, *1901.
> **Jervell and Lange-Nielsen syndrome** – a prolonged Q-T interval recorded in the electrocardiogram of certain congenitally deaf children subject to Adams-Stokes seizures and ventricular fibrillation. *SYN:* surdocardiac syndrome

Jessner, Max, German-U.S. dermatologist, 1887-1978.
> **Jessner chemical peel** – *SYN:* Jessner solution
> **Jessner-Kanof disease** – benign lymphocytic infiltration most often affecting facial skin. *SYN:* Jessner-Kanof lesion
> **Jessner-Kanof lesion** – *SYN:* Jessner-Kanof disease
> **Jessner solution** – Resorcinol (14 g), salicylic acid (14 g), lactic acid (85%; 14 ml), and ethanol (95%; 100 ml). Used for superficial peels for such skin indications as comedonal acne, melasma, skin refreshing, and nonfacial peeling. *SYN:* Jessner chemical peel

Jesuits, Catholic religious order founded by Saint Ignatius Loyola in 1540.
> **Jesuit tea** – tea used by Indians for centuries; first cultivated by the Jesuits in their Paraguayan missions. *SYN:* chenopodium

Jeune, Mathis, French pediatrician, *1910.
> **Jeune syndrome** – hereditary hypoplasia of the thorax, associated with pelvic skeletal abnormality. *SYN:* asphyxiating thoracic dysplasia

Jewett, Eugene Lyon, U.S. orthopedic surgeon, *1900.
> **Jewett bending iron**
> **Jewett bone extractor**
> **Jewett driver**
> **Jewett fracture appliance**
> **Jewett frame**
> **Jewett hip nail**
> **Jewett hyperextension brace**
> **Jewett nail plate** – orthopedic fixation device.

NOTES

Jewett orthosis
Jewett pickup screw
Jewett prosthesis
Jewett reamer
Jewett thoracolumbosacral orthosis

Jewett, Hugh, U.S. urologist, 1903-1990.
  Jewett sound – a short straight sound for dilating the anterior urethra.
  Jewett and Strong staging – staging of bladder carcinoma (O, A through D).

Job, Biblical character in the Old Testament who suffered from skin and bowel disease, from which he recovered.
  Job syndrome – *SYN:* Buckley syndrome

Jobert de Lamballe, Antoine, French surgeon, 1799-1867.
  Jobert de Lamballe fossa – the hollow just above the knee formed by the adductor magnus and the sartorius and gracilis.
  Jobert de Lamballe suture – an interrupted intestinal suture used for invaginating the margins of the intestines in circular enterorrhaphy.

Jobst, Conrad, U.S. engineer.
  Jobst boot – a device used to reduce limb edema. *SYN:* Jobst sleeve
  Jobst sleeve – *SYN:* Jobst boot
  Jobst stocking – an elastic stocking used to treat postphlebitic leg edema.

Jocasta, in Greek mythology, the wife of Laius; she unwittingly married her son Oedipus after Laius was slain.
  Jocasta complex – libidinous fixation on son by mother.

Joest, Ernst, German veterinary pathologist, 1873-1926.
  Joest bodies – intranuclear inclusion bodies (Cowdry type B) produced in certain nerve cells by Borna disease virus.

Joffroy, Alexis, French physician, 1844-1908.
  Joffroy reflex – twitching of the gluteal muscles when firm pressure is made on the buttocks, in cases of spastic paralysis. *SYN:* hip phenomenon
  Joffroy sign – immobility of the facial muscles when the eyeballs are rolled upward, in exophthalmic goiter; disorder of the arithmetical faculty in the early stages of organic brain disease.

Johansson, Sven Christian, Swedish surgeon, 1880-1976.
  Sinding-Larsen-Johansson syndrome – see under Sinding-Larsen

Johne, H. Albert, German physician, 1839-1910.
    Johne bacillus – a species causing Johne disease, a chronic enteritis in cattle. *SYN: Mycobacterium paratuberculosis*
    Johne disease – a disease occurring in cattle and sheep, caused by infection with *Mycobacterium paratuberculosis*. *SYN:* chronic dysentery of cattle; paratuberculosis
    johnin – a diagnostic agent, analogous to tuberculin.

Johnson, Frank B., U.S. pathologist, *1919.
    Dubin-Johnson syndrome – *SYN:* chronic idiopathic jaundice

Johnson, Frank Chambliss, U.S. pediatrician, 1894-1934.
    Stevens-Johnson syndrome – see under Stevens, Albert Mason

Johnson, Harry B., U.S. dentist.
    Johnson method – a method of filling the root canals of teeth by dissolving gutta-percha cones in a chloroform-rosin medium within the root canal. *SYN:* chloropercha method

Johnson, Treat Baldwin, U.S. chemist, 1875-1947.
    Wheeler-Johnson test – see under Wheeler, Henry Lord

Johnston, Christopher, U.S. physician, *1891.
    Johnston organ – organ on fly antennae for sensing air flow during flight.

Jolles, Adolf, Austrian chemist, 1863-1944.
    Jolles test – a test for bile.

Jolly, Friedrich, German neurologist, 1844-1904.
    Jolly reaction – rapid loss of response to faradic stimulation of a muscle with the galvanic response and the power of voluntary contraction retained. *SYN:* Jolly test; myasthenic reaction
    Jolly test – *SYN:* Jolly reaction

Jolly, Justin, French histologist, 1870-1953.
    Howell-Jolly bodies – see under Howell
    Jolly bodies – *SYN:* Howell-Jolly bodies

NOTES

Jones, Ernest, English psychiatrist, 1879-1958.
Ross-Jones test – see under Ross, Sir George W.

Jones, Henry Bence, see under Bence Jones

Jones, Sir Robert, English orthopedic surgeon, 1858-1933.
Jones abduction frame
Jones arm splint
Jones brace
Jones first-toe repair
Jones fracture
Jones metacarpal splint
Jones pin
Jones position – position for treating humeral fracture.
Jones resection arthroplasty
Jones suspension traction
Jones thoracic clamp
Jones towel clamp
Jones transfer
Jones view

Jones, William A., U.S. dentist.
Jones disease – genetic trait resulting in fullness of the face, suggestive of a cherub. *SYN:* cherubism; Jones syndrome
Jones syndrome – *SYN:* Jones disease

Jonnesco, Thomas, Romanian surgeon, 1860-1926.
Jonnesco fossa – a peritoneal recess extending upward behind the superior duodenal fold. *SYN:* superior duodenal recess

Jonston, Johns, Scottish physician in Poland, 1603-1675.
Jonston alopecia – obsolete term for alopecia areata. *SYN:* Jonston area
Jonston area – *SYN:* Jonston alopecia

Jordans, Godefridus H.W., Dutch physician, 1902-1979.
Jordans anomaly – vacuoles in neutrophils and monocytes reported in some families with Erb-type muscular dystrophy.

Jorgenson, Ronald J., U.S. physician, 1841-1911.
Jorgenson syndrome – type of hypohidrotic ectodermal dysplasia, possibly autosomal dominant or X-linked dominant, featuring coarse scalp hair, deciduous teeth with brown spots, short thick nails, and hypohidrosis.

Joseph, surname of one of the families studied in major descriptions of the disease.

Machado-Joseph disease – see under Machado

Joseph, Jacques, German surgeon, 1865-1934.

Joseph chisel

Joseph clamp – used after rhinoplasty to maintain or improve the alignment of the bony support of the nose.

Joseph double-edged knife

Joseph knife – used in rhinoplasty to separate the overlying skin from the nasal dorsum.

Joseph nasal knife

Joseph nasal rasp

Joseph nasal raspatory

Joseph nasal saw

Joseph nasal scissors

Joseph perforator

Joseph periosteal elevator

Joseph punch

Joseph rhinoplasty – reduction and reshaping of the nose.

Joseph ruler

Joseph saw guide

Joseph septal bar

Joseph septal clamp

Joseph septal fracture appliance

Joseph septal frame

Joseph serrated scissors

Joseph single-prong hook

Joseph, R., French pediatrician.

Joseph syndrome – hereditary defect in renal tubules resulting in proteinuria with onset of epilepsy.

Joubert, Marie, 20th century Canadian neurologist.
Joubert syndrome – agenesis of the cerebellar vermis, characterized by tachypnea or prolonged apnea, abnormal eye movements, ataxia, and mental retardation.

Joule, James P., English physicist, 1818-1889.
joule – *SYN:* unit of heat
Joule equivalent – the dynamic equivalent of heat.

Juhlin, L.
Juhlin-Michaelsson syndrome – absence of basophils and eosinophils.

Julien Marie, see under Marie, Julien

Jung, Carl Gustav, Swiss psychiatrist and psychologist, 1875-1961.
jungian psychoanalysis – the theory of psychopathology and the practice of psychotherapy. *SYN:* analytical psychology

Jung, Karl G., Swiss anatomist, 1793-1864.
Jung muscle – an occasional prolongation of the fibers of the tragicus to the spina helicis. *SYN:* pyramidal auricular muscle

Jungbluth, Hermann, 20th century German physician.
Jungbluth vessels – vessels under amnion of embryo.

Jüngling, Adolph O., German surgeon, 1884-1944.
Jüngling disease – an osteitis of tuberculous origin, marked by numerous small cavities in the osseous substance. *SYN:* osteitis tuberculosa multiplex cystica

Junius, Paul, German ophthalmologist, *1871.
Kuhnt-Junius degeneration – see under Kuhnt
Kuhnt-Junius disease – *SYN:* Kuhnt-Junius degeneration

Junod, Victor T., French physician, 1809-1881.
Junod boot – an airtight case used to divert a portion of the blood temporarily from general circulation.

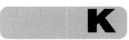

Kabat, Herman, U.S. physiatrist.
    Kabat-Knott method of exercise – *SYN:* Kabat method of exercise
    Kabat method of exercise – system of therapeutic exercises designed for
      those with neuromuscular disabilities. *SYN:* Kabat-Knott method of
      exercise; Knott-Voss method of exercise

Kabuki, highly stylized and sophisticated form of Japanese theater founded in
the 17th century.
    Kabuki makeup syndrome – *SYN:* Niikawa-Kuroki syndrome

Kachemak Bay, one of the world's most important biological marine sites,
located in Alaska.
    Kachemak Bay virus – member of the Bunyaviridae family which infects
      arthropods and vertebrate hosts.

Kader, Bronislaw, Polish surgeon, 1863-1937.
    Kader operation – a form of gastrostomy.

Kaes, Theodor, German neurologist, 1852-1913.
    band of Kaes-Bekhterev – band of horizontal myelinated fibers in the
      most superficial part of the third layer of the isocortex. *SYN:* Bekhterev
      band; layer of Bekhterev; line of Bekhterev; line of Kaes
    line of Kaes – *SYN:* band of Kaes-Bechterew

Kahlbaum, Karl L., German physician, 1828-1899.
    Kahlbaum-Wernicke syndrome

Kahler, Otto, Austrian physician, 1849-1893.
    Kahler bronchial forceps
    Kahler bronchus-grasping forceps
    Kahler disease – disease associated with anemia, hemorrhages,
      recurrent infections, and weakness; considered a malignant neoplasm.
      SYN: MacIntyre disease; multiple myeloma
    Kahler forceps

Kahler laryngeal forceps
Kahler polyp forceps

Kahn, Eugen, German psychologist, *1887.
Kahn Test of Symbol Arrangement – diagnostic psychological test.

Kahn, Reuben, U.S. bacteriologist, *1887.
Kahn test – variation of Wasserman test for syphilis.

Kaiserling, Karl, German pathologist, 1869-1942.
Kaiserling fixative – a method of preserving histologic and pathologic specimens without altering the color.

Kalischer, Siegfried, German physician, *1862.
Sturge-Kalischer-Weber syndrome – *SYN:* Sturge-Weber syndrome

Kalke, Bhagavant, Indian surgical resident who developed a titanium artificial heart valve along with Clarence Walton Lillehei.
Lillehei-Kalke bileaflet valve – see under Lillehei

Kallin, surname of family for which syndrome was named.
Kallin epidermolysis bullosa simplex – type of epidermolysis bullosa simplex, characterized by blistering affecting mainly hands and feet, anodontia, nonscarring alopecia, and dystrophic nails.

Kallmann, Franz Josef, U.S. medical geneticist and psychiatrist, 1897-1965.
Kallmann syndrome – *SYN:* hypogonadism with anosmia

Kamino, H., 20th century U.S. pathologist.
Kamino body – a useful cytologic criterion for Spitz nevi.
Kamino nevus – blue nevus characterized by numerous dendritic melanocytes arranged as solitary units at the dermoepidermal junction.

Kanavel, Allen B., U.S. surgeon, 1874-1938.
Kanavel apparatus – used for finger, wrist, and forearm exercises.
SYN: Kanavel table
Kanavel brain-exploring cannula
Kanavel cock-up splint
Kanavel sign – tenderness of the lateral side of the palm, which may be secondary to bursitis of the ulna.
Kanavel splint
Kanavel table – *SYN:* Kanavel apparatus

Kandel, Eric R., Austrian physician, *1929, joint winner of 2000 Nobel Prize for work related to nervous system signal transduction.

Kandinsky, V.C., Russian psychiatrist, 1827-1899.
Clérambault-Kandinsky complex – see under de Clérambault

Clérambault-Kandinsky syndrome – *SYN:* Clérambault-Kandinsky complex

Kandori, Fumio, Japanese ophthalmologist, *1904.
fleck retina of Kandori – an autosomal recessive disorder of the retinal pigment epithelium occurring among Japanese.

Kanner, Leo, Austrian psychiatrist in U.S., 1894-1991.
Kanner syndrome – a severe emotional disturbance of childhood.
SYN: infantile autism

Kanof, Norman B., U.S. physician.
Jessner-Kanof disease – see under Jessner
Jessner-Kanof lesion – *SYN:* Jessner-Kanof disease

Kantor, John L., U.S. radiologist, 1890-1949.
Kantor string sign – luminal narrowing revealed on x-ray as a thin line of barium terminating at the ileocecal junction.

Kaplan, David M., U.S. physician, 1876-1952.
Kaplan test – test for globulin-albumin in cerebrospinal fluid.

Kaposi, Moritz (born Moritz Kohn), Hungarian dermatologist in Austria, 1837-1902.
Kaposi sarcoma – a multifocal malignant neoplasm. *SYN:* multiple idiopathic hemorrhagic sarcoma
Kaposi varicelliform eruption – a rare complication of vaccinia superimposed on atopic dermatitis, with generalized vesicles and papulovesicles and high fever. *SYN:* eczema vaccinatum

Karmen, Albert, U.S. internist and clinical pathologist, *1930.
Karmen unit – a formerly used enzyme unit.

Karnofsky, D.A., 20th century U.S. physician.
Karnofsky index
Karnofsky scale – a performance scale used to evaluate a patient's progress after a therapeutic procedure.
Karnofsky score

Karplus, Johann P., Austrian physician and physiologist, 1866-1936.
Karplus sign – pleural effusion causes modification in vocal resonance.

Karsch, Johannes, German physician.
Karsch-Neugebauer syndrome – autosomal recessive trait characterized by congenital nystagmus. *SYN:* O'Donnell-Pappas syndrome

Kartagener, Manes, Swiss physician, 1897-1975.
Kartagener syndrome – complete situs inversus associated with bronchiectasis and chronic sinusitis. *SYN:* Kartagener triad; Zivert syndrome
Kartagener triad – *SYN:* Kartagener syndrome

Kasabach, Haig H., U.S. physician, 1898-1943.
Kasabach-Merritt syndrome – capillary hemangioma associated with thrombocytopenic purpura. *SYN:* hemangioma-thrombocytopenia syndrome

Kasai, Morio, 20th century Japanese surgeon.
Kasai operation – an operation for biliary atresia. *SYN:* portoenterostomy

Kasanin, Jacob S., U.S. psychologist, 1897-1946.
Hanfmann-Kasanin Concept Formation Test – see under Hanfmann

Kashida, K., 20th century Japanese physician.
Kashida sign

Kashin, Nikolai I., Russian orthopedist, 1825-1872.
Kashin-Bek disease – a form of generalized osteoarthrosis believed to result from ingestion of wheat infected with the fungus *Fusarium sporotrichiella.*

Kast, Alfred, German physician, 1856-1903.
Kast syndrome – benign neoplasm associated with vascular malformations containing cavernous hemangiomas.

Kasten, Frederick H., U.S. histochemist and cell biologist, *1927.
Kasten fluorescent Feulgen stain – a fluorescent modification of the Feulgen stain.

Kasten fluorescent PAS stain – a fluorescent modification of the periodic acid Schiff stain for polysaccharides that uses one of the Kasten fluorescent Schiff reagents.

Kasten fluorescent Schiff reagents – used in cytochemical detection of DNA.

Katayama, Kunika, Japanese physician, 1856-1931.

Katayama test – a qualitative colorimetric test for the presence of carboxyhemoglobin in the blood.

Katz, Sir Bernard, German-English neurophysiologist and Nobel laureate, *1911.

Goldman-Hodgkin-Katz equation – *SYN:* Goldman equation

Kauffman, E., German physician, 1860-1931.

Aberhalden-Kauffman-Lignac syndrome – see under Aberhalden

Kaufman, Robert L., U.S. physician.

Kaufman syndrome – *SYN:* McKusick-Kaufman syndrome

McKusick-Dungy-Kaufman syndrome – *SYN:* McKusick-Kaufman syndrome

McKusick-Kaufman syndrome – see under McKusick

Kaveggia, E.F.

Opitz-Kaveggia syndrome – see under Opitz, John M.

Kawasaki, Tomisaku, 20th century Japanese pediatrician.

Kawasaki disease – a polymorphous erythematous febrile, sometimes epidemic, disease of unknown etiology occurring in children. *SYN:* Kawasaki syndrome; mucocutaneous lymph node syndrome

Kawasaki syndrome – *SYN:* Kawasaki disease

Kay, Herbert D., English biochemist, *1893.

Jenner-Kay unit – see under Jenner, Harley D.

Kay, Sir Andrew Watt, Scottish professor of surgery.

Kay test – test related to peptic ulcers.

NOTES

Kayser, Bernhard, German ophthalmologist, 1869-1954.

Kayser-Fleischer ring – a greenish-yellow pigmented ring encircling the cornea just within the corneoscleral margin, seen in hepatolenticular degeneration. *SYN:* Fleischer-Strümpell ring

Kazanjian, Varaztad H., Armenian otorhinolaryngologist in the U.S., 1879-1974.

Kazanjian nasal forceps

Kazanjian nasal hump forceps

Kazanjian operation – surgical extension of the vestibular sulcus of edentulous ridges to increase their height and to improve denture retention.

Kazanjian osteotome

Kazanjian scissors

Kazanjian splint

Kearns, Thomas P., U.S. ophthalmologist, *1922.

Kearns-Sayre syndrome – chronic progressive external ophthalmoplegia with associated cardiac conduction defects, short stature, and hearing loss.

Keating-Hart, Walter V., French physician, 1870-1922.

Keating-Hart method – fulguration in the treatment of external cancer or of the field of operation after removal of a malignant growth.

Keen, William W., U.S. surgeon, 1837-1932.

Keen operation – removal of sections of nerves as a cure for torticollis.

Keen sign – increased width at the malleoli in Pott fracture.

Keetley, Charles Robert Bell, English surgeon, 1848-1909.

Keetley-Torek operation – *SYN:* Torek operation

Kegel, A.H., 20th century U.S. gynecologist.

Kegel exercises – alternate contraction and relaxation of perineal muscles for treatment of urinary stress incontinence.

Kehr, Hans, German surgeon, 1862-1916.

Kehr incision

Kehr sign – violent pain in the left shoulder in a case of rupture of the spleen.

Kehr T-tube

Kehrer, Ferdinand A., German neurologist, 1883-1966.

Kehrer reflex – *SYN:* Kisch reflex

Keith, Sir Arthur, Scottish anatomist, 1866-1955.

Keith bundle – modified cardiac muscle fibers. *SYN:* atrioventricular bundle

Keith and Flack node – the mass of specialized cardiac muscle fibers that normally acts as the pacemaker of the cardiac conduction system. *SYN:* Flack node; Keith node; sinuatrial node

Keith node – *SYN:* Keith and Flack node

Keller, William Lordan, U.S. surgeon, 1874-1959.

Keller arthroplasty

Keller bunionectomy – excision of the proximal portion of the proximal phalanx of the first toe.

Keller bunion osteotomy

Keller hallux rigidus operation

Keller hallux valgus operation

Keller operation

Kellie, George, 18th century Scottish anatomist.

Monro-Kellie doctrine – *SYN:* Monro doctrine

Kelly, Adam Brown, English otolaryngologist, 1865-1941.

Paterson-Brown-Kelly syndrome – see under Paterson, Donald Rose

Paterson-Kelly syndrome – *SYN:* Plummer-Vinson syndrome

Kelly, Howard A., U.S. gynecologist, 1858-1943.

Kelly clamp – a curved hemostat without teeth.

Kelly operation – correction of retroversion of the uterus; correction of urinary stress incontinence.

Kelly placenta forceps

Kelly plication

Kelly rectal speculum

Kelly uterine dilator

Kelly uterine scissors

Kelly uterine tenaculum

NOTES

Kelvin, Lord William Thomson, Scottish physicist, 1824-1907.
  kelvin (K) – a unit of thermodynamic temperature equal to 1/273.16 of the thermodynamic temperature of the triple point of water.
  Kelvin scale – temperature scale in which the triple point of water is assigned the value of 273.16 K.
  Kelvin thermometer

Kempner, Walter, U.S. physician, *1903.
  Kempner rice diet – low-salt diet used to treat high blood pressure.

Kendall, Edward C., U.S. biochemist, 1886-1972, joint winner of the 1950 Nobel Prize for research on the hormones of the adrenal cortex.
  Kendall method – test to measure iodine in thyroid tissue.

Kennedy, Edward, U.S. dentist, *1883.
  Kennedy classification – a listing of several forms of partially edentulous jaws in accordance with the distribution of the missing teeth.

Kennedy, Robert Foster, U.S. neurologist, 1884-1952.
  Foster Kennedy syndrome – *SYN:* Kennedy syndrome
  Kennedy syndrome – ipsilateral optic atrophy with central scotoma and contralateral choked disk or papilledema, caused by a meningioma of the ipsilateral optic nerve. *SYN:* Foster Kennedy syndrome

Kennedy, William, U.S. neurologist.
  Kennedy disease – an X-linked recessive disorder characterized by progressive spinal and bulbar muscular atrophy.

Kenny, name of a rehabilitation institute in Minneapolis, MN.
  Kenny rating – *SYN:* Kenny self-care evaluation
  Kenny score – *SYN:* Kenny self-care evaluation
  Kenny self-care evaluation – a system of numeric ratings for evaluating a patient's ability to perform 17 activities. *SYN:* Kenny rating; Kenny score

Kenny, Frederic M., U.S. physician, *1929.
  Kenny syndrome – genetic trait resulting in dwarfism and cortical thickening of tubular bones.

Kenny, Sister Elizabeth, Australian nurse, 1886-1952.
  Kenny crutch – a wooden forearm crutch.
  Kenny treatment – a method for the treatment of anterior poliomyelitis.

Kent, Albert F.S., English physiologist, 1863-1958.
  Kent bundle – *SYN:* His bundle
  Kent-His bundle – *SYN:* His bundle

Kerandel, Jean F., French physician, 1873-1934.

Kerandel sign – a blow to a bony projection causing hyperesthesia and pain.

Kerandel symptom – deep-seated hyperesthesia observed in cases of sleeping sickness.

Kergaradec, Jean Alexandre le Jameau, Vicomte de, French obstetrician-gynecologist, 1788-1877.

Kergaradec sign – soft blowing sound synchronous with cardiac systole of mother, heard on auscultation of gravid uterus. *SYN:* placental souffle; uterine souffle

Kerley, Peter J., English radiologist, 1900-1978.

Kerley B lines – fine peripheral septal lines. *SYN:* costophrenic septal lines

Kernig, Vladimir, Russian physician, 1840-1917.

Kernig sign – a failure of leg extension present in various forms of meningitis.

Kernohan, James W., Irish pathologist, 1897-1981.

Kernohan notch – a notch in the cerebral peduncle due to displacement of the brainstem against the incisura of the tentorium by a transtentorial herniation.

Kernohan-Woltman syndrome – cerebral lesion resulting in same-side hemiparesis. *SYN:* Cruz phenomenon; Woltman-Kernohan syndrome

Woltman-Kernohan syndrome – *SYN:* Kernohan-Woltman syndrome

Kerr, Harry Hyland, U.S. surgeon, 1881-1963.

Parker-Kerr basting suture
Parker-Kerr operation
Parker-Kerr suture – see under Parker, Edward Mason

Kesling, Harold D., U.S. orthodontist, *1901.

Kesling appliance
Kesling spring

Kestenbaum, Alfred, U.S. ophthalmologist, 1890-1961.

Kestenbaum number – the difference between the two pupil diameters when each eye is measured in bright light with the other eye tightly covered.

Kestenbaum sign – a decrease in the number of arterioles crossing optic disk margins as a sign of optic neurtis.

Key, Charles Aston, English cardiologist and surgeon, 1793-1849.

Hodgkin-Key murmur – see under Hodgkin, Thomas

Key, Ernst A.H., Swedish anatomist and physician, 1832-1901.

foramen of Key-Retzius – one of the two lateral openings of the fourth ventricle into the subarachnoid space at the cerebellopontine angle. *SYN:* lateral aperture of the fourth ventricle

Key-Retzius corpuscles – tactile corpuscles, resembling pacinian corpuscles, found in the beak of certain aquatic birds.

sheath of Key and Retzius – the delicate connective tissue enveloping individual nerve fibers within a peripheral nerve. *SYN:* endoneurium

Khorana, Har G., Indian-U.S. chemist, *1922, joint winner of the 1968 Nobel Prize for discovering the process by which enzymes determine cell function in a genetic environment.

Kielland, var. of Kjelland

Kien, Alphonse M.J., 19th century German physician.

Kussmaul-Kien respiration – *SYN:* Kussmaul respiration

Kienböck, Robert, Austrian radiologist, 1871-1953.

Kienböck atrophy – acute atrophy of bone in an extremity following inflammation.

Kienböck disease – osteolysis of the lunate bone following trauma to the wrist. *SYN:* lunatomalacia

Kienböck dislocation – dislocation of semilunar bone.

Kienböck unit – an obsolete unit of x-ray dosage equivalent to 1/10 the erythema dose.

Kiernan, Francis, English physician, 1800-1874.

Kiernan space – interlobular space in the liver.

Kiesselbach, Wilhelm, German laryngologist, 1839-1902.

Kiesselbach area – an area on the anterior portion of the nasal septum rich in capillaries (Kiesselbach plexus) and often the seat of epistaxis. *SYN:* Little area

Kiesselbach plexus

Kiesselbach triangle

Kikuchi, Ichiro, Japanese physician.
   Iso-Kikuchi syndrome – see under Iso

Kikuchi, M., 20th century Japanese physician.
   Kikuchi necrotizing lymphadenitis – nonmalignant disease primarily affecting cervical lymph nodes in females.

Kilian, Hermann F., German gynecologist, 1800-1863.
   Kilian line – a transverse line marking the promontory of the pelvis.

Kiliani, H., German chemist, 1855-1945.
   Kiliani-Fischer reaction – *SYN:* Kiliani-Fischer synthesis
   Kiliani-Fischer synthesis – a synthetic procedure for the extension of the carbon atom chain of aldoses by treatment with cyanide. *SYN:* feedback inhibition; Kiliani-Fischer reaction

Killian, Gustav, German laryngologist, 1860-1921.
   Killian antrum cannula
   Killian bundle – *SYN:* inferior constrictor muscle of pharynx
   Killian cannula
   Killian elevator
   Killian frontal sinus chisel
   Killian frontoethmoidectomy procedure
   Killian gouge
   Killian incision
   Killian nasal speculum
   Killian operation – an operation for frontal sinus disease.
   Killian septal compression forceps
   Killian septal elevator
   Killian septal speculum
   Killian tonsil knife
   Killian triangle – the triangular-shaped area of the cervical esophagus.
      SYN: Laimer triangle
   Killian-Lynch suspension laryngoscope

NOTES

Kimmelstiel, Paul, German pathologist in the U.S., 1900-1970.
  Kimmelstiel-Wilson disease – *SYN:* Kimmelstiel-Wilson syndrome
  Kimmelstiel-Wilson syndrome – nephrotic syndrome and hypertension
    in diabetics, associated with diabetic glomerulosclerosis. *SYN:*
    Kimmelstiel-Wilson disease

Kimura, Tetsuji, 20th century Japanese pathologist.
  Kimura disease – solitary or multiple small benign cutaneous
    erythematous nodules. *SYN:* angiolymphoid hyperplasia with eosinophilia

Kindler, Theresa, Austrian-born dermatologist, 1890-1975.
  Kindler syndrome – rare disorder featuring acral blistering at birth or
    shortly after, followed by progressive poikiloderma and photosensitivity,
    which may improve with age.

Kindler, Werner, German otorhinolaryngologist, *1895.
  Kindler-Zange syndrome – *SYN:* Zange-Kindler syndrome
  Zange-Kindler syndrome – see under Zange

King, Earl J., Canadian biochemist, 1901-1962.
  King-Armstrong unit – *SYN:* King unit
  King unit – the quantity of phosphatase that, acting upon disodium
    phenylphosphate in excess, at pH 9 for 30 minutes, liberates 1 mg of
    phenol. *SYN:* King-Armstrong unit

Kingsbourne, M., English physician.
  Kingsbourne syndrome – neurologic disorder seen in children under the
    age of 3; results in ataxia, nystagmus and myoclonus.

Kingsley, Norman W., U.S. dentist, 1829-1913.
  Kingsley splint – a winged maxillary splint attached to a head appliance
    by elastics. *SYN:* reverse Kingsley splint
  reverse Kingsley splint – *SYN:* Kingsley splint

Kinkiang, city in China.
  Kinkiang fever – schistosomiasis caused by Schistosoma japonicum,
    affecting bowel, liver, and spleen; endemic to Far East.

Kinnier Wilson, see under Wilson, Samuel Alexander Kinnier

Kinyoun, Joseph J., U.S. physician, 1860-1919.
  Kinyoun stain – a method for demonstrating acid-fast microorganisms.

Kirchner, Wilhelm, Austrian otologist, 1849-1936.
  Kirchner diverticulum – eustachian tube diverticulum.

Kirk, Norman Thomas, U.S. Army surgeon, 1888-1960.
   Kirk amputation – amputation at the lower end of the femur, using the tendon of the quadriceps extensor to cover the end of the bone.
   Kirk mallet
   Kirk orthopedic hammer
   Kirk technique

Kirkland, Olin, U.S. periodontist, 1876-1969.
   Kirkland cement
   Kirkland instrument
   Kirkland knife – a heart-shaped knife used in gingival surgery.
   Kirkland periodontal pack

Kirman, H., 20th century English psychiatrist.
   Kirman syndrome – type of ectodermal dysplasia characterized by almost total alopecia, anhidrosis, and severe mental retardation, with normal nails and teeth.

Kirschner, Martin, German surgeon, 1879-1942.
   Kirschner apparatus – *SYN:* Kirschner wire
   Kirschner bone drill
   Kirschner bow
   Kirschner II-C shoulder system
   Kirschner hip replacement system
   Kirschner interlocking intramedullary nail
   Kirschner Medical Dimension hip replacement
   Kirschner pin fixation
   Kirschner skeletal traction
   Kirschner suture
   Kirschner system
   Kirschner total shoulder prosthesis
   Kirschner traction
   Kirschner wire – an apparatus for skeletal traction in long bone fracture. *SYN:* Kirschner apparatus

NOTES

Kirschner wire drill
Kirschner wire fixation
Kirschner wire inserter
Kirschner wire pin
Kirschner wire splint
Kirschner wire spreader
Kirschner wire tightener
Kirschner wire traction

Kirstein, Alfred, German physician, 1863-1922.
Kirstein method – examination of the larynx.

Kisch, Bruno, German physiologist, 1890-1966.
Kisch reflex – closure of the eye in response to stimulation of the skin at the depth of the external auditory meatus. *SYN:* auriculopalpebral reflex; Kehrer reflex

Kitamura, Kaneihiko, Japanese dermatologist, 1899-1989.
Kitamura disease – an autosomal dominant disease featuring reticulate hyperpigmentation beginning on the dorsal hand and spreading to the rest of the body. *SYN:* reticulate acropigmentation of Kitamura
reticulate acropigmentation of Kitamura – *SYN:* Kitamura disease

Kitasato, Baron Shibasaburo, Japanese bacteriologist, 1856-1931.
Kitasato bacillus – *SYN: Yersinia pestis*

Kjeldahl, Johan G.C., Danish chemist, 1849-1900.
Kjeldahl apparatus – an apparatus used in nitrogen analysis.
Kjeldahl method
macro-Kjeldahl method – a procedure for analyzing the content of nitrogenous compounds in urine, serum, or other specimens.
micro-Kjeldahl method – a modification of the macro-Kjeldahl method designed for the analysis of nitrogenous compounds in relatively small quantities.

Kjelland, (Kielland), Christian, Norwegian obstetrician, 1871-1941.
Kjelland blade
Kjelland forceps – an obstetrical forceps having a sliding lock and little pelvic curve.
Kjelland obstetrical forceps
Kjelland rotation

Klapp, Rudolph, German surgeon, 1873-1949.
Klapp creeping treatment – *SYN:* Klapp method
Klapp exercises – *SYN:* Klapp method

Klapp method – treatment of scoliosis by a series of systematic crawling movements whereby the spine is bent laterally and made more flexible. *SYN:* Klapp creeping treatment; Klapp exercises

Klatskin, Gerald, U.S. gastroenterologist, 1910-1988.
Klatskin biliary adenocarcinoma
Klatskin cholangiocarcinoma
Klatskin needle
Klatskin tumor – carcinoma of the bile duct.

Klauder, Joseph Victor, U.S. dermatologist, 1888-1962.
Klauder syndrome – acute inflammation of skin and mucous membranes.

Klebs, Theodor Albrecht Edwin, German physician, 1834-1913.
Klebs disease
Klebsiella – a genus of bacteria (family Enterobacteriaceae) that occurs in the respiratory, intestinal, and urogenital tracts of humans as well as in soil, water, and grain.
Klebsiella oxytoca
Klebsiella pneumoniae – *SYN:* Friedländer bacillus
Klebs-Loeffler bacillus – a species that causes diphtheria and produces a powerful exotoxin causing degeneration of various tissues, notably myocardium. *SYN: Corynebacterium diphtheriae*

Kleigl, name of company manufacturing stage lights.
Kleigl eye – exposure to intense lighting causing conjunctivitis, eyelid edema, tearing, and photophobia. *SYN:* cinema eye

Klein, Edward E., Hungarian histologist, 1844-1925.
Klein-Gumprecht shadow nuclei – shadow nuclei in degenerating lymphoidocytes and macrolymphocytes in leukemia.
Klein muscle – *SYN:* cutaneomucous muscle

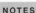

Klein, Jeffrey A., U.S. dermatologist, *1944.
> **Klein needle** – a needle that allows deposition of vasoconstrictive/ anesthetic solution along the paths of the cannula, used in tumescent liposuction.

Kleine, Willi, 20th century German neuropsychiatrist.
> **Kleine-Levin syndrome** – a rare form of periodic hypersomnia associated with bulimia, behavioral disturbances, impaired thought processes, and hallucinations.

Kleinschmidt, Hans, German physician, 1885-1977.
> **Kleinschmidt syndrome** – *SYN: Haemophilus influenzae*, type b

Kleist, Karl, German neurologist, *1879.
> **Kleist apraxia** – inability to draw or write or construct two- and three-dimensional figures using matchsticks. *SYN:* Mayer-Gross apraxia
> **Kleist sign** – when gently raised by examiner, patient's fingers hook into examiner's fingers; indicative of thalamic and frontal lesions.

Klenzak, engineer and machinist, *1956.
> **Klenzak ankle joint** – a type of spring-loaded metal brace joint.
> **Klenzak brace** – brace used for footdrop.
> **Klenzak double-channeled ankle joint**
> **Klenzak joint** – a metal joint used in a brace.
> **Klenzak knee joint**

Kligman, Albert Montgomery, U.S. dermatologist and botanist, *1916.
> **Kligman formula** – formula to lighten hyperpigmented lesions.

Kline, Benjamin S., U.S. pathologist, 1886-1968.
> **Kline test** – a test for syphilis.

Klinefelter, Harry Fitch, Jr., U.S. physician, *1912.
> **Klinefelter syndrome** – a chromosomal anomaly in which patients are male in development but have seminiferous tubule dysgenesis, elevated urinary gonadotropins, variable gynecomastia, and eunuchoid habitus. *SYN:* XXY syndrome

Klinger, (origin unknown).
> **Klinger-Ludwig acid-thionin stain for sex chromosome** – see under Ludwig, Kurt

Klippel, Maurice, French neurologist, 1858-1942.
> **Feil-Klippel syndrome** – *SYN:* Klippel-Feil syndrome
> **Klippel-Feil syndrome** – a congenital defect manifested as a short neck, extensive fusion of the cervical vertebrae, and abnormalities of the

brainstem and cerebellum. *SYN:* cervical fusion syndrome; Feil-Klippel syndrome

Klippel-Trenaunay-Weber syndrome – an anomaly of the extremity in which there is a combination of angiomatosis and anomalous development of the underlying bone and muscle, sometimes associated with localized gigantism. *SYN:* angioosteohypertrophy syndrome; congenital dysplastic angiectasia; hemangiectatic hypertrophy

Kloepfer, H. Warner, 1913-1982.

Kloepfer syndrome – blindness beginning at the age of 2 months, arrested growth at 5 or 6, and progressive mental retardation.

Klotz, Henri P., French physician, *1910.

Klotz syndrome – primary amenorrhea with concomitant poorly developed genitalia and reproductive organs.

Klumpke, Augusta Dejerine-, see under Dejerine-Klumpke.

Klüver, Heinrich, German-born U.S. neurologist, 1897-1979.

Klüver-Barrera Luxol fast blue stain – in combination with cresyl violet, a stain useful for demonstrating myelin and Nissl substance.

Klüver-Bucy syndrome – a syndrome mostly reported in monkeys, characterized by psychic blindness or hyperreactivity to visual stimuli, increased oral and sexual activity, and depressed drive and emotional reactions.

Knapp, Herman J., U.S. ophthalmologist, 1832-1911.

Knapp cataract knife
Knapp eye speculum
Knapp iris hook
Knapp iris knife needle
Knapp iris repositor
Knapp iris scissors
Knapp iris spatula
Knapp lacrimal sac retractor
Knapp lens scoop

NOTES

Knapp lid operation
Knapp pterygium operation
Knapp streaks – striae in Bruch membrane occurring in a variety of systemic disorders affecting elastic tissue. *SYN:* angioid streaks; Knapp striae
Knapp striae – *SYN:* Knapp streaks

Knapp, Karl, German chemist, 1832-1911.
Knapp test – a test for urine glucose.

Knaus, Hermann, Austrian gynecologist, *1892.
Ogino-Knaus rule – see under Ogino

Kneipp, Sebastian, German pastor, 1821-1897.
Kneipp cure – *SYN:* Kneipp treatment
Kneippism – *SYN:* Kneipp treatment
Kneipp treatment – a therapeutic system of treatment consisting of diet, walking barefoot in dewy grass or snow in the early morning, and cold-water applications. *SYN:* Kneipp cure; Kneippism

Knies, Max, German ophthalmologist, 1851-1917.
Knies sign – pupil dilatation related to Graves disease.

Kniest, Wilhelm, 20th century German pediatrician.
Kniest syndrome – a type of metatropic dwarfism.

Knight, James C., U.S. physician, 1810-1887.
Knight brace – a thoracic, lumbar, sacral orthosis with abdominal flexible support. *SYN:* chairback brace

Knoll, Philipp, Bohemian physiologist, 1841-1900.
Knoll glands – glands in the ventricular folds of the larynx (false vocal cords).

Knoop, Hedwig, German physician, *1908.
Knoop theory – related to the catabolism of fatty acids.

Knott, Margaret, U.S. physical therapist, 1913-1978.
Kabat-Knott method of exercise – *SYN:* Kabat method of exercise
Knott-Voss method of exercise – *SYN:* Kabat method of exercise

Knowles, Frederick, U.S. orthopedic surgeon, 1888-1973.
Knowles pin – femoral neck fracture fixation device.
Knowles pin nail
Knowles scissors

Knox, Howard A., U.S. psychiatrist, *1885.
Knox Cube Test – a performance test.

Kobelt, Georg L., German physician, 1804-1857.
   Kobelt cyst
   Kobelt tubules – remnants of the mesonephric tubules in the female.
      SYN: wolffian tubules

Kober, Philip A., U.S. chemist, *1884.
   Kober test – a test for naturally occurring estrogens.

Köbner, H., German dermatologist, 1838-1904.
   Köbner phenomenon – an isomorphic reaction seen in response to
      trauma in previously uninvolved sites of patients with skin diseases.
      SYN: isomorphic response

Koch, Robert, German bacteriologist and Nobel laureate, 1843-1910.
   Koch bacillus – (1) a species that causes tuberculosis.
      SYN: Mycobacterium tuberculosis; (2) a species that causes cholera.
      SYN: Vibrio cholerae
   Koch blue bodies – schizonts of *Theileria parva*, the causative agent of
      East Coast fever.
   Koch law – *SYN:* Koch postulates
   Koch old tuberculin
   Koch original tuberculin
   Koch phenomenon – infection immunity.
   Koch postulates – to establish the specificity of a pathogenic
      microorganism, it must be present in all cases of the disease;
      inoculations of its pure cultures must produce disease in animals, and
      from these it must be again obtained and be propagated in pure
      cultures. *SYN:* Koch law
   Koch-Weeks bacillus – a species found in the respiratory tract; causes
      acute respiratory infections. *SYN: Haemophilus influenzae*; Weeks
      bacillus

NOTES

Koch, Walter, German surgeon, *1880.

   Koch node – the mass of specialized cardiac muscle fibers that normally acts as the "pacemaker" of the cardiac conduction system. *SYN:* sinuatrial node

   Koch triangle – a triangular area of the wall of the right atrium of the heart that marks the situation of the atrioventricular node.

Kocher, E. Theodor, Swiss surgeon and Nobel laureate, 1841-1917.

   Kocher approach

   Kocher artery forceps

   Kocher biliary tract incision

   Kocher bladder retractor

   Kocher clamp – a heavy, straight hemostat.

   Kocher-Debré-Semelaigne syndrome – autosomal recessive inherited athyrotic cretinism associated with muscular pseudohypertrophy. *SYN:* Debré-Semelaigne syndrome

   Kocher dissector

   Kocher elevator

   Kocher forceps

   Kocher goiter dissector

   Kocher hemostat

   Kocher incision – an incision parallel with right costal margin.

   Kocher intestinal forceps

   Kocher kidney-elevating forceps

   Kocher maneuver

   Kocher periosteal dissector

   Kocher retractor

   Kocher sign – in Graves disease, on upward gaze the globe lags behind the movement of the upper eyelid.

   Kocher spoon

   Kocher ureterosigmoidostomy procedure

Kock, Nils G., Swedish surgeon, *1924.

   Kock ileal reservoir

   Kock ileostomy – *SYN:* Kock pouch

   Kock nipple

   Kock nipple valve

   Kock pouch – a continent ileostomy with a reservoir and valved opening fashioned from doubled loops of ileum. *SYN:* Kock ileostomy

Koebner, Heinrich, German dermatologist, 1838-1904.

   Koebner response – psoriasis due to trauma.

Koenen, J.H.O.C., Dutch psychiatrist, 1893-1956.
Koenen tumors – subungual and periungual fibromas associated with tuberous sclerosis.

Koenig, Franz, German surgeon, 1832-1910.
Koenig syndrome – alternating attacks of constipation and diarrhea, with colic, meteorism, and gurgling in the right iliac fossa.

Koerber, Herman, German ophthalmologist, *1878.
Koerber-Salus-Elschnig syndrome – *SYN:* Parinaud I syndrome

Koerte, Werner, German surgeon, 1853-1937.
Koerte-Ballance operation – anastomosis of the facial and hypoglossal nerves for the treatment of facial paralysis.

Koettstorfer, J., 19th century German chemist.
Koettstorfer number – the number of milligrams of KOH required to saponify 1 g of fat. *SYN:* saponification number

Kofferath, Walter, German physician.
Kofferath syndrome – unilateral paralysis in newborns often caused by forceps during delivery.

Kogoj, Franjo, Yugoslavian physician, 1894-1981.
Kogoj abscess
spongiform pustule of Kogoj – an epidermal pustule formed by infiltration of neutrophils into necrotic epidermis in pustular psoriasis.

Köhler, Alban, German radiologist, 1874-1947.
Köhler disease – epiphysial aseptic necrosis of the tarsal navicular bone or of the patella.

Köhler, August, German microscopist, 1866-1948.
Köhler illumination – a method of illumination of microscopic objects.

Köhler, Georges J.F., German immunologist, 1946-1995, joint winner of 1984 Nobel Prize for work related to the immune system.

Kohlmeier, W., German physician.
Kohlmeier-Degos syndrome – vascular occlusive disorder predominantly involving the small arteries of the skin and bowel.

Kohlrausch, Otto L.B., German physician, 1811-1854.
Kohlrausch muscle – the longitudinal muscles of the rectal wall.
Kohlrausch valves – *SYN:* transverse rectal folds

Kohn, Hans N., German pathologist, *1866.
Kohn one-step staining technique
Kohn pores – openings in the interalveolar septa of the lung.
SYN: interalveolar pores

Kohnstamm, Oskar, German physician, 1871-1917.
Kohnstamm phenomenon – a slow, involuntary elevation of the arm after strong pressure against a firm object. *SYN:* after-movement

Kohs, Samuel C., U.S. psychologist, 1890-1977.
Kohs Block Design Test – intelligence test.

Kojewnikoff, Aleksei Y., Russian neurologist, 1836-1902.
Kojewnikoff epilepsy – simple partial motor status epilepticus of the rolandic cortex. *SYN:* epilepsia partialis continua

Kok, O., Dutch physician.
Kok disease – genetic trait associated with hypertonia in newborns.

Kölliker, Rudolph A. von, Swiss histologist, 1817-1905.
Kölliker layer – the layer of connective tissue in the iris.
Kölliker reticulum – non-neuronal cellular elements of the central and peripheral nervous system. *SYN:* neuroglia

Kollmann, Arthur, 19th century German urologist.
Kollmann dilator – a metallic expandable instrument used to dilate urethral strictures.

Kolmer, John Albert, U.S. pathologist, 1886-1962.
Kolmer test – a former standard quantitative method for the Wassermann test, with numerous modifications.

Kolodny, H.
Rebeitz-Kolodny-Richardson syndrome – see under Rebeitz

Kolopp, P., French dermatologist, 1888-1951.
Woringer-Kolopp disease – see under Woringer

Kommerell, B., German radiologist.
Kommerell diverticulum – a descending aorta swelling at origin of aberrant right subclavian artery.

Kondoleon, Emmanuel, Greek surgeon, 1879-1939.
Kondoleon operation – excision of strips of subcutaneous connective tissue for the relief of elephantiasis.

König, Franz, German surgeon, 1832-1910.
König disease – complete or incomplete separation of joint cartilage and underlying bone, usually involving the knee. *SYN:* osteochondritis dissecans

Koplik, Henry, U.S. pediatrician, 1858-1927.
Koplik spots – small red spots on buccal mucosa, occurring early in measles before skin eruption. *SYN:* Filatov spots; Flindt spots

Korff, Karl von, 20th century German anatomist and histologist.
Korff fibers – argyrophilic fibers that pass between odontoblasts at the periphery of the dental pulp and fan out into the dentin.

Kornberg, A., U.S. biochemist and Nobel laureate, *1918.
Kornberg enzyme – DNA polymerase I from *Escherichia coli.*

Kornmehl, Ernest W., U.S. ophthalmologist.
Kornmehl LASIK System

Kornsweig, var. of Kornzweig

Kornzweig, (Kornsweig), Abraham L., U.S. physician, *1900.
Bassen-Kornzweig disease – *SYN:* Bassen-Kornzweig syndrome
Bassen-Kornzweig syndrome – see under Bassen

Korotkoff, Nikolai S., Russian physician, 1874-1920.
Korotkoff sounds – sounds heard over an artery when pressure over it is reduced below systolic arterial pressure, as when blood pressure is determined by the auscultatory method.
Korotkoff test – a test of collateral circulation.

NOTES

Korovnikov, A.F., Russian physician.
Korovnikov syndrome – splenomegaly accompanied by thrombocytosis and gastrointestinal hemorrhage with onset between 20 and 40 years of age.

Korsakoff, (Korsakov), Sergei S., Russian neurologist and psychiatrist, 1853-1900.
Korsakoff psychosis – *SYN:* Korsakoff syndrome
Korsakoff syndrome – an alcohol amnestic syndrome. *SYN:* amnestic psychosis; amnestic syndrome; dysmnesic psychosis; Korsakoff psychosis; polyneuritic psychosis
Wernicke-Korsakoff encephalopathy
Wernicke-Korsakoff syndrome – see under Wernicke

Korsakov, var. of Korsakoff

Koshland, Daniel E., U.S. biochemist, *1920.
Adair-Koshland-Némethy-Filmer model – *SYN:* Koshland-Némethy-Filmer model
Koshland-Némethy-Filmer model – a model to explain the allosteric form of cooperativity. *SYN:* Adair-Koshland-Némethy-Filmer model; induced fit model

Kossa, Julius von, see under von Kossa

Kossel, Albrecht, German physiologist, 1853-1927.
Kossel test – test for hypoxanthine.

Kostmann, Rolf, Swedish pediatrician, *1909.
Kostmann disease – genetic predisposition for developing acute leukemia. *SYN:* Kostmann syndrome
Kostmann syndrome – *SYN:* Kostmann disease

Kovalevsky, Alexander O., Russian embryologist, 1840-1901.
Kovalevsky canal – canal connecting neural tube and archenteron in embryo.

Kowarsky, Albert, 20th century German physician.
Kowarsky test – test for glucose in urine and diabetes in blood.

Koyanagi, Yosizo, Japanese ophthalmologist, 1880-1954.
Vogt-Koyanagi-Harada syndrome – see under Vogt, Alfred
Vogt-Koyanagi syndrome – see under Vogt, Alfred

Krabbe, Knud Haraldsen, Danish neurologist, 1885-1961.
Christensen-Krabbe disease – see under Christensen

Krabbe disease – a metabolic disorder of infancy. *SYN:* globoid cell leukodystrophy

Kraepelin, Emil, German psychiatrist, 1856-1926.
Kraepelin-Morel disease – psychosis of schizophrenia.

Krantz, Kermit E., U.S. obstetrician-gynecologist, *1923.
Marshall-Marchetti-Krantz operation – see under Marshall, Victor F.

Kraske, Paul, German surgeon, 1851-1930.
Kraske operation – removal of the coccyx and excision of the left wing of the sacrum in order to afford approach for resection of the rectum for cancer or stenosis.
Kraske parasacral approach
Kraske position

Krause, Arlington C., U.S. ophthalmologist, *1896.
Krause syndrome – retinopathy of prematurity combined with cerebral dysplasia. *SYN:* encephalo-ophthalmic dysplasia

Krause, Fedor, German surgeon, 1857-1937.
Krause graft – a full-thickness skin graft. *SYN:* Krause-Wolfe graft
Krause method
Krause-Wolfe graft – *SYN:* Krause graft
Wolfe-Krause graft – *SYN:* Wolfe graft

Krause, Karl F.T., German anatomist, 1797-1868.
Krause glands – glands in the mucous membrane of the tympanic cavity.
Krause ligament – the thickened anterior border of the urogenital diaphragm, formed by the fusion of its two fascial layers. *SYN:* transverse perineal ligament
Krause muscle – *SYN:* cutaneomucous muscle

Krause, Wilhelm J.F., German anatomist, 1833-1910.
Krause bone – small bone (secondary ossification center) in the triradiate cartilage between the ilium, the ischium, and the pubic bone in the growing acetabulum.

NOTES

Krause end bulbs – nerve terminals in skin, mouth, conjunctivae, and other parts generally believed to be sensitive to cold. *SYN:* bulboid corpuscles; corpuscula bulboidea

Krause respiratory bundle – a slender, compact fiber bundle composed of primary sensory fibers that enter with the vagus, glossopharyngeal, and facial nerves. *SYN:* solitary tract

Krause valve – *SYN:* Béraud valve

Krebs, Edwin G., U.S. biochemist, *1918, joint winner of 1992 Nobel Prize for work related to protein phosphorylation.

Krebs, Sir Hans Adolph, German biochemist in England and Nobel laureate, 1900-1981.

Krebs cycle – together with oxidative phosphorylation, the main source of energy in the mammalian body and the end toward which carbohydrate, fat, and protein metabolism are directed. *SYN:* tricarboxylic acid cycle

Krebs-Henseleit cycle – the sequence of chemical reactions, occurring primarily in the liver, that results in the production of urea. *SYN:* urea cycle

Krebs-Ringer solution – a modification of Ringer solution.

Kreibig, Wilhelm, German ophthalmologist.

Kreibig opticomalacia – condition that causes unilateral sclerosis of retinal vessels and atrophy of optic nerve, resulting in blindness.

Kretschmann, Friederich, German otologist, 1858-1934.

Kretschmann space – a slight depression in the epitympanic recess below the superior recess of the tympanic membrane.

Kretschmer, Ernst, German psychiatrist, 1888-1964.

Kretschmer types – personality traits related to physical type.

Kreysig, Friedrich L., German physician, 1770-1839.

Heim-Kreysig sign – see under Heim

Kreysig sign – *SYN:* Heim-Kreysig sign

Krishaber, Maurice, French physician, 1836-1883.

Krishaber disease – tachycardia with concomitant vertigo and insomnia.

Krisovski, Max, late 19th century German physician.

Krisovski sign – cicatricial mouth lines seen in cases of congenital syphilis.

Krogh, August, Danish physiologist and Nobel laureate, 1874-1949.

Krogh spirometer – a water-sealed spirometer.

Kromayer, Ernst Ludwig Franz, German dermatologist, 1862-1933.

Aero-Kromayer lamp – air-cooled Kromayer lamp.

Kromayer lamp – a quartz lamp of mercury vapor used in the treatment of skin diseases.

Krompecher, Edmund, German physician, 1870-1926.

Krompecher tumor – slow-growing epithelial tumor derived from basal cells, presenting as a pearly nodule, occasionally with telangiectases.

Kronecker, Karl H., Swiss physiologist, 1839-1914.

Kronecker stain – a 5% sodium chloride stain rendered faintly alkaline with sodium carbonate, used in the examination of fresh tissues under the microscope.

Krönig, Georg, German physician, 1856-1911.

Krönig isthmus – the narrow straplike portion of the resonant field that extends over the shoulder, connecting the larger areas of resonance over the pulmonary apex in front and behind.

Krönig steps – extension of the lower part of the right border of absolute cardiac dullness in hypertrophy of the right heart.

Krönlein, Rudolf U., Swiss surgeon, 1847-1910.

Krönlein hernia – a complicated hernia having a double sac, one part in the inguinal canal, the other projecting from the internal inguinal ring in the subperitoneal tissues. *SYN:* properitoneal inguinal hernia

Krönlein operation – orbital decompression through the anterior lateral wall of the orbit.

Krukenberg, Adolph, German anatomist, 1816-1877.

Krukenberg veins – the terminal branches of the hepatic veins that lie centrally in the hepatic lobules and receive blood from the liver sinusoids. *SYN:* central veins of liver

Krukenberg, Friedrich, German pathologist, 1871-1946.

Krukenberg amputation – a cineplastic amputation at the carpus with the distal end of the forearm.

Krukenberg pigment spindle forceps

NOTES

Krukenberg spindle – a vertical fusiform area of melanin pigmentation on the posterior surface of the central cornea.

Krukenberg sponge

Krukenberg tumor – metastatic carcinoma of the ovary.

Kruse, Walther, German bacteriologist, 1864-1943.

Kruse brush – a bunch of fine platinum wires used to spread material over the surface of a culture medium.

Shiga-Kruse bacillus – *SYN: Shigella dysenteriae*

Kuder, G. Frederic, U.S. psychologist.

Kuder Preference Record – interest inventory test.

Kuersteiner, var. of Kürsteiner

Kufs, Hugo Friedrich, German neuropathologist, 1871-1955.

Kufs disease – cerebral sphingolipidosis, adult type.

Kugelberg, Eric, Swedish neurologist, 1913-1983.

Kugelberg-Welander disease – slowly progressive proximal muscular weakness with fasciculation and wasting. *SYN:* juvenile spinal muscular atrophy; Wohlfart-Kugelberg-Welander disease

Müeller-Kugelberg syndrome – see under Müeller

Wohlfart-Kugelberg-Welander disease – *SYN:* Kugelberg-Welander disease

Kuhlmann, Frederick, U.S. psychologist, 1876-1941.

Kuhlmann-Anderson tests – general intelligence tests.

Kühne, Wilhelm (Willy) F., German physiologist and histologist, 1837-1900.

Kühne fiber – artificial muscle fiber used to demonstrate the contractility of protoplasm.

Kühne methylene blue – methylene blue in absolute alcohol and phenol solution.

Kühne phenomenon – when a constant current is passed through a muscle, an undulation is seen to pass from the positive to the negative pole.

Kühne plate – the endplate of a motor nerve fiber in a muscle spindle.

Kühne spindle – a fusiform end organ in skeletal muscle in which afferent and a few efferent nerve fibers terminate. *SYN:* neuromuscular spindle

Kuhnt, Hermann, German ophthalmologist, 1850-1925.

Kuhnt capsule forceps

Kuhnt dacryostomy

Kuhnt eyelid operation

Kuhnt-Junius degeneration – an obsolete eponym for disciform degeneration. *SYN:* Kuhnt-Junius disease

Kuhnt-Junius disease – *SYN:* Kuhnt-Junius degeneration

Kuhnt spaces – shallow diverticula or recesses between the ciliary body and ciliary zonule that open into the posterior chamber of the eye.

Kulchitsky, Nicholas, Russian histologist, 1856-1925.

Kulchitsky carcinoma – a small cell carcinoma of the esophagus composed of Kulchitsky cells with neurosecretory granules.

Kulchitsky cells – cells scattered throughout the digestive tract believed to produce at least 20 different gastrointestinal hormones and neurotransmitters. *SYN:* enteroendocrine cells

Külz, Rudolph E., German physician, 1845-1895.

Külz cylinder – a renal cast of strongly refracting granules said to be indicative of imminent diabetic coma. *SYN:* coma cast

Kümmell, Hermann, German surgeon, 1852-1937.

Kümmell spondylitis – late posttraumatic collapse of a vertebral body.

Kundrat, Hans, Austrian physician, 1845-1893.

Kundrat disease – lymphoid malignant tumor.

Kunkel, Henry George, U.S. physician, 1916-1983.

Bearn-Kunkel-Slater syndrome – *SYN:* Bearn-Kunkel syndrome

Bearn-Kunkel syndrome – see under Bearn

Kunkel syndrome – *SYN:* Bearn-Kunkel syndrome

Kunkel test

Küntscher, Gerhard, German surgeon, 1902-1972.

Küntscher cloverleaf nail

Küntscher driver

Küntscher femur guide pin

Küntscher intramedullary nail

Küntscher nail – an intramedullary nail used for internal fixation of a fracture.

NOTES

Küntscher nail driver
Küntscher nail extender
Küntscher nail instrument
Küntscher nail set
Küntscher reamer
Küntscher rod
Küntscher shaft reamer
Küntscher traction apparatus

Kuntz, Albert, U.S. professor of histology, 1879-1957.
nerve of Kuntz

Kupffer, Karl W. von, German anatomist, 1829-1902.
Kupffer cells – phagocytic cells of the mononuclear phagocyte series found on the luminal surface of the hepatic sinusoids. *SYN:* stellate cells of liver
Kupffer cell sarcoma

Kurloff, Mikhail G., Russian physician, 1859-1932.
Kurloff bodies – palely basophilic, granular inclusions sometimes observed in the cytoplasm of the large mononuclear leukocytes of guinea pigs and certain other animals.

Kuroki, Yoshikazu, Japanese physician, *1937.
Niikawa-Kuroki syndrome – see under Niikawa

Kürsteiner, (Kuersteiner), W., 19th century German anatomist.
Kürsteiner canals – a fetal complex of vesicular, canalicular, and glandlike structures derived from parathyroid, thymus, or thymic cord.

Kuru, New Guinean word meaning "trembling with fear."
Kuru disease – fatal neurologic disease which existed in Fore tribe in New Guinea, perpetuated by cannibalism until the practice was abolished.

Kurz, Jaromir, Czech ophthalmologist, *1895.
Kurz syndrome – congenital blindness often followed later by mental retardation.

Kurzrock, Raphael, U.S. gynecologist and obstetrician, 1895-1961.
Kurzrock-Miller test – test related to female infertility.

Kurzweil, Raymond C., 20th century U.S. inventor.
Kurzweil reading machine – computerized reading machine.

Kuskokwim, town in Alaska.
Kuskokwim disease – joint stiffness and ankylosis observed in Yupik Eskimos.

Küss, Georges, French physician, 1877-1967.
  Küss disease – sigmoid and rectal stenosis caused by inflammation.

Kussmaul, Adolph, German physician, 1822-1902.
  Kussmaul aphasia – mutism in psychosis.
  Kussmaul breathing
  Kussmaul coma – *SYN:* diabetic coma
  Kussmaul disease – segmental inflammation, with infiltration by
    eosinophils, and necrosis of medium-sized or small arteries.
    SYN: polyarteritis nodosa
  Kussmaul-Kien respiration – *SYN:* Kussmaul respiration
  Kussmaul paradoxical pulse
  Kussmaul pulse – reduction or disappearance of the pulse during
    inspiration.
  Kussmaul respiration – deep, rapid respiration characteristic of diabetic
    or other causes of acidosis. *SYN:* Kussmaul-Kien respiration
  Kussmaul sign – in constrictive pericarditis, a paradoxical increase in
    venous distention and pressure during inspiration. *SYN:* Kussmaul
    symptom
  Kussmaul symptom – *SYN:* Kussmaul sign

Küster, Herman, early 20th century German gynecologist.
  Mayer-Rokitansky-Küster-Hauser syndrome – see under Mayer, Paul
  Rokitansky-Küster-Hauser syndrome – *SYN:* Mayer-Rokitansky-Küster-
    Hauser syndrome

Küstner, Heinz, German gynecologist, *1897.
  Küstner suture
  Küstner uterine tenaculum forceps
  Prausnitz-Küstner antibody – see under Prausnitz
  Prausnitz-Küstner reaction – see under Prausnitz
  reversed Prausnitz-Küstner reaction – see under Prausnitz

Kveim, Morton Ansgar, Norwegian pathologist, 1892-1966.

Kveim antigen – a saline suspension of human sarcoid tissue. *SYN:* Kveim-Stilzbach antigen

Kveim-Stilzbach antigen – *SYN:* Kveim antigen

Kveim-Stilzbach test – *SYN:* Kveim test

Kveim test – an intradermal test for the detection of sarcoidosis. *SYN:* Kveim-Stilzbach test; Nickerson-Kveim test

Nickerson-Kveim test – *SYN:* Kveim test

Kwok, R.H.M., U.S. physician.

Kwok quease – *SYN:* Chinese restaurant syndrome

Kyrle, Josef, Austrian dermatologist, 1880-1926.

Kyrle disease – discrete and confluent horny follicular plugs on crateriform base, often occurring on the arms and legs in diabetics with renal failure. *SYN:* hyperkeratosis follicularis et parafollicularis

Laband, Peter F., U.S. dentist, *1900.
Laband syndrome – fibromatosis of the gingivae associated with hypoplasia of the distal phalanges, nail dysplasia, joint hypermotility, and sometimes hepatosplenomegaly.

Laban von Varalja, Rudolf, German dancer, 1879-1958.
labanotation – dance notation used in physical therapy.

Labbé, Ernest M., French physician, 1870-1939.
Labbé neurocirculatory syndrome – an anxiety neurosis.

Labbé, Leon, French surgeon, 1832-1916.
Labbé triangle – an area where the stomach is normally in contact with the abdominal wall.
Labbé vein – an inconstant vein that passes from the superficial middle cerebral vein posteriorly over the lateral aspect of the temporal lobe to enter the transverse sinus. *SYN:* inferior anastomotic vein

Laborde, Jean B.V., French physician, 1830-1903.
Laborde forceps
Laborde method
Laborde tracheal dilator

Lacan, Jacques, French psychoanalyst, 1901-1981.
Lacanian psychoanalysis – characterized by belief that the unconscious (id) is the ground of being and cannot be controlled by the ego.

Ladd, William E., U.S. pediatric surgeon, 1880-1967.
Ladd band – a peritoneal attachment of an incompletely rotated cecum, causing obstruction of the duodenum, found in malrotation of the intestine.
Ladd calipers
Ladd clamp
Ladd elevator

NOTES

Ladd fiberoptic system
Ladd intracranial pressure sensor
Ladd knife
Ladd operation – division of Ladd band to relieve duodenal obstruction in malrotation of the intestine.
Ladd pressure monitor

Ladd-Franklin, Christine, U.S. psychologist, 1847-1930.
Ladd-Franklin theory – a theory pertaining to color vision. *SYN:* molecular dissociation theory

Laehr, Heinrich, German physician, 1820-1905.
Laehr-Henneberg reflex – *SYN:* Henneberg reflex

Laënnec, René T.H., French physician, 1781-1826.
Laënnec catarrh – asthmatic bronchitis with pearllike expectoration.
Laënnec cirrhosis – cirrhosis in which normal liver lobules are replaced by small regeneration nodules. *SYN:* Laënnec disease; portal cirrhosis
Laënnec disease – *SYN:* Laënnec cirrhosis
Laënnec pearls – obsolete term for small, round, translucent, tenacious bodies in the sputum of some persons with asthma.

Laffer, W.B., U.S. physician.
Laffer-Ascher syndrome

Lafora, Gonzalo Rodriguez, Spanish neurologist, 1887-1971.
Lafora body – an intraneural intracytoplasmic inclusion body seen in familial myoclonus epilepsy.
Lafora body disease – myoclonus epilepsy beginning at 11 to 18 years of age with progressive mental impairment. *SYN:* Lafora disease
Lafora disease – *SYN:* Lafora body disease

Lagrange, Pierre F., French ophthalmologist, 1857-1928.
Lagrange eye scissors
Lagrange sclerectomy

Lahey, Frank H., U.S. surgeon, 1880-1935.
Lahey bag
Lahey carrier
Lahey catheter
Lahey clamp
Lahey dissecting scissors
Lahey drain
Lahey forceps – thyroid forceps used to deliver the uterus in vaginal hysterectomy.

Lahey gall duct forceps
Lahey goiter retractor
Lahey goiter tenaculum
Lahey gouge
Lahey hemostatic forceps
Lahey hook
Lahey incision
Lahey ligature carrier
Lahey needle
Lahey osteotome
Lahey scissors
Lahey score
Lahey tenaculum
Lahey thoracic clamp
Lahey thoracic forceps
Lahey thyroid retractor
Lahey thyroid scissors
Lahey thyroid traction vulsellum forceps
Lahey trephine
Lahey tube
Lahey Y-tube

Lallemand, Claude F., French surgeon, 1790-1853.
   Lallemand bodies – (1) obsolete term for small gelatinoid concretions sometimes observed in seminal fluid; (2) old term for Bence Jones cylinders. *SYN:* Trousseau-Lallemand bodies
   Trousseau-Lallemand bodies – *SYN:* Lallemand bodies (2)

Lallouette, Pierre, French physician, 1711-1792.
   Lallouette pyramid – an inconstant narrow lobe of the thyroid gland that marks the point of continuity with the thyroglossal duct. *SYN:* pyramidal lobe of thyroid gland

NOTES

Lamarck, Jean-Baptiste P.A., French botanist, zoologist, and biological philosopher, 1744-1829.
   lamarckian theory – that acquired characteristics may be transmitted to descendants and that experience, not biology alone, can change and thereby influence genetic transmission.

Lamaze, Fernand, French obstetrician, 1890-1957.
   Lamaze method – a technique of psychoprophylactic preparation for childbirth. *SYN:* Lamaze technique
   Lamaze technique – *SYN:* Lamaze method

Lambert, Edward H., U.S. neurophysiologist, *1915.
   Eaton-Lambert syndrome – *SYN:* Lambert-Eaton syndrome
   Lambert-Eaton syndrome – progressive proximal muscle weakness in patients with carcinoma, caused by antibodies directed against motor-nerve axon terminals. *SYN:* Eaton-Lambert syndrome

Lambert, Johann Heinrich, German mathematician and physicist, 1728-1777.
   Beer-Lambert law – see under Beer, August
   Lambert cosine law – mathematical measure of the intensity of radiation.

Lambl, Wilhelm D.
   lambliasis – giardiasis.

Lambrinudi, Constantine, English orthopedic surgeon, 1890-1943.
   Lambrinudi operation – a form of triple arthrodesis done in such a manner as to prevent footdrop. *SYN:* Lambrinudi triple arthrodesis
   Lambrinudi osteotomy
   Lambrinudi splint
   Lambrinudi technique
   Lambrinudi triple arthrodesis – *SYN:* Lambrinudi operation

Lamy, Maurice Emile Joseph, French physician, 1895-1975.
   Maroteaux-Lamy syndrome – see under Maroteaux

Lancefield, Rebecca Craighill, U.S. bacteriologist, *1895.
   Lancefield classification – a serologic classification dividing hemolytic streptococci into groups which bear a definite relationship to their sources.

Lancereaux, Étienne, French physician, 1829-1910.
   Lancereaux diabetes
   Lancereaux law

Lancisi, Giovanni M., Italian physician, 1654-1720.
   Lancisi sign – a large systolic jugular venous wave.

striae lancisi – the lateral longitudinal stria and the medial longitudinal stria.

Landau, A., German pediatrician.
   Landau reflex – test for hypertonia or hypotonia in infants. *SYN:* Landau response
   Landau response – *SYN:* Landau reflex

Landing, Benjamin Harrison, U.S. pathologist, *1920.
   Norman-Landing syndrome – see under Norman, R.M.

Landis, Eugene M., U.S. physiologist, *1901.
   Landis-Gibbon test – a test for vascular disease.

Landolt, Edmund, French ophthalmologist, 1846-1926.
   Landolt bodies – bipolar nerve cells lying between the retinal rods and cones in amphibia, reptiles, and birds.
   Landolt circles
   Landolt enucleation scissors
   Landolt eye knife
   Landolt eyelid reconstruction
   Landolt keratome
   Landolt operation
   Landolt ring – instrument used for testing of visual acuity.

Landouzy, Louis T.J., French neurologist, 1845-1917.
   Dejerine-Landouzy dystrophy – *SYN:* Landouzy-Dejerine dystrophy
   Dejerine-Landouzy myopathy – *SYN:* Landouzy-Dejerine dystrophy
   Landouzy-Dejerine dystrophy – a relatively benign type of muscular dystrophy commencing in childhood and slowly progressive.
      SYN: Dejerine-Landouzy dystrophy; Dejerine-Landouzy myopathy; facioscapulohumeral muscular dystrophy
   Landouzy-Grasset law – in lesions of one hemisphere, the patient's head is turned to the side of the affected muscles if there is spasticity and to that of the cerebral lesion if there is paralysis. *SYN:* Grasset law

NOTES

Landry, Jean B.O., French physician, 1826-1865.
    Landry-Guillain-Barré syndrome – *SYN:* Landry syndrome
    Landry paralysis – *SYN:* Landry syndrome
    Landry syndrome – marked by paresthesia of the limbs and muscular
        weakness or a flaccid paralysis. *SYN:* acute idiopathic polyneuritis;
        Landry-Guillain-Barré syndrome; Landry paralysis

Landsteiner, Karl, Austrian-U.S. pathologist and Nobel laureate, 1868-1943.
    Donath-Landsteiner cold autoantibody – see under Donath
    Donath-Landsteiner phenomenon – see under Donath
    Landsteiner-Donath test

Landström, John, Swedish surgeon, 1869-1910.
    Landström muscle – microscopic muscle fibers in the fascia behind and
        about the eyeball.

Landzert, T., 19th century German anatomist.
    Gruber-Landzert fossa – see under Gruber, Wenzel L.
    Landzert fossa – a fossa formed by two peritoneal folds enclosing the left
        colic artery and the inferior mesenteric vein at the side of the duodenum

Lane, John Edward, U.S. physician, 1872-1933.
    Lane disease – a hereditary disease of unknown cause characterized by
        symmetric and permanent redness of the palms and soles.

Lane, Sir W. Arbuthnot, English surgeon, 1856-1943.
    Lane band – a congential band on the distal ileum causing stasis.
        SYN: Lane kink
    Lane bone-holding clamp
    Lane bone-holding forceps
    Lane catheter
    Lane clamp
    Lane disease – asymptomatic symmetrical palmar erythema.
        SYN: erythema palmare hereditarium
    Lane dissector
    Lane elevator
    Lane forceps
    Lane kink – *SYN:* Lane band
    Lane mouth gag
    Lane needle
    Lane plates – flattened, narrow, metal plates used to hold the fragments of
        a fractured bone in apposition.
    Lane retractor
    Lane rongeur

Lane screwdriver
Murphy-Lane bone skid

Lang, Basil T., English ophthalmologist, 1880-1928.
Lang dissector
Lang eye speculum
Lang knife
Lang scoop
Lang suture

Langdon Down, see under Down, John Langdon H.

Lange, Carl F.A., German biochemist, 1883-1953.
Lange solution – a colloidal gold solution used to demonstrate protein abnormalities in spinal fluid.
Lange test – an obsolete, nonspecific test for altered proteins in spinal fluid. *SYN:* gold sol test; Zsigmondy test

Lange, Carl G., Danish psychologist, 1834-1900.
James-Lange theory – see under James, William

Lange, Cornelia de, see under de Lange

Langenbeck, Bernhard R.K. von, German surgeon, 1810-1887.
Langenbeck amputation
Langenbeck elevator
Langenbeck flap
Langenbeck forceps
Langenbeck incision
Langenbeck knife
Langenbeck needle holder
Langenbeck periosteal elevator
Langenbeck raspatory
Langenbeck retractor
Langenbeck saw

L

NOTES

Langenbeck triangle – formed by lines drawn from the anterior superior iliac spine to the surface of the great trochanter and to the surgical neck of the femur.

Langendorff, Oscar, German physiologist, 1853-1908.
Langendorff method – perfusion of the isolated mammalian heart by carrying fluid under pressure into the sectioned aorta and thus into the coronary system.

Lange-Nielsen, F., 20th century Norwegian cardiologist.
Jervell and Lange-Nielsen syndrome – see under Jervell

Langer, Karl (Ritter von Edenberg), Austrian anatomist, 1819-1887.
Langer arch – *SYN:* axillary arch muscle
Langer lines – lines which can be extrapolated by connecting linear openings made when a round pin is driven into the skin of a cadaver. *SYN:* cleavage lines
Langer muscle – *SYN:* axillary arch muscle

Langer, Leonard O., Jr., U.S. radiologist, *1928.
Langer-Giedion syndrome – syndrome of mental retardation accompanied by numerous physical abnormalities. *SYN:* Alò-Calò syndrome
Langer-Saldino syndrome – fatal form of neonatal dwarfism.
Langer syndrome – skeletal dysplasia of short-limbed dwarfism.

Langerhans, Paul, German anatomist, 1847-1888.
islets of Langerhans – cellular masses composed of different cell types that comprise the endocrine portion of the pancreas and are the source of insulin and glucagon. *SYN:* islet tissue; Langerhans islands; pancreatic islands; pancreatic islets
Langerhans cell granulomatosis
Langerhans cells – dendritic clear cells in the epidermis that are active participants in cutaneous delayed hypersensitivity.
Langerhans granule – a small membrane-bound granule first reported in Langerhans cells of the epidermis. *SYN:* Birbeck granule
Langerhans islands – *SYN:* islets of Langerhans

Langhans, Theodor, German pathologist, 1839-1915.
Langhans cells – multinucleated giant cells seen in tuberculosis and other granulomas. *SYN:* cytotrophoblastic cells; Langhans-type giant cells
Langhans layer – the inner layer of the trophoblast. *SYN:* cytotrophoblast
Langhans stria – fibrinoid that accumulates on the chorionic plate between the bases of placental villi during the first half of pregnancy.
Langhans-type giant cells – *SYN:* Langhans cells

Langley, John N., English physiologist, 1852-1925.
   Langley granules – granules in serous secreting cells.

Langmuir, Irving, U.S. chemist and Nobel laureate, 1881-1957.
   Langmuir trough – a trough with a movable surface barrier for studying the compression of surface films.

Lannelongue, Odilon M., French surgeon and pathologist, 1840-1911.
   Lannelongue foramina – a number of fossae in the wall of the right atrium, containing the openings of minute intramural veins. *SYN:* foramina of the venae minimae
   Lannelongue ligaments – fibrous bands that pass from the pericardium to the sternum. *SYN:* sternopericardial ligament

Lanquepin, Anne, 20th century French pediatrician.
   Fèvre-Lanquepin syndrome – see under Fèvre

Lanterman, A.J., 19th century U.S. anatomist in Germany.
   Lanterman incisures – *SYN:* Schmidt-Lanterman incisures
   Lanterman segments – the divisions of the nerve fiber between the Schmidt-Lanterman incisures.
   Schmidt-Lanterman clefts – *SYN:* Schmidt-Lanterman incisures
   Schmidt-Lanterman incisures – see under Schmidt, Henry D.

Lanz, Otto, Swiss surgeon in Holland, 1865-1935.
   Lanz incision
   Lanz line – a horizontal plane marking the boundary between the lateral and umbilical regions superiorly and the inguinal and pubic regions inferiorly. *SYN:* interspinal plane
   Lanz low-pressure cuff endotracheal tube
   Lanz operation
   Lanz point
   Lanz tracheostomy tube

L

NOTES

Lapicque, Louis, French physiologist, 1866-1952.
Lapicque law – the chronaxie is inversely proportional to the diameter of an axon.

Laplace, Ernest, U.S. surgeon, 1861-1924.
Laplace forceps – a forceps for approximating intestines during surgical anastomosis.
Laplace liver retractor

Laplace, Pierre S. de, French mathematician, 1749-1827.
Laplace law – the equilibrium relationship between transmural pressure difference, wall tension, and radius of curvature in a concave surface.

Laquer, Ernst, German physiologist, *1910.
Laquer stain for alcoholic hyalin

Laron, Zvi, Israeli pediatric endocrinologist, *1927.
Laron-type dwarfism – dwarfism associated with absent or very low levels of somatomedin C (insulinlike growth factor I) or abnormalities in receptor activity.

Laroyenne, Lucien, French surgeon, 1831-1902.
Laroyenne operation – puncture of Douglas pouch to evacuate pus and to secure drainage in cases of pelvic suppuration.

Larrey, Baron Dominique Jean de, French surgeon, 1766-1842.
Larrey amputation – amputation at the shoulder joint.
Larrey cleft – a muscular defect in the diaphragm between the costal and the sternal portions. *SYN:* trigonum sternocostale
Larrey ligation – a ligation of the femoral artery immediately below the inguinal ligament.
Larrey-Weil disease – *SYN:* Weil disease

Larsen, Loren Joseph, U.S. orthopedic surgeon, *1914.
Larsen syndrome – characterized by multiple congenital dislocations with osseous anomalies, including characteristic flattened facies and cleft soft palate.

Larsson, Tage Konrad Leopold, Swedish scientist, *1905.
Sjögren-Larsson syndrome – see under Sjögren, Karl Gustaf Torsten

Lasègue, Ernest C., French physician, 1816-1883.
Lasègue disease – obsolete eponym for delusions of persecution.
Lasègue maneuver
Lasègue sign – when patient is supine with hip flexed, dorsiflexion of the ankle causes pain or muscle spasm in the posterior thigh indicates lumbar root or sciatic nerve irritation.

Lasègue syndrome – in conversion hysteria, inability to move an anesthetic limb except under control of the sight.

Lash, Abraham Fae, U.S. obstetrician-gynecologist, *1898.
Lash hysterectomy
Lash operation – removal of a wedge of the internal cervical os with suturing of the internal os into a tighter canal structure.
Lash technique

Lassa, town in Yedseram River valley in Nigeria.
Lassa virus – viral hemorrhagic illness, often fatal, caused by an arenavirus.

Lassar, Oskar, German dermatologist, 1849-1907.
Lassar paste – zinc oxide paste with salicylic acid used in the treatment of psoriasis.

Latapi, Fernando, Mexican leprologist, 1902-1989.
Latapi lepromatosis – a form of diffuse nonnodular lepromatous leprosy.

Latarget, André, French anatomist, 1877-1947.
Latarget nerve – terminal branch of anterior vagal trunk which runs along lesser curvature of the stomach. *SYN:* superior hypogastric plexus
Latarget vein – a tributary of the right gastric vein that passes anterior to the pylorus at its junction with the duodenum. *SYN:* prepyloric vein

Latham, Peter M., English physician, 1789-1875.
Latham circle – area of cardiac dullness between left nipple and sternum.

Lato River, river near Apulia, Italy.
Lato River virus – tombusvirus first isolated in irrigation water from Lato River.

Latzko, Wilhelm, Austrian obstetrician, 1863-1945.
Latzko cesarean section
Latzko closure
Latzko colpocleisis
Latzko fistula repair

NOTES

Latzko radical hysterectomy
Latzko repair of vesicovaginal fistula

Lauber, Hans, Swiss ophthalmologist, *1876.
    Lauber disease – defective vision in the presence of bright light associated with white spots in deep layers of retinal tissue.

Laubry, Charles, French cardiologist and founder of French Society of Cardiology, 1872-1960.
    Laubry-Pezzi syndrome – syndrome of congenital heart defect.

Laugier, Stanislas, French surgeon, 1799-1872.
    Laugier hernia – a hernia passing through an opening in the lacunar ligament.
    Laugier sign – in fracture of the lower portion of the radius, the styloid processes of the radius and of the ulna are on the same level.

Laumonier, Jean B.P.N.R., French surgeon, 1749-1818.
    Laumonier ganglion – a small ganglionic swelling on filaments from the internal carotid plexus, lying on the undersurface of the carotid artery in the cavernous sinus. *SYN:* carotid ganglion

Launois, Pierre-Emile, French physician, 1856-1914.
    Launois-Bensaude syndrome – accumulation and progressive enlargement of collections of adipose tissue in the subcutaneous tissue of the head, neck, upper trunk, and upper portions of the upper extremities. *SYN:* multiple symmetric lipomatosis
    Launois-Cléret syndrome – *SYN:* Fröhlich syndrome

Laurence, John Zachariah, English ophthalmologist, 1830-1874.
    Laurence-Moon-Biedl syndrome – mental retardation, pigmentary retinopathy, hypogenitalism, and spastic paraplegia.

Laurer, Johann F., German pharmacologist, 1798-1873.
    Laurer canal – a tube originating on the surface of the ootype of trematodes.

Lauterbur, Paul C., U.S. chemist, *1929, joint winner of 2003 Nobel Prize for work related to magnetic resonance imaging.

Lauth, Ernst A., German physician, 1803-1837.
    Lauth canal – the vascular structure encircling the anterior chamber of the eye and through which the aqueous is returned to the blood circulation. *SYN:* sinus venosus sclerae

Lauth, Thomas, German anatomist and surgeon, 1758-1826.
    Lauth ligament – *SYN:* transverse ligament of the atlas

Lavdovsky, Michail D., Russian histologist, 1846-1902.
    Lavdovsky nucleoid – a set of radiating microtubules extending outward
    from the cytocentrum and centrosphere of a dividing cell. *SYN:*
    astrosphere

Laveran, Charles Louis Alphonse, French protozoologist, 1845-1922, winner
of the 1907 Nobel Prize for physiology and medicine for his discovery of a
protozoan as the cause of malaria.

Lawrence, Robert D., English physician, 1912-1964.
    Lawrence-Seip syndrome – loss of subcutaneous fat associated with
    hepatomegaly, excessive bone growth, and insulin-resistant diabetes.
    SYN: lipoatrophy

Laxová, Renata.
    Neu-Laxová syndrome – see under Neu

Lazarus, the brother of Martha and Mary who was raised from the dead in the
New Testament of the Bible.
    Lazarus complex – psychological sequence observed in survivors of
    cardiac arrest. *SYN:* Lazarus syndrome
    Lazarus sign – spontaneous movement in patients who are brain dead or
    who have suffered spinal cord injury.
    Lazarus syndrome – *SYN:* Lazarus complex

League, Little, see under Little League

Le Bel, Joseph Achille, French chemist, 1847-1930.
    Le Bel-van't Hoff rule – the number of stereoisomers of an organic
    compound is $2n$ where n represents the number of asymmetric carbon
    atoms unless there is an internal plane of symmetry.

Leber, Theodor, German ophthalmologist, 1840-1917.
    amaurosis congenita of Leber – an autosomal recessive cone-rod
    abiotrophy causing blindness or severely reduced vision at birth.
    Leber hereditary optic atrophy – hereditary degeneration of the optic
    nerve and papillomacular bundle, resulting in rapid loss of central vision.

NOTES

Leber idiopathic stellate neuroretinitis – a unilateral neuroretinitis with perifoveal exudates in Henle nerve fiber layer producing a macular star and spontaneous regression in a few months. *SYN:* stellate neuroretinitis

Leber plexus – a small venous plexus in the eye between the venous sinuses of the sclera (of Schlemm) and the spaces of the iridocorneal angle (of Fontana).

Lebombo, region of the Congo, Africa.

Lebombo virus – genus *Orbivirus,* family Reoviridae.

Leboyer, Frederick, French obstetrician.

Leboyer method – babies are allowed to be born without harsh lights and loud noise, placed gently on mother's abdomen, and allowed to take the first breath in their own time, before the umbilical cord is cut. *SYN:* birth without violence

Le Cat, Claude Nicolas, French surgeon, 1700-1768.

Le Cat gulf – hollow of bulbous portion of urethra.

Le Chatelier, Henri, French physical chemist, 1850-1936.

Le Chatelier law – if external factors such as temperature and pressure disturb a system in equilibrium, adjustment occurs in such a way that the effect of the disturbing factors is reduced to a minimum. *SYN:* Le Chatelier principle

Le Chatelier principle – *SYN:* Le Chatelier law

Ledderhose, Georg, German physician, 1855-1925.

Ledderhose syndrome – clawfoot.

Leder, Max, Swiss dermatologist, *1912.

Miescher-Leder syndrome – see under Miescher, Alfred Guido

Lederberg, Joshua, U.S. biochemist, *1925, joint winner of 1958 Nobel Prize for work related to genetics.

Lederer, Max, U.S. pathologist, 1885-1952.

Lederer anemia – obsolete term for a form of acute acquired hemolytic anemia associated with abnormal hemolysins and sometimes with hemoglobinuria.

Ledermann, Sully, French psychiatrist.

Ledermann formula – the formula used to estimate the prevalence of various degrees of alcohol dependency.

Lee, Robert, English physician, 1793-1877.
  Lee ganglion – a gangliated autonomic plexus on each side of the cervix of the uterus, derived from the inferior hypogastric plexus. *SYN:* uterovaginal plexus

Lee, Roger I., U.S. physician, *1881.
  Lee-White method – a method for determining coagulation time of venous blood in tubes of standard bore at body temperature.

Leede, Carl Stockbridge, U.S. physician, *1882.
  Leede-Rumpel phenomenon – *SYN:* Rumpel-Leede phenomenon
  Rumpel-Leede phenomenon – see under Rumpel
  Rumpel-Leede sign – *SYN:* Rumpel-Leede test
  Rumpel-Leede test – see under Rumpel

Leeuwenhoek, Anton van, Dutch microscopist, 1632-1723.
  Leeuwenhoek canals – *SYN:* haversian canals

Lefèvre, Paul, 20th century French dermatologist.
  Papillon-Lefèvre syndrome – see under Papillon

Le Fort, Léon C., French surgeon and gynecologist, 1829-1893.
  Le Fort bougie
  Le Fort catheter
  Le Fort dilator
  Le Fort follower
  Le Fort reconstruction
  Le Fort repair
  Le Fort sound – a curved sound used for dilation of urethral strictures in the male.
  Le Fort speculum
  Le Fort suture

Le Fort, René, French surgeon, 1869-1951.
  Le Fort amputation – a modification of Pirogoff amputation.
  Le Fort classification – classification of bone fractures (I, II, III).

NOTES

Le Fort I fracture – *SYN:* Guérin fracture
Le Fort II fracture – *SYN:* pyramidal fracture
Le Fort III fracture – *SYN:* craniofacial dysjunction fracture
Le Fort osteotomy – osteotomy often done to correct a maxillary skeletal
  deformity.

Legal, Emmo, German physician, 1859-1922.
  Legal test – a test for acetone.

Legendre, Gaston J., French physician, *1887.
  Legendre function
  Legendre sign – in facial hemiplegia of central origin, when the examiner
    raises the lids of the actively closed eyes, the resistance is less on the
    affected side.

Legg, Arthur T., U.S. orthopedic surgeon, 1874-1939.
  Legg-Calvé-Perthes disease – epiphysial aseptic necrosis of the upper
    end of the femur. *SYN:* Calvé-Perthes disease; coxa plana; Perthes
    disease; pseudocoxalgia; quiet hip disease
  Legg osteotome

Legionnaire, the title given to retired servicemen.
  Legionnaire disease – an acute infectious disease characterized by a
    severe and often fatal pneumonia; first outbreak occurred at a
    Legionnaire convention in Philadelphia in 1976.

Lehmann, J.O. Orla, Swedish pathologist, *1927.
  Börjeson-Forssman-Lehmann syndrome – see under Börjeson

Leichtenstern, Otto, German physician, 1845-1900.
  Leichtenstern phenomenon – *SYN:* Leichtenstern sign
  Leichtenstern sign – gently tapping one of the bones of the extremities
    causes the patient to draw back violently in cases of cerebrospinal
    meningitis. *SYN:* Leichtenstern phenomenon

Leigh, Denis, English psychiatrist, *1915.
  Leigh disease – subacute encephalomyelopathy affecting infants.
    SYN: subacute necrotizing encephalomyelopathy; necrotizing
    encephalomyelopathy
  Leigh syndrome

Leiner, Karl, Austrian pediatrician, 1871-1930.
  Leiner disease – severe, extensive seborrheic dermatitis with exfoliative
    dermatitis, generalized lymphadenopathy, and diarrhea in the newborn.
    SYN: erythroderma desquamativum

Leishman, Sir William Boog, Scottish surgeon, 1865-1926.

Leishman chrome cells – basophilic granular leukocytes (basophils) observed in the circulating blood of some persons with blackwater fever.

Leishman-Donovan body – the intracytoplasmic, nonflagellated leishmanial form of certain intracellular parasites. *SYN:* amastigote; L-D body

Leishmania – a genus of digenetic, asexual, protozoan flagellates.

leishmaniasis – tropical disease that is spread by sandflies.

Leishman stain – a polychromed eosin-methylene blue stain used in the examination of blood films.

Leiter, Russell G., U.S. psychologist, *1901.

Leiter International Performance Scale – a nonverbal test for measuring intelligence.

Lejeune, Jerôme J.L.M., French cytogeneticist, *1926.

Lejeune syndrome – a disorder characterized by microcephaly, antimongoloid palpebral fissures, epicanthal folds, micrognathia, strabismus, mental and physical retardation, and a characteristic high-pitched catlike whine. *SYN:* cri-du-chat syndrome

Leksell, Lars, Swedish physician, 1907-1986.

Leksell bone rongeur
Leksell cardiovascular rongeur
Leksell director
Leksell forceps
Leksell frame
Leksell punch
Leksell sternal approximator
Leksell sternal spreader
Leksell trephine

Leloir, Henri Camille, French physician, 1855-1896.

Leloir disease – *SYN:* lupus erythematosus

NOTES

Lembert, Antoine, French surgeon, 1802-1851.
Czerny-Lembert suture – see under Czerny
Lembert suture – an inverting suture for intestinal surgery.

Lemli, Luc, 20th century U.S. pediatrician.
Smith-Lemli-Opitz syndrome – see under Smith, David W.

Lendrum, A.C., 20th century Scottish pathologist.
Fraser-Lendrum stain for fibrin – see under Fraser, Alexander
Lendrum phloxine-tartrazine stain – a stain for demonstrating acidophilic inclusion bodies.

Lenègre, Jean, 20th century French cardiologist.
Lenègre disease – *SYN:* Lenègre syndrome
Lenègre syndrome – isolated damage of the cardiac conduction system as a result of a sclerodegenerative lesion. *SYN:* Lenègre disease

Lenhossék, Michael (Mihály) von, Hungarian anatomist, 1863-1937.
Lenhossék processes – short processes possessed by some ganglion cells.

Lenier, Karl, Austrian physician, 1871-1930.
Lenier dermatitis – skin disorder of newborns.

Lennert, Karl, German histopathologist, *1921.
Lennert classification – classification of non-Hodgkin lymphoma. *SYN:* Kiel classification
Lennert lesion – *SYN:* Lennert lymphoma
Lennert lymphoma – malignant lymphoma with a high proportion of diffusely scattered epithelioid cells, tonsillar involvement, and an unpredictable course. *SYN:* Lennert lesion

Lennhoff, Rudolf, German physician, 1866-1933.
Lennhoff sign – when liver is infected with a tapeworm, a furrow forms between liver cyst and lowest rib on deep inspiration.

Lennox, William G., U.S. neurologist, 1884-1960.
Lennox-Gastaut syndrome – a generalized myoclonic astatic epilepsy in children, with mental retardation. *SYN:* Lennox syndrome
Lennox syndrome – *SYN:* Lennox-Gastaut syndrome

Lenoir, Camille A.H., French anatomist, *1867.
Lenoir facet – the medial articular surface of the patella.

Lenz, Widukind D., German geneticist, 1919-1995.
Lenz-Majewski syndrome – congenital anomalies, mental retardation, sclerosis of the skeletal system.

Lenz syndrome – inherited X-linked trait consisting of multiple abnormalities.

Leonardi, Giuseppe, Italian physician.
Magrassi-Leonardi syndrome – see under Magrassi

Leopold, Christian Gerhard, German gynecologist, 1846-1911.
Leopold maneuvers – four maneuvers employed to determine fetal position.

Lepehne, Georg, German physician, *1887.
Lepehne-Pickworth stain – a staining technique for hemoglobin.

leprechaun, Irish mythological figure, usually depicted as dwarflike and somewhat distorted.
leprechaunism – congenital condition characterized by insulin resistance and growth retardation.

Lerch, Otto, U.S. physician, *1894.
Lerch percussion

Leri, André, French orthopedic surgeon, 1875-1930.
Leri pleonosteosis – *SYN:* dyschondrosteosis
Leri sign – voluntary flexion of the elbow is impossible in a case of hemiplegia when the wrist on that side is passively flexed.
Leri-Weill disease – *SYN:* dyschondrosteosis
Leri-Weill syndrome – *SYN:* dyschondrosteosis
Marie-Leri syndrome – see under Marie, Pierre

Leriche, René, French surgeon, 1879-1955.
Leriche forceps
Leriche operation – sympathetic denervation by arterial decortication. *SYN:* periarterial sympathectomy
Leriche sympathectomy
Leriche syndrome – aortoiliac occlusive disease producing distal ischemic symptoms and signs.

NOTES

Lermoyez, Marcel, French otolaryngologist, 1858-1929.
Lermoyez nasal punch
Lermoyez syndrome – increasing deafness interrupted by a sudden
attack of dizziness after which the hearing improves. *SYN:* labyrinthine
angiospasm

Lerner, I.M., U.S. population geneticist, 1910-1967.
Lerner homeostasis – the restorative mechanisms that tend to correct
perturbations in the genetic composition of a population. *SYN:* genetic
homeostasis

Leroy, Edgar August, French physician, *1883.
Fiessinger-Leroy-Reiter syndrome – *SYN:* Reiter syndrome

Lesch, Michael, U.S. pediatrician, *1939.
Lesch-Nyhan syndrome – a genetic disorder marked by choreoathetosis,
mental retardation, and self-mutilation.

Leschke, Erich Friedrich Wilhelm, German physician, 1887-1933.
Leschke syndrome – syndrome of multiple pigmented macules, asthenia,
sometimes hyperglycemia. *SYN:* Leschke-Ullmann syndrome
Leschke-Ullmann syndrome – *SYN:* Leschke syndrome

Leser, Edmund, German surgeon, 1828-1916.
Leser-Trélat sign – the sudden appearance and rapid increase in the
number and size of seborrheic keratoses with pruritus, associated with
internal malignancy.

Lesser, Ladislaus Leo, German surgeon born in Poland, 1846-1925.
Lesser triangle – the space between the bellies of the digastric muscle
and the hypoglossal nerve.

Lesshaft, Pjotr F., Russian physician, 1836-1909.
Lesshaft triangle – *SYN:* Grynfeltt triangle

Lester, A.M., English physician, 1909-1993.
Lester iris – hyperpigmentation of the papillary margin of the iris observed
in nail-patella syndrome. *SYN:* Lester lines
Lester lines – *SYN:* Lester iris

Letterer, Erich, German pathologist, 1895-1932.
Abt-Letterer-Siwe syndrome – *SYN:* Letterer-Siwe disease
Letterer reticulosis – *SYN:* Letterer-Siwe disease
Letterer-Siwe disease – the acute disseminated form of Langerhans cell
histiocytosis. *SYN:* Abt-Letterer-Siwe syndrome; Letterer reticulosis;
Letterer-Siwe syndrome; nonlipid histiocytosis
Letterer-Siwe syndrome – *SYN:* Letterer-Siwe disease

Letterman, David, 20th century U.S. late-night television host.
  David Letterman sign – on plain film of the wrist, subluxation of scaphoid
    bone resulting in widening of space between scaphoid and lunate carpal
    bones; so called because it is similar to prominent gap between central
    front teeth in this television personality. *SYN:* Lauren Hutton sign; Terry
    Thomas sign

Leudet, Théodor E., French physician, 1825-1887.
  Leudet tinnitus – a dry spasmodic click heard in catarrhal inflammation of
    the eustachian tube.

Lev, Maurice, U.S. pathologist, *1908.
  Lev disease – *SYN:* Lev syndrome
  Lev syndrome – bundle branch block in a patient with normal myocardium
    and normal coronary arteries resulting from fibrosis or calcification
    including the conducting system. *SYN:* Lev disease

Levaditi, Constantin, Romanian bacteriologist in Paris, 1874-1928.
  Levaditi method
  Levaditi stain – a silver nitrate stain for blackening spirochetes in tissue
    sections.

LeVeen, Harry H., U.S. surgeon, *1914.
  LeVeen ascites shunt
  LeVeen catheter
  LeVeen dialysis shunt
  LeVeen endarterectomy
  LeVeen inflation syringe
  LeVeen inflator with pressure gauge
  LeVeen peritoneal shunt
  LeVeen peritoneovenous shunt
  LeVeen shunt – a plastic tube used to transport ascitic fluid from the
    abdomen via a jugular vein to the superior vena cava.
  LeVeen valve

NOTES

Leventhal, Michael Leo, U.S. obstetrician-gynecologist, 1901-1971.
  Stein-Leventhal syndrome – see under Stein, Irving Freiler, Sr.

Lévi, E. Leopold, French endocrinologist, 1868-1933.
  dominantly inherited Lévi disease – dominantly inherited dwarfism
    characterized by low birth weight, snub nose, and stocky build.
    SYN: snub-nose dwarfism
  Lorain-Lévi dwarfism – see under Lorain
  Lorain-Lévi infantilism – *SYN:* Lorain-Lévi dwarfism
  Lorain-Lévi syndrome – *SYN:* Lorain-Lévi dwarfism

Levi-Montalcini, Rita, Italian neurobiologist, *1909, joint winner of 1986
Nobel Prize for work related to growth factors.

Levin, Abraham, U.S. physician, 1880-1940.
  Levin tube – a tube introduced through the nose into the upper alimentary
    canal to facilitate intestinal decompression.
  Levin tube catheter

Levin, Max, U.S. neurologist, *1901.
  Kleine-Levin syndrome – see under Kleine

Levine, Samuel A., U.S. cardiologist, 1891-1966.
  Lown-Ganong-Levine syndrome – see under Lown

Levret, André, French obstetrician, 1703-1780.
  Levret forceps – a modification of the Chamberlen forceps, curved to
    correspond to the curve of the parturient passage.
  Mauriceau-Levret maneuver – *SYN:* Mauriceau maneuver

Lévy, Gabrielle, French neurologist, 1886-1935.
  Roussy-Lévy disease – see under Roussy
  Roussy-Lévy syndrome – *SYN:* Roussy-Lévy disease

Lewandowski, Felix, German dermatologist, 1879-1921.
  Jadassohn-Lewandowski syndrome – see under Jadassohn
  nevus elasticus of Lewandowski – obsolete term for plaques now known
    to be a collagenous nevus.

Lewars, P.H.D., 20th century English oral surgeon.
  Lewars disease – chronic mandibular periostitis affecting mainly denture
    wearers, caused by embedded vegetable matter.

Lewey, var. of Lewy

Lewis, Edward B., joint winner of 1995 Nobel Prize for work related to
genetics and early development of embryo.

Lewis, Gilbert N., U.S. chemist, 1875-1946.
   Lewis acid – an acid that is an electron pair acceptor.

Lewisohn, Richard, U.S. surgeon, 1875-1961.
   Lewisohn method – method of preventing coagulation of blood outside
   the body, resulting in development of modern transfusion techniques.

Lewy, (Lewey), Frederic H., German neurologist in the U.S., 1885-1950.
   Lewy bodies – intracytoplasmic inclusion bodies especially noted in
   pigmented brainstem neurons and seen in Parkinson disease.

Leyden, Ernst V. von, German physician, 1832-1910.
   Charcot-Leyden crystals – see under Charcot
   Leyden ataxia – *SYN:* Westphal-Leyden syndrome
   Leyden crystals – *SYN:* Charcot-Leyden crystals
   Leyden disease
   Leyden-Möbius muscular dystrophy – *SYN:* limb-girdle muscular
   dystrophy
   Leyden neuritis – fatty degeneration of the fibers of the affected nerve.
   Westphal-Leyden syndrome – see under Westphal

Leydig, Franz von, German anatomist, 1821-1908.
   Leydig cell adenoma – small benign tumors of the testis that often
   produce testosterone, causing endocrine symptoms. *SYN:* interstitial cell
   tumor of testis
   Leydig cells – cells between the seminiferous tubules of the testis that
   secrete testosterone. *SYN:* interstitial cells
   Leydig drain
   Leydig duct – embryonic duct which becomes ductus deferens in males.

Lhermitte, Jean, French neurologist, 1877-1959.
   Lhermitte sign – sudden electriclike shocks extending down the spine on
   flexing the head.

NOTES

Li, Frederick Pei, epidemiologist, *1940.
  Li-Fraumeni cancer syndrome – familial breast cancer in young women,
  with soft tissue sarcomas in children and other cancers in close
  relatives.

Libman, Emanuel, U.S. physician, 1872-1946.
  Libman-Sacks endocarditis – verrucous endocarditis sometimes
  associated with disseminated lupus erythematosus. *SYN:* atypical
  verrucous endocarditis; Libman-Sacks syndrome; nonbacterial
  verrucous endocarditis
  Libman-Sacks syndrome – *SYN:* Libman-Sacks endocarditis

Liborius, Paul, 19th century Russian bacteriologist.
  Liborius method – a method for culturing anaerobic bacteria.

Lichtenstein, Louis, U.S. physician, 1906-1977.
  Jaffe-Lichtenstein disease – see under Jaffe, Henry Lewis

Lichtheim, Ludwig, German physician, 1845-1928.
  Dejerine-Lichtheim phenomenon – *SYN:* Lichtheim sign
  Lichtheim sign – in subcortical aphasia, the patient can indicate by use of
  the fingers the number of syllables of a word but cannot speak. *SYN:*
  Dejerine-Lichtheim phenomenon
  Lichtheim syndrome

Liddell, Edward G.T., English neurophysiologist, 1895-1981.
  Liddell-Sherrington reflex – tonic contraction of the muscles in response
  to a stretching force due to stimulation of muscle proprioceptors.
  SYN: myotatic reflex

Lieberkuhn, var. of Lieberkühn

Lieberkühn, (Lieberkuhn), Johann N., German anatomist and physician,
1711-1756.
  lieberkühn – concave reflector on a microscope; directs a concentrated
  beam of light on the material being examined.
  Lieberkühn crypts – *SYN:* Lieberkühn glands
  Lieberkühn follicles – *SYN:* Lieberkühn glands
  Lieberkühn glands – the tubular glands in the mucous membrane of the
  small and large intestines. *SYN:* intestinal glands; Lieberkühn crypts;
  Lieberkühn follicles

Liebermann, Leo von S., Hungarian physician, 1852-1926.
  Burchard-Liebermann reaction – see under Burchard
  Liebermann-Burchard test – a calorimetric test for unsaturated sterols,
  notably cholesterol.

Liebermeister, Carl von, German physician, 1833-1901.
Liebermeister rule – in adult febrile tachycardia, about eight pulse beats correspond to an increase of 1°C.

Liebig, Baron Justus von, German chemist, 1803-1873.
Liebig theory – that the hydrocarbons that oxidize readily and burn are nutritive material that produce the greatest quantity of animal heat.

Liebow, Averill A., Austrian-U.S. pulmonary pathologist, 1911-1978.
usual interstitial pneumonia of Liebow – a progressive inflammatory condition of the lung. *SYN:* fibrosing alveolitis; Hamman-Rich syndrome; idiopathic interstitial fibrosis

Liéou, Y.C., French physician.
Barré-Liéou syndrome – see under Barré
Liéou-Barré syndrome – *SYN:* Barré-Liéou syndrome

Liepmann, Hugo K., German neurologist, 1863-1925.
Liepmann disease – *SYN:* apraxia

Liesegang, Ralph E., German chemist, 1869-1947.
Liesegang rings – colored rings of precipitated silver chromate formed when a drop of concentrated silver nitrate is added to the surface of a gel containing potassium dichromate.

Lieutaud, Joseph, French anatomist and pathologist, 1703-1780.
Lieutaud body – *SYN:* Lieutaud trigone
Lieutaud triangle – *SYN:* Lieutaud trigone
Lieutaud trigone – a triangular smooth area at the base of the bladder between the openings of the two ureters and that of the urethra. *SYN:* Lieutaud body; Lieutaud triangle; trigone of bladder
Lieutaud uvula – a slight projection into the cavity of the bladder marking the location of the middle lobe of the prostate. *SYN:* uvula of bladder

Lightwood, Reginald Cyril, English pediatrician, 1898-1985.
Lightwood disease – hypercalciuria in infants.
Lightwood syndrome – tubular acidosis of the kidney.

NOTES

Lignac, George O.E., Dutch pediatrician, 1891-1954.
   Aberhalden-Kauffman-Lignac syndrome – see under Aberhalden
   Lignac disease
   Lignac-Fanconi syndrome – the most common of a group of diseases
      with characteristic renal tubular dysfunction disorders. *SYN:* cystinosis

Likert, Rensis, U.S. social psychologist, *1903.
   Likert scale – a method of measuring attitudes.

Lillehei, Clarence Walton, U.S. surgeon, 1918-1999.
   Lillehei-DeWall oxygenator – oxygenator for use during open-heart
      surgery. *SYN:* helix oxygenator
   Lillehei-Kalke bileaflet valve – prosthetic heart valve that was the
      precursor to the St. Jude valve.
   Lillehei-Nakib toroidal valve – mechanical heart valve usually used to
      replace the mitral valve.

Lillie, Ralph D., U.S. pathologist, 1896-1979.
   Glenner-Lillie stain for pituitary – see under Glenner
   Lillie allochrome connective tissue stain
   Lillie azure-eosin stain
   Lillie-Crow test
   Lillie ferrous iron stain
   Lillie sulfuric acid Nile blue stain

Lilliput, a mythical land inhabited by little people, described in Gulliver's
Travels, a novel by Jonathan Swift.
   Lilliputian hallucination – people, animals, and objects appear smaller
      than they would be normally in real life.

Lilly, John C., U.S. physiologist, *1915.
   Silverman-Lilly pneumotachograph – see under Silverman, Leslie

Lindau, Arvid Wilhelm, Swedish pathologist, 1892-1958.
   Lindau disease – *SYN:* von Hippel-Lindau syndrome
   Lindau tumor – a benign cerebellar neoplasm. *SYN:* hemangioblastoma
   von Hippel-Lindau syndrome – see under von Hippel

Lindbergh, Charles A., U.S. aviator, 1902-1974.
   Carrel-Lindbergh pump – see under Carrel

Lindemann, Edward E., U.S. surgeon, 1879-1919.
   Lindemann cannula – a cannula used in blood transfusion.

Lindner, Karl, Austrian ophthalmologist, 1883-1961.
   Lindner bodies – initial bodies resembling inclusion bodies found in
      scrapings of epithelial cells infected with trachoma.

Lindner corneoscleral suture
Lindner cyclodialysis spatula
Lindner cyclodialysis spoon
Lindner sclerotomy
Lindner spatula

Lindqvist, Johan Torsten, Swedish physician, *1906.
Fahraeus-Lindqvist effect – see under Fahraeus

Lindsay, P.G., 20th century U.S. physician.
Lindsay nails – the distal portion of the fingernails develops brown pigmentation due to chronic renal failure. *SYN:* half-and-half nails

Lineweaver, Hans, U.S. physical chemist, *1907.
Lineweaver-Burk equation – rearrangement of the Michaelis-Menten equation.
Lineweaver-Burk plot – graphical representation of enzyme kinetic data. *SYN:* double-reciprocal plot; Woolf-Lineweaver-Burk plot

Ling, Per Henrik, Swedish hygienist, 1776-1839.
lingism – *SYN:* Ling method
Ling method – gymnastic exercises without the use of apparatus. *SYN:* lingism

Linné, Carl von, Swedish botanist and physician, 1707-1778.
linnaean system of nomenclature – the system of nomenclature in which the names of species are composed of genus and species. *SYN:* binary nomenclature

Lipmann, Fritz A., German biochemist in the U.S. and Nobel laureate, 1899-1986.
Warburg-Lipmann-Dickens-Horecker shunt – *SYN:* Dickens shunt

Lipschütz, Benjamin, Austrian physician, 1878-1931.
Lipschütz cell – a cell whose protoplasm contains single and double granules of varying size, stainable with hematoxylin. *SYN:* centrocyte
Lipschütz erythema – *SYN:* Afzelius erythema

L

NOTES

Lipschütz ulcer – a simple acute ulceration of the vulva or lower vagina of nonvenereal origin. *SYN:* ulcus vulvae acutum

Lisa, Mona, subject of world-famous painting by Leonardo Da Vinci, known for her smile.

Mona Lisa syndrome – contracture of facial muscle, associated with Bell palsy.

Lisch, Karl, Austrian ophthalmologist, 1907-1999.

Lisch nodule – iris hamartomas typically seen in type 1 neurofibromatosis. *SYN:* Sakurai-Lisch nodule

Sakurai-Lisch nodule – *SYN:* Lisch nodule

Lisfranc, Jacques, French surgeon, 1790-1847.

Lisfranc amputation – amputation of the foot at the tarsometatarsal joint, the sole being preserved to make the flap. *SYN:* Lisfranc operation

Lisfranc dislocation

Lisfranc fracture

Lisfranc joints – the three synovial joints between the tarsal and metatarsal bones. *SYN:* tarsometatarsal joints

Lisfranc ligaments – ligaments that pass from the cuneiform bones to the metatarsals, the one from the first cuneiform to the second metatarsal being the strongest. *SYN:* interosseous cuneometatarsal ligaments

Lisfranc operation – *SYN:* Lisfranc amputation

scalene tubercle of Lisfranc – a small spine on the inner edge of the first rib, giving attachment to the scalenus anterior muscle. *SYN:* scalene tubercle

Lison, Lucien, Belgian scientist, *1907.

Lison-Dunn stain – a technique using leuco patent blue V and hydrogen peroxidase to demonstrate hemoglobin peroxidase on time sections and smears.

Lison, Michael, Israeli physician.

Lison syndrome – genetic trait resulting in premature graying of hair, sharp facial features, vitiligo, and other abnormalities.

Lissauer, Heinrich, German neurologist, 1861-1891.

column of Spitzka-Lissauer – *SYN:* Spitzka marginal tract

Lissauer bundle – *SYN:* Lissauer fasciculus

Lissauer column – *SYN:* Lissauer fasciculus

Lissauer fasciculus – a longitudinal bundle of thin, unmyelinated and poorly myelinated fibers capping the apex of the posterior horn of the spinal gray matter. *SYN:* dorsolateral fasciculus; Lissauer bundle; Lissauer column; Lissauer marginal zone; Lissauer tract

Lissauer marginal zone – *SYN:* Lissauer fasciculus
Lissauer paralysis
Lissauer tract – *SYN:* Lissauer fasciculus
Lissauer zone

Lisser, Hans, U.S. physician, *1888.
Escamilla-Lisser-Shepardson syndrome
Escamilla-Lisser syndrome – see under Escamilla

Lister, Joseph (Lord Lister), English surgeon, 1827-1912.
Lister dressing – the first type of antiseptic dressing, one of gauze impregnated with carbolic acid.
Listerella – in bacteriology, a rejected generic name sometimes cited as a synonym of *Listeria*; the type species is *Listerella hepatolytica*.
Lister forceps
Listeria – a genus of aerobic to microaerophilic, motile, peritrichous bacteria.
Listerine – antiseptic mouthwash.
listerism – *SYN:* Lister method
Lister knife
Lister method – antiseptic surgery as first advocated by Lister in 1867. *SYN:* listerism
Lister scissors
Lister tubercle – a small prominence on the dorsal aspect of the distal end of the radius that serves as a trochlea or pulley for the tendon. *SYN:* dorsal tubercle of radius

Listing, Johann B., German physiologist, 1808-1882.
Listing law – when the eye leaves one object and fixes upon another it revolves about an axis perpendicular to a plane cutting both the former and the present lines of vision.
Listing reduced eye – a representation that simplifies calculations of retinal imagery.

NOTES

Liston, Robert, English surgeon, 1794-1847.
Liston bone-cutting forceps
Liston knives – long-bladed knives of various sizes used in amputations.
Liston shears – strong shears for cutting plaster of Paris bandages.
Liston splint – a long splint extending from the axilla to the sole of the foot.

Little, James, U.S. surgeon, 1836-1885.
Little area – *SYN:* Kiesselbach area

Little, Sir Ernest Gordon Graham, English dermatologist, 1867-1950.
Graham Little syndrome – *SYN:* Little syndrome
Little syndrome – syndrome featuring patchy scarring alopecia of scalp, loss of pubic and axillary hair, and keratosis pilaris. *SYN:* Graham Little syndrome; lichen planopilaris

Little, William J., English surgeon, 1810-1894.
Little disease – a type of cerebral palsy in which there is bilateral spasticity, with the lower extremities more severely affected. *SYN:* spastic diplegia

Little League, organized sports group for children.
Little League elbow – elbow pain due to repetitive throwing motion. *SYN:* medial apophysitis

Litton, Clyde, 20th century U.S. plastic surgeon.
Litton formula – formula consisting of phenol, glycerin, croton oil, and water, developed in 1962 for use in facial rejuvenation.

Littré, Alexis, French anatomist, 1658-1726.
Littré glands – numerous mucous glands in the wall of the penile urethra. *SYN:* glands of the male urethra
Littré hernia – a hernia in which only a portion of the wall of the intestine is engaged. *SYN:* parietal hernia

Litzmann, Karl K.T., German gynecologist, 1815-1890.
Litzmann obliquity – inclination of the fetal head so that the posterior parietal bone presents to the parturient canal. *SYN:* posterior asynclitism

Livernois, R., ophthalmologist.
Livernois lens-folding forceps

Livierato, P., Italian physician, 1860-1936.
Livierato sign – cardiac sign.

Lobo, Jorge, Brazilian physician, 1900-1979.
Lobo disease – a chronic localized mycosis of the skin. *SYN:* lobomycosis
lobomycosis – *SYN:* Lobo disease

Lobry de Bruyn, Cornelius A., Dutch chemist, 1857-1904.
Lobry de Bruyn-van Ekenstein transformation – the base-catalyzed interconversion of an aldose and a ketose.

Lobstein, Johann F.G., German pathologist, 1777-1835.
Lobstein ganglion – a small sympathetic ganglion often present in the course of the greater splanchnic nerve. *SYN:* splanchnic ganglion

Locke, Frank S., English physiologist, 1871-1949.
Cabot-Locke murmur – see under Cabot
Locke-Ringer solution – a solution used in the laboratory for physiological and pharmacological experiments.
Locke solutions – solutions used for irrigating and culturing mammalian heart and other tissues in laboratory experiments.

Lockwood, Charles B., English anatomist and surgeon, 1858-1914.
ligament of Lockwood – *SYN:* suspensory ligament of eyeball
Lockwood clamp
Lockwood forceps
Lockwood ligament – *SYN:* suspensory ligament of eyeball
Lockwood tendon

Loeb, Leo, U.S. pathologist, 1869-1959.
Loeb deciduoma – mass of decidual tissue produced in the uterus, in the absence of a fertilized ovum, by means of mechanical or hormonal stimulation.

Loeffler, (Löffler), Friedrich A.J., German bacteriologist and surgeon, 1852-1915.
Klebs-Loeffler bacillus – see under Klebs
Loeffler bacillus – a species that causes diphtheria. *SYN: Corynebacterium diphtheriae*
Loeffler blood culture medium – a culture medium for the isolation of *Corynebacterium diphtheriae.*
Loeffler caustic stain – a stain for flagella, utilizing an aqueous solution of tannin and ferrous sulfate with the addition of an alcoholic fuchsin stain.

NOTES

Loeffler methylene blue – a stain for diphtheria organisms.

Loeffler stain – a stain for flagella.

Loevit, Moritz, Austrian pathologist, 1851-1918.

Loevit cell – originally a term denoting all forms of human red blood cells containing a nucleus, both pathologic and normal. *SYN:* erythroblast

Loewenthal, Wilhelm, German physician, 1850-1894.

Loewenthal bundle – a bundle of thick, heavily myelinated fibers that ends in the medial region of the anterior horn of the cervical spinal cord and appears to be involved in head movements during visual and auditory tracking. *SYN:* Loewenthal tract; tectospinal tract

Loewenthal reaction – the agglutinative reaction in relapsing fever.

Loewenthal tract – *SYN:* Loewenthal bundle

Loewi, Otto, German-U.S. physiologist and pharmacologist, 1873-1961, joint winner of 1936 Nobel prize for work related to nerve impulse chemical transmission.

Löffler, var. of Loeffler

Löffler, Wilhelm, Swiss physician, 1887-1972.

Löffler disease – *SYN:* Löffler endocarditis

Löffler endocarditis – fibroplastic parietal endocarditis with eosinophilia, an endocarditis of obscure cause characterized by progressive congestive heart failure, multiple systemic emboli, and eosinophilia. *SYN:* Löffler disease; Löffler syndrome (2)

Löffler parietal fibroplastic endocarditis – sclerosis of the endocardium in the presence of a high eosinophil count.

Löffler pneumonia – eosinophilic pneumonia.

Löffler syndrome – (1) *SYN:* simple pulmonary eosinophilia; (2) *SYN:* Löffler endocarditis

Löfgren, Sven Halvar, Swedish physician, 1910-1978.

Löfgren syndrome – related to sarcoidosis.

Logan, William H.G., early 20th century U.S. plastic surgeon.

Logan bow – heavy stainless steel wire bent in an arc and taped to both cheeks to protect the incision and to relieve tension on a freshly repaired cleft lip.

Lohlein, Max Herman Friedrich, German physician, 1877-1921.

Baehr-Lohlein lesion – see under Baehr

Lohlein-Baehr lesion – *SYN:* Baehr-Lohlein lesion

Lohuizen, Cato H.J. Van, Dutch physician.
Lohuizen disease – flat or depressed netlike erythema of the skin, resulting in marble pattern.

Løken, Aagot Christie, 20th century Norwegian physician.
Senior-Løken syndrome – see under Senior

Lombard, Etienne, French physician, 1868-1920.
Lombard voice-reflex test – a test useful in assessing functional hearing loss.

Lombroso, Cesare, Italian criminologist and professor, 1835-1909.
characterology – Lombroso was a proponent of the theory that attempted to establish a correlation between physical characteristics and criminal behavior.

Londe, P.F.L., French neurologist, 1865-1944.
Fazio-Londe atrophy – see under Fazio
Fazio-Londe disease – *SYN:* Fazio-Londe atrophy

London, Fritz, German-U.S. physicist, 1900-1954.
London forces – *SYN:* van der Waals forces

Long, John H., U.S. physician, 1856-1927.
Long coefficient – *SYN:* Long formula
Long formula – a formula for estimating from the specific gravity of a specimen of urine the approximate amount of solids in grams per liter. *SYN:* Long coefficient

Longmire, William P., Jr., U.S. surgeon, *1913.
Longmire anastomosis
Longmire operation – intrahepatic cholangiojejunostomy with partial hepatectomy for biliary obstruction.

Looney, Joseph M., U.S. biochemist, *1896.
Folin-Looney test – see under Folin

NOTES

Looser, Emil, Swiss physician, 1877-1936.
　Looser lines – radiolucent bands in the cortex of a bone. *SYN:* Looser zones
　Looser zones – *SYN:* Looser lines

Lorain, Paul, French physician, 1827-1875.
　Lorain disease – dwarfism generally associated with hypogonadism. *SYN:* idiopathic infantilism
　Lorain-Lévi dwarfism – a rare form of dwarfism caused by the absence of a functional anterior pituitary gland. *SYN:* Lorain-Lévi infantilism; Lorain-Lévi syndrome; pituitary dwarfism
　Lorain-Lévi infantilism – *SYN:* Lorain-Lévi dwarfism
　Lorain-Lévi syndrome – *SYN:* Lorain-Lévi dwarfism

Lorenz, Adolf, Austrian surgeon, 1854-1946.
　Lorenz sign – an obsolete term for stiffness of the thoracic spine in early pulmonary tuberculosis.

Lorenz, Konrad, Austrian zoologist, *1903, joint winner of 1973 Nobel Prize for work related to social behavior.

Loschmidt, Joseph (Johann), Czech chemist and physicist, 1821-1895.
　Loschmidt number – N equals the number of atoms in a gram-atom or the number of molecules in a gram-molecule.

Lotheissen, Georg, Austrian surgeon, 1868-1941.
　Lotheissen herniorrhaphy
　Lotheissen operation

Lou Gehrig, see under Gehrig, Henry Louis

Louis, Pierre C.A., French physician, 1787-1872.
　Louis angle – the angle between the manubrium and the body of the sternum at the manubriosternal junction. *SYN:* sternal angle
　Louis law – tuberculosis in any organ is associated with tuberculosis in the lung.

Louis-Bar, Denise, mid-20th century Belgian neuropathologist.
　Louis-Bar syndrome – an autosomal recessive disorder characterized by cerebellar ataxia and telangiectasia. *SYN:* ataxia telangiectasia

Lovén, Otto C., Swedish physician, 1835-1904.
　Lovén reflex – a reaction in which a local dilation of vessels accompanies a general vasoconstriction.

Lovibond, J.L., 20th century English dermatologist.
Lovibond angle – angle located at the junction between the nail plate and proximal nail fold, and which is normally less than 160 degrees. In clubbing, the angle exceeds 180 degrees.
Lovibond profile sign – *SYN:* Lovibond angle

Low, George C., English physician, 1872-1952.
Castellani-Low sign – see under Castellani

Lowe, Charles U., U.S. pediatrician, *1921.
Lowe syndrome – a congenital syndrome with hydrophthalmia, cataracts, mental retardation, aminoaciduria, reduced ammonia production by the kidney, and vitamin D-resistant rickets. *SYN:* Lowe-Terrey-MacLachlan syndrome; oculocerebrorenal syndrome
Lowe-Terrey-MacLachlan syndrome – *SYN:* Lowe syndrome

Löwenberg, Benjamin B., French laryngologist, 1836-1905.
Löwenberg canal – *SYN:* cochlear duct
Löwenberg forceps – forceps for the removal of adenoid growths in the nasopharynx.
Löwenberg scala – *SYN:* cochlear duct

Löwenstein, L.W.
Buschke-Löwenstein tumor – see under Buschke

Lower, Richard, English anatomist and physiologist, 1631-1691.
Lower ring – one of four fibrous rings that form part of the fibrous skeleton of the heart. *SYN:* fibrous ring of heart
Lower tubercle – the slight projection on the wall of the right atrium between the orifices of the venae cavae. *SYN:* intervenous tubercle

Lowman, Charles LeRoy, U.S. orthopedist, 1879-1977.
Lowman bone-holding clamp
Lowman bone-holding forceps
Lowman clamp
Lowman flatfoot procedure

L

NOTES

Lowman forceps
Lowman retractor
Lowman rongeur
Lowman sling procedure

Lown, Bernard, U.S. cardiologist, *1921.
Lown cardioverter
Lown-Ganong-Levine syndrome – electrocardiographic syndrome of a short P-R interval with normal duration of the QRS complex.
Lown technique

Lowry, Oliver H., U.S. biochemist, *1910.
Lowry-Folin assay – *SYN:* Lowry protein assay
Lowry protein assay – a method for determining protein concentrations using the Folin-Ciocalteu reagent. *SYN:* Lowry-Folin assay

Lowry, R. Brian, 20th century Irish medical geneticist in Canada.
Coffin-Lowry syndrome – *SYN:* Coffin-Siris syndrome

Lowsley, Oswald S., U.S. urologist, 1884-1955.
Lowsley forceps
Lowsley hemostat
Lowsley lithotrite
Lowsley needle
Lowsley nephropexy
Lowsley prostate retractor
Lowsley retractor
Lowsley ribbon-gut needle
Lowsley stone crusher
Lowsley tractor – instrument used in perineal prostatectomy.
Lowsley urethroscope

Lubarsch, Otto, German pathologist, 1860-1933.
Lubarsch crystals – intracellular crystals in the testis resembling sperm crystals.

Luc, Henri, French laryngologist, 1855-1925.
Caldwell-Luc operation – see under Caldwell, George W.
Luc forceps
Luc operation – *SYN:* Caldwell-Luc operation
Ogston-Luc operation – see under Ogston

Lucas, Richard C., English anatomist and surgeon, 1846-1915.
Lucas groove – a faint groove occasionally caused by the chorda tympani nerve on the spine of the sphenoid. *SYN:* stria spinosa

Lucas-Champonnière, Justin M.M., French surgeon, 1843-1913.
Lucas-Champonnière disease – a form of bronchitis.

Luciani, Luigi, Italian physiologist, 1842-1919.
Luciani syndrome – syndrome of the cerebellum associated with lack of muscle tone, lack of strength, and incoordination. *SYN:* Luciani triad
Luciani triad – *SYN:* Luciani syndrome

Lucio, Raphael, Mexican physician, 1819-1866.
Lucio leprosy – an acute form occurring in pure diffuse lepromatous leprosy. *SYN:* lazarine leprosy; Lucio leprosy phenomenon
Lucio leprosy phenomenon – *SYN:* Lucio leprosy

Lucké, Balduin, U.S. pathologist, 1889-1954.
Lucké adenocarcinoma – *SYN:* Lucké carcinoma
Lucké carcinoma – a herpes virus-associated adenocarcinoma of the kidney in adult frogs. *SYN:* Lucké adenocarcinoma
Lucké virus – a herpesvirus associated with Lucké carcinoma.

Lücke, George A., German surgeon, 1829-1894.
Lücke test – a test for hippuric acid.

Ludloff, Karl, German surgeon, 1864-1945.
Ludloff sign – (1) swelling and ecchymosis appearing at the base of Scarpa triangle; (2) inability to raise the thigh in the sitting posture.

Ludwig, Daniel, German anatomist, 1625-1680.
Ludwig angle – the angle between the manubrium and the body of the sternum at the manubriosternal junction. *SYN:* sternal angle

Ludwig, Karl F.W., German anatomist and physiologist, 1816-1895.
depressor nerve of Ludwig – *SYN:* Ludwig nerve
Ludwig ganglion – a small collection of parasympathetic nerve cells in the interatrial septum.
Ludwig labyrinth – proximal and distal convoluted tubules and the associated renal corpuscles supplied by branches of the interlobular arteries. *SYN:* convoluted part of kidney lobule

NOTES

Ludwig nerve – a branch of the vagus which ends in the aortic arch and base of the heart. *SYN:* aortic nerve; depressor nerve of Ludwig

Ludwig stromuhr – one of the first devices for measuring flow in blood vessels.

Ludwig, Kurt, German anatomist, *1922.

Klinger-Ludwig acid-thionin stain for sex chromatin – a method using a preliminary acid treatment on buccal smears prior to staining with buffered thionin, to differentiate Barr body.

Ludwig, Wilhelm Friedrich von, German surgeon, 1790-1865.

Ludwig angina – cellulitis, usually of odontogenic origin, bilaterally involving the submaxillary, sublingual, and submental spaces.

Ludwig applicator

Ludwig sinus applicator

Luebering, J.

Rapoport-Luebering shunt – see under Rapoport, Samuel Mitja

Luer, German instrument maker, d. 1883.

Luer curette

Luer forceps

Luer-Lok syringe – *SYN:* Luer syringe

Luer needle

Luer reconstruction plate

Luer retractor

Luer rongeur

Luer scoop

Luer speculum

Luer suction cannula adapter

Luer syringe – a glass syringe used for hypodermic and intravenous purposes. *SYN:* Luer-Lok syringe

Luer tracheal cannula

Luer tube

Luetscher, John A., U.S. physician, *1913.

Luetscher syndrome – excessive aldosterone causing renal, liver, and heart disease.

Luft, John H., U.S. histologist, *1927.

Luft potassium permanganate fixative – a fixative useful in electron microscopy for cytologic preservation of lipoprotein complexes in membranes and myelin, because of its oxidative properties.

Luft, Rolf, 20th century Swedish endocrinologist.
Luft disease – a metabolic disease.

Lugol, Jean Guillaume Auguste, French physician, 1786-1851.
Lugol iodine solution – an iodine-potassium iodide solution used as an oxidizing agent, for removal of mercurial fixation artifacts, and also in histochemistry and to stain amebas.

Lumsden, Thomas W., English physician, 1874-1953.
Lumsden pneumotoxic center

Luna, Lee G., 20th century U.S. medical technologist.
Luna-Ishak stain – a staining method using celestine blue and acid fuchsin in which bile canaliculi stain pink to red.

Luria, Salvador E., Italian-U.S. biologist, 1912-1991, joint winner of 1969 Nobel Prize for work related to viruses.

Luschka, Hubert, German anatomist, 1820-1875.
foramen of Luschka – one of the two lateral openings of the fourth ventricle into the subarachnoid space at the cerebellopontine angle. *SYN:* lateral aperture of the fourth ventricle
Luschka bursa – a cystic notochordal remnant found inconstantly in the posterior wall of the nasopharynx at the lower end of the pharyngeal tonsil. *SYN:* pharyngeal bursa
Luschka cartilage – a small cartilaginous nodule sometimes found in the anterior portion of the vocal cord.
Luschka crypt
Luschka cystic glands – small mucous tubuloalveolar glands in the mucosa of the larger bile ducts, especially in the neck of the gallbladder. *SYN:* glands of biliary mucosa
Luschka ducts – glandlike tubular structures in the wall of the gallbladder, especially in the part covered with peritoneum.
Luschka ganglion
Luschka gland – *SYN:* Luschka tonsil

L

Luschka joints – small synovial joints between adjacent lateral lips of the bodies of the lower cervical vertebrae. *SYN:* uncovertebral joints

Luschka ligaments – fibrous bands that pass from the pericardium to the sternum. *SYN:* sternopericardial ligament

Luschka muscles

Luschka nerve

Luschka sinus – venous sinus in the petrosquamous suture.

Luschka tonsil – a collection of more or less closely aggregated lymphoid nodules on the posterior wall and roof of the nasopharynx. *SYN:* Luschka gland; pharyngeal tonsil

Luse, Sarah A., 20th century U.S. physician.

Luse bodies – collagen fibers with abnormally long spacing between electron-dense bands.

Lust, Franz A., 20th century German pediatrician.

Lust phenomenon – abduction with dorsal foot flexion related to latent tetany. *SYN:* Lust sign; peroneal nerve phenomenon; peroneal sign

Lust sign – *SYN:* Lust phenomenon

Lutembacher, René, French cardiologist, 1884-1916.

Lutembacher syndrome – a congenital cardiac abnormality consisting of a defect of the interatrial septum, mitral stenosis, and enlarged right atrium.

Lutz, Alfredo, Brazilian physician, 1855-1940.

Lutz-Splendore-Almeida disease – a chronic mycosis caused by *Paracoccidioides brasiliensis. SYN:* paracoccidioidomycosis

Luys, Jules B., French physician, 1828-1897.

centre médian de Luys – *SYN:* centromedian nucleus

corpus luysi – *SYN:* subthalamic nucleus

Luys body – *SYN:* subthalamic nucleus

Luys body syndrome

nucleus of Luys – *SYN:* subthalamic nucleus

Lwoff, André, French virologist and microbiologist, 1902-1994, joint winner of 1965 Nobel Prize for work related to synthesis of viruses and enzymes.

Lyell, Alan, 20th century Scottish dermatologist.

Lyell disease – a disease affecting infants in which large areas of skin peel off as a result of upper respiratory staphylococcal infection. *SYN:* Ritter disease; Ritter syndrome; staphylococcal scalded skin syndrome

Lyell syndrome – a syndrome in which a large portion of the skin becomes intensely erythematous with epidermal necrosis, and peels off. *SYN:* toxic epidermal necrolysis

Lyme, city in Connecticut where disease was first recognized.
Lyme arthritis – the arthritic manifestations of Lyme disease.
Lyme disease – infectious disease spread by tick.

Lynch, Henry T., U.S. oncologist, *1928.
Lynch syndrome I – familial predisposition to colon cancer.
Lynch syndrome II – familial predisposition for other primary cancers in addition to the predisposition for colon cancer; site is often female reproductive organs.

Lynen, Feodor, German biochemist, 1911-1979, joint winner of 1964 Nobel Prize for work related to cholesterol and metabolism of fatty acids.

Lyon, B.B. Vincent, U.S. physician, 1880-1953.
Meltzer-Lyon test – see under Meltzer, Samual J.

Lyon, Mary F., English cytogeneticist, *1925.
Lyon hypothesis – *SYN:* lyonization
lyonization – the normal phenomenon that wherever there are two or more haploid sets of X-linked genes in each cell, all but one of the genes are inactivated, apparently at random, and have no phenotypic expression. *SYN:* Lyon hypothesis; X-inactivation

L

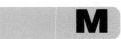

MacCallum, William George, U.S. pathologist, 1874-1944.

MacCallum patch – found in deep layers of the endocardium in patients with rheumatic fever.

MacCallum plaque – irregular thickness usually found in the left atrium in patients with rheumatic fever.

MacConkey, Alfred Theodore, English bacteriologist, 1861-1931.

MacConkey agar – a medium used to identify gram-negative bacilli and characterize them according to their status as lactose fermenters. *SYN:* MacConkey medium

MacConkey medium – *SYN:* MacConkey agar

Macewen, Sir William, Scottish surgeon, 1848-1924.

Macewen classification

Macewen drill

Macewen herniorrhaphy

Macewen operation

Macewen osteotomy

Macewen saw

Macewen sign – percussion of the skull gives a cracked-pot sound in cases of hydrocephalus. *SYN:* Macewen symptom

Macewen symptom – *SYN:* Macewen sign

Macewen triangle – *SYN:* suprameatal triangle

Mach, Ernst Waldfried Josef Wenzel, Austrian scientist, 1838-1916.

Mach band – a relatively bright or dark band.

Mach number – the ratio between the speed of an object moving through a fluid medium and the speed of sound in the same medium.

Mach, Rene Sigmund, Swiss physician, *1904.

Mach syndrome – adrenal hyperplasia.

NOTES

Machado, surname of one of the two families studied in major descriptions of the disease.
  Machado-Joseph disease – a rare form of hereditary ataxia, characterized by the onset in early adult life of progressive disease, found primarily in people of Azorean ancestry.

Mache, Heinrich, Austrian physicist, 1876-1954.
  Mache unit – a measurement of radioactivity.

Machiavelli, Niccolo, Italian author and statesman, 1469-1527.
  machiavellianism – a personality trait of one who manipulates others to achieve goals.
  Mach scale – used to determine an individual's use of manipulation.

Machover, Karen Alper, U.S. psychologist, 1902-1996.
  Machover draw-a-person test – a test used in psychology and psychiatry.

Macintosh, Charles, Scottish chemist, 1766-1843.
  Macintosh blockers – a system of tubes used during thoracic operations to block one lung or lobe from the other.

MacIntyre, William, English physician, 1791-1857.
  MacIntyre disease – *SYN:* Kahler disease

Mackay, Ralph Stuart, U.S. physicist, *1924.
  Mackay-Marg tonometer – a recording electronic applanation tonometer.

Mackenrodt, Alwin Karl, German gynecologist, 1859-1925.
  Mackenrodt incision
  Mackenrodt ligament – *SYN:* cardinal ligament
  Mackenrodt operation

Mackenzie, Richard James, Scottish surgeon, 1821-1854.
  Mackenzie amputation – a modification of Syme amputation at the ankle joint, the flap being taken from the inner side. *SYN:* Mackenzie operation
  Mackenzie operation – *SYN:* Mackenzie amputation

Mackenzie, Sir James, Scottish physician in England, 1853-1925.
  Mackenzie polygraph – an instrument formerly used in the clinical investigation of cardiac arrhythmias.

MacLachlan, Elsie A., 20th century researcher.
  Lowe-Terrey-MacLachlan syndrome – *SYN:* Lowe syndrome

MacLean, Charles Murray, West African physician, 1788-1824.
  MacLean-Maxwell disease – a chronic calcaneal condition.

Maclennan, Alexander, English physician.
  Maclennan syndrome – sphincter pain. *SYN:* Thaysen syndrome

MacLeod, John James Richard, joint winner of 1923 Nobel Prize for discovering insulin.

Macleod, Roderick, Scottish physician, 1795-1852.
> **Macleod rheumatism** – rheumatoid arthritis with abundant serous effusion in the affected joints.

Macleod, William Mathieson, English physician, 1911-1977.
> **Macleod syndrome** – *SYN:* Swyer-James syndrome (1)
> **Swyer-James-Macleod syndrome** – *SYN:* Swyer-James syndrome (2)

MacNeal, Ward J., U.S. bacteriologist, 1881-1946.
> **MacNeal tetrachrome blood stain** – for blood smears.
> **Novy and MacNeal blood agar** – see under Novy

MacQuarrie, Thomas William, U.S. psychologist.
> **MacQuarrie test for mechanical ability** – test used in psychology and psychiatry.

MacWilliams, John Alexander, English physician, 1857-1937.
> **MacWilliams test** – a urine test for albumin and other proteolytic digestion products.

Maddox, Ernest E., English ophthalmologist, 1860-1933.
> **Maddox prism**
> **Maddox rod**
> **Maddox rod occluder**
> **Maddox rod test** – used to test eye muscle balance.

Madelung, Otto Wilhelm, German surgeon, 1846-1926.
> **Madelung deformity** – a distal radial ulnar subluxation due to relative deficiency of axial growth of the medial side of the distal radius. *SYN:* carpus curvus
> **Madelung disease** – accumulation and progressive enlargement of adipose tissue in the subcutaneous tissue of the head, neck, upper trunk, and upper portions of the upper extremities. *SYN:* multiple symmetric lipomatosis

NOTES

Madelung lipoma – fatty tumor.
Madelung neck – multiple symmetric lipomatosis confined to the neck.
Madelung subluxation – incomplete dislocation or luxation.

Madlener, Max, German surgeon, 1868-1951.
Madlener operation – tubal sterilization by clamp and tie.

Madsen, Thorvald J.M., 1870-1957.
Arrhenius-Madsen theory – see under Arrhenius

Madura, a district in India where the condition was first described in 1842.
Madura foot – infectious fungal disease localized predominantly in the foot, having discharge from the exposed area. *SYN:* Ballingall disease; maduromycosis
maduromycosis – *SYN:* Madura foot

Maffucci, Angelo, Italian physician, 1847-1903.
Maffucci syndrome – enchondromatosis with multiple cavernous hemangiomas. *SYN:* dyschondroplasia with hemangiomas

Magee, Kenneth Raymond, U.S. physician, *1926.
Shy-Magee syndrome – see under Shy

Magendie, François, French physiologist, 1783-1855.
Bell-Magendie law – *SYN:* Bell law
Magendie foramen – *SYN:* medial aperture of the fourth ventricle
Magendie-Hertwig sign – skew deviation of the eyes in acute cerebellar lesions. *SYN:* Magendie-Hertwig syndrome
Magendie-Hertwig syndrome – *SYN:* Magendie-Hertwig sign
Magendie law – *SYN:* Bell law
Magendie spaces – space between the pia and arachnoid at the level of the fissures of the brain.

Magenis, Ellen, 20th century U.S. physician.
Smith-Magenis syndrome – see under Smith, Ann C.M.

Magill, Sir Ivan Whiteside, English anesthesiologist, 1888-1986.
Magill band
Magill catheter
Magill circuit
Magill endotracheal tube
Magill forceps
Magill laryngoscope
Magill Pain Questionnaire

Magnan, Valentin Jacques Joseph, French psychiatrist, 1835-1916.
Magnan sign – paresthesia in the psychosis of cocaine addicts.

Magnan trombone movement – involuntary forward and back movement of the tongue when it is drawn out of the mouth in several basal ganglia disorders.

Magnus, I.A.
Magnus syndrome – protoporphyrin in bone marrow.

Magnus, Rudolph, German physiologist, 1873-1927.
Magnus sign – an obsolete sign: after death, constriction of a limb or one of its segments is not followed by venous congestion of the distal part.

Magoss, I.V., U.S. physician.
Magoss-Walshe syndrome – preaortic renal vein compression.

Magrassi, Flaviano, Italian physician, *1908.
Magrassi-Leonardi syndrome – eosinophilic pneumonia.

Mahaim, Ivan, French cardiologist, 1897-1965.
Mahaim fibers – paraspecific fibers originating from the A-V node, the His bundle, or the bundle branches and inserting into the ventricular myocardium. *SYN:* nodoventricular fibers

Mahler, Richter A., German obstetrician, 1863-1941.
Mahler baseline dyspnea index
Mahler sign – indication of thrombosis with increase in pulse rate and no elevation of temperature.

Mahorner, Howard Raymond, U.S. surgeon, *1903.
Ochsner-Mahorner test – see under Ochsner, Edward William Alton

Maier, Rudolf Robert, German physician, 1824-1888.
Maier sinus – an infundibuliform depression on the internal surface of the lacrimal sac which receives the lacrimal canaliculi.

Main, Thomas Forrest, English psychiatrist.
Main syndrome – psychotic female health professional who exploits her background to obtain health care.

Mainzer, Frank, U.S. radiologist, *1939.
Saldino-Mainzer syndrome – see under Saldino

Maisonneuve, Jules Germain François, French surgeon, 1809-1897.
Maisonneuve amputation
Maisonneuve bandage
Maisonneuve fracture
Maisonneuve sign
Maisonneuve urethrotome

Maissiat, Jacques H., French anatomist, 1805-1878.
Maissiat band – a fibrous reinforcement of the fascia lata on the lateral surface of the thigh. *SYN:* iliotibial tract
Maissiat ligament

Maixner, Emmerich, Austrian physician, 1847-1920.
Maixner cirrhosis – hemorrhagic liver cirrhosis.

Majewski, Frank, German pediatrician and human geneticist, *1941.
Lenz-Majewski syndrome – see under Lenz
Majewski syndrome – fatal form of neonatal dwarfism.
Mohr-Majewski syndrome – see under Mohr, Otto Lous

Majocchi, Domenico, Italian dermatologist, 1849-1929.
Majocchi disease – asymptomatic anular lesions, principally of the lower extremities of adolescent males. *SYN:* purpura annularis telangiectodes; Majocchi syndrome
Majocchi granulomas – erythematous papules due to a deep follicular fungal infection, most frequently seen on shaved legs of women. *SYN:* tinea profunda
Majocchi purpura
Majocchi syndrome – *SYN:* Majocchi disease

Makai, Endre, 20th century Hungarian surgeon.
Rothmann-Makai syndrome – see under Rothmann

Makeham, William Matthew, English actuary, d. 1892.
Makeham hypothesis – assumption that death is the consequence of two generally coexisting causes: (1) chance; (2) a deterioration or increased inability to withstand destruction.

Malacarne, Michele V.G., Italian surgeon, 1744-1816.
Malacarne pyramid – a lobule on the undersurface of the cerebellum, the posterior portion of the vermis.
Malacarne space – the bottom of the interpeduncular fossa at the base of the midbrain. *SYN:* posterior perforated substance

Malan, Edmond, U.S. physician.
Malan **syndrome** – vascular disorder of the foot and leg.

Malassez, Louis Charles, French physiologist, 1842-1910.
Malassez **disease** – testicular cyst.
Malassez **epithelial rests** – epithelial remains of Hertwig root sheath in the periodontal ligament.
Malassezia – a genus of fungi (family Cryptococcaceae) of low pathogenicity.

Maldonado, (origin unknown).
Maldonado-San Jose stain – method for staining pancreatic islet cells.

Malecot, Achille-Etienne, French surgeon, *1852.
Malecot **catheter** – a two- or four-winged catheter.
Malecot **drain**
Malecot **tube**

Malgaigne, Joseph François, French surgeon, 1806-1865.
Malgaigne **amputation** – amputation of the foot in which only the astragalus is retained. *SYN:* subastragalar amputation
Malgaigne **apparatus**
Malgaigne **bulging**
Malgaigne **clamp**
Malgaigne **fossa** – a space containing the bifurcation of the common carotid artery. *SYN:* carotid triangle; Malgaigne triangle
Malgaigne **fracture**
Malgaigne **hernia** – infantile inguinal hernia prior to the descent of the testis.
Malgaigne **hook**
Malgaigne **luxation** – longitudinal subluxation of the radial head from the anular ligament. *SYN:* nursemaid's elbow
Malgaigne **swelling**
Malgaigne **triangle** – *SYN:* Malgaigne fossa

NOTES

Malherbe, Albert, French physician, 1845-1915.

    Malherbe calcifying epithelioma – a benign solitary hair follicle tumor. *SYN:* Malherbe-Chenantais epithelioma; pilomatrixoma

    Malherbe-Chenantais epithelioma – *SYN:* Malherbe calcifying epithelioma

Mali, J.W.H., 1918-1996.

    angiodermatitis of Mali – violaceous, brown-black papules covering the feet and legs due to proliferation of existing vasculature.

Mall, Franklin Paine, U.S. anatomist and embryologist, 1862-1917.

    Mall formula – the age in days of a human embryo calculated as the square root of its length.

    Mall ridges – rarely used term for pulmonary ridges.

    periportal space of Mall – a tissue space between the limiting lamina and the portal canal in the liver.

Mallory, Frank Burr, U.S. pathologist, 1862-1941.

    Mallory aniline blue stain – *SYN:* Mallory trichrome stain

    Mallory bodies II – large, poorly defined accumulations of eosinophilic material in the cytoplasm of damaged hepatic cells in certain forms of cirrhosis. *SYN:* alcoholic hyaline bodies

    Mallory collagen stain

    Mallory iodine stain

    Mallory phloxine stain

    Mallory phosphotungstic acid hematoxylin stain

    Mallory stain for actinomyces

    Mallory stain for hemofuchsin

    Mallory trichrome stain – a method especially suitable for studying connective tissue. *SYN:* Mallory aniline blue stain; Mallory triple stain

    Mallory triple stain – *SYN:* Mallory trichrome stain

    picro-Mallory trichrome stain – a modification of Mallory trichrome stain that involves the addition of picric acid.

Mallory, George Kenneth, U.S. pathologist, *1900.

    Mallory syndrome – gastroesophageal junction mucosal laceration.

    Mallory-Weiss lesion – laceration of the gastric cardia, as seen in the Mallory-Weiss syndrome. *SYN:* Mallory-Weiss tear

    Mallory-Weiss syndrome – laceration of the lower end of the esophagus, associated with bleeding, caused usually by severe retching and vomiting.

    Mallory-Weiss tear – *SYN:* Mallory-Weiss lesion

Malpighi, Marcello, Italian anatomist, histologist, and embryologist, 1628-1694.

malpighian bodies – small nodular masses of lymphoid tissue attached to the sides of the smaller arterial branches. *SYN:* malpighian glands; malpighian nodules; splenic lymph follicles

malpighian capsule – *SYN:* glomerular capsule

malpighian cell – a cell of the stratum spinosum of the epidermis.

malpighian corpuscles – *SYN:* renal corpuscle

malpighian glands – *SYN:* malpighian bodies

malpighian glomerulus – a tuft formed of capillary loops at the beginning of each nephric tubule in the kidney. *SYN:* malpighian tuft

malpighian layer – *SYN:* malpighian stratum

malpighian nodules – *SYN:* malpighian bodies

malpighian pyramid – *SYN:* renal pyramid

malpighian rete – *SYN:* malpighian stratum

malpighian stigmas – the points of entrance of smaller veins into the larger veins of the spleen.

malpighian stratum – the living layer of epidermis comprising the stratum basale, stratum spinosum, and stratum granulosum. *SYN:* malpighian layer; malpighian rete

malpighian tubules – in insects, slender tubular or hairlike excretory structures.

malpighian tuft – *SYN:* malpighian glomerulus

malpighian vesicles – the minute air-filled vesicles on the surface of an expanded lung.

Malta, an island in the Mediterranean Sea south of Sicily.

Malta fever – *SYN:* brucellosis

Malthus, Thomas R., English statistician and clergyman, 1766-1834.

malthusianism – the theory that the world's population will outgrow the food supply.

M

Manchester, city in England, where the operation was developed.
   Manchester operation – a vaginal operation for prolapse of the uterus, consisting of cervical amputation and parametrial fixation (cardinal ligaments) anterior to the uterus. *SYN:* Fothergill operation

Manhold, John H., U.S. dentist, *1919.
   Volpe-Manhold Index – see under Volpe

Mankovskii, var. of Mankowsky

Mankowsky, (Mankovskii), Boris Nikitich, Russian physician, 1883-1962.
   Mankowsky syndrome – familial bone disorders. *SYN:* familial dysplastic osteopathy

Mann, Frank C., U.S. surgeon, 1887-1962.
   Mann-Bollman fistula – used in experimental investigations of the digestive tract.
   Mann-Williamson operation – an operation performed on experimental animals in research on peptic ulcer.
   Mann-Williamson ulcer – the ulcer that develops in the jejunum after the Mann-Williamson operation.

Mann, Henry Berthold, U.S. mathematician, *1905.
   Mann-Whitney test – rank sum test.

Mann, John Dixon, English physician, 1840-1912.
   Dixon Mann sign – *SYN:* Mann sign
   Mann sign – seen in Graves disease. *SYN:* Dixon Mann sign

Mann, Ludwig, German physician, 1866-1936.
   Mann syndrome – brain contusion accompanied by coordination disorders.
   Wernicke-Mann hemiplegia – see under Wernicke
   Wernicke-Mann paralysis – *SYN:* Wernicke-Mann hemiplegia

Mannkopf, Emil W., German physician, 1836-1918.
   Mannkopf sign – acceleration of the pulse when a painful point is pressed upon.

Mansfield, Sir Peter, English physics professor, *1933, joint winner of 2003 Nobel Prize for work related to magnetic resonance imaging.

Manson, Sir Patrick, English authority on tropical medicine, 1844-1922.
   Manson disease – *SYN:* schistosomiasis mansoni
   Mansonella – a genus of filaria, widely distributed in tropical Africa and South America.

Manson eye worm – a widely distributed spiruroid nematode parasite of fowl. *SYN: Oxyspirura mansoni*

Mansonia – a genus of brown or black medium-sized mosquitoes.

Manson pyosis – obsolete term for a superficial pyogenic infection. *SYN:* pemphigus contagiosus

Manson schistosomiasis – *SYN:* schistosomiasis mansoni

Manson syndrome – pulmonary obliterative arteriolitis.

Oxyspirura mansoni – *SYN:* Manson eye worm

Schistosoma mansoni – a disease-causing parasite transmitted by snails.

schistosomiasis mansoni – infection with *Schistosoma mansoni. SYN:* intestinal schistosomiasis; Manson disease; Manson schistosomiasis

Mantel, Nathan, U.S. biostatistician, 1919-2002.
Mantel-Haenszel test – a summary chi-square test for stratified data, used when controlling for confounding.

Mantoux, Charles, French physician, 1877-1947.
Mantoux method
Mantoux pit – shallow depressions of the palms and soles in basal cell nevus syndrome.

Maranon, Gregorio, Spanish endocrinologist, 1887-1960.
Maranon I syndrome – spinal disorder.
Maranon II syndrome – muscle lipomas.
Maranon III syndrome – thyrotoxic state.
Maranon IV syndrome – testicular hypertrophy and gynecomastia.

Marburg, city in Germany.
Marburg disease – characterized by a prominant rash and hemorrhages in many organs, often fatal. *SYN:* African hemorrhagic disease; green monkey disease; Marburg virus
Marburg virus – *SYN:* Marburg disease

NOTES

Marcacci, Arturo, Italian physiologist, 1854-1915.
Marcacci muscle – a sheet of smooth muscle fibers underlying the areola and nipple of the mammary gland.

Marchand, Felix Jacob, German pathologist, 1846-1928.
Marchand adrenals – small collections of accessory adrenal tissue in the broad ligament of the uterus or in the testes. *SYN:* Marchand rest
Marchand cell
Marchand rest – *SYN:* Marchand adrenals
Marchand syndrome – liver cirrhosis.
Marchand wandering cell – a cell of the mononuclear phagocyte system.

Marchant, Gérard T.J., French surgeon, 1850-1903.
Marchant zone – the area on the sphenoid and occipital bones at the base of the skull.

Marchesani, Oswald, German ophthalmologist, 1900-1952.
Marchesani syndrome – recessive autosomal inheritance disorder.
SYN: Weill-Marchesani syndrome
Weill-Marchesani syndrome – *SYN:* Marchesani syndrome

Marchetti, Andrew A., U.S. obstetrician and gynecologist, 1901-1970.
Marchetti operation
Marshall-Marchetti-Krantz operation – see under Marshall, Victor F.

Marchi, Vittorio, Italian physician, 1851-1908.
Marchi fixative – used to demonstrate degenerating myelin.
Marchi reaction – failure of the myelin sheath of a nerve to blacken when submitted to the action of osmic acid.
Marchi stain – a method for demonstrating fat and degenerating nerve fibers.
Marchi tract – a bundle of thick, heavily myelinated fibers originating in the deep layers of the superior colliculus. *SYN:* tectospinal tract

Marchiafava, Ettore, Italian pathologist, 1847-1935.
Marchiafava-Bignami disease – a disorder consisting of demyelination of the corpus callosum and cortical laminar necrosis involving the frontal and temporal lobes. *SYN:* Marchiafava syndrome
Marchiafava-Micheli anemia – *SYN:* Marchiafava-Micheli syndrome
Marchiafava-Micheli syndrome – an infrequent disorder with insidious onset and chronic course, characterized by episodes of hemolytic anemia, hemoglobinuria, pallor, icterus or bronzing of the skin, a moderate degree of splenomegaly, and sometimes hepatomegaly.
SYN: Marchiafava-Micheli anemia; paroxysmal nocturnal hemoglobinuria
Marchiafava syndrome – *SYN:* Marchiafava-Bignami syndrome

Marcille, Maurice, 1871-1941.
 Marcille triangle – an area bounded by the medial border of the psoas major, the lateral margin of the vertebral column, and the iliolumbar ligament below.

Marcus Gunn, see under Gunn, Robert Marcus

Marden, Philip M., U.S. physician.
 Marden-Walker syndrome – autosomal recessive trait.

Marek, Josef, Hungarian veterinarian and pathologist, 1867-1952.
 Marek disease – *SYN:* avian lymphomatosis
 Marek disease virus – the herpesvirus that causes avian lymphomatosis. *SYN:* avian neurolymphomatosis virus

Marey, Étienne Jules, French physiologist, 1830-1904.
 Marey law – the pulse rate varies inversely with the blood pressure.

Marfan, Antoine Bernard-Jean, French pediatrician, 1858-1942.
 Dennie-Marfan syndrome – see under Dennie
 Marfan disease – *SYN:* Marfan syndrome
 Marfan law – the healing of localized tuberculosis protects against subsequent development of pulmonary tuberculosis.
 Marfan syndrome – a syndrome of congenital changes in the mesodermal and ectodermal tissues, skeletal changes, ectopia lentis, and vascular defects. *SYN:* Marfan disease

M

Marg, Elwin, U.S. physicist, *1918.
 Mackay-Marg tonometer – see under Mackay

Marghescu, S., German physician.
 Marghescu syndrome – congenital poikiloderma; autosomal recessive trait.

Margolis, Emmanuel, 20th century Israeli geneticist.
 Ziprkowski-Margolis syndrome – see under Ziprkowski

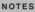
NOTES

Marie, Julien, French pediatrician, *1899.
    Julien Marie syndrome – *SYN:* Marie syndrome
    Marie syndrome – a form of reticuloendotheliosis that affects infants.
    SYN: Julien Marie syndrome

Marie, Pierre, French neurologist, 1853-1940.
    Bamberger-Marie disease – *SYN:* Bamberger-Marie syndrome
    Bamberger-Marie syndrome – see under Bamberger, Eugen
    Brissaud-Marie syndrome – see under Brissaud
    Charcot-Marie-Tooth disease – see under Charcot
    Debré-Marie syndrome – see under Debré
    Foix-Cavany-Marie syndrome – see under Foix
    Marie ataxia – obsolete term for a variety of non-Friedreich hereditary
        ataxias.
    Marie-Leri syndrome – swelling of deformed joints.
    Marie-Sainton syndrome – excessive head development. *SYN:*
        cleidocranial dysplasia; cleidocranial dysostosis
    Marie-Strümpell disease – *SYN:* Strümpell-Marie disease
    Marie I syndrome – *SYN:* Menzel syndrome
    Marie II syndrome – endocrine and neurologic disorders.
    Nonne-Marie syndrome – *SYN:* Menzel syndrome
    Strümpell-Marie disease – see under Strümpell

Marie Unna, see under Unna, Marie

Marin Amat, Manuel, Spanish ophthalmologist, *1879.
    Marin Amat syndrome – involuntary eye closure.

Marinesco, Georges, Romanian neurologist, 1863-1938.
    Marinesco-Radovici reflex – *SYN:* Radovici sign
    Marinesco-Sjögren-Garland syndrome – a rare neurologic disorder
        characterized by cerebellolental degeneration with mental retardation.
        SYN: cataract-oligophrenia syndrome; Torsten Sjögren syndrome
    Marinesco-Sjögren syndrome – development and mental retardation.
        SYN: Garland-Moorhouse syndrome; hereditary oligophrenic
        cerebellolental degeneration; oligophrenic cerebellolenticular
        degeneration; Sjögren syndrome; Torsten syndrome
    Marinesco succulent hand – edema of the hand with coldness and lividity
        of the skin, observed in syringomyelia. *SYN:* main succulente

Marion, Georges, French urologist, 1869-1932.
    Marion disease – a congenital obstruction of the posterior urethra.

Mariotte, Edmé, French physicist, 1620-1684.

    Mariotte blind spot – an oval area of the ocular fundus devoid of light receptors where the axons of the retinal ganglion cell converge to form the optic nerve head. *SYN:* optic disk

    Mariotte bottle – a stoppered bottle with bottom outlet, used as a reservoir for constant infusions.

    Mariotte experiment – an experiment that proves the absence of photoreceptors where the optic nerve enters the eye.

    Mariotte law – *SYN:* Boyle law

Marjolin, Jean Nicolas, French physician, 1780-1850.

    Marjolin syndrome – *SYN:* Marjolin ulcer

    Marjolin ulcer – well-differentiated but aggressive squamous cell carcinoma occurring in cicatricial tissue at the epidermal edge of a sinus draining underlying osteomyelitis. *SYN:* epidermoid ulcer; Marjolin syndrome

Markoe, Thomas Masters, U.S. physician, 1819-1901.

    Markoe abscess – chronic bone abscess.

Markoff, var. of Markov

Markov, (Markoff), Andrei, Russian mathematician, 1865-1922.

    Markov chain – number of steps or events in sequence.

    Markov chaining – a theory used in psychiatry.

    Markov process – a process such that the conditional probability distribution for the state at any future instant, given the present state, is unaffected by any additional knowledge of the past history of the system.

Markovits, A.S.

    Markovits syndrome – ocular pain.

Marlow, Frank William, U.S. ophthalmologist, 1858-1942.

    Marlow test – a test for heterophoria.

NOTES

Marmor, Leonard, U.S. physician.
Marmor modular knee prosthesis

Maroteaux, Pierre, French medical geneticist, *1926.
Maroteaux-Lamy syndrome – an error of mucopolysaccharide metabolism characterized by excretion of dermatan sulfate in the urine, growth retardation, and skeletal deformities. *SYN:* polydystrophic dwarfism; type VI mucopolysaccharidosis
Maroteaux-Spranger-Wiedemann syndrome – genetic defects.
Maroteaux syndrome – metaphyseal dysostosis of the knees.

Marsh, James, English chemist, 1789-1846.
Marsh test – for detection of arsenic.

Marsh, Sir Henry, Irish physician, 1790-1860.
Marsh disease – *SYN:* Graves disease

Marshall, Don, U.S. ophthalmologist, *1905.
Marshall syndrome – midface hypoplasia, cataract, sensorineural hearing loss, and hypohidrosis.

Marshall, Eli K., U.S. pharmacologist, 1889-1966.
Marshall method – a quantitative procedure for estimating free and conjugated sulfanilamide in body fluids.

Marshall, John, English anatomist, 1818-1891.
Marshall oblique vein – a small vein on the posterior wall of the left atrium that merges with the great cardiac vein to form the coronary sinus. *SYN:* oblique vein of left atrium
Marshall syndrome – inflamed edematous papules.
Marshall vestigial fold – a pericardial fold containing the obliterated remains of the left superior vena cava. *SYN:* fold of left vena cava

Marshall, Richard E., U.S. physician.
Marshall-Smith syndrome – *SYN:* Marshall syndrome
Marshall syndrome – clinical growth disorder. *SYN:* Marshall-Smith syndrome

Marshall, Victor F., U.S. urologist, *1913.
Marshall-Marchetti-Krantz operation – an operation for urinary stress incontinence, performed retropubically.

Marshall, Wallace, U.S. physician.
Marshall-White syndrome – ischemic angiospastic spots on the palms of the hands. *SYN:* Bier spots; Bier syndrome

Martegiani, J., 19th century Italian anatomist.
    Martegiani area – *SYN:* Martegiani funnel
    Martegiani funnel – the funnel-shaped dilation on the optic disk that
        indicates the beginning of the hyaloid canal. *SYN:* Martegiani area

Martin, A.
    Bosviel-Martin syndrome – *SYN:* Martin syndrome
    Martin syndrome – hemorrhage of the uvula. *SYN:* apoplexia uvulae;
        Bosviel-Martin syndrome; staphylohematoma

Martin, August E., German gynecologist, 1847-1933.
    Martin-Albright syndrome – hereditary defects. *SYN:* Albright IV syndrome
    Martin-Gruber anastomosis – a nerve anomaly in the forearm, consisting
        of a median-to-ulnar nerve communication.
    Martin tube – a drainage tube with a cross piece near the extremity to
        keep it from slipping out of a cavity.

Martin, Henry A., U.S. surgeon, 1824-1884.
    Martin bandage – a roller bandage of soft rubber used to make
        compression on a limb in the treatment of varicose veins or ulcers.
    Martin cartilage clamp
    Martin disease – a periosteoarthritis of the foot from excessive walking.
    Martin incision
    Martin vigorimeter

Martin, J.E.
    Thayer-Martin agar – see under Thayer
    Thayer-Martin medium – *SYN:* Thayer-Martin agar

Martin, J. Purdon, 20th century English physician.
    Martin-Bell syndrome – *SYN:* fragile X syndrome

Martin, Peter Guy Cutlack, English surgeon.
    Martin pump – accelerated blood transfusion rotary pump.

NOTES

Martin de Gimard, Jules Louis Alexandre, French physician, *1858.
  Martin de Gimard syndrome – necrotic purpura in children. *SYN:* de
  Gimard syndrome; Gimard syndrome

Martin du Pan, Charles, Swiss physician, 1878-1948.
  Martin du Pan-Rutishauser syndrome – joint ankylosis. *SYN:* laminar
  osteochondritis

Martinotti, Giovanni, Italian physician, 1857-1928.
  Martinotti cell – a small multipolar nerve cell of the cerebral cortex.

Martius, Karl A., German chemist, *1920.
  martius yellow – an acid dye used as a stain in plant and animal histology
  and as a light filter for photomicrography.

Martorell, Fernando Otzet, Spanish vascular surgeon, 1906-1984.
  Martorell syndrome – atheromatous and/or thrombotic obliteration of the
  branches of the aortic arch. *SYN:* aortic arch syndrome

Martorell, R.
  Martorell I syndrome – above-the-ankle ulceration. *SYN:* hypertensive
  ischemic ulcer

Marzola, Mario, Australian physician.
  Marzola lateral scalp lift – a technique based on the paramedian scalp
  reduction incision, resulting in minimal stretch-back.

Mashburn, Neely Cornelius, U.S. physician, *1886.
  Mashburn complex coordinator – instrument used in measuring eye-
  hand and foot coordination

Masini, Giulio, Italian physician, 1874-1937.
  Masini sign – a marked degree of dorsal extension of the fingers on the
  metacarpals and of the toes on the metatarsals, noted in children with
  mental instability.

Maslow, Abraham H., U.S. psychologist, 1908-1970.
  Maslow hierarchy – a ranking of needs that a human presumably fills
  successively in the order of lowest to highest: physiological needs, love
  and belonging, self-esteem, and self-actualization.
  Maslow pyramid of needs
  Maslow theory of human motivation

Mason, Edward E., U.S. surgeon, *1920.
  Mason operation – high division of the stomach used for treatment of
  morbid obesity. *SYN:* gastric bypass

Masselon, M. Julián, French physician, 1844-1917.
Masselon glasses
Masselon spectacles – keep the upper eyelid raised above the pupil in cases of paralytic blepharoptosis. *SYN:* lid crutch spectacles

Masset, Alfred Auguste, French physician, *1870.
Masset test – shows the presence of bile pigments.

Masshoff, Johann Wilhelm, German physician, *1908.
Masshoff syndrome – mesenteric lymphadenitis.

Masson, Claude L. Pierre, Canadian pathologist, 1880-1959.
Fontana-Masson silver stain – *SYN:* Masson-Fontana ammoniacal silver stain
Masson argentaffin stain
Masson body – macrophages and fibrin found in pulmonary alveoli in organizing pneumonia.
Masson-Fontana ammoniacal silver stain – a stain used to demonstrate melanin and argentaffin granules. *SYN:* Fontana-Masson silver stain

Masson, W., scientist.
Masson disk – measures threshold of brightness vision.

Master, Arthur Matthew, U.S. physician, 1895-1973.
Master test – requires the subject to ascend and descend two nine-inch steps repeatedly, the number of trips determined from age- and sex-specific tables. *SYN:* Master two-step exercise test
Master two-step exercise test – *SYN:* Master test

Masters, William Howell, U.S. gynecologist, 1915-2001.
Allen-Masters syndrome – see under Allen, Willard Myron

Masugi, Matazo, Japanese pathologist, 1896-1947.
Masugi nephritis – glomerulonephritis produced by injecting into rats a rabbit antiserum prepared against rat kidney tissue suspensions.

Matas, Rudolph, U.S. surgeon, 1860-1957.
Matas operation – obsolete term for aneurysmoplasty.

Mathes, Paul, Austrian physician, 1871-1923.
  Mathes syndrome – breast pain with nursing. *SYN:* puerperal mastitis

Matsoukas, J.
  Matsoukas syndrome – genetic defects.

Mattox, Kenneth L., U.S. surgeon, *1938.
  Mattox maneuver – technique used in repair of abdominal traumatic injury.

Matzenauer, Rudolf, Austrian dermatologist, *1861.
  Matzenauer-Pollard syndrome – spontaneous inflammatory skin lesions
    affecting women with dysmenorrhea. *SYN:* dermatitis symmetrica
    dysmenorrhagica

Mauchart, Burkhard D., German anatomist, 1696-1751.
  Mauchart ligaments

Maugeri, Salvatore, Italian physician, *1905.
  Maugeri syndrome – cardiopulmonary symptoms associated with silicate
    exposure. *SYN:* silicotic mediastinopathy

Maumené, Edme Jules, French chemist, 1818-1891.
  Maumené test – urine test for glucose.

Maumenee, A.E.
  Maumenee syndrome – opacified and thickened corneas.

Maunoir, Jean Pierre, French physician, 1768-1861.
  Maunoir hydrocele – serous dilatation of cervical cleft, duct, or cervical
    lymph space. *SYN:* cervical hydrocele
  Maunoir iris scissors
  Maunoir scissors

Maurer, Georg, German physician in Sumatra, *1909.
  Maurer clefts – *SYN:* Maurer dots
  Maurer dots – finely granular precipitates or irregular cytoplasmic particles
    that usually occur diffusely in red blood cells infected with the
    trophozoites of *Plasmodium falciparum. SYN:* Maurer clefts

Mauriac, Charles Marie Tamarelle, French physician, 1832-1905.
  Mauriac syndrome – tertiary syphilis manifestation. *SYN:* erythema
    nodosum syphiliticum

Mauriac, Leonard Pierre, French physician, *1882.
  Mauriac syndrome – complications of juvenile-onset diabetes mellitus.
    SYN: Pierre Mauriac syndrome
  Pierre Mauriac syndrome – *SYN:* Mauriac syndrome

Mauriceau, François, French obstetrician, 1637-1709.
 Mauriceau-Levret maneuver – *SYN:* Mauriceau maneuver
 Mauriceau maneuver – a method of assisted breech delivery.
  SYN: Mauriceau-Levret maneuver

Mauthner, Ludwig, Austrian ophthalmologist, 1840-1894.
 Mauthner cell – a large neuron of the spinal cord with its cell body located
 in the metencephalon of fish and amphibia.
 Mauthner fiber – an axon.
 Mauthner sheath – the plasma membrane of the axon. *SYN:* axolemma
 Mauthner test – an obsolete test for color perception.

Maxcy, Kenneth Fuller, U.S. bacteriologist, *1889.
 Maxcy disease – a type of typhoid fever endemic in the southern United
 States.

Maxim, Charles Hiram, U.S. physician, 1839-1887.
 Maxim-Gilbert sequencing – a method of sequencing DNA using
 dimethyl sulfate and hydrazinolysis.

Maximow, Alexander A., Russian physician in U.S., 1874-1928.
 Maximow stain for bone marrow

Maxwell, James Clerk, Scottish physicist and mathematician, 1831-1879.
 Maxwell law – a law of distribution of velocities.

Maxwell, James Laidlaw, Taiwanese physician, 1836-1921.
 MacLean-Maxwell disease – see under MacLean
 maxwell – magnetic flux unit.

Maxwell, Patrick William, Irish ophthalmologist, 1856-1917.
 Maxwell ring – a small faint ring in the visual field.

May, Duane L., 20th century U.S. physician.
 May-White syndrome – autosomal dominant trait causing progressive
 myoclonus epilepsy with lipomas, deafness, and ataxia.

NOTES

May, Richard, German physician, 1863-1936.
    May-Hegglin anomaly – *SYN:* Hegglin anomaly
    May-Hegglin syndrome – *SYN:* Hegglin syndrome

Maydl, Karl, Austrian physician, 1853-1903.
    Maydl colostomy
    Maydl disease
    Maydl hernia
    Maydl operation
    Maydl pessary

Mayer, Karl, Austrian neurologist, 1862-1932.
    Mayer reflex – apposition and adduction of the thumb. *SYN:* basal joint reflex

Mayer, Karl W., German gynecologist, 1795-1868.
    Mayer pessary – elastic ring pessary. *SYN:* Dumontpallier pessary
    Mayer position
    Mayer speculum

Mayer, Paul, German histologist, 1848-1923.
    Mayer hemalum stain – a progressive nuclear stain also used as a counterstain.
    Mayer mucicarmine stain
    Mayer mucihematein stain
    Mayer-Rokitansky-Küster-Hauser syndrome – congenital absence of the vagina. *SYN:* Rokitansky-Küster-Hauser syndrome

Mayer-Gross, Willi, German neurologist, *1889.
    Mayer-Gross apraxia – *SYN:* Kleist apraxia

Mayo, Charles Horace, U.S. surgeon, 1865-1939.
    Mayo bunionectomy – excision of the head of the first metatarsal.
    Mayo cannula
    Mayo carpal instability classification
    Mayo carrier
    Mayo clamp
    Mayo elbow prosthesis
    Mayo forceps
    Mayo-Gibbon heart-lung machine
    Mayo-Hegar needle holder
    Mayo hemostat
    Mayo herniorrhaphy
    Mayo hook
    Mayo instrument table

Mayo knife
Mayo needle
Mayo needle holder
Mayo nerve block
Mayo probe
Mayo resection arthroplasty
Mayo retractor
Mayo scissors
Mayo scoop
Mayo semiconstrained elbow prosthesis
Mayo stripper
Mayo suture
Mayo total ankle prosthesis
Mayo total elbow arthroplasty

Mayo, William J., U.S. surgeon, 1861-1939.
    Mayo operation – radical cure of umbilical hernia.
    Mayo vein – *SYN:* prepyloric vein

Mayo-Robson, Sir Arthur W., English surgeon, 1853-1933.
    Mayo-Robson point – a point just above and to the right of the umbilicus,
      where tenderness on pressure exists in disease of the pancreas.
    Mayo-Robson position – a supine position used in gallbladder operations.

Mayou, Marmaduke Stephen, English ophthalmologist, 1876-1934.
    Batten-Mayou disease – *SYN:* Batten disease

Mazza, Salvador, Argentinian physician, 1886-1946.
    Chagas-Mazza disease – *SYN:* Chagas disease

Mazzini, L.Y., U.S. serologist, 1894-1973.
    Mazzini test – slide test for detection of early, latent, and congenital
      syphilis and for the detection of false-positive cases.

Mazzoni, Vittorio, Italian physician, 1880-1940.
    Golgi-Mazzoni corpuscle – see under Golgi

NOTES

Mazzoni corpuscle – a tactile corpuscle apparently identical with Krause end bulb.

Mazzotti, Luigi, Mexican parasitologist, 1900-1971.
Mazzotti reaction – *SYN:* Mazzotti test
Mazzotti test – diagnostic test of onchocerciasis. *SYN:* Mazzotti reaction

McArdle, Brian, English neurologist, d. 2002.
McArdle disease – *SYN:* McArdle syndrome
McArdle-Schmid-Pearson disease – *SYN:* McArdle syndrome
McArdle syndrome – glycogenosis due to muscle glycogen phosphorylase deficiency, resulting in accumulation of glycogen of normal chemical structure in muscle. *SYN:* Cori syndrome; McArdle disease; McArdle-Schmid-Pearson syndrome; type 5 glycogenosis

McBride, Earl D., U.S. orthopedic surgeon, 1891-1975.
McBride bunionectomy – removal of a bunion. *SYN:* McBride bunion repair; McBride operation
McBride bunion repair – *SYN:* McBride bunionectomy
McBride cup
McBride femoral prosthesis
McBride operation – *SYN:* McBride bunionectomy
McBride pin
McBride plate
McBride procedure
McBride prosthesis
McBride tripod
McBride tripod pin traction

McBurney, Charles, U.S. surgeon, 1845-1913.
McBurney incision – an incision parallel with the course of the external oblique muscle, one or two inches cephalad to the anterior superior spine of the ilium.
McBurney inguinal herniorrhaphy – *SYN:* McBurney operation
McBurney operation – surgery to repair inguinal hernia. *SYN:* McBurney inguinal herniorrhaphy
McBurney point – a point where pressure elicits tenderness in acute appendicitis.
McBurney retractor
McBurney sign – tenderness at site two-thirds of the distance between the umbilicus and the anterior-superior iliac spine seen in appendicitis.

McCall, M.L., 20th century U.S. gynecologist.
McCall culdoplasty

McCarthy, Daniel J., U.S. neurologist, 1874-1958.

McCarthy reflexes – (1) contraction of the adductors of the thigh upon tapping the spinal column. *SYN:* spinoadductor reflex; (2) contraction of the orbicularis oculi muscle induced by tapping the supraorbital nerve. *SYN:* supraorbital reflex

McCarthy scales of children's abilities – used to test children's comprehension between 2-1/2 and 8-1/2 years of age.

McCarthy, Joseph Francis, U.S. urologist, 1874-1965.

McCarthy catheter

McCarthy coagulation electrode

McCarthy cystoscope

McCarthy electrotome

McCarthy evacuator

McCarthy forceps

McCarthy panendoscope

McCarthy resectoscope

McCarthy telescope

McClintock, Barbara, winner of 1983 Nobel Prize for work related to genetics.

McCrea, Lowrain E., U.S. urologist, *1896.

McCrea cystoscope

McCrea sound

McCune, Donovan James, U.S. pediatrician, 1902-1976.

McCune-Albright syndrome – polyostotic fibrous dysplasia with irregular brown patches of cutaneous pigmentation and endocrine dysfunction, especially precocious puberty in girls. *SYN:* Albright disease; Albright syndrome (2)

McDonald, Ellice, U.S. gynecologist, 1876-1955.

McDonald cerclage

McDonald clamp

NOTES

McDonald maneuver – measurement of uterus to approximate gestational age in weeks.
McDonald measurement
McDonald pelvimetry
McDonald procedure
McDonald rule – to determine the lunar months of pregnancy.

McEvedy, Peter George, English surgeon, 1890-1951.
McEvedy approach – used in femoral herniorrhaphy.

McFarlane, D.C.
Oliver-McFarlane syndrome – see under Oliver, G.L.

McGill University, university in Montreal, Canada, where questionnaire was developed.
McGill Pain Questionnaire – used to quantify location, type, and magnitude of pain.

McGinn, Sylvester, U.S. cardiologist, *1904.
McGinn-White sign – EKG evidence of right ventricle dilatation due to pulmonary embolism.

McGoon, Dwight C., U.S. surgeon, *1925.
McGoon technique – plastic reconstruction of an incompetent mitral valve.

McIndoe, Sir Archibald Hector, English surgeon, 1900-1960.
McIndoe chisel
McIndoe elevator
McIndoe forceps
McIndoe incision
McIndoe operation
McIndoe rasp
McIndoe retractor
McIndoe scissors
McIndoe vaginal creation
McIndoe vaginal reconstruction

McIntosh, James, English pathologist and bacteriologist, *1916.
McIntosh-Fildes jar – anaerobic bacterial culture receptacle.

McKee, George Kenneth, English orthopedic surgeon, *1930.
McKee brace
McKee-Farrar acetabular cup
McKee-Farrar hip prosthesis
McKee femoral prosthesis

McKee line
McKee prosthesis
McKee table
McKee totally constrained elbow prosthesis
McKee tri-fin nail

McKittrick, Leland Sterling, U.S. physician, *1892.
  McKittrick syndrome – colon and rectal villous adenoma, with electrolyte imbalance. *SYN:* McKittrick-Wheelock syndrome
  McKittrick-Wheelock syndrome – *SYN:* McKittrick syndrome

McKusick, Victor Almon, U.S. physician, *1921.
  Cross-McKusick-Breen syndrome – *SYN:* Cross syndrome
  Esterly-McKusick syndrome – see under Esterly
  McKusick-Cross syndrome – *SYN:* McKusick syndrome
  McKusick-Dungy-Kaufman syndrome – *SYN:* McKusick-Kaufman syndrome
  McKusick-Kaufman syndrome – autosomal recessive trait characterized by multiple anomalies. *SYN:* Kaufman syndrome; McKusick-Dungy-Kaufman syndrome

McLean, Malcolm, U.S. obstetrician, 1848-1924.
  Tucker-McLean forceps – see under Tucker

McMurray, Thomas Porter, English surgeon, 1887-1949.
  McMurray knife
  McMurray maneuver
  McMurray osteotomy
  McMurray sign
  McMurray test – rotation of the tibia on the femur.

McNemar, Quinn, U.S. psychologist and statistician, *1900.
  Terman-McNemar test of mental ability – see under Terman

McPhail, M.K., Canadian physiologist, *1907.
  McPhail test – for progesterone.

McPheeters, Herman Oscar, 20th century U.S. physician.
McPheeters treatment – varicose ulcer treatment.

McQuarrie, I.
McQuarrie syndrome – signs of hypoglycemia.

McReynolds, John O., U.S. ophthalmologist, 1865-1942.
McReynolds eye spatula
McReynolds keratome
McReynolds operation
McReynolds pterygium knife
McReynolds pterygium scissors
McReynolds pterygium transplant
McReynolds technique

McVay, Chester B., U.S. surgeon, *1911.
McVay herniorrhaphy – *SYN:* McVay operation
McVay incision
McVay operation – repair of inguinal and femoral hernias. *SYN:* McVay
herniorrhaphy

MD Anderson, Cancer Center in Houston, Texas.
MD Anderson grading system

M'Dowel, Benjamin G., Irish anatomist, 1829-1885.
frenulum of M'Dowel – tendinous fasciculi passing from the tendon of the
pectoralis major muscle across the bicipital groove.

Meadows, William Robert, U.S. cardiologist, *1919.
Meadows syndrome – postpartum myocardiopathy.

Mean, James Howard, U.S. endocrinologist, 1885-1967.
Mean sign – lag of the eyeball on upward gaze.

Meara, R.H., 20th century English dermatologist.
Dowling-Meara syndrome – see under Dowling

Mechnikov, Ilya Ilyich, joint winner of 1908 Nobel Prize for work related to
immunology.

Meckel, Johann Friedrich, the elder, German anatomist and obstetrician,
1714-1774.
Meckel band – the portion of the anterior ligament of the malleus that
extends from the base of the anterior process through the petrotympanic
fissure, to attach to the spine of the sphenoid. *SYN:* Meckel ligament
Meckel cave
Meckel cavity – *SYN:* Meckel space

Meckel ganglion – a small parasympathetic ganglion in the upper part of the pterygopalatine fossa. *SYN:* pterygopalatine ganglion

Meckel ligament – *SYN:* Meckel band

Meckel space – the cleft in the meningeal layer of dura of the middle cranial fossa that encloses the roots of the trigeminal nerve and the trigeminal ganglion. *SYN:* Meckel cavity; trigeminal cave

Meckel sphenopalatine ganglionectomy

Meckel, Johann Friedrich, the younger, German anatomist and embryologist, 1781-1833.

Meckel cartilage – a temporary supporting structure in the embryonic mandible. *SYN:* mandibular cartilage

Meckel diverticulum – the remains of the yolk stalk of the embryo.

Meckel-Gruber syndrome – a malformation syndrome.
SYN: dysencephalia splanchnocystica; Meckel syndrome

Meckel plane – a craniometric plane cutting the alveolar and the auricular points.

Meckel scan – use of technetium-99m pertechnetate in a scan of the gastric mucosa to detect ectopic gastric mucosa in Meckel diverticulum.

Meckel syndrome – *SYN:* Meckel-Gruber syndrome

Medawar, Sir Peter Brian, joint winner of 1960 Nobel Prize for work related to immunology.

Medea, from Greek mythology: Medea killed the children fathered by Jason after he left her for a younger woman.

Medea complex – a mother's compulsion to kill her children as revenge against their father.

Medin, Karl O., Swedish physician, 1847-1927.

Medin poliomyelitis

Medjugorje, a Yugoslavian village in which six teenagers were said to have seen the Virgin Mary. They received daily messages of peace by looking toward a hilltop behind which there was a setting sun.

Medjugorje maculopathy

NOTES

Medusa, in Greek mythology, a Gorgon who turned men to stone.
  caput Medusae – (1) varicose veins radiating from the umbilicus; (2)
    dilated ciliary arteries girdling the corneoscleral limbus in rubeosis iridis.
    SYN: head of Medusa
  head of Medusa – *SYN:* caput Medusae

Meeh, K., 19th century German physiologist.
  Meeh-DuBois formula – for predicting surface area. *SYN:* Meeh formula
  Meeh formula – *SYN:* Meeh-Dubois formula

Meekeren, Job van, Dutch surgeon, 1611-1666.
  Meekeren-Ehlers-Danlos syndrome – *SYN:* Ehlers-Danlos syndrome

Mees, R.A., 20th century Dutch physician.
  Mees lines – horizontal white bands of the nails seen in chronic arsenic
    poisoning and occasionally in leprosy. *SYN:* Mees stripes
  Mees stripes – *SYN:* Mees lines

Meesmann, Alois, German ophthalmologist, 1888-1969.
  Meesmann dystrophy – corneal dystrophy; autosomal dominant trait.
    SYN: Meesmann syndrome; Meesmann-Wilke disease; Meesmann-Wilke
    syndrome
  Meesmann syndrome – *SYN:* Meesmann dystrophy
  Meesmann-Wilke disease – *SYN:* Meesmann dystrophy
  Meesmann-Wilke syndrome – *SYN:* Meesmann dystrophy

Méglin, J.A., French physician, 1756-1824.
  Méglin point – where the greater palatine nerve emerges from the great
    palatine foramen.

Meibom, Hendrik (Heinrich), Dutch anatomist and physician 1638-1700.
  meibomian conjunctivitis – obsolete term for a conjunctivitis associated
    with chronic inflammation of the meibomian glands, with swollen tarsal
    plates and frothy seborrheic secretion. *SYN:* seborrheic
    blepharoconjunctivitis
  meibomian cyst – a chronic inflammatory granuloma of a meibomian
    gland. *SYN:* chalazion
  meibomian glands – sebaceous glands embedded in the tarsal plate of
    each eyelid, discharging at the edge of the lid near the posterior border.
    SYN: tarsal glands
  meibomian sty – an acute purulent infection of a meibomian (tarsal)
    gland. *SYN:* hordeolum internum

Meier, Georg, German serologist, *1875.
  Porges-Meier test – see under Porges

Meier, Norman Charles, U.S. psychologist, 1893-1967.
   Meier art judgment test – used to determine an individual's artistic abilities.

Meige, Henri, French physician, 1866-1940.
   Meige disease – autosomal dominant lymphedema with onset at about the age of puberty.
   Nonne-Milroy-Meige syndrome – see under Nonne

Meigs, Arthur V., U.S. physician, 1850-1912.
   Meigs capillaries – located in the myocardium.

Meigs, Joseph Vincent, U.S. gynecologist, 1892-1963.
   Demons-Meigs syndrome – *SYN:* Meigs syndrome
   Meigs-Cass syndrome – *SYN:* Meigs syndrome
   Meigs curette
   Meigs hemostat
   Meigs operation
   Meigs retractor
   Meigs-Salmon syndrome – *SYN:* Meigs syndrome
   Meigs suture
   Meigs syndrome – fibromyoma of the ovary associated with hydroperitoneum and hydrothorax. *SYN:* Demons-Meigs syndrome; Meigs-Cass syndrome; Meigs-Salmon syndrome

Meinicke, Ernst, German physician, 1878-1945.
   Meinicke test – the first successful application of immune precipitation to diagnosis of syphilis, now obsolete.

Meirowsky, Emil, German-U.S. dermatologist, 1876-1960.
   Meirowsky phenomenon – temporary darkening of the skin that occurs immediately after exposure to ultraviolet A.

Meissner, Georg, German anatomist and physiologist, 1829-1905.
   Meissner corpuscle – *SYN:* tactile corpuscle
   Meissner ganglion

Meissner plexus – a gangliated plexus of unmyelinated nerve fibers. *SYN:* submucosal plexus

Melchior, Johannes Christian, Danish pediatrician, 1923-1995.
Dyggve-Melchior-Clausen syndrome – see under Dyggve

Meleney, Frank L., U.S. surgeon, 1889-1963.
Meleney gangrene – *SYN:* Meleney ulcer
Meleney infection
Meleney ulcer – undermining ulcer of the skin and subcutaneous tissues, usually following an operation. *SYN:* Meleney gangrene; progressive bacterial synergistic gangrene

Melkersson, Ernst Gustaf, Swedish physician, 1898-1932.
Melkersson-Rosenthal syndrome – cheilitis granulomatosum, fissured tongue, and facial nerve paralysis. *SYN:* Melkersson syndrome; Miescher cheilitis
Melkersson syndrome – *SYN:* Melkersson-Rosenthal syndrome

Melnick, John C., U.S. radiologist, *1928.
Melnick-Needles syndrome – a generalized skeletal dysplasia with prominent forehead and small mandible. *SYN:* osteodysplasty

Melnick, M., 20th century U.S. orofacial geneticist.
Melnick-Fraser syndrome – autosomal dominant syndrome characterized by branchial fistulae, preauricular pits, hearing loss, and renal dysplasia.

Melotte, George W., U.S. dentist, 1835-1915.
Melotte metal – a soft, fusable alloy.

Meltzer, Martin, U.S. physician, *1930.
Meltzer syndrome – vascular, renal, and arthritic disturbances.

Meltzer, Samuel J., U.S. physiologist, 1851-1920.
Meltzer law – all living functions are continually controlled by two opposite forces: augmentation and inhibition. *SYN:* law of contrary innervation
Meltzer-Lyon test – used in diagnosis of gallbladder conditions.
Meltzer sign – loss of second sound on auscultation of the heart after swallowing.

Mende, Irmgard, German physician.
Mende syndrome – congenital syndrome combining partial albinism, deafness, mongoloid facies, chronic blepharitis, cleft lip, and occasionally mental retardation. *SYN:* type IV acrocephalosyndactyly; Waardenburg syndrome

Mendel, Gregor Johann, Austrian geneticist, 1822-1884.
Mendel first law – factors that affect development retain their individuality from generation to generation, do not become contaminated when mixed in a hybrid, and become sorted out from one another when the next generation of gametes is formed. *SYN:* law of segregation
mendelian character – an inherited character under the control of a single locus.
mendelian inheritance – inheritance in which stable and undecomposable characters controlled by a single genetic locus are transmitted over many generations. *SYN:* alternative inheritance
mendelian ratio – the ratio of progeny with a particular phenotype or genotype expected in accordance with Mendel law among the offspring of matings specified as to genotype or phenotype.
Mendel second law – different hereditary factors assort independently when the gametes are formed. *SYN:* law of independent assortment

Mendel, Kurt, German neurologist, 1874-1946.
Bekhterev-Mendel reflex – see under Bekhterev
Mendel-Bekhterev reflex – *SYN:* Bekhterev-Mendel reflex
Mendel instep reflex – the foot being firmly supported on its inner side, a sharp tap on the dorsal tendons causes extension of the second to the fifth toes. *SYN:* back of foot reflex

Mendeléeff, Dimitri (Dmitri) I., Russian chemist, 1834-1907.
Mendeléeff law – the properties of elements are periodical functions of their atomic weights. *SYN:* periodic law
mendelevium – an element, atomic No. 101, atomic weight 258.1, prepared in 1955 by bombardment of einsteinium with alpha particles.

Mendelson, Curtis Lester, U.S. obstetrician, *1913.
Mendelson syndrome – aspiration pneumonia in obstetrical patients.

Mendenhall, Edgar N., U.S. family practitioner, 1891-1970.
Rabson-Mendenhall syndrome – see under Rabson

NOTES

Mendes Da Costa, Samuel, Dutch dermatologist, 1862-1941.
  Mendes Da Costa syndrome – edema.

Ménétrier, Pierre E., French physician, 1859-1935.
  Ménétrier disease – gastric mucosal hyperplasia. *SYN:* giant hypertrophy of
    gastric mucosa; hypertrophic gastritis; Ménétrier syndrome
  Ménétrier syndrome – *SYN:* Ménétrier disease

Menge, Karl, German gynecologist, 1864-1945.
  Menge operation
  Menge pessary – a ring pessary.

Mengo, a region of Uganda where the virus was discovered in animals in
1948.
  Mengo encephalomyelitis – *SYN:* Mengo virus
  Mengo virus – a strain of encephalomyocarditis. *SYN:* Mengo
    encephalomyelitis

Ménière, Prosper, French physician, 1799-1862.
  Ménière disease – characterized by vertigo, nausea, vomiting, tinnitus,
    and progressive deafness due to swelling of the endolymphatic duct.
    SYN: auditory vertigo; endolymphatic hydrops; labyrinthine vertigo;
    Ménière syndrome
  Ménière syndrome – *SYN:* Ménière disease

Menkes, John H., U.S. pediatric neurologist, *1928.
  Menkes disease – *SYN:* kinky-hair syndrome
  Menkes syndrome – *SYN:* kinky-hair syndrome

Mennell, James Beaver, English physician, 1880-1957.
  Mennell sign – a test for spinal problems.

Mensendieck, Bess M., U.S. physician, 1861-1957.
  Mensendieck exercises – physical education system.

Menten, Maud Leonora, Canadian pathologist in U.S., 1879-1960.
  Michaelis-Menten constant – *SYN:* Michaelis constant
  Michaelis-Menten equation – see under Michaelis
  Michaelis-Menten hypothesis – see under Michaelis
  Victor-Michaelis-Menten equation – *SYN:* Michaelis-Menten equation

Menzel, P.
  Menzel syndrome – cerebellar ataxia. *SYN:* Marie I syndrome; Nonne-
    Marie syndrome; Sanger Brown syndrome

Mercier, Louis Auguste, French urologist, 1811-1882.
  median bar of Mercier – *SYN:* Mercier bar

Mercier bar – a fold of mucous membrane extending from the orifice of the ureter of one side to that of the other side. *SYN:* interureteric fold; median bar of Mercier

Mercier catheter

Mercier sound – a catheter the beak of which is short and bent almost at a right angle.

Mercier valve – an occasional fold of mucosa of the bladder partially occluding the ureteral orifice.

Merendino, K. Alvin, U.S. surgeon, 1914-1985.

Merendino technique – plastic reconstruction of an incompetent mitral valve.

Meretoja, J., 20th century Finnish physician.

Meretoja syndrome – interstitial amyloid accumulation. *SYN:* amyloidosis

Merkel, Friedrich Sigmund, German anatomist and physiologist, 1845-1919.

Merkel cell tumor – a rare malignant cutaneous tumor. *SYN:* primary neuroendocrine carcinoma of the skin; trabecular carcinoma

Merkel corpuscle – a specialized tactile sensory nerve ending in the epidermis. *SYN:* Merkel tactile cell; Merkel tactile disk; tactile meniscus

Merkel tactile cell – *SYN:* Merkel corpuscle

Merkel tactile disk – *SYN:* Merkel corpuscle

Merkel, Julius, German psychologist.

Merkel law – principle used in psychology.

Merkel, Karl L., German anatomist and laryngologist, 1812-1876.

Merkel filtrum ventriculi – a groove between the two prominences in each lateral wall of the vestibule of the larynx. *SYN:* filtrum ventriculi

Merkel fossa – a groove in the posterolateral wall of the vestibule of the larynx between the corniculate and cuneiform cartilages.

Merkel muscle – a fasciculus from the posterior cricoarytenoid muscle inserted into the inferior horn of the thyroid cartilage. *SYN:* ceratocricoid muscle

Merrifield, R. Bruce, U.S. biochemist and Nobel laureate, *1921.
   Merrifield synthesis – the synthesis of peptides and proteins via an automated system on carrier polymers.

Merritt, Katharine Krom, U.S. pediatrician, *1886.
   Kasabach-Merritt syndrome – see under Kasabach

Merten, David F., U.S. radiologist.
   Singleton-Merten syndrome – see under Singleton

Merwarth, H.R.
   Merwarth syndrome – progressive hemiplegia due to venous occlusion.
      SYN: cerebral venous thrombosis

Méry, Jean, French anatomist, 1645-1722.
   Méry gland – one of two small compound racemose glands that discharge through a small duct into the spongy portion of the urethra.
      SYN: bulbourethral gland

Merzbacher, Ludwig, German physician in Argentina, 1875-1942.
   Merzbacher-Pelizaeus disease – *SYN:* Pelizaeus-Merzbacher disease
   Pelizaeus-Merzbacher disease – see under Pelizaeus

Mesmer, Franz Anton, Austrian physician, 1733-1815.
   mesmeric crisis – reaction technique. *SYN:* grand crisis; magnetic crisis
   mesmerism – the use of hypnotism as practiced by Mesmer.

Metchnikoff, Elie, Russian biologist in France and Nobel laureate, 1845-1916.
   Metchnikoff theory – the body is protected against infection by leukocytes and other cells.

Mett, Emil Ludwig Paul, German physician, *1867.
   Mett test – for digestion.
   Mett tube – glass tube filled with coagulated egg white.

Meyenburg, H. von, Swiss pathologist, *1877.
   Meyenburg-Altherr-Uehlinger syndrome – *SYN:* Meyenburg disease
   Meyenburg complex – clusters of small bile ducts occurring in polycystic livers, separate from the portal areas.
   Meyenburg disease – a degenerative disease of cartilage.
      SYN: Meyenburg-Altherr-Uehlinger syndrome; relapsing polychondritis; von Meyenburg disease
   von Meyenburg disease – *SYN:* Meyenburg disease

Meyer, Adolf, U.S. psychiatrist, 1866-1950.
Meyer-Archambault loop – the fibers of the visual radiation that loop around the tip of the temporal horn.
Meyer temporal loop

Meyer, Edmund V., German laryngologist, 1864-1931.
Meyer cartilages – the anterior sesamoid cartilages at the anterior attachments of the vocal ligaments.

Meyer, Georg H., Swiss anatomist, 1815-1892.
Meyer line – a line through the axis of the big toe and passing the midpoint of the heel.
Meyer posture – normal posture of a standing subject.
Meyer sinus – a small concavity in the floor of the external auditory canal near the tympanic membrane.

Meyer, Hans H., German pharmacologist, 1853-1939.
Meyer-Overton rule – because inhalation agents act through the central nervous system cells, anesthetic potency increases with lipid solubility.
Meyer-Overton theory of narcosis – that narcotic efficiency parallels the coefficient of partition between oil and water, and that lipoids in the cell and on the cell membrane absorb the drug because of this affinity.
SYN: lipoid theory of narcosis

Meyer, Willy, U.S. surgeon, 1854-1932.
Meyer reagent – a solution to detect minute traces of blood.

Meyer-Betz, Friedrich, 20th century German physician.
Meyer-Betz disease – *SYN:* Meyer-Betz syndrome
Meyer-Betz syndrome – excretion of myoglobin in the urine resulting from muscle degeneration. *SYN:* Meyer-Betz disease; myoglobinuria

Meyerhof, Otto F., German-U.S. biochemist and Nobel laureate, 1884-1951.
Embden-Meyerhof-Parnas pathway – *SYN:* Embden-Meyerhof pathway
Embden-Meyerhof pathway – see under Embden

M

NOTES

Meyerhof oxidation quotient – an index for the effect of oxygen on glycolysis and on fermentation.

Meyer-Schwickerath, Gerhard Rudolph Edmund, German ophthalmologist, *1920.
Meyer-Schwickerath coagulator

Meyerson, L.B., 20th century U.S. dermatologist.
Meyerson nevus – *SYN:* Meyerson phenomenon
Meyerson phenomenon – an eczematous, papulosquamous reaction around a melanocytic nevus. *SYN:* halo dermatitis; Meyerson nevus

Meynert, Theodor H., Austrian neurologist, 1833-1892.
Meynert cells – solitary pyramidal cells found in the cortex in the region of the calcarine fissure.
Meynert commissures – the commissural fibers that lie above and behind the optic chiasm. *SYN:* commissurae supraopticae
Meynert decussation
Meynert fasciculus – a compact bundle of fibers in the midbrain.
SYN: Meynert retroflex bundle; retroflex fasciculus
Meynert layer – layer three of the cortex cerebri. *SYN:* pyramidal cell layer
Meynert retroflex bundle – *SYN:* Meynert fasciculus

Meynet, Paul Claude Hyacinthe, French physician, 1831-1892.
Meynet nodes – nodules in joint capsules and tendons in rheumatic disorders.

Mibelli, Vittorio, Italian dermatologist, 1860-1910.
Mibelli angiokeratomas – telangiectatic small papules of the extremities, common in adolescent girls.
Mibelli disease – *SYN:* Mibelli syndrome
Mibelli syndrome – eruption of miliary translucent papules. *SYN:* Mibelli disease; porokeratosis

Michaelis, Leonor, German-U.S. chemist and physician, 1875-1949.
Michaelis buffer
Michaelis constant – the true dissociation constant for the enzyme-substrate binary complex in a single-substrate rapid equilibrium enzyme-catalyzed reaction. *SYN:* Michaelis-Menten constant
Michaelis-Gutmann body – a rounded homogenous body containing calcium and iron found within macrophages in the bladder wall in malacoplakia.
Michaelis-Menten constant – *SYN:* Michaelis constant
Michaelis-Menten equation – an initial-rate equation for a single-substrate noncooperative enzyme-catalyzed reaction relating the initial

velocity to the initial substrate concentration. *SYN:* Victor-Michaelis-Menten equation

Michaelis-Menten hypothesis – that a complex is formed between an enzyme and its substrate (the O'Sullivan-Tompson hypothesis), which complex then decomposes to yield free enzyme and the reaction products (Brown hypothesis), the latter rate determining the overall rate of substrate-product conversion.

Victor-Michaelis-Menten equation – *SYN:* Michaelis-Menten equation

Michaelsson, G.
Juhlin-Michaelsson syndrome – see under Juhlin

Michel, Benno, 20th century U.S. dermatopathologist.
Michel medium – maintains tissue-fixed immunoreactants of skin biopsy specimen that is to be examined with direct immunofluorescence or immunoelectron microscopy.

Michel, Gaston, French surgeon, 1874-1937.
Michel clip
Michel deformity
Michel forceps
Michel malformation
Michel mirror
Michel pick
Michel spur
Michel trephine

Micheli, Ferdinando, Italian physician, 1872-1936.
Marchiafava-Micheli anemia – *SYN:* Marchiafava-Micheli syndrome
Marchiafava-Micheli syndrome – see under Marchiafava

Michotte, L.J., French physician.
Michotte syndrome – *SYN:* Baastrup syndrome

Middeldorpf, K., German physician.
Middeldorpf splint

NOTES

Middeldorpf triangle
Middeldorpf tumor – congenital sacral tumor.

Miehlke, A.
Miehlke-Partsch syndrome – deformities of neonates which are caused by thalidomide. *SYN:* thalidomide-induced phocomelia

Mierzejewski, Jan Lucian, Polish neurologist and psychiatrist, 1839-1908.
Mierzejewski effect – development of excessive gray brain matter.

Miescher, Alfred Guido, Swiss dermatologist, 1877-1961.
Miescher cheilitis – *SYN:* Melkersson-Rosenthal syndrome
Miescher-Leder syndrome – reddish granulomatous plaques.
SYN: granuloma disciformis; necrobiosis maculosa
Miescher I syndrome – benign velvety warty growths. *SYN:* acanthosis nigricans
Miescher II syndrome – inflammatory granulomas of the lips.
SYN: granulomatous cheilitis

Miescher, Johann F., Swiss pathologist, 1811-1887.
Miescher elastoma – circinate groups of hyperkeratotic papules associated with pseudoxanthoma elasticum.
Miescher granuloma – an anular eruption on sun-exposed skin.
SYN: actinic granuloma
Miescher tubes – elongate fusiform or cylindrical bodies forming the encapsulated cystic intramuscular stage of the protozoan *Sarcocystis*.

Mietens, Carl, German physician.
Mietens-Weber syndrome – autosomal recessive defects.

Migula, Walter, German naturalist, 1863-1938.
Migula classification – a bacteria classification.

Mikaelian, 20th century Lebanese physician.
Mikaelian syndrome – probable autosomal recessive trait characterized by deafness and other anomalies.

Mikity, Victor G., U.S. radiologist, *1919.
Wilson-Mikity syndrome – see under Wilson, Miriam

Mikulicz, Johannes (Jan) von-Radecki, Polish surgeon in Germany, 1850-1905.
Heineke-Mikulicz herniorrhaphy
Heineke-Mikulicz pyloroplasty – see under Heineke
Mikulicz angle
Mikulicz aphthae – a severe form of aphthae. *SYN:* aphthae major
Mikulicz clamp

Mikulicz crusher

Mikulicz disease – benign swelling of the lacrimal, and usually also of the salivary glands, in consequence of an infiltration of and replacement of the normal gland structure by lymphoid tissue.

Mikulicz drain

Mikulicz forceps

Mikulicz incision

Mikulicz mask – gauze-covered frame, worn over the nose and mouth while performing surgery.

Mikulicz operation

Mikulicz pack

Mikulicz pad

Mikulicz retractor

Mikulicz sponge

Mikulicz syndrome – symptoms characteristic of Mikulicz disease occurring as a complication of some other disease, such as lymphoma or leukemia.

Mikulicz-Vladimiroff amputation – an osteoplastic resection of the foot. *SYN:* Vladimiroff-Mikulicz amputation

Vladimiroff-Mikulicz amputation – *SYN:* Mikulicz-Vladimiroff amputation

Miles, William E., English surgeon, 1869-1947.

Miles clamp

Miles clip

Miles operation – combined abdominoperineal resection for rectal carcinoma. *SYN:* Miles resection

Miles punch biopsy forceps

Miles resection – *SYN:* Miles operation

Miles retractor

Milian, Gaston Auguste, French physician, 1871-1945.

Milian disease – *SYN:* Milian syndrome

Milian erythema – *SYN:* Milian syndrome

Milian syndrome – reaction to arsenophenamine compounds. *SYN:* Milian disease; Milian erythema; ninth-day erythema

Milkman, Louis Arthur, U.S. radiologist, 1895-1951.
Milkman fracture
Milkman syndrome – osteomalacia with multiple pseudofractures.

Millar, John, Scottish physician, 1733-1805.
Millar asthma – stridorous laryngismus.

Millard, Auguste L.J., French physician, 1830-1915.
Millard-Gubler syndrome – *SYN:* Gubler syndrome

Millard, Henry B., U.S. physician, 1832-1893.
Millard test – for albumin.

Miller, Grier.
Kurzrock-Miller test – see under Kurzrock

Miller, James Q., U.S. physician.
Miller-Dieker syndrome – arrested brain development. *SYN:* lissencephaly; Norman-Roberts syndrome

Miller, Marvin, 20th century U.S. pediatrician.
Miller syndrome – facial and limb defects at birth. *SYN:* postaxial acrofacial dysostosis

Miller, Thomas Grier, U.S. internist, 1886-1981.
Miller-Abbott catheter – *SYN:* Miller-Abbott tube
Miller-Abbott tube – a double-lumen tube used for intestinal decompression. *SYN:* Abbott tube; Miller-Abbott catheter

Miller, Willoughby D., U.S. dentist, 1853-1907.
Miller theory – that dental caries is caused by microorganisms of the mouth fermenting dietary carbohydrates and producing acids that demineralize the teeth.

Millikan, Clark Harold, U.S. neurologist, *1915.
Millikan-Siekert syndrome – stenosis of proximal subclavian artery. *SYN:* basilar artery insufficiency

Millin, Terence John, English and Irish surgeon, 1890-1980.
Millin clamp
Millin forceps
Millin operation
Millin prostatectomy
Millin retractor
Millin tube

Millon, Auguste N.E., French chemist, 1812-1867.
  Millon-Nasse test – for protein.
  Millon reaction – used to test for proteins.
  Millon reagent – mercuric nitrate and nitric acid as used in the Millon reaction.

Mills, Charles Karsner, U.S. physician, 1845-1931.
  Mills disease – slowly progressive paralysis. *SYN:* ascending hemiplegia

Mills, Hiram F., U.S. engineer, 1836-1921.
  Mills-Reincke phenomenon – water purification results in fewer deaths from all diseases.

Milroy, William Forsyth, U.S. physician, 1855-1942.
  Milroy disease – congenital type of autosomal dominant lymphedema.
  Nonne-Milroy-Meige syndrome – see under Nonne

Milstein, César, Argentinian-English immunologist, joint winner of 1984 Nobel Prize for work related to immune system.

Milton, John Laws, English dermatologist, 1820-1898.
  Milton disease – *SYN:* Quincke edema
  Milton urticaria – *SYN:* Quincke edema

Mims, Leroy C., 20th century U.S. pediatrician.
  Feuerstein-Mims-Schimmelpenning syndrome –
    SYN: Schimmelpenning-Feuerstein-Mims syndrome
  Feuerstein-Mims syndrome – *SYN:* Schimmelpenning-Feuerstein-Mims syndrome
  Schimmelpenning-Feuerstein-Mims syndrome – see under Schimmelpenning

Minamata, bay in Japan where condition was first observed.
  Minamata syndrome – paresthesias and degenerative changes caused by ingestion of fish contaminated by methyl mercury. *SYN:* alkyl mercury poisoning

NOTES

Minerva, Roman goddess of warfare and memory.
Minerva cast
Minerva collar
Minerva jacket – plaster cast made for stabilization of the vertebra.

Minin, A.V., 20th century Russian surgeon.
Minin light – produces violet or ultraviolet light.

Minkowski, (Minkowsky), Oskar, German physician, 1858-1931.
Minkowski-Chauffard syndrome – familial blood disorder; autosomal dominant trait.

Minkowsky, var. of Minkowski

Minnesota, 32nd state admitted to the Union in 1858.
Minnesota Mechanical Ability Test – test developed in the 1920s at the University of Minnesota; subject is required to reassemble a mechanical object from its disassembled parts. *SYN:* Heidbreder test

Minor, Lazar Salomonovich, Russian physician, 1855-1942.
Minor-Oppenheim syndrome – *SYN:* Minor syndrome
Minor syndrome – paralysis caused by hemorrhage into the spinal cord. *SYN:* central hematomyelia; Minor-Oppenheim syndrome

Minot, George Richards, U.S. physician and Nobel laureate, 1885-1950.
Minot-Murphy diet – the use of large amounts of raw liver in the treatment of pernicious anemia.

Mirizzi, P.L., 20th century Argentinian physician.
Mirizzi syndrome – stenosis of hepatic duct. *SYN:* hepatic duct obstruction

Mishima, Yutaka, 20th century Japanese dermatologist.
Mishima dual pathway theory – a theory of dual origin of malignant melanoma to explain why different types show different growth rates.

Mitchell, Charles L., U.S. orthopedic surgeon, *1901.
Mitchell bunionectomy
Mitchell distal osteotomy
Mitchell operation
Mitchell osteotomy

Mitchell, Silas Weir, U.S. neurologist, poet, and novelist, 1829-1914.
Gerhardt-Mitchell disease – see under Gerhardt, Carl
Mitchell disease – *SYN:* Gerhardt-Mitchell disease
Mitchell treatment – treatment of mental illness by rest, nourishing diet, and a change of environment. *SYN:* Weir Mitchell therapy; Weir Mitchell treatment

Weir Mitchell disease – *SYN:* Gerhardt-Mitchell disease
Weir Mitchell therapy – *SYN:* Mitchell treatment
Weir Mitchell treatment – *SYN:* Mitchell treatment

Mitrofanoff, Paul, French pediatric surgeon, *1934.
   Mitrofanoff principle

Mitsuda, Kensuke, Japanese physician, 1876-1964.
   Mitsuda antigen – an autoclaved suspension of human tissue naturally
     infected with *Mycobacterium leprae.*
   Mitsuda reaction – a delayed hypersensitivity lepromin reaction in the
     form of erythematous papular nodules at the site of intradermal injection
     of Mitsuda antigen in a lepromin test.
   Mitsuda test – lepromin test by intradermal injection.

Mitsuo, Gentaro, Japanese ophthalmologist, 1876-1913.
   Mitsuo phenomenon – restoration of the normal color of the fundus with
     dark adaptation in Oguchi disease.

Miura, Noboru, Japanese dentist.
   Cooperman-Miura syndrome – see under Cooperman
   Miura-Cooperman syndrome – *SYN:* Cooperman-Miura syndrome

Mixter, Samuel Jason, U.S. surgeon, 1855-1926.
   Mixter clamp
   Mixter dilating probe
   Mixter dilator
   Mixter forceps
   Mixter hemostat
   Mixter irrigating probe
   Mixter needle
   Mixter-Paul hemostatic forceps
   Mixter probe
   Mixter punch
   Mixter scissors
   Paul-Mixter tube

M

NOTES

Miyagawa, Yoneji, Japanese bacteriologist, 1885-1959.
   Miyagawa bodies – a term previously used to refer to *Chlamydia trachomatis* (*Miyagawanella lymphogranulomatosis*), the elementary bodies that develop in the intracytoplasmic microcolonies of lymphogranuloma venereum.
   Miyagawanella – formerly considered a genus of Chlamydiaceae, but now synonymous with *Chlamydia*.

M'Naghten, Daniel, English criminal, tried in March, 1843.
   M'Naghten rule – the classic English test of criminal responsibility.

Mobitz, Woldemar, German cardiologist, *1889.
   Mobitz type I atrioventricular block – the dropped beat of the Wenckebach phenomenon.
   Mobitz type II atrioventricular block – a dropped cardiac cycle that occurs without alteration in the conduction of the preceding intervals.

Möbius, Paul J., German physician, 1853-1907.
   Leyden-Möbius muscular dystrophy – *SYN:* limb-girdle muscular dystrophy
   Möbius sign – impairment of ocular convergence in Graves disease.
   Möbius I syndrome – moderate migraine accompanied by extraocular palsy. *SYN:* occasional oculomotor paralysis; ophthalmoplegic migraine
   Möbius II syndrome – a developmental bilateral facial paralysis usually associated with oculomotor or other neurological disorders. *SYN:* congenital facial diplegia; developmental bilateral facial paralysis

Moe, John H., U.S. surgeon, *1905.
   Moe alar hook
   Moe hook
   Moe impactor
   Moe intertrochanteric plate – *SYN:* Moe plate
   Moe nail
   Moe plate – plate used for internal fixation of intertrochanteric femoral fracture. *SYN:* Moe intertrochanteric plate
   Moe procedure
   Moe rod
   Moe spinal fusion
   Moe system

Moeller, Alfred, German bacteriologist, *1868.
   Moeller grass bacillus – a species found in soil and dust and on plants. *SYN:* *Mycobacterium phlei*

Moeller, Julius Otto Ludwig, German surgeon, 1819-1887.
    Moeller glossitis – *SYN:* Moeller-Hunter syndrome
    Moeller-Hunter syndrome – red, swollen, and painful tongue. *SYN:* atrophic
        glossitis; Hunter glossitis; Moeller glossitis

Moenckeberg, var. of Mönckeberg

Moersch, Frederick Paul, U.S. physician.
    Moersch-Woltmann syndrome – prodromal occasional aching and
        tightness of muscles. *SYN:* stiff man syndrome

Mohr, Francis, 19th century U.S. pharmacist.
    Mohr test – test for stomach contents containing hydrochloric acid.

Mohr, Otto Lous, Norwegian geneticist, 1886-1967.
    Mohr finger splint
    Mohr-Majewski syndrome – fatal dwarfism with multiple congenital
        anomalies.

Mohrenheim, Joseph J. Freiherr von, Austrian-Russian surgeon, 1755-1799.
    Mohrenheim fossa – a triangular depression bounded by the clavicle and
        the adjacent borders of the deltoid and pectoralis major muscles.
        SYN: infraclavicular fossa; Mohrenheim space
    Mohrenheim space – *SYN:* Mohrenheim fossa

Mohs, Frederick E., U.S. surgeon, 1910-2002.
    Mohs chemosurgery – a microscopically controlled technique for removal
        of skin tumors. *SYN:* microscopically controlled surgery; Mohs
        micrographic surgery; Mohs surgery
    Mohs fresh tissue chemosurgery technique – chemosurgery in which
        superficial cancers are excised after fixation in vivo.
    Mohs micrographic surgery – *SYN:* Mohs chemosurgery
    Mohs surgery – *SYN:* Mohs chemosurgery
    Mohs technique

Mohs, Friedrich, German mineralogist, 1773-1839.
    Mohs hardness number – a number on a mineralogic scale.

Mohs scale – a qualitative scale in which minerals are classified in order of their increasing hardness. *SYN:* hardness scale

Molisch, Hans, Austrian chemist, 1856-1937.
Molisch test – a color test for sugar.

Moll, Jacob Anton, Dutch oculist, 1832-1914.
Moll glands – a number of modified apocrine sudoriferous glands in the eyelids, with ducts that usually open into the follicles of the eyelashes. *SYN:* ciliary glands

Mollaret, Pierre, French neurologist, 1898-1987.
Mollaret meningitis – *SYN:* Mollaret syndrome
Mollaret syndrome – recurrent benign viral infection. *SYN:* Mollaret meningitis; recurrent meningitis

Moloney, John B., 20th century U.S. oncologist.
Moloney virus – a lymphoid leukemia retrovirus of mice, in the subfamily Oncovirinae.

Moloney, Paul J., Canadian physician, 1870-1939.
Moloney test – detects a high degree of sensitivity to diphtheria toxoid.

Moloy, Howard C., U.S. obstetrician, 1903-1953.
Caldwell-Moloy classification – see under Caldwell, William E.

Monakow, Constantin von, Swiss histologist, 1853-1930.
Monakow bundle – *SYN:* Monakow tract
Monakow fasciculus – *SYN:* Monakow tract
Monakow fibers – *SYN:* Monakow tract
Monakow nucleus – a cell group lateral to the cuneate nucleus which receives posterior root fibers corresponding to the proprioceptive innervation of the arm and hand. *SYN:* accessory cuneate nucleus
Monakow syndrome – contralateral hemiplegia, hemianesthesia, and homonymous hemianopsia due to occlusion of the anterior choroidal artery.
Monakow tract – indirect increase in flexor muscle tone. *SYN:* Monakow bundle; Monakow fasciculus; Monakow fibers; rubrospinal tract

Mona Lisa, see under Lisa, Mona

Mönckeberg, (Moenckeberg), Johann G., German pathologist, 1877-1925.
Mönckeberg arteriosclerosis – involves the peripheral arteries with deposition of calcium in the medial coat but with little or no encroachment on the lumen. *SYN:* medial arteriosclerosis; Mönckeberg

calcification; Mönckeberg degeneration; Mönckeberg medial
calcification; Mönckeberg sclerosis; Mönckeberg syndrome
Mönckeberg calcification – *SYN:* Mönckeberg arteriosclerosis
Mönckeberg degeneration – *SYN:* Mönckeberg arteriosclerosis
Mönckeberg medial calcification – *SYN:* Mönckeberg arteriosclerosis
Mönckeberg sclerosis – *SYN:* Mönckeberg arteriosclerosis
Mönckeberg syndrome – *SYN:* Mönckeberg arteriosclerosis

Moncrieff, Alan Aird, English physician, *1901.
  Moncrieff cannula
  Moncrieff discission
  Moncrieff irrigator
  Moncrieff operation
  Moncrieff syndrome – autosomal recessive trait. *SYN:* Moncrieff-Wilkinson
    syndrome
  Moncrieff-Wilkinson syndrome – *SYN:* Moncrieff syndrome

Mondini, C., Italian physician, 1729-1803.
  Mondini deafness – congenital deafness.
  Mondini deformity

Mondonesi, Filippo, Italian physician.
  Mondonesi reflex – in the case of coma from severe apoplexy, pressure
    on the eyeballs causes contraction of the facial muscles of expression
    on the side opposite to the lesion; in coma due to diabetes, uremia, or
    other toxic cause, the reflex is present on both sides. *SYN:* bulbomimic
    reflex

Mondor, Henri Jean Justin, French surgeon, 1885-1962.
  Mondor disease – *SYN:* Mondor syndrome
  Mondor phlebitis – *SYN:* Mondor syndrome
  Mondor syndrome – thoracoepigastric vein phlebitis. *SYN:* Mondor
    disease; Mondor phlebitis; thrombophlebitis of the breast and chest wall

NOTES

Monge Medrano, Carlos, Peruvian professor of medicine and high altitude specialist, 1884-1970.
> **Monge disease** – loss of high-altitude tolerance after prolonged exposure. *SYN:* chronic mountain sickness; Monge syndrome
> **Monge syndrome** – *SYN:* Monge disease

Monheit, Gary D., 20th century U.S. dermatologist.
> **Monheit combination peel** – degreasing Jessner solution plus 35% trichloroacetic acid peel used to treat actinic keratoses, lentigines, and seborrheic keratoses.

Moniz, Antonio Caetano de Abgreu Freire Egas, Portuguese neurosurgeon and diplomat, 1874-1955, joint winner of 1949 Nobel Prize for work related to prefrontal lobotomy for treatment of certain psychoses.

Monneret, Jules Auguste Edward, French physician, 1810-1868.
> **Monneret pulse** – slow, soft, and full pulse.

Monod, Jacques L., French biochemist and Nobel laureate, 1910-1976.
> **Monod-Wyman-Changeux model** – used to explain the allosteric form of cooperativity. *SYN:* concerted model

Monro, Alexander, Jr., Scottish anatomist, 1733-1817.
> **Monro doctrine** – states that the cranial cavity is a closed box and that a change in the quantity of intracranial blood can occur only through the displacement of or replacement by cerebrospinal fluid. *SYN:* Monro-Kellie doctrine
> **Monro foramen** – the short passage that connects the third ventricle of the diencephalon with the lateral ventricles of the cerebral hemispheres. *SYN:* interventricular foramen
> **Monro-Kellie doctrine** – *SYN:* Monro doctrine
> **Monro line** – *SYN:* Monro-Richter line
> **Monro-Richter line** – passes from the umbilicus to the anterior superior iliac spine. *SYN:* Monro line; Richter-Monro line
> **Monro sulcus** – *SYN:* hypothalamic sulcus
> **Richter-Monro line** – *SYN:* Monro-Richter line

Monro, Alexander, Sr., Scottish anatomist and surgeon, 1697-1767.
> **bursa of Monro** – *SYN:* intratendinous bursa of elbow

Monsel, L., 19th century French army pharmacist.
> **Monsel solution** – ferric subsulfate solution used for hemostasis.

Monson, George S., U.S. dentist, 1869-1933.
> **anti-Monson curve** – in dentistry, a curve of occlusion which is convex upward. *SYN:* reverse curve

Monson curve – the curve of occlusion in which each cusp and incisal edge touches or conforms to a segment of the surface of a sphere 8 inches in diameter, with its center in the region of the glabella.

Monteggia, Giovanni Battista, Italian surgeon, 1762-1815.
Monteggia dislocation
Monteggia fracture – fracture of the ulna with dislocation of the radial head.
Monteggia lesion
reverse Monteggia fracture

Montessori, Maria, Italian psychiatrist and educator, 1870-1952.
Montessori school – program on self-education with emphasis on practical living.

Montgomery, H.
Montgomery disease – rare, benign, normolipemic condition featuring hundreds of yellowish papules on the skin and sometimes mucous membranes.

Montgomery, William Featherstone, Irish obstetrician, 1797-1859.
Montgomery follicles – *SYN:* Montgomery glands
Montgomery glands – a number of small mammary glands forming small rounded projections from the surface of the areola of the breast.
SYN: areolar glands; Montgomery follicles
Montgomery strap
Montgomery tubercles – elevated reddened areolar glands.
Montgomery vaginal speculum

Moon, Henry, English dental surgeon, 1845-1892.
Moon molars – small dome-shaped first molar teeth occurring in congenital syphilis.

Moon, Robert C., U.S. ophthalmologist, 1844-1914.
Laurence-Moon-Biedl syndrome – see under Laurence

NOTES

Moon, William, English inventor, 1818-1894.
Moon system – a touch-type alphabet for the blind. *SYN:* Moon type
Moon type – *SYN:* Moon system

Moore, Austin Talley, U.S. orthopedist and surgeon, 1899-1963.
Austin Moore arthroplasty
Austin Moore extractor
Austin Moore prosthesis

Moore, Charles H., English surgeon, 1821-1870.
Moore method – treatment of aneurysm.

Moore, Edward Mott, U.S. physician, 1814-1902.
Moore approach
Moore bone drill
Moore bone retractor
Moore driver
Moore elevator
Moore extractor
Moore forceps
Moore fracture
Moore hip prosthesis
Moore hollow chisel
Moore nail
Moore pin
Moore rasp
Moore stem
Moore technique
Moore template
Moore tube

Moore, Matthew T., U.S. neuropsychiatrist, *1901.
Moore syndrome – painful abdominal symptoms that may be followed by
seizures. *SYN:* abdominal epilepsy; visceral epilepsy

Moore, Robert Foster, English ophthalmologist, 1878-1963.
Moore lightning streaks – photopsia manifested by vertical flashes of
light caused by the involutional shrinkage of vitreous humor.

Mooren, Albert, German ophthalmologist, 1828-1899.
Mooren ulcer – chronic inflammation of the peripheral cornea that slowly
progresses centrally with corneal thinning and sometimes perforation.

Moorhouse, D.
Garland-Moorhouse syndrome – *SYN:* Marinesco-Sjögren syndrome

Mooser, Hermann, Swiss pathologist in Mexico, 1891-1971.
  Mooser bodies – a term used to refer to the rickettsiae found in the exudate and in tissue from the tunica vaginalis in endemic typhus fever (caused by *Rickettsia typhi*).
  Mooser cell

Morand, Sauveur F., French surgeon, 1697-1773.
  Morand foot – a foot having eight toes.
  Morand spur – the lower of two elevations on the medial wall of the posterior horn of the lateral ventricle of the brain. *SYN:* calcar avis

Morax, Victor, French ophthalmologist, 1866-1935.
  Morax-Axenfeld conjunctivitis – conjunctivitis caused by diplobacillus.
  Morax-Axenfeld diplobacillus – *SYN: Moraxella lacunata*
  Moraxella – a genus of obligately aerobic nonmotile bacteria (family Neisseriaceae) parasitic on the mucous membranes of humans and other mammals.
  Moraxella anatipestifer
  Moraxella bovis
  Moraxella lacunata – a species causing conjunctivitis. *SYN:* Morax-Axenfeld diplobacillus
  Moraxella liquefaciens
  Moraxella lwoffi
  Morax keratoplasty
  Morax operation

Morel, Bénédict A., French psychiatrist, 1809-1873.
  Kraepelin-Morel disease – see under Kraepelin
  Morel disease – alcohol withdrawal. *SYN:* delirium tremens
  Morel ear – a large, misshapen, outstanding auricle with obliterated grooves and thinned edges.
  Stewart-Morel syndrome – *SYN:* Morgagni syndrome

Morel, Ferdinand, Swiss physician, 1888-1957.
  Morel-Wildi syndrome – frontal cerebral cortex dysgenesis.

NOTES

Morelli, F., 20th century Italian physician.
    Morelli test – *SYN:* Moritz test

Morgagni, Giovanni Battista, Italian anatomist and pathologist, 1682-1771.
    frenulum of Morgagni – a fold running from the junction of the two commissures of the ileocecal valve on either side along the inner wall of the cecocolic junction. *SYN:* frenulum of ileocecal valve; Morgagni frenum; Morgagni retinaculum
    Morgagni-Adams-Stokes syndrome – *SYN:* Adams-Stokes syndrome
    morgagnian cyst – a vestigial remnant of the embryonic mesonephric duct. *SYN:* vesicular appendices of uterine tube
    Morgagni appendix – an inconstant narrow lobe of the thyroid gland. *SYN:* pyramidal lobe of thyroid gland
    Morgagni cartilage – a small nonarticulating rod of elastic cartilage in the aryepiglottic fold anterolateral and somewhat superior to the corniculate cartilage. *SYN:* cuneiform cartilage; Morgagni tubercle
    Morgagni caruncle – middle lobe of prostate.
    Morgagni cataract – a hypermature cataract in which the nucleus gravitates within the capsule. *SYN:* sedimentary cataract
    Morgagni columns – a number of vertical ridges in the mucous membrane of the upper half of the anal canal. *SYN:* anal columns
    Morgagni concha – the upper thin, spongy, bony plate projecting from the lateral wall of the nasal cavity, separating the superior meatus from the sphenoethmoidal recess. *SYN:* superior nasal concha
    Morgagni crypts – the grooves between the anal columns. *SYN:* anal sinuses
    Morgagni disease – *SYN:* Adams-Stokes syndrome
    Morgagni foramen – congenital defect in the fusion of sternal and costal elements of the diaphragmatic anlage that is the site of a parasternal hernia. *SYN:* foramen cecum of tongue
    Morgagni fossa – the terminal dilated portion of the urethra in the glans penis. *SYN:* Morgagni fovea; navicular fossa of the urethra
    Morgagni fovea – *SYN:* Morgagni fossa
    Morgagni frenum – *SYN:* frenulum of Morgagni
    Morgagni globules – vesicles beneath the capsule and between lens fibers in an early cataract. *SYN:* Morgagni spheres
    Morgagni hernia
    Morgagni humor – *SYN:* Morgagni liquor
    Morgagni hydatid – a vestigial remnant of the embryonic mesonephric duct. *SYN:* vesicular appendices of uterine tube

Morgagni lacuna – one of a number of little recesses in the mucous membrane of the spongy urethra into which empty the ducts of the urethral glands. *SYN:* urethral lacuna

Morgagni liquor – a fluid found postmortem between the epithelium and the fibers of the lens, resulting from the liquefaction of a semifluid material existing there during life. *SYN:* Morgagni humor

Morgagni nodule – a nodule at the center of the free border of each semilunar valve at the beginning of the pulmonary artery and aorta. *SYN:* nodule of semilunar valve

Morgagni prolapse – chronic inflammation of laryngeal ventricle.

Morgagni retinaculum – *SYN:* frenulum of Morgagni

Morgagni sinus – *SYN:* anal sinuses; laryngeal ventricle; prostatic utricle

Morgagni spheres – *SYN:* Morgagni globules

Morgagni syndrome – hyperostosis frontalis interna in elderly women, with obesity and neuropsychiatric disorders. *SYN:* metabolic craniopathy; Stewart-Morel syndrome

Morgagni tubercle – *SYN:* Morgagni cartilage

Morgagni valves – delicate crescent-shaped mucosal folds that pass between the lower ends of neighboring anal columns. *SYN:* anal valves

Morgagni ventricle – the recess in each lateral wall of the larynx between the vestibular and vocal folds and into which the laryngeal sacculus opens. *SYN:* laryngeal ventricle

Morgan, Campbell De, see under De Morgan

Morgan, D.B., 20th century U.S. dermatologist.
Dennie-Morgan fold – *SYN:* Morgan fold
Dennie-Morgan line – *SYN:* Morgan fold
Morgan fold – a double infraorbital fold seen in many atopic patients. *SYN:* Dennie-Morgan fold; Dennie-Morgan line; Morgan line
Morgan line – *SYN:* Morgan fold

Morgan, Harry de R., English physician, 1863-1931.
　Morgan bacillus – type (and only) species of the genus *Morganella.*
　　SYN: Morganella morganii

Morgan, Thomas Hunt, U.S. zoologist, 1866-1945, 1933 Nobel Prize winner for work related to chromosomes and their relation to heredity.

Mori, O., 20th century Japanese pathologist.
　Harada-Mori filter paper strip culture – filter paper, fecal specimen, and tap water placed in a centrifuge tube.

Morison, James Rutherford, English surgeon, 1853-1939.
　Morison incision
　Morison method
　Morison pouch – the deep recess of the peritoneal cavity on the right side. *SYN:* hepatorenal recess

Morita, Shomei, 20th century Japanese physician.
　Morita therapy – psychotherapy based on elements of conduct in Zen Buddhism.

Moritz, Friedrich Heinrich Ludwig, German physician, 1861-1938.
　Moritz reaction – *SYN:* Moritz test
　Moritz test – determines the difference between a transudate and an exudate. *SYN:* Morelli test; Moritz reaction; Rivalta reaction

Mörner, Karl A.H., Swedish chemist, 1855-1917.
　Mörner test – for cysteine and tyrosine.

Moro, Ernst, German physician, 1874-1951.
　Moro reflex – the reflex response of an infant when allowed to drop a short distance through the air or startled by a sudden noise or jolt. *SYN:* startle reflex

Morquio, Louis, Uruguayan physician, 1867-1935.
　Brailsford-Morquio disease – *SYN:* Morquio syndrome
　Morquio disease – *SYN:* Morquio syndrome
　Morquio sign
　Morquio syndrome – an error of mucopolysaccharide metabolism characterized by severe skeletal defects. *SYN:* Brailsford-Morquio disease; Morquio disease; Morquio-Ullrich disease; type IV A, B mucopolysaccharidosis
　Morquio-Ullrich disease – *SYN:* Morquio syndrome

Morris, Sir Henry, English surgeon, 1844-1926.
　Morris biphase screw
　Morris cannula

Morris catheter
Morris clamp
Morris drain
Morris incision
Morris retractor
Morris splint

Morrison, Ashton B., Irish pathologist in the U.S., *1922.
Verner-Morrison syndrome – see under Verner

Morrow, Prince Albert, U.S. physician, 1846-1913.
Morrow-Brooke syndrome – *SYN:* Brooke disease (2)

Morsier, G. de, see under de Morsier

Mortensen, Ole, Danish physician.
Mortensen syndrome – *SYN:* Di Guglielmo syndrome (2)

Mortimer, Mrs., female patient for whom the malady is named.
Mortimer disease – *SYN:* Mortimer malady
Mortimer malady – skin disease. *SYN:* Mortimer disease

Morton, Dudley J., U.S. orthopedist, 1884-1960.
Morton syndrome – congenital shortening of the first metatarsal, causing metatarsalgia.

Morton, Richard, English physician, 1637-1698.
Morton cough – associated with tuberculosis.

Morton, Samuel G., U.S. physician, 1799-1851.
Morton plane – passes through the summits of the parietal and occipital protuberances.

Morton, Thomas George, U.S. physician, 1835-1903.
Morton bandage
Morton disease – *SYN:* Morton neuralgia
Morton foot – *SYN:* Morton neuralgia
Morton interdigital neuroma

M

NOTES

Morton nerve entrapment syndrome – *SYN:* Morton neuralgia
Morton neuralgia – neuralgia of an interdigital nerve. *SYN:* Morton disease; Morton foot; Morton neuroma; Morton nerve entrapment syndrome; Morton toe
Morton neuroma – *SYN:* Morton neuralgia
Morton ophthalmoscope
Morton sign
Morton test
Morton toe – *SYN:* Morton neuralgia
Morton toe support

Morvan, Augustin Marie, French physician, 1819-1897.
Morvan chorea – continuous involuntary quivering of muscles at rest. *SYN:* myokymia
Morvan disease – the presence of longitudinal cavities in the spinal cord. *SYN:* Morvan syndrome; syringomyelia
Morvan syndrome – *SYN:* Morvan disease

Moschcowitz, Alexis Victor, U.S. surgeon, 1865-1933.
Moschcowitz enterocele repair
Moschcowitz operation – femoral hernia repair.

Moschcowitz, Eli, U.S. physician, 1879-1964.
Moschcowitz disease – *SYN:* hemolytic thrombocytopenic purpura
Moschcowitz-Singer-Symmers syndrome – *SYN:* Moschcowitz syndrome
Moschcowitz syndrome – acute febrile pleiochromic anemia with hyaline thrombosis of terminal arterioles and capillaries *SYN:* Baehr-Schiffrin disease; Moschcowitz-Singer-Symmers syndrome
Moschcowitz test – for arteriosclerosis.

Mosenthal, Herman Otto, U.S. physician, 1878-1954.
Mosenthal test – to evaluate renal concentrating ability.

Mosher, Clelia D., U.S. physician, 1863-1940.
Mosher exercises – for dysmenorrhea.

Mosler, Karl F., German physician, 1831-1911.
Mosler diabetes – inosituria with excretion of large quantities of water.
Mosler sign – tenderness over the sternum in a patient with acute myeloblastic anemia.

Moss, Gerald, U.S. physician, 1931-1973.
Moss decompression feeding catheter
Moss G-tube PEG kit
Moss PEG kit

Moss T-anchor needle
Moss tube

Moss, Melvin Lionel, U.S. oral pathologist, *1923.
    Gorlin-Chaudhry-Moss syndrome – see under Gorlin, Robert James

Moss, William Lorenzo, U.S. physician, 1876-1957.
    Moss classification – a classification of ABO blood types.

Mosse, Max, German internist, 1873-1936.
    Mosse polycythemia – *SYN:* Mosse syndrome
    Mosse syndrome – cirrhosis of the liver with polycythemia vera.
       SYN: liver cirrhosis; Mosse polycythemia

Mosso, Angelo, Italian physiologist, 1846-1910.
    Mosso ergograph – an instrument used to obtain a graphic record of
    flexion of a finger, hand, or arm.
    Mosso sphygmomanometer – an apparatus for measuring the blood
    pressure in the digital arteries.

Moszkowicz, Ludwig, Austrian surgeon, 1873-1945.
    Moszkowicz test – for arteriosclerosis. *SYN:* hyperemia test

Motais, Ernst, French ophthalmologist, 1845-1913.
    Motais operation – transplantation of the middle third of the tendon of the
    superior rectus muscle of the eyeball into the upper lid to supplement the
    action of the levator muscle in ptosis.

Mounier-Kuhn, P., 20th century French physician.
    Mounier-Kuhn syndrome – congenital widening of the trachea and
    bronchi. *SYN:* tracheobronchomegaly

Mount, Lester Adrian, U.S. physician, *1910.
    Mount-Reback syndrome – autosomal dominant disorder, with multiple
    anomalies. *SYN:* familial paroxysmal choreoathetosis; paroxysmal
    kinesigenic choreoathetosis

M

NOTES

Moynahan, E.J., 20th century English physician.
  Moynahan syndrome – familial congenital disorder characterized by multiple anomalies. *SYN:* progressive cardiomyopathic lentiginosis

Moynihan, Lord Berkeley George Andrew, English surgeon, 1865-1936.
  Moynihan clamp
  Moynihan clip
  Moynihan forceps
  Moynihan gutter – right paracolic gutter.
  Moynihan incision
  Moynihan position
  Moynihan probe
  Moynihan respirator
  Moynihan scoop
  Moynihan speculum

Mozart, Wolfgang Amadeus, Austrian composer, 1756-1791.
  Mozart ear – fusion of the large portion of the anthelix with the helix.

Much, Hans C.R., German physician, 1880-1932.
  Much bacillus – the form present in the tuberculous skin lesions.

Mucha, Victor, Austrian dermatologist, 1877-1919.
  Mucha-Habermann disease – an acute dermatitis affecting children and young adults. *SYN:* Mucha-Habermann syndrome; pityriasis lichenoides et varioliformis acuta
  Mucha-Habermann syndrome – *SYN:* Mucha-Habermann disease

Muckle, Thomas James, 20th century Canadian pediatrician.
  Muckle-Wells syndrome – a syndrome characterized by familial amyloidosis.

Muehrcke, Robert C., U.S. nephrologist, d. 2003.
  Muehrcke lines – white lines parallel with the lunula and separated from each other by normal pink areas, associated with hypoalbuminemia.

Müeller, R.
  Müeller-Kugelberg syndrome – muscle degeneration caused by steroid use. *SYN:* steroid myopathy

Muir, Edward G., English surgeon, 1906-1973.
  Muir-Torre syndrome – *SYN:* Torre syndrome

Mulder, Gerardus Johann, Dutch chemist, 1802-1880.
  Mulder test – for glucose. *SYN:* xanthoproteic reaction

Mulder, Johannes, Dutch anatomist, 1769-1810.
Mulder angle – a facial angle.

Mules, Philip H., English ophthalmologist, 1843-1905.
Mules eye implant
Mules graft
Mules operation – evisceration of the eyeball followed by the insertion within the sclera of a spherical prosthesis to support an artificial eye.
Mules prosthesis
Mules scoop

Müller, Friedrich von, German physician, 1858-1941.
Müller sign – rhythmic movements of the uvula, accompanied by redness and swelling of the velum palati and tonsils in aortic insufficiency.

Müller, Heinrich, German anatomist, 1820-1864.
Müller fibers – (1) circular fibers; (2) sustentacular neuroglial cells of the retina. *SYN:* Müller radial cells
Müller muscle – *SYN:* circular fibers; orbitalis muscle; superior tarsal muscle
Müller radial cells – *SYN:* Müller fibers (2)
Müller trigone – the floor of the supraoptic recess of the third ventricle.

Müller, Hermann F., German histologist, 1866-1898.
formol-Müller fixative – contains 2% commercial formalin.

Muller, Hermann Joseph, U.S. biologist and geneticist, 1890-1967, winner of the 1947 Nobel Prize for work related to x-ray mutations.
Muller-Hinton agar – medium containing beef infusion, peptone, and starch.

Müller, Johannes P., German anatomist, physiologist, and pathologist, 1801-1858.
Müller capsule – the expanded beginning of a nephron composed of an inner and outer layer. *SYN:* glomerular capsule

M

NOTES

Müller duct – either of the two paired embryonic tubes extending along the mesonephros. *SYN:* paramesonephric duct

Müller law – each type of sensory nerve ending gives rise to its own specific sensation. *SYN:* law of specific nerve energies

Müller maneuver – the reverse of the Valsalva maneuver.

Müller tubercle – the first evidence of the embryonic uterus and vagina. *SYN:* sinus tubercle

Müller, Peter, German obstetrician, 1836-1922.
  Hillis-Müller maneuver – see under Hillis

Müller, Walther, 20th century German physicist.
  Geiger-Müller counter – see under Geiger
  Geiger-Müller tube

Mulvihill, John J., 20th century U.S. pediatrician.
  Mulvihill-Smith syndrome – an autosomal recessive syndrome characterized by delayed physical and mental development, premature aging, birdlike facies, multiple pigmented nevi, and late immunodeficiency.

Münchausen, Baron Karl Friedrich Hieronymus von, German soldier and adventurer, 1720-1797.
  Münchausen by proxy syndrome – a parent, usually knowledgeable about or experienced in health care, harming a child in order to gain the attention of healthcare providers.
  Münchausen syndrome – repeated fabrication of clinically convincing simulations of disease for the purpose of gaining medical attention. *SYN:* Albatross syndrome

Munchmeyer, Ernst, German physician, 1846-1880.
  Munchmeyer disease – diffuse and progressive ossifying polymyositis.

Mundinger, F., German neurosurgeon, *1924.
  Riechert-Mundinger apparatus – see under Riechert
  Riechert-Mundinger technique – see under Riechert

Munk, Fritz, German physician, *1879.
  Munk disease – kidney disease.

Munro, John C., U.S. surgeon, 1858-1910.
  Munro point – a point at the right edge of the rectus abdominis muscle where pressure elicits tenderness in appendicitis.

Munro, William John, Australian dermatologist, 1863-1903.
  Munro abscess – *SYN:* Munro microabscess

Munro microabscess – microscopic collection of polymorphonuclear leukocytes found in the stratum corneum in psoriasis. *SYN:* Munro abscess

Munro Kerr, John Martin, Scottish obstetrician and gynecologist, 1868-1955.
Munro Kerr cesarean section – *SYN:* Munro Kerr section
Munro Kerr incision
Munro Kerr maneuver
Munro Kerr section – cesarean section that opens the lower uterine segment transversely without displacing the bladder. *SYN:* Munro Kerr cesarean section

Munsell, Albert Henry, U.S. painter, 1858-1918.
Farnsworth-Munsell color test – see under Farnsworth
Munsell color system – method of color notation.

Munsell, Hazel E., U.S. chemist, *1891.
Sherman-Munsell unit – see under Sherman, Henry C.

Munson, Edward Sterling, U.S. ophthalmologist, *1933.
Munson sign – abnormal bulging of the lower eyelid.

Münzer, Egmont, Austrian physician, 1865-1924.
tract of Münzer and Wiener – a fiber bundle arising in the superior colliculus and ending in the lateral part of the gray matter of the ventral part of the pons. *SYN:* tectopontine tract

Murad, Ferid, U.S. physician, *1936, joint winner of 1998 Nobel Prize for work related to nitric oxide as a signal molecule in biological systems.

Murat, Louis, French physician, *1874.
Murat sign – in tuberculosis patients.

Murchison, Charles, English physician, 1830-1879.
Murchison-Pel-Ebstein syndrome – multiple symptoms of fever, sweats, etc., generally related to malignancy.

M

Muret, Paul-Louis, French physician, *1878.
  Quénu-Muret sign – see under Quénu

Murphy, John B., U.S. surgeon, 1857-1916.
  Murphy approach
  Murphy bone lever
  Murphy bone skid
  Murphy brace
  Murphy button – mechanical device used for intestinal anastomosis.
  Murphy chisel
  Murphy dilator
  Murphy drip – *SYN:* proctoclysis
  Murphy forceps
  Murphy gouge
  Murphy hook
  Murphy knife
  Murphy-Lane bone skid
  Murphy light
  Murphy method
  Murphy needle
  Murphy percussion – *SYN:* piano percussion
  Murphy punch
  Murphy reamer
  Murphy retractor
  Murphy scissors
  Murphy sign – right upper quadrant pain on inspiration.
  Murphy splint
  Murphy tube

Murphy, William Parry, U.S. physician, *1892, joint winner of 1934 Nobel Prize for work related to anemia.
  Minot-Murphy diet – see under Minot

Murray, John, English physician, 1843-1873.
  Murray-Puretic-Drescher syndrome – autosomal recessive trait characterized by albinism, bleeding tendency, and other related abnormalities.

Murray, Joseph E., U.S. plastic surgeon, *1919, joint winner of 1990 Nobel Prize for work related to cell and organ transplantation.

Murray Valley, location in Australia where epidemics occurred in 1950 and 1951.
  Murray Valley disease – *SYN:* Murray Valley encephalitis

Murray Valley encephalitis – a severe encephalitis with high mortality. *SYN:* Australian X disease; Australian X encephalitis; Murray Valley disease

Murray Valley virus – a group B arbovirus that causes Murray Valley encephalitis. *SYN:* Australian X disease virus; MVE virus

Murri, A.

Murri disease

Murri syndrome – cerebellar degeneration. *SYN:* cerebellar ataxia

Musset, L.C. Alfred de, French poet, 1810-1857.

de Musset sign – *SYN:* Musset sign

Musset sign – in incompetence of the aortic valve, rhythmical nodding of the head, synchronous with the heart beat. *SYN:* de Musset sign

Mustard, William T., Canadian thoracic surgeon, 1914-1987.

Mustard operation – correction at the atrial level of hemodynamic abnormality due to transposition of the great arteries. *SYN:* Mustard procedure

Mustard procedure – *SYN:* Mustard operation

Myerson, Abraham, U.S. neurologist, 1881-1948.

Myerson sign – a sign of Parkinson disease.

Naboth, Martin, German anatomist and physician, 1675-1721.
  nabothian cyst – a retention cyst that develops when a mucous gland of the cervix uteri is obstructed. *SYN:* nabothian follicle
  nabothian follicle – *SYN:* nabothian cyst
  nabothian gland

Naegeli, Oskar, Swiss physician, 1885-1959.
  Naegeli syndrome – reticular skin pigmentation, diminished sweating, hypodontia, and hyperkeratosis of the palms and soles.
  SYN: Franceschetti-Jadassohn syndrome

Naegeli, Otto, Swiss physician, 1871-1938.
  Glanzmann-Naegeli syndrome – *SYN:* Glanzmann thrombasthenia
  Naegeli monocytic leukemia – a variant of granulocytic leukemia with monocytosis in the peripheral blood. *SYN:* myelomonocytic leukemia

Naffziger, Howard C., U.S. surgeon, 1884-1961.
  Naffziger operation – orbital decompression for severe malignant exophthalmos.
  Naffziger syndrome – *SYN:* Adson syndrome (1); scalenus-anticus syndrome
  Naffziger test

Nagel, Willibald A., German ophthalmologist and physiologist, 1870-1911.
  Nagel test – a test for color vision.

Nägele, Franz K., German obstetrician, 1777-1851.
  Nägele maneuver
  Nägele obliquity – inclination of the fetal head in cases of flat pelvis, the anterior parietal bone presenting to the parturient canal. *SYN:* anterior asynclitism
  Nägele pelvis – an obliquely contracted or unilateral synostotic pelvis.

NOTES

Nägele rule – estimates date of delivery by counting back three months from the first day of the last menstrual period and adding seven days.

Nageotte, Jean, French histologist, 1866-1948.
Babinski-Nageotte syndrome – see under Babinski
Nageotte bracelets
Nageotte cells – found in the cerebrospinal fluid.

Nager, Felix Robert, Swiss otorhinolaryngologist, 1877-1959.
Nager acrofacial dysostosis
Nager-de Reynier syndrome – *SYN:* Treacher Collins syndrome
Nager sign

Nagler, F.P.O., 20th century Australian bacteriologist.
Nagler reaction

Nagler, Joseph, Austrian radiologist, *1910.
Nagler effect
Nagler test

Nagyrapolt, Albert Szent-György von, winner of 1937 Nobel Prize for work related to regulation of respiration.

Najjar, Victor A., U.S. physician and biochemist, *1914.
Crigler-Najjar disease – *SYN:* Crigler-Najjar syndrome
Crigler-Najjar syndrome – see under Crigler

Nakagawa, K., Japanese dermatologist.
Nakagawa angioma – rare type of angioma, with onset during infancy.

Nakanishi, Kazuhiro, Japanese physician, *1945.
Nakanishi stain – a method for vital staining of bacteria.

Nakib, Ahmad, Lebanese medical resident who developed a mechanical heart valve with Clarence Walton Lillehei.
Lillehei-Nakib toroidal valve – see under Lillehei

Nance, Walter E., U.S. physician.
Nance deafness – *SYN:* Nance syndrome
Nance dwarfism – *SYN:* Nance-Sweeney syndrome
Nance-Horan syndrome – X-linked trait with multiple congenital abnormalities. *SYN:* X-linked cataract-dental syndrome
Nance-Sweeney syndrome – autosomal recessive inheritance. *SYN:* Nance dwarfism
Nance syndrome – X-linked characteristic of multiple otologic abnormalities. *SYN:* Nance deafness

Nanta, Andre, French dermatologist, 1883-1966.

Gandy-Nanta disease – see under Gandy

Napalkov, A.V., Russian neurophysiologist.
Napalkov phenomenon – conditioned reflex response in which fear increases instead of decreases when stimulus is removed.

Napier, John, Scottish mathematician, 1550-1617.
napier – unit for comparing the magnitude of two powers, usually in electricity or acoustics; it is one half of the natural logarithm of the ratio of the two powers. *SYN:* neper (Np)

Narcissus, Greek mythological youth who refused all offers of love.
narcissism – self-love, which may include sexual attraction toward oneself. *SYN:* self-love

Nasmyth, Alexander, English dentist, 1789-1849.
Nasmyth cuticle – two extremely thin layers covering the entire crown of newly erupted teeth and subsequently abraded by mastication. *SYN:* enamel cuticle; Nasmyth membrane
Nasmyth membrane – *SYN:* Nasmyth cuticle

Nasse, Christian Friedrich, German physician, 1788-1851.
Millon-Nasse test – see under Millon

Nasu, T., Japanese pathologist, 1915-1996.
Nasu disease – autosomal recessive disorder characterized by lipodystrophy, sclerosing leukoencephalopathy, and skeletal abnormalities. *SYN:* membranous lipodystrophy; Nasu-Hakola disease
Nasu-Hakola disease – *SYN:* Nasu disease

Nathans, Daniel, joint winner of 1978 Nobel Prize for work related to restriction of enzymes.

Nauheim, from Bad Nauheim, a German spa.
Nauheim bath – *SYN:* Nauheim treatment
Nauheim treatment – treatment of certain cardiac affections by baths in water through which carbonic acid gas is bubbling, followed by resistance exercises. *SYN:* Nauheim bath; Schott treatment

NOTES

Nauta, Walle J.H., U.S. neuroscientist, *1916.
Nauta stain – for degenerating axons.

Nazzaro, P., Italian dermatologist, 1921-1975.
Nazzaro syndrome – paraneoplastic syndrome with clinical findings of pityriasis rubra pilaris and keratosis pilaris.

Necker, Louis, Swiss physicist and mathematician, 1730-1804.
Necker cube – line drawing in which 12 angles of the cube are visible.

Needles, Carl F., U.S. pediatrician, *1935.
Melnick-Needles syndrome – see under Melnick, John C.

Needles, J.W., U.S. dentist.
Needles split cast method – a procedure for placing indexed casts on an articulator to facilitate their removal and replacement on the instrument. *SYN:* split cast method

Neel, A.V., Scandinavian physician.
Bing-Neel syndrome – see under Bing, J.

Neelsen, Friedrich K.A., German pathologist, 1854-1894.
Ziehl-Neelsen stain – see under Ziehl

Neftel, William B., U.S. neurologist, 1830-1906.
Neftel disease – paresthesia of the head and trunk and extreme discomfort in any but the recumbent position.

Negri, Adelchi, Italian physician, 1876-1912.
Negri bodies – pathognomonic inclusion bodies found in the cytoplasm of certain nerve cells containing the rabies virus. *SYN:* Negri corpuscles
Negri corpuscles – *SYN:* Negri bodies

Negro, Camillo, Italian neurologist, 1861-1927.
Negro cogwheel rigidity – *SYN:* Negro phenomenon
Negro phenomenon – a sudden brief halt in usually smooth respiration or other motor activity. *SYN:* cogwheel phenomenon; Negro cogwheel rigidity; Negro rigidity
Negro rigidity – *SYN:* Negro phenomenon

Neher, Erwin, German biophysicist, *1944, joint winner of 1991 Nobel Prize for work related to ion channels in the cell.

Neisser, Albert Ludwig S., German physician, 1855-1916.
Neisser coccus – *SYN: Neisseria gonorrhoeae*
Neisser diplococcus
Neisseria – a genus of aerobic to facultatively anaerobic bacteria (family Neisseriaceae) that are parasites of animals.

Neisseria catarrhalis
Neisseria flavescens
Neisseria gonorrhoeae – a species that causes gonorrhea in humans.
   SYN: Neisser coccus
Neisseria lactamica
Neisseria meningitidis
Neisseria mucosa
Neisseria sicca
Neisseria subflava
Neisser syringe – a urethral syringe used in treatment of gonococcal
   urethritis.

Neisser, Max, German bacteriologist, 1869-1938.
   Neisser stain – for the polar nuclei of the diphtheria bacillus.

Nélaton, Auguste, French surgeon, 1807-1873.
   Nélaton bullet probe
   Nélaton catheter
   Nélaton dislocation – wedging of the astragalus between the widely
      separated tibia and fibula, usually complicated with fracture.
   Nélaton drain
   Nélaton fibers – *SYN:* Nélaton sphincter
   Nélaton fold
   Nélaton line – a line drawn from the anterior superior iliac spine to the
      tuberosity of the ischium. *SYN:* Roser-Nélaton line
   Nélaton operation
   Nélaton sphincter – the middle rectal fold. *SYN:* Nélaton fibers
   Nélaton syndrome – hereditary neuropathy. *SYN:* Denny-Brown syndrome
   Roser-Nélaton line – *SYN:* Nélaton line

Nelson, Don H., U.S. internist, *1925.
   Nelson syndrome – hyperpigmentation, third nerve damage, and
      enlarging sella turcica caused by pituitary adenomas that become
      symptomatic following adrenalectomy. *SYN:* postadrenalectomy syndrome

N

NOTES

Nelson tumor – a pituitary tumor causing the symptoms of Nelson syndrome.

Nelson, R.S., 20th century U.S. physician.
Sprinz-Nelson syndrome – *SYN:* Dubin-Johnson syndrome

Némethy, George, Hungarian-U.S. biochemist, *1934.
Adair-Koshland-Némethy-Filmer model – *SYN:* Koshland-Némethy-Filmer model
Koshland-Némethy-Filmer model – see under Koshland

Nencki, Marcellus von, Polish physician, 1847-1901.
Nencki test – for indole.

Néri, Vincenzo, Italian neurologist, *1882.
Néri sign – a sign of organic hemiplegia.

Nernst, Walther, German physicist and Nobel laureate, 1864-1941.
Nernst equation – the equation relating the electrical potential and concentration gradient of an ion across a permeable membrane at equilibrium.
Nernst potential
Nernst theory – that the passage of an electric current through tissues causes a dissociation of the ions.

Nessler, A., German chemist, 1827-1905.
Nessler reagent – a solution of potassium hydroxide, mercuric iodide, and potassium iodide.

Netherton, Earl Weldon, U.S. dermatologist, *1893.
Comèl-Netherton syndrome – *SYN:* Netherton syndrome
Netherton syndrome – brittle hair; atopic manifestations. *SYN:* Comèl-Netherton syndrome; congenital ichthyosiform erythroderma

Nettleship, Edward, English ophthalmologist and dermatologist, 1845-1913.
Nettleship dilator
Nettleship iris repositor
Nettleship syndrome – pigmented nodules or macules. *SYN:* urticaria pigmentosa

Neu, Richard L., U.S. scientist.
Neu-Laxová syndrome – multiple birth defects. *SYN:* Neu syndrome
Neu syndrome – *SYN:* Neu-Laxová syndrome

Neubauer, Johann E., German anatomist, 1742-1777.
Neubauer artery – *SYN:* thyroid ima artery
Neubauer ruled hemacytometer

Neufeld, Alonzo John, U.S. orthopedic surgeon, *1906.
Neufeld apparatus
Neufeld cast
Neufeld driver
Neufeld dynamic method
Neufeld femoral nail plate
Neufeld nail
Neufeld pin
Neufeld plate
Neufeld screw
Neufeld traction
Neufeld tractor

Neufeld, Ferdinand, German bacteriologist, 1869-1945.
Neufeld capsular swelling – increase in opacity and visibility of the capsule of capsulated organisms exposed to specific agglutinating anticapsular antibodies. *SYN:* Neufeld quellung reaction; Neufeld reaction; quellung phenomenon; quellung reaction; quellung test
Neufeld quellung reaction – *SYN:* Neufeld capsular swelling
Neufeld reaction – *SYN:* Neufeld capsular swelling

Neugebauer, H., German physician.
Karsch-Neugebauer syndrome – see under Karsch

Neuhauser, Edward Blaine, U.S. physician, *1908.
Neuhauser-Berenberg syndrome – excessive vomiting in children. *SYN:* cardioesophageal relaxation syndrome

Neumann, Ernst F.C., German histologist, anatomist, and pathologist, 1834-1918.
Neumann cells – nucleated cells in the bone marrow developing into red blood cells.
Neumann sheath – a layer of tissue relatively resistant to the action of acids, which forms the walls of the dentinal tubules. *SYN:* dentinal sheath

N

Neumann syndrome – muscle cell tumor in infants *SYN:* neonatal myoblastoma

Rouget-Neumann sheath – see under Rouget, Charles M.B.

Neumann, Franz E., German physicist, 1798-1895.

Charcot-Neumann crystals – *SYN:* Charcot-Leyden crystals

Neumann law – in compounds of analogous chemical constitution, the molecular heat, or the product of the specific heat by the atomic weight, is always the same.

Neumann, Isidor Edler von Heilwart, Austrian dermatologist, 1832-1906.

Neumann disease – a form of pemphigus vulgaris in which vegetations develop on the eroded surfaces left by ruptured bullae. *SYN:* pemphigus vegetans

Neumann, M.A.

Neumann syndrome – inherited dementia. *SYN:* familial dementia

Neumann-Neurode, Detleff, German physical educator, 1879-1945.

Neumann-Neurode exercises – exercises for children from the age of 4 months.

Neusser, Edmund von, Austrian physician, 1852-1912.

Neusser granules – tiny basophilic granules sometimes observed in an indistinct zone about the nucleus of a leukocyte.

Neve, Ernest Frederic, English physician, 1861-1941.

Neve cancer – epithelioma caused by heat and substances of kangri when worn against the skin. *SYN:* kangri burn cancer

Newcastle, a community in England near the location where Newcastle disease was first observed.

Newcastle disease – an influenzalike disease of birds that is transmissible to man if in contact with diseased birds. *SYN:* avian influenza; Ranikhet disease

Newton, Sir Isaac, English physicist, 1642-1727.

newton – derived unit of force in the SI system.

Newton disk – a disk on which there are seven colored sectors, which, when rapidly rotated, appear white.

newtonian aberration – the difference in focus or magnification of an image arising because of a difference in the refraction of different wavelengths composing white light. *SYN:* chromatic aberration

newtonian constant of gravitation – a universal constant relating the gravitational force, attracting two masses toward each other when they are separated by a distance.

newtonian flow – the type of flow characteristic of a newtonian fluid.

newtonian fluid – a fluid in which flow and rate of shear are always proportional to the applied stress.

newtonian viscosity – the viscosity characteristics of a newtonian fluid.

Newton law – the attractive force between any two bodies is proportional to the product of their masses and inversely proportional to the square of the distance between their centers. *SYN:* law of gravitation

Newton rings – colored rings on thin surfaces.

Nezelof, C., French pathologist, *1922.

Nezelof syndrome – type of thymic alymphoplasia. *SYN:* cellular immunodeficiency with abnormal immunoglobulin synthesis

Nickerson, Walter J., U.S. microbiologist.

Nickerson-Kveim test – *SYN:* Kveim antigen

Nicol, William, Scottish physicist, 1768-1851.

Nicol prism – transmits only polarized light.

Nicolas, Joseph, French physician, 1868-1960.

Favre-Durand-Nicolas disease – *SYN:* Durand disease

Nicolas-Favre disease – venereal infection usually caused by *Chlamydia trachomatis*. *SYN:* venereal lymphogranuloma

Nicolas-Moutot-Charlet syndrome – congenital mucocutaneous disease.

Nicolau, Stefan George, Romanian physician

Nicolau syndrome – accidental intra-arterial injection resulting in embolization. *SYN:* embolia cutis medicamentosa

Nicolle, J.H., French microbiologist and Nobel laureate, 1866-1936.

Nicolle stain for capsules – mixture of a saturated solution of gentian violet in alcohol-phenol.

Nicolle white mycetoma – mycetoma caused by a species of *Aspergillus*.

Nielsen, Holger, Danish army officer, 1866-1955.

Nielsen method – a method of artificial respiration.

Nielsen, Johannes Mygaard, U.S. physician, 1890-1969.
Nielsen I syndrome – excessive weakness caused by physical exhaustion. *SYN:* neuromuscular exhaustion
Nielsen II syndrome – apathy, akinesia, mutism, and incontinence.

Niemann, Albert, German physician, 1880-1921.
Niemann disease – *SYN:* Niemann-Pick disease
Niemann-Pick cell – *SYN:* Pick cell
Niemann-Pick disease – lipid histiocytosis that occurs most commonly in Jewish infants and leads to early death. *SYN:* Niemann disease; sphingomyelin lipidosis
Niemann splenomegaly – enlargement of spleen occurring in Niemann-Pick disease.

Nierhoff, H.
Nierhoff-Huebner syndrome – convulsion, somnolence, and muscular flaccidity. *SYN:* endochondral dysostosis

Nievergelt, Kurt, Swiss physician, *1913.
Nievergelt-Erb syndrome – *SYN:* Nievergelt syndrome
Nievergelt-Pearlman syndrome – *SYN:* Nievergelt syndrome
Nievergelt syndrome – rare bone disease characterized by multiple deformities. *SYN:* Nievergelt-Erb syndrome; Nievergelt-Pearlman syndrome

Niewenglowski, Gaston H., 19th century French scientist.
Niewenglowski rays – radiation emitted from a phosphorescent body after exposure to sunlight.

Niikawa, Norio, Japanese geneticist and physician, *1942.
Niikawa-Kuroki syndrome – causes facial characteristics that are similar in appearance to traditional Kabuki theater makeup. *SYN:* Kabuki makeup syndrome

Nikiforoff, Mikhail, Russian dermatologist, 1858-1915.
Nikiforoff method – for the fixing of blood films.

Nikolsky, Pyotr V., Russian dermatologist, 1858-1940.
Nikolsky sign – a peculiar vulnerability of the skin in pemphigus vulgaris.

Nipah, village in Malaysia where the first human case was detected in 1999.
Nipah virus – a paramyxovirus with features of encephalitis and meningitis; spread from swine to humans.

Nirenberg, Marshall W., U.S. biochemist, *1927, joint winner of 1968 Nobel Prize for work related to genetic code.

Nisbet, William, English physician, 1759-1822.
Nisbet chancre – chancre with lymphangitis; abscesses of the penis.

Nishimoto, A., Japanese physician.
Nishimoto disease – vascular syndrome. *SYN:* Nishimoto-Takeuchi syndrome
Nishimoto-Takeuchi syndrome – *SYN:* Nishimoto disease

Nissen, Rudolf, Swiss surgeon, 1896-1981.
Nissen forceps
Nissen fundoplication
Nissen gastrectomy
Nissen hiatal hernia repair
Nissen operation
Nissen procedure
Nissen rib spreader
Nissen suture

Nissl, Franz, German neurologist, 1860-1919.
Nissl bodies – *SYN:* Nissl substance
Nissl degeneration –cell body degeneration occurring after transection of the axon.
Nissl granules – *SYN:* Nissl substance
Nissl methods – staining techniques.
Nissl stain – a method for staining nerve cells.
Nissl substance – the material consisting of granular endoplasmic reticulum and ribosomes that occurs in nerve cell bodies and dendrites. *SYN:* basophil substance; Nissl bodies; Nissl granules; substantia basophilia; tigroid bodies

Nitabuch, Raissa, 19th century German physician.
Nitabuch layer – *SYN:* Nitabuch membrane
Nitabuch membrane – a layer of fibrin between the boundary zone of compact endometrium and the cytotrophoblastic shell in the placenta. *SYN:* Nitabuch layer; Nitabuch stria

NOTES

Nitabuch stria – *SYN:* Nitabuch membrane

Noack, Margot, German physician, *1909.
Noack syndrome – multiple congenital malformations.
SYN: acrocephalopolysyndactyly

Nobel, Alfred B., Swedish chemist and philanthropist, 1833-1896.
nobelium (No) – an unstable transuranium element, atomic no. 102.
Nobel Prize – award to honor contributions to world peace, literature, economics, physiology, medicine, chemistry, and physics.

Noble, Charles P., U.S. gynecologist, 1863-1935.
Noble position – patient standing and bent slightly forward.

Noble, Robert L., Canadian physiologist, *1910.
Noble-Collip procedure – obsolete procedure in which shock in rats is induced by rotating them in a drum.

Nocard, Edmund I.E., French veterinarian, 1850-1903.
Nocardia – a genus of aerobic nonmotile actinomycetes (family Nocardiaceae, order Actinomycetales), transitional between bacteria and fungi, which are mainly saprophytic but may produce disease in human beings and other animals.
Nocardia brasiliensis
Nocardiaceae – a family of acid-fast, gram-positive, aerobic bacteria (order Actinomycetales) that includes the genus *Nocardia*.
Nocardia **dacryoliths** – white pseudoconcretions, composed of masses of *Nocardia* species found in the lacrimal canaliculi. *SYN:* Desmarres dacryoliths
Nocardiasis bovine farcy
nocardiosis – a pulmonary or brain infection that is caused by *Nocardia asteroides*.
Preisz-Nocard bacillus – see under Preisz

Noguchi, Hideyo, Japanese pathologist, 1876-1928.
Noguchia – a genus of aerobic to facultatively anaerobic, motile, peritrichous bacteria.
Noguchia granulosis – a bacterial species sometimes regarded as a cause of trachoma in humans.
Noguchi test – for globulin.

Nomarski, Georges, 20th century French optical inventor.
Nomarski optics – system for differential interference contrast microscopy.

Nonne, Max, German physician, 1861-1959.
Nonne-Marie syndrome – *SYN:* Menzel syndrome

Nonne-Milroy-Meige syndrome – ankle edema. *SYN:* congenital elephantiasis; tropholymphedema

Nonnenbruch, Wilhelm, German physician, 1887-1955.
Nonnenbruch syndrome – oliguria. *SYN:* extrarenal kidney syndrome

Noonan, C.D.
Saldino-Noonan syndrome – see under Saldino

Noonan, Jacqueline A., U.S. pediatric cardiologist, *1921.
Noonan syndrome – the male phenotype of Turner syndrome, characterized by congenital heart disease.

Nordau, Max Simon, German scientist, 1849-1923.
Nordau disease – degeneration of the mind and body.

Nordhausen, a town in Saxony where the acid was first prepared.
Nordhausen sulfuric acid – contains sulfurous acid gas in solution.
SYN: fuming sulfuric acid

Norman, Margaret G., Canadian physician.
Norman-Roberts syndrome – *SYN:* Miller-Dieker syndrome

Norman, R.M., English physician.
Norman-Landing syndrome – genetic defects. *SYN:* beta-galactosidase deficiency

Norrie, Gordon, Danish ophthalmologist, 1855-1941.
Norrie disease – congenital bilateral masses of tissue arising from the retina or vitreous and resembling glioma, usually with atrophy of iris and development of cataract, associated mental retardation and deafness.
SYN: Norrie syndrome; Norrie-Warburg syndrome
Norrie syndrome – *SYN:* Norrie disease
Norrie-Warburg syndrome – *SYN:* Norrie disease

Norris, Richard, English physiologist, 1831-1916.
Norris corpuscles – decolorized red blood cells that are invisible or almost invisible in the blood plasma unless they are appropriately stained.

N

NOTES

Norton, Larry, 20th century U.S. oncologist.
Norton-Simon hypothesis – a tumor is composed of populations of faster growing cells, which are sensitive to therapy, and slower growing, more resistant cells.

Norton, U.F., U.S. obstetrician.
Norton operation – extraperitoneal cesarean section by a paravesical approach.

Norum, K.R.
Norum syndrome – corneal defects.

Norwalk, city in Ohio where the agent was first identified.
Norwalk agent – a calicivirus that is responsible for over half the reported cases of epidemic viral gastroenteropathy.

Norwood, O'Tar T., 20th century U.S. dermatologist.
Hamilton-Norwood classification – *SYN:* Norwood classification
Norwood classification – system for classifying male pattern baldness. *SYN:* Hamilton classification; Hamilton-Norwood classification

Nothnagel, C.W. Hermann, Austrian physician, 1841-1905.
Nothnagel acroparesthesia – abnormal sensation in the extremities accompanied by circulatory disorders. *SYN:* vasomotor acroparesthesia
Nothnagel syndrome – dizziness, staggering, and rolling gait, with irregular forms of oculomotor paralysis and often nystagmus, seen in cases of tumor of the midbrain.

Novy, Frederick G., U.S. bacteriologist, 1864-1957.
Novy and MacNeal blood agar – a nutrient agar suitable for the cultivation of a number of trypanosomes.
Novy rat disease – a viral disease among experimental rats.

Nuck, Anton, Dutch anatomist, 1650-1692.
canal of Nuck – a persistent processus vaginalis in the female.
Nuck diverticulum – a peritoneal diverticulum in the embryonic lower anterior abdominal wall. *SYN:* processus vaginalis of peritoneum
Nuck hydrocele – accumulation of serous fluid in the labium majus or in Nuck canal. *SYN:* hydrocele feminae

Nuel, Jean P., Belgian ophthalmologist and otologist, 1847-1920.
Nuel space – an interval in the spiral organ (of Corti) between the outer pillar cells on one side and the phalangeal cells and hair cells on the other.

Nuhn, Anton, German anatomist, 1814-1889.
    Nuhn gland – one of the small mixed glands deeply placed near the apex of the tongue on each side of the frenulum. *SYN:* anterior lingual gland

Nuremberg, city in Germany in which code was established following World War II.
    Nuremberg Code – protects the rights of individuals who participate in medical research.

Nurse, Sir Paul M., English scientist, *1949, joint winner of 2001 Nobel Prize for work related to key regulators of cell cycles.

Nussbaum, Johann von, German surgeon, 1829-1890.
    Nussbaum bracelet – an appliance designed for use with writer's cramp.

Nussbaum, Moritz, German histologist, 1850-1915.
    Nussbaum experiment – exclusion of the glomeruli of the kidney from the circulation by ligation of the renal artery.

Nüsslein-Volhard, Christiane, joint winner of 1995 Nobel Prize for work related to genetics and early development of an embryo.

Nygaard, Kaare Kristiaan, U.S. physician.
    Nygaard-Brown syndrome – *SYN:* Trousseau syndrome

Nyhan, William Leo, U.S. pediatrician, *1926.
    Lesch-Nyhan syndrome – see under Lesch
    Sakati-Nyhan syndrome – see under Sakati
    Sakati-Nyhan-Tisdale syndrome – *SYN:* Sakati-Nyhan syndrome

Nyssen, Rene, Belgian physician.
    Nyssen-van Bogaert-Meyer syndrome – autosomal recessive trait, with multiple defects.

Nysten, Pierre Hubert, French physician, 1771-1818.
    Nysten law – rigor mortis affects first the muscles of the head and spreads toward the feet.

N

NOTES

Obal, Adalbert, U.S. physician.
 Obal syndrome – ocular disorders associated with severe malnutrition. *SYN:* camp eyes; nutritional amblyopia; polydeficiency retrobulbar neuritis syndrome

O'Beirne, James, Irish surgeon, 1786-1862.
 O'Beirne sphincter – a circular band of muscular fibers at the rectosigmoid junction. *SYN:* rectosigmoid sphincter
 O'Beirne tube

Ober, Frank Roberts, U.S. orthopedic surgeon, 1881-1960.
 Ober anterior transfer
 Ober exercise – developed to stretch a tight fascia lata.
 Ober incision
 Ober operation
 Ober posterior drainage
 Ober release
 Ober technique
 Ober tendon passer
 Ober test – used to determine the degree of tightness of the fascia lata.

Obermayer, Friedrich, Austrian physician, 1861-1925.
 Obermayer test – for indican.

Obermeier, Otto H.F., German physician, 1843-1873.
 Obermeier spirillum – a species causing relapsing fever, transmitted by bedbugs and lice. *SYN: Borrelia recurrentis*

Obersteiner, H., Austrian neurologist, 1847-1922.
 Obersteiner-Redlich line – *SYN:* Obersteiner-Redlich zone
 Obersteiner-Redlich zone – marks the true boundary between the central and the peripheral nervous system. *SYN:* Obersteiner-Redlich line

Oblomov, Ilya Ilych, character from a 19th century novel.

NOTES

Oblomov syndrome – the refusal to become normally active after an illness.

O'Brien, Cecil Starling, U.S. ophthalmologist, 1889-1977.
O'Brien akinesia
O'Brien block
O'Brien scissors

O'Brien, John Patrick, Australian dermatopathologist, *1914.
O'Brien granuloma – anular lesion occurring on sun-exposed skin, showing giant cell reaction and solar elastosis.

Obrinsky, William, U.S. physician, *1913.
Obrinsky syndrome – aplasia or hypoplasia of the abdominal wall.
SYN: prune belly syndrome

Occam, William (William of Ockham [original spelling]), English philosopher, 1300-1341.
Occam razor – in principle of scientific parsimony, the simplest explanation is always preferable.

Ochoa, Severo, Spanish-U.S. biochemist and Nobel laureate, 1905-1993.
Ochoa law – the content of the X-chromosome tends to be phylogenetically conserved.

Ochsner, Albert John, U.S. surgeon, 1858-1925.
Ochsner cartilage forceps
Ochsner clamp – a straight hemostat with teeth.
Ochsner forceps
Ochsner hemostat
Ochsner hook
Ochsner method – obsolete treatment for appendicitis.
Ochsner muscle
Ochsner retractor
Ochsner ring
Ochsner scissors
Ochsner-Sherren regime – nonoperative treatment of appendiceal mass.
Ochsner tissue forceps
Ochsner trocar
Ochsner tube

Ochsner, Edward William Alton, U.S. surgeon, 1896-1981.
Ochsner-Mahorner test – modification of Perthes test.
Ochsner test – for median nerve injury.

Oddi, Ruggero, Italian physician, 1864-1913.
  sphincter of Oddi – the smooth muscle sphincter of the hepatopancreatic ampulla within the duodenal papilla. *SYN:* sphincter of hepatopancreatic ampulla

Odelberg, Axel Axelsson, Swedish physician, *1892.
  Odelberg disease – *SYN:* Van Neck disease
  Van Neck-Odelberg disease – *SYN:* Van Neck disease
  Van Neck-Odelberg syndrome – *SYN:* Van Neck disease

Odland, George, 20th century U.S. dermatologist.
  Odland body – membrane-bound organelle found in cells of the upper spinous layer and stratum granulosum, containing lipids that are dispersed into the intercellular space and that form a permeability barrier. *SYN:* keratinosome; lamellar granule; membrane-coating granule

O'Donnell, F.E., Jr.
  O'Donnell-Pappas syndrome – *SYN:* Karsch-Neugebauer syndrome

O'Dwyer, Joseph P., U.S. physician, 1841-1898.
  O'Dwyer tube – a metal tube formerly used for intubation of the larynx in diphtheria.

Oeckerman, P.A.
  Oeckerman syndrome – multiple genetic defects.

Oedipus, King Oedipus of Thebes, mythical Greek hero.
  oedipism (1) self-infliction of injury to the eyes; (2) manifestation of the Oedipus complex.
  Oedipus complex – a phase of psychosexual development in which the child is erotically attached to the parent of the opposite sex and has feelings of aggression toward the same-sex parent.
  Oedipus period – the time of a child's development characterized by erotic attachment to the parent of the opposite sex.

Oehl, Eusebio, Italian anatomist, 1827-1903.
Oehl muscles – strands of muscle fibers in the chordae tendineae of the left atrioventricular valve.

Oehler, Johannes, German physician, *1879.
Oehler symptom – a sudden pallor and coldness in the arm, with slight disability, occurring on lifting a heavy weight.

Oersted, Hans-Christian, Danish physicist, 1777-1851.
oersted (Oe) – a unit of magnetic field intensity.

Oertel, Max J., German ENT surgeon, 1835-1897.
Oertel treatment – cardiovascular disease treatment by diet, fluid restriction, and weight control.

Ofuji, Shigeo, 20th century Japanese dermatologist.
Ofugi disease I – pruritic circinate plaques studded with follicular papules or pustules, seen primarily in Japanese adults.
Ofugi disease II – intensely pruritic sheets of coalescent erythematous papules, sparing compressed abdominal folds. *SYN:* papuloerythroderma of Ofuji
papuloerythroderma of Ofuji – *SYN:* Ofuji disease II

Ogden, Frank Nevin, U.S. physician, *1895.
Zuelzer-Ogden syndrome – see under Zuelzer

Ogilvie, Sir William Heneage, English surgeon, 1887-1971.
Ogilvie herniorrhaphy
Ogilvie syndrome – motility disturbance of the intestines.

Ogino, Kyusaka, 20th century Japanese physician.
Ogino-Knaus rule – the basis for the rhythm method of contraception.

Ogston, Sir Alexander, Scottish surgeon, 1844-1929.
Ogston line – a guide to resection of the medial condyle for genu valgum.
Ogston-Luc operation – an operation for frontal sinus disease.

Oguchi, Chuta, Japanese ophthalmologist, 1875-1945.
Oguchi disease – a rare congenital, nonprogressive night blindness.

Ogura, Joseph H., U.S. otolaryngologist, *1915.
Ogura cartilage forceps
Ogura fossa
Ogura operation – orbital decompression by removal of the floor of the orbit through an opening made in the supradental fossa.
Ogura saw
Ogura technique

Ogura tissue forceps

O'Hara, Michael, Jr., U.S. surgeon, 1869-1926.
O'Hara forceps – two slender clamp forceps used in intestinal anastomosis.
O'Hara operation

Ohara, Shoichiro, 20th century Japanese physician.
Ohara disease – *SYN:* tularemia

Ohm, Georg Simon, German physicist, 1787-1854.
ohm – the practical unit of electrical resistance.
Ohm law – in an electric current passing through a wire, the intensity of the current in amperes equals the electromotive force in volts divided by the resistance in ohms.

Okazaki, Reiji, Japanese biochemist, 1930-1975.
Okazaki fragment – short pieces of DNA formed during DNA synthesis.

Oken, Lorenz, German physiologist, 1779-1851.
canal of Oken – *SYN:* wolffian body
corpus of Oken – *SYN:* wolffian body

Oldfield, Michael C., 20th century English physician.
Oldfield syndrome – familial colon polyposis.

Oliver, C.P., 20th century U.S. pediatrician.
Adams-Oliver syndrome – see under Adams, Robert

Oliver, G.L.
Oliver-McFarlane syndrome – genetic defects.

Oliver, William Silver, English physician, 1836-1908.
Oliver sign – tracheal tugging.
Oliver test – for albumin.

Ollendorf, Helene, German dermatologist.
Buschke-Ollendorf syndrome – see under Buschke

NOTES

Ollier, Louis Xavier Edouard Léopold, French surgeon, 1830-1900.
Ollier approach
Ollier disease – proliferation of cartilage in the metaphyses of several bones, causing distorted growth in length or pathological fractures. *SYN:* enchondromatosis
Ollier graft – a thin split-thickness graft, usually in small pieces. *SYN:* Ollier-Thiersch graft; Thiersch graft
Ollier incision
Ollier layer
Ollier method
Ollier operation
Ollier rake retractor
Ollier raspatory
Ollier retractor
Ollier technique
Ollier theory – a theory of compensatory growth.
Ollier-Thiersch graft – *SYN:* Ollier graft

Olmsted, H.C., 20th century U.S. pediatrician.
Olmsted syndrome – congenital palmar, plantar, and periorificial keratoderma leading to flexion contractures and digital spontaneous amputation, hyperkeratotic plaques around body orifices, and onychodystrophy. *SYN:* mutilating palmoplantar keratoderma with periorificial keratotic plaques

Olshausen, Robert von, German obstetrician, 1835-1915.
Olshausen operation – surgery done for retroversion of the uterus.
Olshausen sign
Olshausen suspension

Olshevsky, Dimitry E., U.S. physician, *1900.
Olshevsky tube

Olszewski, Jerzy, Polish-Canadian neuropathologist, 1913-1966.
Steele-Richardson-Olszewski disease – *SYN:* Steele-Richardson-Olszewski syndrome
Steele-Richardson-Olszewski syndrome – see under Steele

Ombrédanne, Louis, French surgeon, 1871-1956.
Ombrédanne forceps
Ombrédanne mallet
Ombrédanne operation – *SYN:* transseptal orchiopexy

Omenn, Gilbert Stanley, U.S. internist, *1941.

Omenn syndrome – a rapidly fatal autosomal recessive immunodeficiency disease.

Ommaya, Ayub Khan, U.S. neurosurgeon, *1930.

Ommaya cerebrospinal fluid reservoir
Ommaya intraventricular reservoir system
Ommaya reservoir
Ommaya reservoir implant material
Ommaya reservoir prosthesis
Ommaya reservoir transensor
Ommaya retromastoid reservoir
Ommaya shunt
Ommaya side-port flat-bottomed reservoir
Ommaya suboccipital reservoir
Ommaya tube
Ommaya ventricular reservoir

Ondine, a water nymph in German mythology.

Ondine curse – alveolar hyperventilation.

Onodi, Adolf, Hungarian laryngologist, 1857-1920.

Onodi cell – a variant of a posterior ethmoidal air cell in intimate relationship with the optic nerve just distal to the optic chiasm.

Onufrowicz, Wladislaus, Swiss anatomist, 1836-1900.

Onuf nucleus – small somatic motor neurons in the ventral horn of the spinal cord at level S2.

Oorthuys, J.W.E., Dutch geneticist, 1943-1992.

Delleman-Oorthuys syndrome – *SYN:* Delleman syndrome

Opalski, Adam, Polish physician, 1897-1963.

Opalski cell – a characteristically altered glial cell in the basal ganglia and thalamus, found in hepatocerebral degeneration and Wilson disease.

O

Opie, Eugene L., U.S. pathologist, 1873-1971.
  Opie paradox – necrotizing local anaphylaxis.

Opitz, John Marius, U.S. pediatrician, *1935.
  Opitz-Frias syndrome – males affected from birth; swallowing problems with recurrent aspiration, stridorous breathing, and hoarse cry.
  Opitz-Kaveggia syndrome – in males; X-linked recessive syndrome of multiple congenital anomalies and mental retardation.
  Smith-Lemli-Opitz syndrome – see under Smith, David W.

Opitz, Z.
  Opitz syndrome – thrombophlebitis of the splenic vein.

Oppenheim, Hermann, German neurologist, 1858-1919.
  Minor-Oppenheim syndrome – *SYN:* Minor syndrome
  Oppenheim brace
  Oppenheim congenital hypotonia
  Oppenheim disease – *SYN:* Oppenheim syndrome
  Oppenheim gait
  Oppenheim reflex – extension of the toes induced by scratching of the inner side of the leg, a sign of cerebral irritation.
  Oppenheim sign – suggests pyramidal tract disease.
  Oppenheim splint
  Oppenheim spring wire splint
  Oppenheim stroke test
  Oppenheim syndrome – congenital atonic pseudoparalysis, observed especially in infants. *SYN:* amyotonia congenita; Oppenheim disease
  Ziehen-Oppenheim disease – see under Ziehen

Oppenheim, Moriz, Austrian-U.S. dermatologist, 1876-1949.
  Oppenheim-Urbach disease – skin condition usually observed in diabetic patients. *SYN:* Urbach-Oppenheim disease
  Urbach-Oppenheim disease – *SYN:* Oppenheim-Urbach disease

Oppenheimer, A.
  Oppenheimer syndrome – limitation of spinal motion. *SYN:* physiologic vertebral ligamentous calcification

Oppler, Bruno, German physician, d. 1932.
  Boas-Oppler bacillus

Oram, Samuel, 20th century English cardiologist.
  Holt-Oram syndrome – see under Holt, Mary

Orbeli, Leon Algarovich, Russian physiologist, 1882-1958.

Orbeli effect – the fatigue of a muscle stimulated by its nerve is reduced by concurrent stimulation of sympathetic fibers to the muscle. *SYN:* Orbeli phenomenon

Orbeli phenomenon – *SYN:* Orbeli effect

Ormond, John Kelso, U.S. urologist, *1886.

Ormond disease – *SYN:* retroperitoneal fibrosis

Ornish, Dean, U.S. physician, *1953.

Ornish reversal diet – designed to reverse coronary artery disease.

Oroya, region of Peru where disease was first discovered.

Oroya fever – *SYN:* Carrión disease

Orr, Hiram Winnett, U.S. orthopedic surgeon, 1877-1956.

Orr forceps
Orr incision
Orr method
Orr technique
Orr treatment

Orsi, Francesco, Italian physician, 1828-1890.

Orsi-Grocco method – palpatory percussion of the heart.

Orth, Johannes J., German pathologist, 1847-1923.

Orth fixative – formalin added to Müller fixative, used for bringing out chromaffin, studying early degenerative processes and necrosis, and for demonstrating rickettsiae and bacteria.

Orth stain – a lithium carmine stain for nerve cells and their processes.

Ortner, Norbert, Austrian physician, 1865-1935.

Ortner syndrome – laryngeal paralysis that is associated with heart disease.

Ortolani, Marius, 20th century Italian orthopedic surgeon.

Ortolani click
Ortolani maneuver

NOTES

Ortolani sign
Ortolani test – test for congenital hip dislocation.

Orton, Samuel T., U.S. neurologist, 1879-1975.
Wolf-Orton bodies – see under Wolf

Orzechowski, K.
Orzechowski syndrome – involuntary oscillations of the eyes in horizontal and vertical directions; tremulousness; sign of encephalitis.

Osebold, W.R.
Osebold-Remondini syndrome – middle phalanges of all digits are hypoplastic or absent; autosomal dominant inheritance.
SYN: brachydactyly

Osgood, Robert B., U.S. orthopedic surgeon, 1873-1956.
Osgood femoral supracondylar osteotomy
Osgood modified technique
Osgood operation
Osgood rotational osteotomy
Osgood-Schlatter disease – epiphysial aseptic necrosis of the tibial tubercle. *SYN:* apophysitis tibialis adolescentium; Schlatter disease; Schlatter-Osgood disease
Schlatter-Osgood disease – *SYN:* Osgood-Schlatter disease

Osler, Sir William, Canadian physician in U.S. and England, 1849-1919.
Osler disease – a chronic form of polycythemia. *SYN:* polycythemia vera
Osler node – a tender cutaneous lesion characteristic of subacute bacterial endocarditis.
Osler sign – in acute bacterial endocarditis, circumscribed painful erythematous swelling in the skin and subcutaneous tissues of the hands and feet.
Osler II syndrome – recurrent episodes of colic pain. *SYN:* ball-valve gallstone
Osler triad
Rendu-Osler-Weber syndrome – see under Rendu

Österreicher, W.
Österreicher-Fong syndrome – *SYN:* Fong lesion

Ostertag, B.
Ostertag syndrome – *SYN:* hereditary amyloid nephropathy

Ostrum, Herman William, U.S. physician, *1893.
Ostrum-Furst syndrome – congenital tribasilar synostosis.

Ostwald, Friedrich Wilhelm, German physical chemist and Nobel laureate, 1853-1932.

Ostwald solubility coefficient – the milliliters of gas dissolved per milliliter of liquid and per atmosphere partial pressure of the gas at any given temperature.

Osuntokun, B.O., Nigerian physician.

Osuntokun syndrome – autosomal recessive trait characterized by auditory imperception and indifference to pain. *SYN:* auditory imperception syndrome; congenital pain asymbolia

Ota, Masao T., Japanese dermatopathologist, 1885-1945.

Ota nevus – pigmentation of the conjunctiva and skin around the eye, usually unilateral. *SYN:* oculodermal melanocytosis; Ota syndrome

Ota syndrome – *SYN:* Ota nevus

Othello, one of Shakespeare's characters.

Othello syndrome – delusions of infidelity of one's sexual partner; onset usually in 4th decade of life; may be a feature of depressive psychosis, epilepsy, or alcoholism. *SYN:* erotic jealousy

Otis, Arthur Brooks, U.S. respiratory physiologist, *1913.

Rahn-Otis sample – see under Rahn

Otto, Adolph W., German surgeon, 1786-1845.

Otto disease – characterized by an inward bulging of the acetabulum into the pelvic cavity, resulting from arthritis of the hip joints. *SYN:* arthrokatadysis; Otto pelvis; protrusio acetabuli

Otto forceps

Otto pelvis – *SYN:* Otto disease

Ottoson, David, Swedish physiologist, *1918.

Ottoson potential – an electronegative wave of potential occurring on the surface of the olfactory epithelium in response to stimulation by an odor. *SYN:* electroolfactogram

O

NOTES

Ouchterlony, Orjan, Swedish bacteriologist, *1914.
    Ouchterlony immunodiffusion
    Ouchterlony method – *SYN:* Ouchterlony test
    Ouchterlony technique – *SYN:* Ouchterlony test
    Ouchterlony test – double (gel) diffusion test in two dimensions. *SYN:*
        Ouchterlony method; Ouchterlony technique

Oudin, Paul, French electrotherapist, 1851-1923.
    Oudin current – a high-frequency current.
    Oudin resonator – a special wire coil.

Overton, Charles E., German biologist in Sweden, 1865-1933.
    Meyer-Overton rule – see under Meyer, Hans H.
    Meyer-Overton theory of narcosis – see under Meyer, Hans H.

Owen, Sir Richard, English anatomist, 1804-1892.
    contour lines of Owen – *SYN:* Owen lines
    interglobular space of Owen – one of a number of irregularly branched
        spaces near the periphery of the dentin of the crown of a tooth.
        SYN: interglobular space
    Owen lines – accentuated incremental lines in the dentin thought to be
        due to disturbances in the mineralization process. *SYN:* contour lines of
        Owen

Owren, Paul Arnor, Norwegian hematologist, *1905.
    Owren disease – congenital deficiency of factor V, resulting in
        prolongation of prothrombin time and coagulation time.

Paas, Herman R., German physician, *1900.
    Paas disease – familial skeletal deformities.

Pacchioni, Antonio, Italian anatomist, 1665-1726.
    pacchionian bodies – tufted prolongations of pia-arachnoid.
        SYN: arachnoid granulations; pacchionian corpuscles; pacchionian glands; pacchionian granulations
    pacchionian corpuscles – *SYN:* pacchionian bodies
    pacchionian depressions – pits on the inner surface of the skull in which are lodged the arachnoidal granulations. *SYN:* granular pits
    pacchionian glands – *SYN:* pacchionian bodies
    pacchionian granulations – *SYN:* pacchionian bodies

Pachon, Michel V., French physiologist, 1867-1938.
    Pachon method – cardiography with the patient lying on the left side.
    Pachon test – in a case of aneurysm, determination of the collateral circulation by estimation of the blood pressure.

Pacini, Filippo, Italian anatomist, 1812-1883.
    pacinian corpuscles – *SYN:* Vater corpuscles
    Pacini bodies
    Vater-Pacini corpuscles – *SYN:* Vater corpuscles

Padgett, Earl Calvin, U.S. surgeon, 1893-1946.
    Padgett blade
    Padgett cannula
    Padgett dermatome
    Padgett graft
    Padgett implant
    Padgett prosthesis

NOTES

Page, Irvin H., U.S. physician, 1901-1991.
Page syndrome – periodic appearance of blotchy flushes covered by beads of perspiration on the face, upper chest, and abdomen.

Pagenstecher, Alexander, German ophthalmologist, 1828-1879.
Pagenstecher circle – around the point of attachment of a freely movable abdominal tumor.

Paget, Sir James, English surgeon, 1814-1899.
extramammary Paget disease – *SYN:* Paget disease
Paget abscess syndrome – an abscess recurrence at the same site after apparent cure.
Paget associated osteogenic sarcoma
Paget cells – relatively large neoplastic epithelial cells.
Paget disease – an intraepidermal form of mucinous adenocarcinoma, most commonly in the anogenital region. *SYN:* extramammary Paget disease
Paget disease of bone – osteitis deformans. *SYN:* Paget II syndrome
Paget disease of the nipple – ductal carcinoma.
Paget disease of the penis – carcinoma that develops after balanitis.
Paget juvenile syndrome – *SYN:* familial osteoectasia
Paget quiet necrosis – necrosis in the superficial layers of the shaft of a long bone.
Paget I syndrome – relationship to or possible extension of mammary duct carcinoma.
Paget II syndrome – *SYN:* Paget disease of bone
Paget test – to determine whether a mass is a solid tumor or a cyst.
Paget-von Schrötter syndrome – stress thrombosis or spontaneous thrombosis of the subclavian or axillary vein. *SYN:* effort-induced thrombosis

Paget, Sir Richard, English physical scientist, 1869-1955.
Paget-Gorman sign language – *SYN:* Paget sign language
Paget sign language – a sign language for the hearing impaired. *SYN:* Paget-Gorman sign language

Pagon, R.A.
Pagon syndrome – anemia from birth (in males); ataxia evident by age 1 year; clonus and positive Babinski sign. *SYN:* sideroblastic anemia; spinocerebellar ataxia

Pahvant Valley, valley in Utah where first cases of the fever were reported.
Pahvant Valley fever – tularemia. *SYN:* Pahvant Valley plague
Pahvant Valley plague – *SYN:* Pahvant Valley fever

Paine, R.S.
> **Paine-Efron syndrome** – pain in the back and thigh followed by slowly progressive ataxia. *SYN:* ataxia-telangiectasia variant
> **Paine retinaculatome**
> **Paine syndrome** – males only; onset at birth; physical and mental retardation; seizures. *SYN:* microcephaly

Pajot, Charles, French obstetrician, 1816-1896.
> **Pajot hook**
> **Pajot law** – a law governing a fetus' rotating movements during labor.
> **Pajot maneuver** – obsolete term for method to bring the fetal head down in the axis of the birth canal.

Pal, Jacob, Austrian physician, 1863-1936.
> **Pal stain** – used to study myelinated nerves.

Palade, George Emil, Romanian-U.S. cell biologist and Nobel laureate, *1912.
> **Palade granule** – a granule of ribonucleoprotein, the site of protein synthesis from aminoacyl-tRNAs as directed by mRNAs. *SYN:* ribosome
> **Weibel-Palade bodies** – see under Weibel

Palfyn, Jean, Belgian surgeon and anatomist, 1650-1730.
> **Palfyn sinus** – a space within the crista galli of the ethmoid communicating with the ethmoidal and frontal sinuses.
> **Palfyn suture**

Pallister, P.D.
> **Pallister syndrome** – autosomal dominant inheritance affecting both sexes.

Palmaz, J.C., 20th century U.S. vascular surgeon.
> **Palmaz stent** – an intravascular stent.

Palmer, Walter L., U.S. physician, *1896.
> **Palmer acid test for ulcer** – in duodenal ulcer, the administration of acid by duodenal tube causes severe pain.

NOTES

Pan, Greek mythological god of the forest.
   panic – extreme and unreasoning anxiety and fear.

Panacea, in Greek mythology, one of the daughters of Aesculapius.
   panacea – a remedy for all diseases.

Pancoast, Henry Khunrath, U.S. radiologist, 1875-1939.
   Pancoast syndrome – lower trunk brachial plexopathy and Horner
      syndrome due to malignant tumor in the region of the superior
      pulmonary sulcus. *SYN:* Hare syndrome
   Pancoast tumor – adenocarcinoma of a lung apex causing Pancoast
      syndrome. *SYN:* superior pulmonary sulcus tumor

Pancoast, Joseph, U.S. surgeon, 1805-1882.
   Pancoast operation
   Pancoast suture – in plastic surgery, union of two edges by a tongue-and-
      groove arrangement.

Pander, Heinrich Christian, German anatomist, 1794-1865.
   Pander islands – cords of corpuscular matter in an embryo that develops
      into blood and blood vessels.
   Pander layer – a layer of the mesoblast.

Pandy, Kalman, Hungarian neurologist, 1868-1945.
   Pandy reaction – a test to determine the presence of proteins in the spinal
      fluid. *SYN:* Pandy test
   Pandy test – *SYN:* Pandy reaction

Paneth, Josef, Austrian physician, 1857-1890.
   Paneth granular cells – cells located at the base of intestinal glands of the
      small intestine that contain large acidophilic refractile granules and may
      produce lysozyme. *SYN:* Davidoff cells

Panizza, Bartolomeo, Italian anatomist, 1785-1867.
   Panizza plexus – lymph vessel plexuses located in the prepuce's lateral
      fossae.

Panner, Hans J., Danish radiologist, 1871-1930.
   Panner disease – epiphyseal aseptic necrosis of the capitellum of the
      humerus.

Pansch, Adolf, German anatomist, 1841-1887.
   Pansch fissure – a sulcus cerebral fissure running from the lower
      extremity of the central fissure nearly to the end of the occipital lobe.

Panum, Peter L., Danish physiologist, 1820-1885.
    Panum area – the area in and about the macula retinae in which stimulation of noncorresponding retinal points results in stereoscopic vision. *SYN:* fusion area

Papanicolaou, George N., Greek-U.S. physician, anatomist, and cytologist, 1883-1962.
    Papanicolaou examination
    Papanicolaou smear – *SYN:* Pap smear
    Papanicolaou smear test – *SYN:* Pap test
    Papanicolaou stain – a multichromatic stain used in cancer screening, especially of gynecologic smears.
    Papanicolaou test – *SYN:* Pap test
    Pap smear – vaginal or cervical cells obtained for cytological study. *SYN:* Papanicolaou smear
    Pap test – examination of cells stained with Papanicolaou stain. *SYN:* Papanicolaou smear test; Papanicolaou test

Papas, C.V., Greek physician.
    Bartsocas-Papas syndrome – see under Bartsocas

Papez, James W., U.S. anatomist, 1883-1958.
    Papez circle – network of nerve fibers and centers.
    Papez circuit – a long circuitous conduction chain in the mammalian forebrain.
    Papez theory of emotions – theory that emotions are controlled by Papez circle.

Papillon, M.M., 20th century French dermatologist.
    Papillon-Lefèvre syndrome – a congenital hyperkeratosis of the palms and soles, with progressive destruction of alveolar bone about the deciduous and permanent teeth.

Papillon-Léage, E., 20th century French dentist.
    Papillon-Léage and Psaume syndrome – an inherited, lethal syndrome in males, with varying combinations of defects of the oral cavity, face,

NOTES

P

and hands, and, frequently, mental retardation. *SYN:* orodigitofacial dysostosis

Pappas, H.R.
O'Donnell-Pappas syndrome – *SYN:* Karsch-Neugenbauer syndrome

Pappenheim, Artur, German physician, 1870-1916.
Pappenheim stain – a method for differentiating tubercle and smegma bacilli.
Unna-Pappenheim stain – see under Unna, Paul G.

Pappenheimer, Alwin M., U.S. pathologist, 1878-1955.
Pappenheimer bodies – phagosomes containing ferruginous granules, found in red blood cells in diseases such as sideroblastic anemia, hemolytic anemia and sickle cell disease.

Paracelsus, Aureolus Theophrastus Bombastus von Hohenheim, Swiss physician, 1493-1541.
paracelsian method – the use of chemical agents only in the treatment of disease.

Pardee, Harold Ensign Bennett, U.S. physician, 1886-1973.
Pardee sign – ST segment elevation on electrocardiogram.

Paré, Ambroise, French surgeon, 1510-1590.
Paré suture – the approximation of the edges of a wound by pasting strips of cloth to the surface and stitching them instead of the skin.

Parenti, Gian Carlo, Italian physician.
Parenti-Fraccaro syndrome – *SYN:* type IB achondrogenesis

Parham, Frederick William, U.S. surgeon, 1856-1927.
Parham band – a metallic ribbon used to repair fractured long bones.
Parham support

Parinaud, Henri, French ophthalmologist, 1844-1905.
Parinaud conjunctivitis – a chronic necrotic inflammation of the conjunctiva characterized by large, irregular, reddish follicles and regional lymphadenopathy.
Parinaud oculoglandular syndrome – unilateral conjunctival granuloma with preauricular adenopathy in tularemia, chancre, and tuberculosis.
Parinaud ophthalmoplegia – *SYN:* Parinaud syndrome
Parinaud syndrome – paralysis of conjugate upward gaze with a lesion at the level of the superior colliculi. *SYN:* Parinaud ophthalmoplegia
Parinaud I syndrome – retraction nystagmus; systemic hypertension; Babinski sign; extraocular palsy; pupils usually normal in size but have

poor reaction to light and near vision. *SYN:* divergence paralysis; Koerber-Salus-Elsching syndrome

Paris, city in France.

plaster of Paris – a gypsum material used for making casts.

Park, Henry, English surgeon, 1744-1831.

Park aneurysm – an arteriovenous aneurysm in which the brachial artery communicates with the brachial and median basilic veins.

Park, William H., U.S. bacteriologist, 1863-1939.

Park-Williams bacillus – a special strain of *Corynebacterium diphtheriae* used for toxin production.

Park-Williams fixative – a fixative for spirochetes, comprised of a 2% solution of osmic acid.

Parker, Edward Mason, U.S. surgeon, 1860-1941.

Parker clamp

Parker discission knife

Parker fixation forceps

Parker-Heath anterior chamber syringe

Parker-Heath cautery

Parker-Heath electrocautery

Parker-Heath piggyback probe

Parker incision

Parker-Kerr basting suture

Parker-Kerr operation

Parker-Kerr suture – a continuous inverting suture used to close an open end of intestine.

Parker needle

Parker retractor

Parker serrated discission knife

Parker, George Howard, U.S. zoologist, 1864-1955.

Parker fluid – formaldehyde and alcohol.

NOTES

Parker, R.W.

Parker syndrome – onset under the age of 10 years; possible association with various congenital deformities. *SYN:* adrenal medullary neuroblastoma

Parkinson, James, English physician, 1755-1824.

Parkinson disease – a neurological disorder usually resulting from deficiency of dopamine as the consequence of degenerative, vascular, or inflammatory changes in the basal ganglia. *SYN:* parkinsonism (1)

Parkinson facies – the expressionless or masklike facies characteristic of parkinsonism. *SYN:* masklike face; Parkinson sign

parkinsonism – (1) *SYN:* Parkinson disease; (2) syndrome similar to Parkinson disease appearing as a side effect of certain drugs.

Parkinson sign – *SYN:* Parkinson facies

Parkinson triangle

Parkinson, Sir John, English cardiologist, *1885.

Wolff-Parkinson-White syndrome – see under Wolff, Louis

Parnas, Jakob Karol, Polish physiologic chemist, 1884-1955.

Embden-Meyerhof-Parnas pathway – *SYN:* Embden-Meyerhof pathway

Parona, Francesco, Italian surgeon, 1861-1910.

Parona space – a space between the pronator quadratus deep and the overlying flexor tendons of the forearm.

Parrot, Jules Marie, French physician, 1829-1883.

Bednar-Parrot syndrome – *SYN:* Parrot I syndrome

Parrot atrophy of the newborn

Parrot nodes – *SYN:* Parrot sign

Parrot pseudoparalysis – syphilitic osteochondritis in newborns causing pseudoparalysis in one or more extremities. *SYN:* syphilitic pseudoparalysis

Parrot sign – indicates congenital syphilis in newborns. *SYN:* Parrot nodes

Parrot I syndrome – pseudoparalysis; periarticular swelling, onset seldom after 3 months of age. *SYN:* Bednar-Parrot syndrome; Parrot syphilitic osteochondritis

Parrot II syndrome – failure to thrive, emaciation, edema, dry skin, with subcutaneous fat loss, abdomen flat or distended, hypothermia, slow pulse, decreased metabolic rate. *SYN:* marasmus; infantile atrophy; inanition; athrepsia

Parrot syphilitic osteochondritis – *SYN:* Parrot I syndrome

Parrot ulcer – seen in stomatitis or thrush.

Parry, Caleb Hillier, English physician, 1755-1822.
Parry disease – *SYN:* Graves disease

Partsch, C.J., German physician.
Miehlke-Partsch syndrome – see under Miehlke

Pascal, Blaise, French scientist, 1623-1662.
pascal – a derived unit of pressure or stress in the SI system.
Pascal law – fluids at rest transmit pressure equally in every direction.

Pascheff, Constantin (Konstantin), Bulgarian ophthalmologist, 1873-1961.
Pascheff conjunctivitis – a unilateral, suppurative, necrotic inflammation
of the conjunctiva. *SYN:* necrotic infectious conjunctivitis

Paschen, Enrique, German pathologist, 1860-1936.
Paschen bodies – particles of virus observed in relatively large numbers
in squamous cells of the skin. *SYN:* Paschen corpuscles; Paschen
granules
Paschen corpuscles – *SYN:* Paschen bodies
Paschen granules – *SYN:* Paschen bodies

Pasini, Agostino, Italian dermatologist, 1875-1944.
atrophoderma of Pasini and Pierini – a form of slate-colored atrophy of
the skin occurring in discrete 2-cm or larger lesions.
Pasini-Pierini syndrome – slight depression below the level of normal
skin of different shapes, colors, and dimensions. *SYN:* atrophic morphea
variant
Pasini syndrome – small, firm, white perifollicular papules that appear
primarily on the lumbosacral region. *SYN:* albopapuloid epidermolysis
bullosa
Pasini variant

Pasqualini, R.Q.
Pasqualini syndrome – having no libido or potency.
SYN: pseudoeunuchoidism

NOTES

P

Passavant, Philippas G., German physician, 1815-1893.
  Passavant bar – *SYN:* Passavant cushion
  Passavant cushion – a prominence on the posterior wall of the
    nasopharynx formed by contraction of the superior constrictor of the
    pharynx during swallowing. *SYN:* Passavant bar; Passavant pad;
    Passavant ridge
  Passavant pad – *SYN:* Passavant cushion
  Passavant ridge – *SYN:* Passavant cushion

Passey, R.D., 20th century English pathologist.
  Harding-Passey melanoma – see under Harding

Passow, Arnold von, German ophthalmologist, 1888–1966.
  Passow syndrome – multiple congenital anomalies.

Passwell, J.H., 20th century Israeli physician.
  Passwell syndrome – ichthyosis, mental retardation, and dwarfism from
    birth.

Pasteur, Louis, French chemist and bacteriologist, 1822-1895.
  Pasteur effect – the inhibition of fermentation by oxygen, first observed by
    Pasteur.
  Pasteurella
  Pasteurella aerogenes – species found in swine that can cause human
    wound infections following a pig bite.
  Pasteurella multocida – bacterial species associated with dogs and cats.
  Pasteurella pestis – *SYN: Yersinia pseudotuberculosis*
  Pasteurella "SP" – a rarely encountered organism that can cause
    infection after a guinea pig bite.
  Pasteurella tularensis – *SYN: Francisella tularensis*
  pasteurellosis – infection with bacteria of *Pasteurella*.
  pasteurization – bacteria destruction process.
  pasteurizer – pasteurization apparatus.
  Pasteur pipette – a cotton-plugged, glass tube drawn out to a fine tip,
    used for the sterile transfer of small volumes of fluid.
  Pasteur vaccine

Pastia, Constantin Chessec, Romanian physician, 1883-1926.
  Pastia lines
  Pastia sign – the presence of pink or red transverse lines at the bend of
    the elbow in the preeruptive stage of scarlatina. *SYN:* Thomson sign

Patau, Klaus, 20th century German-born U.S. physician.
  Bartholin-Patau syndrome – *SYN:* Patau syndrome

Patau syndrome – usually fatal within two years, characterized by mental retardation, malformed ears, and multiple organ anomalies. *SYN:* Bartholin-Patau syndrome; trisomy 13 syndrome

Patein, G., French physician, 1857-1928.
Patein albumin – a substance resembling serum albumin but soluble in acetic acid. *SYN:* acetosoluble albumin

Patella, Vincenzo, Italian physician, 1856-1928.
Patella disease – pyloric stenosis in tuberculosis patients.

Paterson, Donald Rose, English otolaryngologist, 1863-1939.
Paterson-Brown-Kelly syndrome – limited elevation of the eye in adduction, due to fascia contracting the superior oblique muscle on the same side. *SYN:* tendon sheath syndrome
Paterson cannula
Paterson forceps
Paterson-Kelly syndrome – *SYN:* Plummer-Vinson syndrome

Patey, David H., English surgeon, 1899-1977.
Patey axillary node dissection
Patey mastectomy
Patey modified radical mastectomy
Patey operation – modified radical mastectomy.

Patrick, Hugh T., U.S. neurologist, 1860-1938.
Patrick drill
Patrick maneuver
Patrick sign
Patrick test – determines the presence or absence of sacroiliac disease.
Patrick trigger area

NOTES

P

Paul, Constantin C.T., French physician, 1833-1896.
Paul sign – inflammation of the pericardium may create difficulty in feeling the apex beat, though precordial activity is felt.

Paul, Frank Thomas, English surgeon, 1851-1941.
Mixter-Paul hemostatic forceps
Paul-Mixter tube

Paul, Gustav, Austrian physician, 1859-1935.
Paul reaction – formerly a test for smallpox. *SYN:* Paul test
Paul test – *SYN:* Paul reaction

Paul, John Rodman, U.S. pathologist, 1893-1971.
Paul-Bunnell test – for infectious mononucleosis.

Pauli, Wolfgang, Austrian-U.S. physicist and Nobel laureate, 1900-1958.
Pauli exclusion principle – the theory limiting the number of electrons in the orbit or shell of an atom.

Pauling, Linus C., U.S. chemist and Nobel laureate, 1901-1994.
Pauling-Corey helix – the helical form present in many proteins. *SYN:* α helix
Pauling theory – a theory of narcosis pertaining to nonhydrogen-bonding agents. *SYN:* hydrate microcrystal theory of anesthesia

Pautrier, Lucien M.A., French dermatologist, 1876-1959.
Pautrier abscess – *SYN:* Pautrier microabscess
Pautrier microabscess – a microscopic lesion in the epidermis, seen in mycosis fungoides. *SYN:* Pautrier abscess

Pauzat, Jean E., 19th century French physician.
Pauzat disease – osteoplastic periostitis or fatigue fractures of the metatarsal bones, caused by excessive marching.

Pavlov, Ivan, Russian physiologist and Nobel laureate, 1849-1936.
Pavlov behavioral theory
pavlovian conditioning – a type of conditioning in which a previously neutral stimulus elicits a response as a result of pairing it a number of times with an unconditioned stimulus for that response. *SYN:* respondent conditioning
Pavlov method – the method of studying conditioned reflex activity by the observation of a motor indicator, such as the salivary or electroencephalographic response.
Pavlov pouch – a section of the stomach of a dog used in studies of gastric secretions. *SYN:* miniature stomach; Pavlov stomach

Pavlov reflex – peripheral vasoconstriction and a rise in blood pressure in response to a fall in pressure in the great veins. *SYN:* auriculopressor reflex

Pavlov stomach – *SYN:* Pavlov pouch

Pavlov theory of schizophrenia – belief that symptoms of schizophrenia result from an inhibited state of the cerebral cortex.

Pavy, Fredrick W., English physician, 1829-1911.

Pavy disease – cyclic or recurrent physiologic albuminuria.

Paxton, Francis Valentine, English physician, 1840-1924.

Paxton disease – *Corynebacterium* infection of axillary and pubic hairs. *SYN:* trichomycosis axillaris

Payne, J. Howard, U.S. surgeon, *1916.

Payne operation – a jejunoileal bypass for morbid obesity.

Payne retractor

Payr, Erwin, German surgeon, 1871-1946.

Payr clamp – a clamp used in gastrectomy or enterectomy.

Payr disease – constipation, with left upper quadrant pain. *SYN:* splenic flexure syndrome

Payr forceps

Payr gastrectomy

Payr membrane – a fold of peritoneum that crosses over the left flexure of the colon.

Payr rectractor

Payr sign – pain on pressure over the sole of the foot, a sign of thrombophlebitis.

Payr syndrome – occurs in approximately 20% of patients with irritable bowel, usually postprandially.

Péan, Jules Émile, French surgeon, 1830-1898.

Péan amputation

Péan clamp

Péan forceps

NOTES

Péan incision
Péan operation
Péan position
Péan scissors

Pearl, Raymond, U.S. biologist, 1879-1940.
Pearl index – the number of failures of a contraceptive method per 100 woman years of exposure.

Pearlman, Hubert S., U.S. orthopedic surgeon.
Nievergelt-Pearlman syndrome – see under Nievergelt

Pearson, H.A.
Pearson syndrome – refractory sideroblastic anemia; malabsorption or other pancreatic exocrine insufficiency.

Pearson, Karl, English mathematician, 1857-1936.
McArdle-Schmid-Pearson disease – *SYN:* McArdle syndrome
Poisson-Pearson formula – see under Poisson

Pecquet, Jean, French anatomist, 1622-1674.
Pecquet cistern – *SYN:* Pecquet reservoir
Pecquet duct – the largest lymph vessel in the body. *SYN:* thoracic duct
Pecquet reservoir – a dilated sac at the lower end of the thoracic duct into which the intestinal trunk and two lumbar lymphatic trunks open.
SYN: cisterna chyli; Pecquet cistern; receptaculum pecqueti
receptaculum pecqueti – *SYN:* Pecquet reservoir

Pedersen, E.
Pedersen syndrome – abrupt onset of vertigo, nausea, vomiting.
SYN: neurolabyrinthitis

Peiffer, J., German physician, *1922.
Hirsch-Peiffer stain – used for cytologic demonstration of metachromatic leukodystrophy.

Pel, Pieter Klasses, Dutch physician, 1852-1919.
Murchison-Pel-Ebstein syndrome – see under Murchison
Pel crises – ocular crises.
Pel-Ebstein disease – *SYN:* Pel-Ebstein fever
Pel-Ebstein fever – the remittent fever common in Hodgkin disease.
SYN: Pel-Ebstein disease

Pelger, Karel, Dutch physician, 1885-1931.
Huët-Pelger anomaly – *SYN:* Pelger-Huët nuclear anomaly
Pelger-Huët nuclear anomaly – congenital inhibition of lobulation in the nuclei of neutrophilic leukocytes. *SYN:* Huët-Pelger anomaly

Pelizaeus, Friedrich, German neurologist, 1850-1917.
Merzbacher-Pelizaeus disease – *SYN:* Pelizaeus-Merzbacher disease
Pelizaeus-Merzbacher disease – a sudanophilic leukodystrophy with a tigroid appearance of the myelin resulting from patchy demyelination. *SYN:* Merzbacher-Pelizaeus disease

Pellegrini, Augusto, Italian surgeon, *1877.
Pellegrini disease – a calcific density in the medial collateral ligament and/or bony growth at the internal condyle of the femur. *SYN:* Pellegrini-Stieda disease
Pellegrini-Stieda disease – *SYN:* Pellegrini disease

Pellizzari, Pietro, Italian dermatologist, 1823-1892.
Jadassohn-Pellizzari anetoderma – see under Jadassohn

Pellizzi, G.B., 19th-20th century Italian physician.
Pellizzi syndrome – a disorder in which gonadal maturation and the adolescent growth spurt in bodily height occur in the first decade of life. *SYN:* macrogenitosomia praecox

Pemberton, John de J., U.S. surgeon, 1887-1967.
Pemberton sign – in patients with upper mediastinal obstruction secondary to tumor, retrosternal goiter, or lymphoma, venous congestion occurs when the arms are raised above the head.

Pena, S.D.J.
Pena-Shokeir II syndrome – onset from birth of vomiting, failure to thrive.

Pendred, Vaughan, English surgeon, 1869-1946.
Pendred syndrome – a type of familial goiter.

Penfield, W.
Penfield syndrome – onset 6 to 7 years of age, primarily in males, of seizures accompanied by vegetative manifestations.

Penrose, Charles B., U.S. gynecologist, 1862-1925.
Penrose drain – a soft tube-shaped rubber drain.
Penrose tourniquet

NOTES

Penrose tube

Penzoldt, Franz, German physician, 1849-1927.
Penzoldt test – for acetone.

Pepper, William, Jr., U.S. physician, 1874-1947.
Pepper syndrome – obsolete term for neuroblastoma of the adrenal gland with metastases in the liver.

Pereyra, Armand Joseph, U.S. gynecologist and obstetrician, *1904.
Pereyra bladder suspension
Pereyra cannula
Pereyra needle
Pereyra operation – *SYN:* Pereyra procedure
Pereyra paraurethral suspension
Pereyra procedure – surgical procedure for the correction of incontinence.
   SYN: Pereyra operation; Pereyra technique
Pereyra technique – *SYN:* Pereyra procedure
Pereyra vesicourethral suspension

Perez, Bernard, French physician, 1836-1903.
Perez reflex – running a finger down the spine of an infant held supported in a prone position will normally cause the whole body to become extended.

Perez, George V., Spanish physician, d. 1920.
Perez sign – rales common in cases of fibrous mediastinitis and also of aneurysm of the aortic arch.

Perheentupa, Jaakko, Finish physician.
Perheentupa syndrome – failure to grow, amblyopia. *SYN:* Mulibrey (muscle, liver, brain, eye) nanism

Perkins, Elisha, U.S. physician, 1741-1799.
perkinism – a form of quackery purporting to treat disease by applying metals with magnetic and magic properties.

Perkins, George, English orthopedic surgeon, 1892-1979.
Perkins elevator
Perkins formula
Perkins line
Perkins retractor
Perkins test
Perkins tonometer
Perkins traction
Perkins tractor

Perkoff, G.T.
  Perkoff syndrome – poststeroid myopathy. *SYN:* Slocumb syndrome

Perlia, Richard, 19th century German ophthalmologist.
  convergence nucleus of Perlia – *SYN:* Perlia nucleus
  Perlia nucleus – a small cell group located between the somatic cell
    columns of the oculomotor nuclei. *SYN:* convergence nucleus of Perlia;
    Spitzka nucleus

Perlman, M., 20th century Israeli physician.
  Perlman syndrome – fatal autosomal recessive disorder.

Perls, Max, German pathologist, 1843-1881.
  Perls Prussian blue stain – for ferric iron.
  Perls test – for hemosiderin, utilizing Perls Prussian blue stain.

Perlstein, Meyer Aaron, U.S. pediatrician, 1902-1969.
  Perlstein brace – *SYN:* Perlstein orthosis
  Perlstein joint – *SYN:* Perlstein orthosis
  Perlstein orthosis – children's ankle-foot orthosis. *SYN:* Perlstein brace;
    Perlstein joint

Perrin, Maurice, French surgeon, 1826-1889.
  Perrin-Ferraton disease – hip snap.

Perroncito, Aldo, Italian histologist, 1882-1929.
  Perroncito apparatus – fibrils in the form of spirals which occur during
    nerve regeneration. *SYN:* Perroncito spirals
  Perroncito spirals – *SYN:* Perroncito apparatus

Perry, Murle, 20th century U.S. colostomy patient.
  Perry bag – a type of colostomy bag.

Persian Gulf, location of war where the syndrome was first experienced.
  Persian Gulf syndrome – various symptoms experienced by veterans of
    the Persian Gulf War.

NOTES

Perthes, Georg C., German surgeon, 1869-1927.
Calvé-Perthes disease – *SYN:* Legg-Calvé-Perthes disease
Legg-Calvé-Perthes disease – see under Legg
Perthes disease – *SYN:* Legg-Calvé-Perthes disease
Perthes incision
Perthes lesion
Perthes sling – used primarily for patients with Legg-Calvé-Perthes disease to support the leg in partial flexion.
Perthes test – for patency of the deep femoral vein.

Pertik, Otto, Hungarian pathologist, 1852-1913.
Pertik diverticulum – an abnormally deep pharyngeal recess.

Peters, Albert, German physician, 1862-1938.
Peters anomaly – a congenital disorder originating from faulty separation of embryonic structures. *SYN:* anterior chamber cleavage syndrome

Peters, Hubert, Austrian obstetrician, 1859-1934.
Peters ovum – one of very few young human embryos recovered in good condition; its study furnished many facts regarding early embryonic changes.
Peters tissue forceps

Petersen, Christian F., German surgeon, 1845-1908.
Petersen bag – an obsolete device consisting of a rubber bag introduced into the rectum and inflated to push up the bladder to facilitate suprapubic cystotomy.
Petersen lithotomy
Petersen operation

Petit, Alexis T., French physicist, 1791-1820.
Dulong-Petit law – see under Dulong

Petit, Antoine, French surgeon and anatomist, 1718-1794.
Petit ligament – a fold of peritoneum containing the rectouterine muscle. *SYN:* sacrouterine fold

Petit, François du, French surgeon and anatomist, 1664-1741.
Petit canals – the spaces between the fibers of the ciliary zonule at the equator of the lens of the eye. *SYN:* zonular spaces
Petit sinus – the space between the superior aspect of each cusp of the aortic valve and the dilated portion of the wall of the ascending aorta. *SYN:* aortic sinus

Petit, Jean L., French surgeon, 1674-1750.
Petit hernia – lumbar hernia occurring in Petit triangle.

Petit herniotomy – herniotomy without incision into the sac.
Petit ligament
Petit lumbar triangle – an area in the posterior abdominal wall.
    SYN: lumbar triangle

Petit, Paul, French anatomist, *1889.
    Petit aponeurosis – the posterior layer of the broad ligament of the uterus.

Pétrequin, Joseph Pierre Eléonor, French surgeon, 1809-1896.
    Pétrequin ligament

Petri, Julius, German bacteriologist, 1852-1921.
    Petri dish – a small shallow plate used especially in microbiology for the cultivation of microorganisms on solid media. *SYN:* Petri plate
    Petri plate – *SYN:* Petri dish
    Petri test – for proteins.

Pette, H.H., German neuropathologist, 1887-1964.
    Pette-Döring disease – a form of subacute sclerosing panencephalitis.
    SYN: nodular panencephalitis

Pettenkofer, Max Josef von, German chemist, 1818-1901.
    Pettenkofer test – for bile acids in urine.

Pettit, Auguste, French physician, 1869-1939.
    Bachman-Pettit test – see under Bachman

Petzetakis, M.
    Petzetakis syndrome – possible virus of *Chlamydia.* *SYN:* cat-scratch fever
    Petzetakis-Takos syndrome – keratitis, eyelid edema, and other eye ailments caused by severe malnutrition.

Peutz, Johnnes Laurentius Augustinus, Dutch physician, 1886-1957.
    Jeghers-Peutz syndrome – *SYN:* Peutz-Jeghers syndrome
    Peutz-Jeghers syndrome – generalized hamartomatous multiple polyposis of the intestinal tract, consistently involving the jejunum, associated with melanin spots of the lips, buccal mucosa, and fingers.
    SYN: Jeghers-Peutz syndrome; Peutz syndrome

NOTES

Peutz syndrome – *SYN:* Peutz-Jeghers syndrome

Peyer, Johann Conrad, Swiss anatomist, 1653-1712.
Peyer glands – *SYN:* Peyer patches
Peyer nodules – solitary lymph nodes.
Peyer patches – collections of many lymphoid follicles closely packed together, forming oblong elevations on the mucous membrane of the small intestine. *SYN:* aggregate glands; aggregate lymphatic follicles; aggregate lymphatic nodules; agmen peyerianum; folliculi lymphatici aggregati; Peyer glands

Peyronie, François de la, French surgeon, 1678-1747.
Peyronie disease – plaques or strands of dense fibrous tissue surrounding the corpus cavernosum of the penis, causing deformity and painful erection. *SYN:* penile fibromatosis; van Buren disease
Peyronie-like plaque

Peyrot, Jean J., French surgeon, 1843-1918.
Peyrot thorax – an obliquely oval deformity of the chest in cases of a very large pleural effusion.

Pezzer, Oscar M.B. de, see under de Pezzer

Pezzi, Cesare, Italian physician.
Laubry-Pezzi syndrome – see under Laubry

Pfannenstiel, Hermann Johann, German gynecologist, 1862-1909.
Pfannenstiel incision – an incision made transversely and through the external sheath of the recti muscles, about an inch above the pubes.
Pfannenstiel transverse approach

Pfaundler, Meinhard von, German physician, 1872-1947.
Pfaundler-Hurler syndrome – *SYN:* Hurler syndrome

Pfeiffer, Emil, German physician, 1846-1921.
Pfeiffer disease – infectious mononucleosis. *SYN:* glandular fever

Pfeiffer, Richard F.J., German physician, 1858-1945.
Pfeiffer bacillus – a species found in the respiratory tract that causes acute respiratory infection, acute conjunctivitis, bacterial meningitis, and purulent meningitis. *SYN: Haemophilus influenzae*
Pfeiffer blood agar – solid agar, with a few drops of human blood smeared on the surface.
Pfeifferella – an obsolete genus of bacteria.
Pfeiffer phenomenon – bacteriolysis.
Pfeiffer syndrome – *SYN:* type V acrocephalosyndactyly

Pflüger, Eduard F.W., German anatomist and physiologist, 1829-1910.
    Pflüger cords – ovarian tubes. *SYN:* Pflüger tubes
    Pflüger law – a given segment of a nerve is irritated by the development of catelectrotonus and the disappearance of anelectrotonus, but the reverse does not hold. *SYN:* law of polar excitation
    Pflüger tubes – *SYN:* Pflüger cords

Pfuhl, Eduard, German physician, 1852-1905.
    Pfuhl sign – the pressure of pus within a subphrenic abscess rises during inspiration and falls during expiration, the reverse of what happens in the case of a purulent collection above the diaphragm.

Phalen, George S., U.S. orthopedist, *1911.
    Phalen maneuver – a maneuver done to check for carpal tunnel abnormality. *SYN:* Phalen sign; Phalen test
    Phalen position
    Phalen sign – *SYN:* Phalen maneuver
    Phalen test – *SYN:* Phalen maneuver

Phelps, Abel Mix, U.S. surgeon, 1851-1902.
    Phelps brace
    Phelps gracilis test
    Phelps operation – surgery for talipes.
    Phelps orthosis
    Phelps splint

Phelps, Winthrop Morgan, U.S. orthopedic surgeon, 1894-1971.
    Phelps method of exercise – a method of exercise used to treat individuals with central nervous system lesions.
    Phelps neurectomy
    Phelps partial resection
    Phelps scalpulectomy

Phemister, Dallas B., U.S. surgeon, 1882-1951.
    Phemister acromioclavicular pin fixation
    Phemister approach

NOTES

P

Phemister biopsy trephine
Phemister brace
Phemister elevator
Phemister graft – an autogenous onlay bone graft used in treating delayed union of fractures.
Phemister incision
Phemister medial approach
Phemister onlay bone graft
Phemister punch
Phemister rasp
Phemister raspatory
Phemister reamer
Phemister splint

Philadelphia, city in Pennsylvania.
Philadelphia chromosome – an abnormal minute chromosome formed by a rearrangement of chromosomes 9 and 22.
Philadelphia cocktail – *SYN:* Rivers cocktail
Philadelphia collar – head and neck orthosis.

Philip, Sir Robert W., Scottish physician, 1857-1939.
Philip glands – enlarged deep glands just above the clavicle.

Philippe, Claudien, French pathologist, 1866-1903.
Philippe triangle

Phillips, Charles, French urologist, 1809-1871.
Phillips bougie
Phillips catheter – a urethral catheter with a filiform guide for the urethra.
Phillips clamp
Phillips dilator
Phillips forceps

Phocas, B. Gerasime, French surgeon, 1861-1937.
Phocas disease – chronic glandular mastitis.

Physick, Philip Syng, U.S. surgeon, 1768-1837.
Physick operation
Physick pouches – proctitis with mucous discharge and burning pain, involving especially the sacculations between the rectal valves.

Pick, Arnold, Czech psychiatrist, 1851-1924.
Arnold Pick syndrome – inability to focus reflexively on objects due to apperceptive blindness.

Pick bundle – nerve fibers recurring rostralward from the pyramidal tract in the medulla oblongata and believed to consist of corticonuclear fibers.

Pick, Friedel, German physician, 1867-1926.
  Pick atrophy – *SYN:* Pick disease
  Pick bodies – intracytoplasmic argentophilic inclusion bodies seen in neurons in Pick disease.
  Pick disease – a rare type of cerebral degenerative disorder manifested primarily as dementia. *SYN:* Pick atrophy; Pick syndrome; progressive circumscribed cerebral atrophy
  Pick syndrome – *SYN:* Pick disease

Pick, Ludwig, German physician, 1868-1935.
  Niemann-Pick cell – *SYN:* Pick cell
  Niemann-Pick disease – see under Niemann
  Pick cell – a relatively large mononuclear cell widely distributed in the spleen and other tissues in Niemann-Pick disease. *SYN:* Niemann-Pick cell
  Pick tubular adenoma – a testicular tumor. *SYN:* androblastoma

Pickles, William, English physician, 1885-1969.
  Pickles chart – day-by-day plots of new cases of infectious disease used to demonstrate the progress of an epidemic in a relatively isolated population.

Pickworth, F.A.
  Lepehne-Pickworth stain – see under Lepehne

Pierini, Luigi, 20th century Argentinian dermatologist.
  atrophoderma of Pasini and Pierini – see under Pasini
  Pasini-Pierini syndrome – see under Pasini

Pierre Mauriac, see under Mauriac, Leonard Pierre

Pierre Robin, see under Robin, Pierre

Piersol, George Arthur, U.S. anatomist, 1856-1924.
  Piersol point – shows the location of the vesical orifice.

NOTES

P

Pignet, Maurice-C.J., French surgeon, *1871.
  Pignet formula

Pilcz, Alexander, Austrian neurologist, 1871-1954.
  Pilcz reflex – pupillary consensual light reflex.

Piltz, Jan, Polish neurologist, 1870-1931.
  Piltz reflex – a pupil's attention reflex.
  Piltz sign – constriction of both pupils when an effort is made to close
    eyelids forcibly held apart. *SYN:* eye-closure pupil reaction; Westphal-Piltz
    phenomenon; Westphal pupillary reflex
  Westphal-Piltz phenomenon – *SYN:* Piltz sign

Pinard, Adolphe, French obstetrician, 1844-1934.
  Pinard fetoscope
  Pinard maneuver – for management of a frank breech presentation.
  Pinard sign

Pindborg, Jens J., Danish oral pathologist, *1921.
  Pindborg tumor – a benign epithelial odontogenic neoplasm.
    SYN: calcifying epithelial odontogenic tumor

Pinel, Philippe, French psychiatrist, 1745-1826.
  Haslam-Pinel syndrome – see under Haslam
  Pinel-Haslam syndrome – *SYN:* Haslam-Pinel syndrome
  Pinel system – the abolition of forcible restraint in the treatment of mental
    hospital patients.

Pinkus, Felix, German-U.S. dermatologist, 1868-1947.
  Pinkus disease – benign asymptomatic, flat-topped, skin-colored papules
    mainly affecting children and young adults.

Pinkus, Hermann Karl Benno, German-U.S. dermatologist, 1905-1985.
  Pinkus disease – boggy plaque in which degenerating hair follicles
    contain pools of mucin. *SYN:* alopecia mucinosa; follicular mucinosis;
    mucinous alopecia
  Pinkus epithelioma – *SYN:* Pinkus fibroepithelioma
  Pinkus fibroepithelioma – a pedunculated, dome-shaped tumor,
    considered to be a form of basal cell carcinoma. *SYN:* Pinkus epithelioma;
    premalignant fibroepithelioma

Piñol Aguadé, Joaquin, Spanish physician, *1917.
  Vilanova-Piñol Aguadé syndrome – see under Vilanova

Pins, Emil, Austrian physician, 1845-1913.
  Pins sign – *SYN:* Ewart sign

Pins syndrome – dullness, diminution of fremitus and of the vesicular murmur, and a slight distant blowing sound heard in the posteroinferior region of the left chest in cases of pericardial effusion.

Pintner, Rudolf, U.S. psychologist, 1884-1942.
Pintner-Paterson scale of performance tests – series of 15 performance tests.

Piotrowski, Aleksanda, German neurologist, *1878.
Piotrowski reflex – plantar flexion of the ankle and toes, occurs by tapping the anterior tibial muscle. *SYN:* Piotrowski sign
Piotrowski sign – *SYN:* Piotrowski reflex

Piper, E.B., U.S. obstetrician-gynecologist, 1881-1935.
Piper forceps – obstetrical forceps used to facilitate delivery of the head in breech presentation.
Piper lateral wall retractor

Pirie, George A., Scottish radiologist, 1864-1929.
Pirie bone – an anomalous bone of the foot located near the head of the talus. *SYN:* dorsal talonavicular bone

Pirogoff, Nikolai I., Russian surgeon, 1810-1881.
Pirogoff amputation – amputation of the foot.
Pirogoff angle – the junction of the internal jugular and subclavian veins; in neuroradiology, the angle of union of the superior thalamostriate vein with the internal cerebral vein. *SYN:* venous angle
Pirogoff operation
Pirogoff triangle – a triangle formed by the intermediate tendon of the digastric muscle, the posterior border of the mylohyoid muscle, and the hypoglossal nerve.

Pirquet von Cesenatico, Clemens P., Austrian physician, 1874-1929.
Pirquet reaction – *SYN:* Pirquet test
Pirquet test – a cutaneous tuberculin test. *SYN:* dermotuberculin reaction; Pirquet reaction

NOTES

P

Piskacek, Ludwig, Austrian obstetrician, 1854-1933.
Piskacek sign – asymmetrical enlargement of the corpus uteri.

Pitkin, George, U.S. surgeon, 1885-1934.
Pitkin dermatome
Pitkin needle – *SYN:* Pitkin syringe
Pitkin syringe – a self-filling syringe used to administer anesthesia.
SYN: Pitkin needle

Pitot, Henri, French engineer, 1695-1771.
Pitot tube – a stationary L-shaped tube inserted in a fluid stream and used for measuring the velocity of fluid movement.

Pitres, Jean A., French physician, 1848-1927.
Pitres area – prefrontal cortex of the cerebral hemisphere.
Pitres rule – a multilingual person who recovers from aphasia will recover the language that was most fluent at the time of the event.
Pitres section – six coronal sections through the brain.
Pitres sign – diminished sensation in the testes and scrotum in tubes dorsalis; pain is caused by slight touch. *SYN:* haphalgesia

Placido da Costa, Antonio, Portuguese ophthalmologist, 1848-1916.
Placido da Costa disk – an instrument marked with lines or circles, used to observe the corneal reflex. *SYN:* Placido disk; Placido keratoscope
Placido disk – *SYN:* Placido da Costa disk
Placido keratoscope – *SYN:* Placido da Costa disk

Planck, Max, German physicist and Nobel laureate, 1858-1947.
Planck constant – a natural constant occurring in many physical formulas.
Planck theory – that energy can be emitted, transmitted, and absorbed only in discrete quantities. *SYN:* quantum theory

Plateau, Joseph Antoine Ferdinand, Belgian physicist, 1801-1883.
Plateau-Talbot law – when successive light stimuli follow each other sufficiently rapidly to become fused, their apparent brightness is diminished.

Plato, Greek philosopher, 427-347 B.C.
platonic love – a love in which there is no sexual desire.

Platt, Sir Harry, English surgeon, *1886.
Putti-Platt arthroplasty
Putti-Platt director
Putti-Platt instrumentation
Putti-Platt operation – see under Putti
Putti-Platt procedure – *SYN:* Putti-Platt operation

Putti-Platt shoulder procedure
reverse Putti-Platt procedure

Plaut, Hugo Karl, German physician, 1858-1928.
  Plaut bacillus – *SYN: Fusobacterium nucleatum*

Pleasure, Max A., U.S. dentist. 1903-1965.
  Pleasure curve – a curve of occlusion which, when viewed in sagittal
    section, conforms to a line that is convex upward, except for the last
    molars.

Plimmer, Henry G., English protozoologist, 1857-1918.
  Plimmer bodies – obsolete term for cancer bodies.

Plotz, Harry, U.S. physician, 1890-1947.
  Plotz bacillus – a small, gram-positive bacterium suggested as the
    pathogenic agent of typhus fever.

Plugge, Pieter Cornelis, Dutch biochemist, 1847-1897.
  Plugge test – for phenol.

Plummer, Henry Stanley, U.S. physician, 1874-1937.
  Plummer bag – *SYN:* Plummer dilator
  Plummer bougie
  Plummer dilator – an instrument for dilating the lower end of the
    esophagus in cardiospasm. *SYN:* Plummer bag
  Plummer disease – hyperthyroidism resulting from a nodular toxic goiter,
    usually not accompanied by exophthalmos.
  Plummer sign – a sign of Graves disease.
  Plummer-Vinson syndrome – iron deficiency anemia, dysphagia,
    esophageal web, and atrophic glossitis. *SYN:* Paterson-Kelly syndrome;
    sideropenic dysphagia

Plutarch, Greek philosopher, ca. 46-119 A.D.
  Appian-Plutarch syndrome – see under Appian of Alexandria

NOTES

P

Pohl, John F., U.S. orthopedic surgeon, 1903-1981.
method of Pohl – locomotor rehabilitation system for individuals with central nervous system lesions.

Pohl, Julius Heinrich, late 19th century German pharmacologist.
Pohl test – for globulins.

Poirier, Paul J., French surgeon, 1853-1907.
Poirier gland – a lymph node on the uterine artery where it crosses the ureter.
Poirier line – extends from the nasion to the lambda.
space of Poirier

Poiseuille, Jean Léonard Marie, French physiologist and physicist, 1797-1869.
poise – the unit of viscosity equal to 1 dyne-second per square centimeter and to 0.1 pascal-second.
Poiseuille equation
Poiseuille law – describes the volume flow rate of a liquid through a tube.
Poiseuille space – *SYN:* still layer
Poiseuille viscosity coefficient – an expression of the viscosity as determined by the capillary tube method.

Poisson, Siméon Denis, French mathematician, 1781-1840.
Poisson distribution – a discontinuous distribution important in statistical work.
Poisson-Pearson formula – determines the statistical error in calculating the endemic index of malaria.
Poisson ratio

Poland, (Polland), Alfred, English physician, 1820-1872.
Poland anomaly – *SYN:* Poland syndrome
Poland syndrome – absence of a portion of the pectoralis major muscle and syndactyly. *SYN:* Poland anomaly

Politzer, Adam, Austrian otologist, 1835-1920.
Politzer bag – a pear-shaped rubber bag used for forcing air through the eustachian tube by the Politzer method.
Politzer ear perforator
politzerization – *SYN:* Politzer method
Politzer knife
Politzer luminous cone – a triangular area at the anterior inferior part of the tympanic membrane. *SYN:* pyramid of light

Politzer method – inflation of the eustachian tube and tympanum by forcing air into the nasal cavity at the instant the patient swallows. *SYN:* politzerization

Politzer operation

Politzer otoscope

Politzer speculum

Politzer test – a test for deafness in one ear.

Polland, var. of Poland

Polya, var. of Pólya

Pólya, Jenö (Eugene Polya), Hungarian surgeon, 1876-1944.

Hofmeister-Pólya anastomosis

Pólya anastomosis

Pólya femoral herniorrhaphy

Pólya gastrectomy – partial gastrectomy with retrocolic anastomosis of the full width of stomach to jejunum. *SYN:* Pólya operation

Pólya gastroenterostomy

Pólya gastrojejunostomy

Pólya operation – *SYN:* Pólya gastrectomy

Pólya technique

Reichel-Pólya stomach resection – see under Reichel, Friedrich P.

Pomeroy, Ralph H., U.S. obstetrician-gynecologist, 1867-1925.

Pomeroy operation – excision of a ligated portion of the fallopian tubes.

Pomeroy salpingectomy

Pomeroy sterilization

Pomeroy syringe

Pomeroy tubal ligation

Pompe, Johann C., 20th century Dutch physician.

Pompe disease – glycogenosis due to lysosomal alpha-1,4-glucosidase deficiency. *SYN:* Pompe syndrome; type 2 glycogenosis

Pompe syndrome – *SYN:* Pompe disease

NOTES

Poncet, Antonin, French surgeon, 1849-1913.
Poncet disease – *SYN:* Poncet rheumatism
Poncet rheumatism – tuberculous arthritis. *SYN:* Poncet disease

Ponfick, Emil, German pathologist, 1844-1913.
Ponfick shadow – a hypochromic, crescent-shaped erythrocyte.
SYN: achromocyte

Pontiac, city in Michigan, where an outbreak of Legionella occurred in 1968.
Pontiac fever – a strain of *Legionella pneumophila.*

Pool, Eugene H., U.S. surgeon, 1874-1949.
Pool phenomenon – in tetany, spasm of the extensor muscles of the knee
and of the calf muscles when the extended leg is flexed at the hip; in
tetany, contraction of the arm muscles following the stretching of the
brachial plexus resembles the contraction resulting from stimulation of
the ulnar nerve. *SYN:* Pool-Schlesinger sign; Schlesinger sign
Pool-Schlesinger sign – *SYN:* Pool phenomenon

Porges, Otto, Austrian bacteriologist, 1879-1968.
Porges-Meier test – an early flocculation test for syphilis.
Porges method – a method of destroying the capsule of bacteria by
heating with N/4 hydrochloric acid and neutralizing with NaOH.

Porro, Edoardo, Italian obstetrician, 1842-1902.
Porro cesarean hysterectomy – *SYN:* Porro hysterectomy
Porro hysterectomy – cesarean section followed by hysterectomy.
SYN: Porro cesarean hysterectomy; Porro operation
Porro operation – *SYN:* Porro hysterectomy

Porter, Curt C., U.S. biochemist, *1914.
Porter-Silber chromogens – used chiefly to determine plasma cortisol
concentrations and the urinary output of 17-hydroxycorticoids.
Porter-Silber chromogens test – a urine test used as a measure of
adrenocortical function. *SYN:* 17-hydroxycorticosteroid test
Porter-Silber reaction – the basis of the 17-hydroxycorticosteroid test.

Porter, Rodney R., English biochemist, 1917-1985, joint winner of 1972 Nobel
Prize for work related to antibodies.

Porter, Thomas C., English scientist, 1860-1933.
Ferry-Porter law – see under Ferry
Porter law – a principle that critical flicker frequency increases with
brightness of stimulus independent of stimulus wavelength.

Porter, W.B.
Porter syndrome – idiopathic benign pericarditis.

Porter, William H., Irish surgeon, 1790-1861.
    Porter fascia – the layer of fascia investing the infrahyoid muscles and contributing to the formation of the carotid sheath. *SYN:* pretracheal fascia
    Porter tugging – tracheal tugging.

Porteus, M.E.M., 20th century English geneticist.
    Porteus syndrome – an X-linked disorder characterized by mental retardation, short stature, high-pitched voice, high forehead, alopecia, and receding hairline.

Porteus, Stanley David, U.S. psychologist, 1883-1972.
    Porteus maze – an original intelligence test.

Posadas, Alejandro, Argentinian parasitologist, 1870-1902.
    Posadas disease – a variable, benign, severe, or fatal systemic mycosis due to inhalation of dust particles containing arthroconidia of *Coccidioides immitis*. *SYN:* coccidioidomycosis

Posner, Carl, German urologist, 1854-1929.
    Posner gonioprism
    Posner procedure
    Posner test – for the source of albumin in urine.

Potain, Pierre C.E., French physician, 1825-1901.
    Potain sign – in dilation of the aorta, dullness on percussion.

Poth, D.O., U.S. physician.
    Poth keratosis – self-healing skin disorder that resembles squamous cell carcinoma.

Pott, Sir Percivall, English surgeon, 1713-1788.
    Pott abscess – tuberculous abscess of the spine.
    Pott aneurysm – dilation and tortuosity of a vein resulting from an acquired communication with an adjacent artery. *SYN:* aneurysmal varix
    Pott curvature – a gibbous deformity, i.e., a sharp angulation of the spine, occurring in Pott disease. *SYN:* angular curvature

NOTES

P

Pott disease – tuberculous infection of the spine associated with a sharp angulation of the spine at the point of disease. *SYN:* tuberculous spondylitis

Pott eversion osteotomy

Pott fracture – fracture of the lower part of the fibula and of the malleolus of the tibia, with outward displacement of the foot.

Pott gangrene – dry gangrene occurring in the aged in consequence of occlusion of an artery, particularly affecting the extremities. *SYN:* senile gangrene

Pott paralysis – *SYN:* Pott paraplegia

Pott paraplegia – paralysis of the lower part of the body and the extremities due to pressure on the spinal cord as the result of tuberculous spondylitis. *SYN:* Pott paralysis

Pott puffy tumor – a circumscribed swelling of the scalp indicating an underlying osteitis of the skull or an extradural abscess.

Pott spinal curvature

Pott I syndrome – *SYN:* Dupuytren fracture

Pott II syndrome – dry gangrene caused by arterial obstruction. *SYN:* senile gangrene

Potter, Edith L., U.S. perinatal pathologist, *1901.

Potter classification of polycystic kidney

Potter disease – *SYN:* Potter facies

Potter facies – characteristic facies seen in severe renal malformations. *SYN:* Potter disease

Potter syndrome – renal agenesis, with hypoplastic lungs and associated neonatal respiratory distress.

Potter, Irving White, U.S. obstetrician, 1868-1956.

Potter version – obsolete term for an internal version to a breech presentation.

Potts, Willis J., U.S. pediatric surgeon, 1895-1968.

Potts anastomosis – *SYN:* Potts operation

Potts aortic clamp

Potts bronchial forceps

Potts bulldog forceps

Potts cardiovascular clamp

Potts clamp – a fine-toothed, multiple-point, vascular fixation clamp that imparts limited trauma to the vessel while securely holding it.

Potts coarctation clamp

Potts coarctation forceps

Potts dilator
Potts dissector
Potts elevator
Potts expansile dilator
Potts expansile knife
Potts forceps
Potts ligature
Potts needle
Potts operation – direct side-to-side anastomosis between the aorta and pulmonary artery as a palliative procedure in congenital malformation of the heart. *SYN:* Potts anastomosis
Potts patent ductus clamp
Potts rib shears
Potts scissors
Potts shunt
Potts-Smith bipolar forceps
Potts splint
Potts tenaculum
Potts valvulotome
Potts vascular scissors

Pötzl, Otto, Austrian psychiatrist, *1877.
Pötzl phenomenon – an appearance in dreams.
Pötzl syndrome – a form of alexia.

Poulet, Alfred, French physician, 1848-1888.
Poulet disease – rheumatoid osteoperiostitis.

Poupart, François, French anatomist, 1616-1708.
Poupart inguinal ligament
Poupart ligament – a fibrous band that forms the floor of the inguinal canal. *SYN:* inguinal ligament
Poupart ligament shelving edge

NOTES

P

Poupart line – a vertical line that marks off the hypochondriac, lumbar, and iliac from the epigastric, umbilical, and hypogastric regions, respectively.

Powassan, city in Ontario, Canada, where disease was first reported.
Powassan encephalitis – an acute disease of children, transmitted by ixodid ticks.
Powassan virus – causes Powassan encephalitis.

Pozzi, Samuel J., French gynecologist and anatomist, 1846-1918.
Pozzi forceps
Pozzi muscle – a short extensor muscle of the fingers of rare occurrence, comparable to the short extensor of the toes. *SYN:* extensor digitorum brevis muscle of hand
Pozzi operation
Pozzi syndrome – leukorrhea and backache, occasionally affiliated with endometriosis.
Pozzi tenaculum

Prader, Andrea, Swiss pediatrician, *1919.
Prader-Willi syndrome – a congenital syndrome of unknown etiology characterized by short stature, mental retardation, polyphagia with marked obesity, and sexual infantilism.

Pratt, Joseph H., U.S. physician, 1872-1956.
Pratt anoscope
Pratt curette
Pratt dilator
Pratt director
Pratt forceps
Pratt hook
Pratt open reduction
Pratt probe
Pratt proctoscope
Pratt scissors
Pratt sound
Pratt speculum
Pratt symptom – rigidity in the muscles of an injured limb preceding the occurrence of gangrene.
Pratt T-clamp
Pratt technique

Prausnitz, Otto Carl W., German hygienist, 1876-1963.
Prausnitz-Küstner antibody – one of the IgE class of antibodies first demonstrated by passive transfer to the skin. *SYN:* atopic reagin

Prausnitz-Küstner reaction – formerly the standard method of demostrating IgE.

reversed Prausnitz-Küstner reaction – the appearance of an urticarial reaction at the site of injection when serum containing reaginic antibody is injected into the skin of a person in whom the allergen is already present.

Prehn, D.T., 20th century U.S. physician.
Prehn sign – confirms testicular torsion.

Preiser, Georg Karl Felix, German orthopedic surgeon, 1879-1913.
Preiser disease – atrophy or osteoporosis due to osteoporosis or fracture that has not been properly treated.

Preisz, Hugo von, Hungarian bacteriologist, 1860-1940.
Preisz-Nocard bacillus – a species found in necrotic areas in sheep kidney, in caseous lymphadenitis in sheep, and in ulcerative lesions in warm-blooded animals. *SYN: Corynebacterium pseudotuberculosis*

Prentice, Charles F., U.S. optician, 1854-1946.
Prentice rule – each centimeter of decentration of a lens results in 1 prism diopter of deviation of light for each diopter of lens power.

Prévost, Jean Louis, Swiss physician, 1838-1927.
Prévost law – the head turns toward a lateral cerebral lesion.
Prévost sign – seen in hemiplegia where there is conjugate deviation of the head and eyes.

Preyer, Thierry Wilhelm, German physiologist, 1841-1897.
Preyer reflex – *SYN:* auricle reflex
Preyer test – for carbon monoxide in the blood.

Pribnow, David, 20th century U.S. molecular biologist.
Pribnow box – a highly conserved DNA sequence of about 180 base pairs near the 3′ end of specific homeotic genes.

Price, Ernest Arthur, English biochemist, *1882.
Carr-Price reaction – see under Carr

NOTES

Price-Jones, Cecil, English hematologist, 1863-1943.
Price-Jones curve – distribution curve of the measured diameters of red blood cells.

Priessnitz, Vinzenz, Silesian peasant, 1799-1851.
Priessnitz compresses – the use of cold water as packs, showers, or baths as a therapeutic system.
Priessnitz method of treatment – the use of physical work, fresh air, diet, and exercise; may also include Priessnitz compresses.

Priestley, John Gillies, English physiologist, 1880-1941.
Haldane-Priestley sample – see under Haldane

Princeteau, L.R., French physician, *1884.
Princeteau tubercle – a slight prominence on the temporal bone near the apex of the petrous part where the superior petrosal sinus begins.

Pringle, John James, English dermatologist, 1855-1922.
Bourneville-Pringle disease – see under Bourneville
Pringle disease – obsolete misnomer for a hamartoma occurring on the face. *SYN:* adenoma sebaceum

Prinzmetal, Myron, U.S. cardiologist, 1908-1994.
Prinzmetal angina – a form of angina pectoris. *SYN:* angina inversa; variant angina pectoris
Prinzmetal II syndrome – precordial anginal attacks. *SYN:* angina pectoris variant

Pritikin, Nathan, U.S. physician, d. 1985.
Pritikin diet – stresses consumption of whole grains, vegetables, and small amounts of lean meat and fish coupled with daily aerobic exercise.

Proetz, Arthur Walter, U.S. otolaryngologist, 1888-1966.
Proetz test – for sense of smell acuity.

Profeta, Giuseppe, Italian dermatologist, 1840-1910.
Profeta law – the subject of congenital syphilis is immune against the acquired disease.

Profichet, Georges Charles, French physician, *1873.
Profichet syndrome – calcareous deposits, primarily affecting extremities. *SYN:* calcinosis circumscripta; calcinosis cutis

Proskauer, Bernhard, German bacteriologist, 1851-1915.
Voges-Proskauer reaction – see under Voges

Proust, Louis J., French chemist, 1755-1826.
   Proust law – the relative weights of the several elements forming a chemical compound are invariable. *SYN:* law of definite proportions

Proust, T., 19th century French physician.
   Proust space – a pocket formed by the deflection of the peritoneum from the rectum to the bladder in the male. *SYN:* rectovesical pouch

Prowazek, Stanislas J.M. von, German protozoologist, 1876-1915.
   Halberstaedter-Prowazek bodies – *SYN:* Prowazek-Greeff bodies
   Prowazek bodies – obsolete term for either of two types of inclusion bodies associated with certain diseases.
   Prowazek-Greeff bodies – distinctive, complex, intracytoplasmic forms found in the conjunctival epithelial cells of persons in the acute phase of trachoma. *SYN:* Halberstaedter-Prowazek bodies; trachoma bodies
   Prowazekia – a genus of coprozoic flagellate protozoans.

Prusiner, Stanley B., winner of 1997 Nobel Prize for work related to infection.

Prussak, Alexander, Russian otologist, 1839-1897.
   Prussak fibers – elastic and connective tissue fiber bounding the pars flaccida membranae tympani.
   Prussak pouch – *SYN:* superior recess of tympanic membrane
   Prussak space – *SYN:* superior recess of tympanic membrane

Psaume, J., 20th century French physician.
   Papillon-Léage and Psaume syndrome – see under Papillon-Léage

Puchtler, H.
   Puchtler-Sweat stain – (1) for basement membranes; (2) for hemoglobin and hemosiderin.

Pudenz, Robert H., U.S. neurosurgeon, 1911-1998.
   Heyer-Pudenz valve – see under Heyer
   Pudenz reservoir
   Pudenz-Schulte thecoperitoneal shunt
   Pudenz shunt

P

Pudenz tube
Pudenz valve – *SYN:* Heyer-Pudenz valve
Pudenz ventricular catheter

Pudlak, P., 20th century Czech physician.
Hermansky-Pudlak syndrome – see under Hermansky

Puestow, Charles B., U.S. surgeon, 1902-1973.
Puestow anastomosis
Puestow biliary tract procedure
Puestow dilator
Puestow guide wire
Puestow procedure – longitudinal pancreatic jejunostomy.
Puestow wire

Pumphrey, Robert E., U.S. physician, *1933.
Bart-Pumphrey syndrome – see under Bart, Robert S.

Punnett, Reginald Crundall, English geneticist, 1875-1967.
Punnett square – a grid used in genetics. *SYN:* checkerboard

Purdy, Charles Wesley, U.S. physician, 1846-1901.
Purdy test – urine test for albumin.

Puretic, S., Croatian dermatologist, 1922-1971.
Murray-Puretic-Drescher syndrome – see under Murray, John

Purkinje, Johannes E. von (Jan E. Purkyne), Bohemian anatomist and physiologist, 1787-1869.
Purkinje afterimage – *SYN:* Bidwell ghost
Purkinje cells – large nerve cells of the cerebellar cortex with a piriform cell body and dendrites arranged in a plane transverse to the folium. *SYN:* Purkinje corpuscles
Purkinje conduction – conduction of the cardiac impulse through the Purkinje system.
Purkinje corpuscles – *SYN:* Purkinje cells
Purkinje effect – *SYN:* Purkinje phenomenon
Purkinje fibers – interlacing fibers formed of modified cardiac muscle cells that are the terminal ramifications of the conducting system of the heart found beneath the endocardium of the ventricles.
Purkinje figures – shadows of the retinal vessels seen as dark lines on a reddish field when a light enters the eye through the sclera and not the pupil.
Purkinje image tracker
Purkinje images – *SYN:* Purkinje-Sanson images

Purkinje layer – the layer of Purkinje cells between the molecular and granular layers of the cerebellar cortex. *SYN:* piriform neuron layer

Purkinje network – the network formed by Purkinje fibers beneath the endocardium.

Purkinje phenomenon – in the light-adapted eye, the region of maximal brightness is in the yellow; in the dark-adapted eye, the region of maximal brightness is in the green. *SYN:* Purkinje effect; Purkinje shift

Purkinje-Sanson images – the two images formed by the anterior and posterior surfaces of the cornea, and the two images formed by the anterior and posterior surfaces of the lens. *SYN:* catatropic images; Purkinje images; Sanson images

Purkinje shift – *SYN:* Purkinje phenomenon

Purkinje system – terminal ramifications in the ventricles of the specialized conducting system of the heart.

Purkyne, var. of Purkinje

Purmann, Matthaeus G., German surgeon, 1648-1721.
Purmann method – treatment of an aneurysm by extirpation of the sac.

Purtscher, Othmar, German ophthalmologist, 1852-1927.
Purtscher disease – *SYN:* Purtscher retinopathy
Purtscher retinopathy – traumatic retinal angiopathy which causes transient visual impairment. *SYN:* Purtscher disease; Purtscher syndrome
Purtscher syndrome – *SYN:* Purtscher retinopathy

Putnam, James J., U.S. neurologist, 1846-1918.
Putnam-Dana syndrome – subacute combined degeneration of the spinal cord.

Putti, Vittorio, Italian surgeon, 1880-1940.
Putti approach
Putti arthroplasty gouge
Putti bone rasp
Putti frame
Putti gouge

NOTES

Putti knee arthrodesis
Putti operation
Putti-Platt arthroplasty
Putti-Platt director
Putti-Platt instrumentation
Putti-Platt operation – a procedure for recurrent dislocation of shoulder joint. *SYN:* Putti-Platt procedure
Putti-Platt procedure – *SYN:* Putti-Platt operation
Putti-Platt shoulder procedure
Putti rasp
Putti shoulder arthrodesis
Putti splint
Putti technique
reverse Putti-Platt procedure

Puusepp, Lyudvig M., Estonian neurosurgeon, 1879-1942.
Puusepp reflex – light stroking of the outer sole of the foot causes slow abduction of the fifth toe.

Pygmalion, Greek mythological character.
Pygmalion effect – self-fulfilling prophecy. *SYN:* Rosenthal effect
pygmalionism – rarely used term for the state of being in love with an object of one's own creation.

Pyle, S. Idell, radiologist.
Greulich and Pyle atlas – see under Greulich

Pym, Sir William, English physician, 1772-1861.
Pym fever – an infectious but not contagious disease occurring in the Balkan Peninsula and other parts of Southern Europe, apparently caused by the bite of the sandfly. *SYN:* phlebotomus fever

Quain, Sir Richard, English physician, 1816-1898.
  Quain fatty heart – fatty tissue around the heart, or fatty degeneration of the heart. *SYN:* cor adiposum

Quant, C.A.J., early 20th century Dutch physician.
  Quant sign – a T-shaped depression found in the occipital bone.

Quasimodo, fictional character in the novel *The Hunchback of Notre Dame.*
  Quasimodo complex – personality disorder in which there is abnormal concern about a defect in one's physical appearance.

Quatrefages de Breau, Jean L.A. de, French naturalist, 1810-1892.
  Quatrefages angle – formed by the meeting of the prolongation of two lines tangential to the most prominent part of the zygomatic arch and to the parietofrontal suture on each side. *SYN:* parietal angle

Queckenstedt, Hans, German physician, 1876-1918.
  Queckenstedt maneuver – *SYN:* Queckenstedt-Stookey test
  Queckenstedt phenomenon – *SYN:* Queckenstedt-Stookey test
  Queckenstedt sign – *SYN:* Queckenstedt-Stookey test
  Queckenstedt-Stookey test – when there is a block of subarachnoid channels, compression of the jugular vein causes little or no increase of pressure in the cerebrospinal fluid. *SYN:* Queckenstedt maneuver; Queckenstedt phenomenon; Quekenstedt sign; Queckenstedt test
  Queckenstedt test – *SYN:* Queckenstedt-Stookey test

Quénu, Eduard A.V.A., French surgeon and anatomist, 1852-1933.
  Quénu hemorrhoidal plexus – lymphatic plexuses in the skin about the anus.
  Quénu-Muret sign – in aneurysm, well-maintained collateral circulation is indicated by issue of blood when the main artery of the limb is compressed and a puncture is made at the periphery.

NOTES

Quervain, Fritz de, see under de Quervain

Quetelet, Lambert Adolphe Jacques, Belgian mathematician and anthropologist, 1796-1874.
    Quetelet index of constitution – weight over height.
    Quetelet rule – body weight in kilograms equals height in centimeters minus 100.

Queyrat, L. Auguste, French dermatologist, 1856-1933.
    erythroplasia of Queyrat – carcinoma in situ of the glans penis.
    Queyrat syndrome – painless thickening of external genitalia; has also been described in the mouth and on the tongue.

Quick, Armand James, U.S. physician, 1894-1978.
    Quick method – *SYN:* prothrombin test
    Quick test – *SYN:* prothrombin test

Quincke, Georg, German physicist, 1834-1924.
    Quincke tubes – glass tubes used in the study of hearing thresholds.

Quincke, Heinrich Irenaeus, German physician, 1842-1922.
    Quincke capillary pulsation – *SYN:* Quincke pulse
    Quincke disease – *SYN:* Quincke edema
    Quincke edema – recurrent, large, circumscribed areas of subcutaneous edema of sudden onset, usually disappearing within 24 hours. *SYN:* angioedema; Milton disease; Milton urticaria; Quincke disease; Quincke I syndrome
    Quincke meningitis – intracranial hypertension of unknown origin.
    Quincke needle
    Quincke pulse – capillary pulsation, a sign of arteriolar dilation and especially well seen in severe aortic insufficiency. *SYN:* Quincke capillary pulsation; Quincke sign
    Quincke puncture – a puncture into the subarachnoid space of the lumbar region to obtain spinal fluid for diagnostic or therapeutic purposes. *SYN:* lumbar puncture
    Quincke sign – *SYN:* Quincke pulse
    Quincke spinal needle
    Quincke I syndrome – *SYN:* Quincke edema

Quinquad, Charles Eugene, French physician, 1842-1894.
    Quinquad disease – pustules of the scalp's hair follicles.
    Quinquad phenomenon – sideways movement of the fingers seen in those with tremors. *SYN:* Quinquad sign
    Quinquad sign – *SYN:* Quinquad phenomenon

Quinton, Wayne E., 20th century U.S. nephrologist.
    Quinton biopsy catheter
    Quinton catheter
    Quinton dual lumen catheter
    Quinton Q-Port catheter
    Quinton Q-Port vascular access port
    Quinton-Scribner shunt – an arteriovenous shunt inserted for
       hemodialysis.
    Quinton tube

NOTES

Rabson, Salem M., U.S. pathologist, 1901-1984.
Rabson-Mendenhall syndrome – diabetes mellitus that is insulin resistant.

Radford, Edward P., Jr., U.S. physiologist, *1922.
Radford nomogram – used to predict necessary tidal volume for artificial respiration on the basis of respiratory rate, body weight, and sex.

Radovici, André, 20th century French physician.
Marinesco-Radovici reflex – *SYN:* Radovici sign
Radovici reflex – *SYN:* Radovici sign
Radovici sign – chin twitching that is caused by scratching the palm. *SYN:* Marinesco-Radovici reflex; palm-chin reflex; palmomental reflex; Radovici reflex

Raeder, Georg Johan, Norwegian ophthalmologist, 1889-1956.
Raeder paratrigeminal syndrome – a postganglionic Horner syndrome associated with trigeminal nerve dysfunction, caused by involvement of the carotid sympathetic plexus.

Rahe, Richard H., U.S. psychiatrist, *1936.
Holmes-Rahe questionnaire – *SYN:* Rahe-Holmes questionnaire
Rahe-Holmes questionnaire – a survey to measure the stressfulness of various life events. *SYN:* Holmes-Rahe questionnaire

Rahn, Hermann, U.S. respiratory physiologist, *1912.
Rahn-Otis sample – an approximation of alveolar gas continuously provided by a simple device that admits just the latter part of each expiration.

Raimiste, Johann M., early 20th century German neurologist.
Raimiste sign – indicates paresis of the hand.

Rainey, George, English anatomist, 1801-1884.
Rainey corpuscles – spores or bradyzoites found within the elongated cysts of the protozoan *Sarcocystis*.
Rainey tube – sarcocyst. *SYN:* Rainey tubule
Rainey tubule – *SYN:* Rainey tube

Ralfe, Charles Henry.
Ralfe test – for acetone in the urine.

Raman, Sir Chandrasekhara Venkata, Indian physicist and Nobel laureate, 1888-1970.
Raman effect – a change in frequency undergone by monochromatic light scattered in passage through a transparent substance whose characteristics determine the amount of change. *SYN:* Raman shift
Raman shift – *SYN:* Raman effect
Raman spectrum – the characteristic array of light produced by the Raman effect.

Ramirez, Oscar M., U.S. plastic surgeon, *1949.
Ramirez EndoFacelift[TM] **dissector**
Ramirez EndoFacelift[TM] **elevator**
Ramirez EndoFacelift[TM] **needle holder**
Ramirez EndoForehead[TM] **A/M dissector**
Ramirez EndoForehead[TM] **A/M scissors**
Ramirez EndoForehead[TM] **dissector, curved**
Ramirez EndoForehead[TM] **dissector, straight**
Ramirez EndoForehead[TM] **dissector**
Ramirez EndoForehead[TM] **flap dissector**
Ramirez EndoForehead[TM] **forceps**
Ramirez EndoForehead[TM] **grasper**
Ramirez EndoForehead[TM] **parietal elevator**
Ramirez EndoForehead[TM] **protector, right and left**
Ramirez EndoForehead[TM] **punch**
Ramirez EndoForehead[TM] **scissors**
Ramirez EndoForehead[TM] **spreader**
Ramirez EndoForehead[TM] **suction coagulator**
Ramirez EndoForehead[TM] **T dissector**
Ramirez telescoping cannula

Ramon, Gaston, French bacteriologist, 1886-1963.
Ramon flocculation test – determines amount of antitoxin necessary to neutralize a toxin. *SYN:* Ramon test
Ramon test – *SYN:* Ramon flocculation test

Ramond, Louis, French internist, 1879-1952.
Ramond point
Ramond sign – a rigidity in the erectus spinae muscle, which occurs with effusive pleurisy.

Rampley, surname of an English surgery technician in the 1880's.
Rampley sponge-holding forceps

Ramsay Hunt, see under Hunt, James Ramsay

Ramsden, Jesse, English optician, 1735-1800.
Ramsden eyepiece
Ramsden ocular – an eyepiece of a microscope, consisting of two planoconvex lenses with convexities turned to each other.

Ramstedt, Conrad, German surgeon, 1867-1963.
Fredet-Ramstedt operation – *SYN:* Ramstedt operation
Ramstedt clamp
Ramstedt dilator
Ramstedt operation – longitudinal incision through the anterior wall of the pyloric canal to the level of the submucosa, to treat hypertrophic pyloric stenosis. *SYN:* Fredet-Ramstedt operation; pyloromyotomy; Ramstedt procedure; Ramstedt pyloromyotomy
Ramstedt procedure – *SYN:* Ramstedt operation
Ramstedt pyloromyotomy – *SYN:* Ramstedt operation
Ramstedt pyloroplasty

Rancho Los Amigos Hospital, medical facility in Downey, California.
Rancho Los Amigos feeder
Rancho Los Amigos Level of Cognitive Functioning Scale
Rancho Los Amigos orthosis
Rancho Los Amigos splint

Rand, Gertrude, U.S. visual psychologist, 1886-1970.
Hardy-Rand-Ritter test – see under Hardy, LeGrand

R

NOTES

Rand, M.J., 20th century pharmacologist.
Burn and Rand theory – see under Burn, J.H.

Randall, Alexander, U.S. urologist, 1885-1951.
Randall curette
Randall endometrial biopsy curette
Randall operation
Randall plaques – minute stones of urinary salts found on erosions of renal papillae.
Randall stone forceps – used to extract calculi from the renal pelvis or calices.

Randolph, Nathaniel Archer, U.S. physician, 1858-1887.
Randolph test – for peptones in the urine.

Ranikhet, town in northern India.
Ranikhet disease – *SYN:* Newcastle disease

Ranke, Johannes, German anthropologist and physician, 1836-1916.
Ranke angle – a facial angle.

Ranke, Karl E. von, German chemist, 1870-1926.
Ranke complex
Ranke formula – for determining the amount of albumin in serous fluid.
Ranke stage

Rankin, Fred Wharton, U.S. surgeon, 1886-1954.
Rankin clamp – a three-bladed clamp used in resection of colon.
Rankin forceps
Rankin hemostat
Rankin hemostatic forceps
Rankin intestinal clamp
Rankin operation
Rankin prostatic retractor
Rankin retractor
Rankin suture

Rankine, William J. McQ., Scottish physicist, 1820-1870.
Rankine scale – a thermometer scale with its zero point at absolute zero.

Ransohoff, Joseph, U.S. surgeon, 1853-1921.
Ransohoff sign – yellow pigmentation in the umbilical region in rupture of the common bile duct.

Ranvier, Louis A., French pathologist, 1835-1922.
nodes of Ranvier – short intervals in the myelin sheaths of nerve fibers.

Ranvier crosses – black or brown figures in the shape of a cross, marking Ranvier nodes in the longitudinal section of a nerve stained with silver nitrate.

Ranvier disks – tactile nerve endings of cupped disklike form in the skin. *SYN:* Ranvier tactile disks

Ranvier membrane

Ranvier plexus – a subbasal stroma plexus of the cornea.

Ranvier segment – the portion of a myelinated nerve fiber between two successive nodes. *SYN:* internodal segment

Ranvier tactile disks – *SYN:* Ranvier disks

Raoult, François M., French physicist, 1830-1899.

Raoult law – the vapor pressure exerted by a component in a solution is directly proportional to its mole-fraction in the solution.

Rapoport, Abraham, Canadian urologist, 1926-1977.

Rapoport test – a differential ureteral catheterization test used to evaluate suspected renovascular hypertension.

Rapoport, Samuel Mitja, Russian biochemist, 1912-1977.

Rapoport-Luebering shunt – part of the glycolytic pathway characteristic of human erythrocytes.

Rapp, R.S.

Rapp-Hodgkin syndrome – autosomal dominant inheritance, with cleft palate and lip deformities. *SYN:* anhidrotic ectodermal dysplasia

Rappaport, Henry, U.S. pathologist, *1913.

Rappaport classification – a classification of non-Hodgkin lymphomas.

Rapunzel, legendary young woman whose long hair allowed her to escape from a tower in which she was held captive.

Rapunzel syndrome – internal matter that has formed a compact body that occasionally assumes the appearance of strands of twisted hair that extend from a bezoar through the intestine. *SYN:* bezoar

Rasmussen, Fritz W., Danish physician, 1834-1881.

Rasmussen aneurysm – aneurysmal dilation of a branch of a pulmonary artery in a tuberculous cavity.

Rasmussen, Grant L., U.S. neuroanatomist, *1904.

bundle of Rasmussen – *SYN:* olivocochlear tract

Rasmussen encephalitis – antibodies to a stimulatory glutamate receptor in the CNS are found and are perhaps autoimmune. *SYN:* Rasmussen syndrome

Rasmussen syndrome – *SYN:* Rasmussen encephalitis

Rastelli, Gian Carlo, Italian cardiovascular surgeon, 1933-1970.

Rastelli graft

Rastelli implant

Rastelli operation – for repair of transposition of the great arteries.

Rastelli prosthesis

Rathbone, Josephine Langworthy Rathbone-Karpovich, U.S. physical educator, 1899-1982.

Rathbone relaxation method – a method of relaxation used in physical education.

Rathke, Martin H., German anatomist, physiologist, and pathologist, 1793-1860.

Rathke bundles – muscular bundles on the lining walls of the ventricles of the heart. *SYN:* trabeculae carneae

Rathke cleft cyst – an intrasellar or suprasellar cyst lined by cuboidal epithelium derived from remnants of Rathke pouch. *SYN:* Rathke cyst

Rathke column

Rathke cyst – *SYN:* Rathke cleft cyst

Rathke diverticulum – a tubular outgrowth of ectoderm from the stomodeum of the embryo. *SYN:* pituitary diverticulum; Rathke pocket; Rathke pouch

Rathke duct

Rathke fold – two fetal folds of mesoderm.

Rathke pocket – *SYN:* Rathke diverticulum

Rathke pouch – *SYN:* Rathke diverticulum

Rathke pouch tumor – a suprasellar neoplasm, usually cystic, that develops from the nests of epithelium derived from Rathke pouch. *SYN:* craniopharyngioma

Rathke punch

Rau, Johann J., Dutch anatomist, 1668-1719.

processus ravii – *SYN:* Rau process

Rau process – a slender spur running anterior from the neck of the malleus toward the petrotympanic fissure. *SYN:* anterior process of malleus; processus ravii

Rauber, August A., German anatomist, 1841-1917.
Rauber layer – the thinned-out trophoblastic membrane over the embryonic disk in developing carnivores and ungulates.

Rauch, S.
Rauch syndrome – occurs in young women at onset of puberty; bilateral swelling of parotid and occasionally of submandibular glands, with slow progression of obesity over a five-year period.

Rauchfuss, Karl Andreyevich, Russian pediatrician, 1835-1915.
Rauchfuss sling
Rauchfuss sling splint
Rauchfuss triangle – an area of dullness affiliated with Grocco sign.

Rauscher, Frank J., U.S. virologist, *1931.
Rauscher leukemia virus – an RNA retrovirus associated with leukemia in rodents. *SYN:* Rauscher virus
Rauscher virus – *SYN:* Rauscher leukemia virus

Rauwolf, Leonhard, German botanist, 1535-1596.
Rauwolfia serpentina – the dried roots of a tropical shrub whose extracts are used as hypotensive drugs and sedatives.

Ravenna, F.
Ravenna syndrome – evident at birth or within the third year of life; slow growth eventually determining mild disproportionate dwarfism. *SYN:* atypical achondroplasia

Ray, Isaac, U.S. psychiatrist, 1807-1881.
Ray mania – moral insanity.

Rayer, Pierre François Olive, French physician, 1793-1867.
Rayer disease – xanthomatosis with hypercholesterolemia, resulting from biliary cirrhosis. *SYN:* biliary xanthomatosis

NOTES

Rayleigh, Lord John W.S., English physicist and Nobel laureate, 1842-1919.
rayl – unit of acoustic impedance.
Rayleigh equation – a ratio of red to green required by each observer to match spectral yellow. *SYN:* Rayleigh test
Rayleigh test – *SYN:* Rayleigh equation

Raymond, Fulgence, French neurologist, 1844-1910.
Raymond apoplexy – a type of stroke in evolution.

Raynaud, Maurice, French physician, 1834-1881.
Raynaud disease – *SYN:* Raynaud syndrome
Raynaud gangrene – *SYN:* Raynaud syndrome
Raynaud phenomenon – spasm of the digital arteries, with blanching and numbness or pain of the fingers, often precipitated by cold.
Raynaud sign – *SYN:* acrocyanosis
Raynaud syndrome – idiopathic paroxysmal bilateral cyanosis of the digits. *SYN:* Raynaud disease; Raynaud gangrene; symmetric asphyxia

Read, Grantley Dick-, see under Dick-Read

Réaumur, René A.F. de, French physicist, 1683-1757.
Réaumur scale – a thermometer scale.

Reback, S., 20th century U.S. physician.
Mount-Reback syndrome – see under Mount, Lester Adrian

Rebeitz, J.J.
Rebeitz-Kolodny-Richardson syndrome – possible metabolic failure at the cellular level, clumsiness or slowness of limbs, impairment in control of muscle movements, with involuntary muscle movement.

Récamier, Joseph C.A., French gynecologist, 1774-1852.
Récamier curette
Récamier operation – curettage of the uterus.
Récamier procedure

Recklinghausen, Friedrich Daniel von, German histologist and pathologist, 1833-1910.
central Recklinghausen disease type II – congenital disorder characterized by café-au-lait spots, intertriginous freckling, iris hamartomas, and multiple skin neurofibromas.
Recklinghausen-Applebaum disease – a condition of hemochromatosis.
Recklinghausen disease of bone – increased osteoclastic resorption of calcified bone with replacement by fibrous tissue due to primary hyperparathyroidism or other causes of the rapid mobilization of mineral salts. *SYN:* osteitis fibrosa cystica

Recklinghausen disease type I – *SYN:* von Recklinghausen disease
Recklinghausen disease type II – *SYN:* von Recklinghausen disease
Recklinghausen tonometer
Recklinghausen tumor – a small benign tumor of the male epididymis
and female genital tract. *SYN:* adenomatoid tumor
von Recklinghausen disease – two distinct major hereditary disorders:
type I (neurofibromatosis type II), and central type II (neurofibromatosis
type I). *SYN:* neurofibromatosis
von Recklinghausen neurofibromatosis

Reclus, Paul, French surgeon, 1847-1914.
Reclus disease – benign cystic growths in the breast.

Redi, F., Italian physician, 1626-1697.
redia – intramolluscan development stage of a digenetic trematode.

Redlich, Emil, Austrian neurologist, 1866-1930.
Obersteiner-Redlich line – *SYN:* Obersteiner-Redlich zone
Obersteiner-Redlich zone – see under Obersteiner

Reed, Dorothy M., U.S. pathologist, 1874-1964.
Dorothy Reed cells – *SYN:* Reed-Sternberg cells
Reed cells – *SYN:* Reed-Sternberg cells
Reed-Sternberg cells – large transformed lymphocytes, generally
regarded as pathognomonic of Hodgkin disease. *SYN:* Dorothy Reed
cells; Reed cells; Sternberg cells; Sternberg-Reed cells
Sternberg-Reed cells – *SYN:* Reed-Sternberg cells

Reed, Walter, U.S. army surgeon, 1851-1902.
Reed-Frost model – mathematical model of infectious disease
transmission and herd immunity.

Reenstierna, John, Swedish dermatologist, *1882.
Ito-Reenstierna test – *SYN:* Ducrey test

Rees, George Owen, English physician, 1813-1889.
Rees test – for albumin.

NOTES

Rees, H. Maynard, 20th century U.S. physician.
Rees-Ecker fluid – an aqueous solution of sodium citrate, sucrose, and brilliant cresyl blue used in platelet counts.

Reese, Algernon B., U.S. ophthalmologist, 1896-1981.
Cogan-Reese syndrome – see under Cogan
Reese dermatome
Reese forceps
Reese knife
Reese ptosis operation

Refetoff, S.
Refetoff syndrome – a condition characterized by goiter and elevated serum level of thyroid hormones, without manifestations of thyrotoxicosis.

Refsum, Sigvald Bernhard, Norwegian neurologist, 1907-1991.
Refsum disease – a rare hereditary degenerative disorder characterized by retinitis pigmentosa, demyelinating polyneuropathy, deafness, nystagmus, and cerebellar signs. *SYN:* heredopathia atactica polyneuritiformis; Refsum syndrome
Refsum syndrome – *SYN:* Refsum disease

Regaud, Claude, French radiologist, 1870-1940.
Regaud fixative – used to preserve mitochondria but not fat.
residual body of Regaud – the excess cytoplasm that separates from the spermatozoon during spermiogenesis.

Regen, Eugene M., U.S. orthopedic surgeon, *1900.
Regen exercise – exercise done to emphasize the convexity of the lumbar spine. *SYN:* squatting exercise
Regen flexion exercise

Rehberg, P.B., Danish physiologist, *1895.
Rehberg test – creatinine clearance test.

Rehfuss, Martin E., U.S. physician, 1887-1964.
Rehfuss method – fractional method to test gastric activity.
Rehfuss stomach tube – a tube with a calibrated syringe.

Reichel, Friedrich P., German gynecologist and surgeon, 1858-1934.
Reichel chondromatosis
Reichel cloacal duct
Reichel-Pólya stomach resection – retrocolic anastomosis of the full circumference of the open stomach to the jejunum.

Reichel, P.

Reichel syndrome – swelling and motion limitation of knee, hip, elbow, or shoulder. *SYN:* synovial chondromatosis

Reichert, F.L.

Reichert syndrome – paroxysm of stabbing pain in the external auditory meatus associated with other pain in the face and postauricular area. *SYN:* Jacobson neuralgia

Reichert, Karl Bogislaus, German anatomist, 1811-1884.

Reichert camera

Reichert canal

Reichert cartilage – embryonic cartilage.

Reichert cochlear recess – *SYN:* cochlear recess

Reichert-Meissl number – an index of the volatile acid content of a fat.

Reichert radius gauge

Reichert scar

Reichert slit lamp

Reichert substance – one of several steroids.

Reichert tonometer

Reichmann, Mikola, Polish physician, 1851-1918.

Reichmann disease – *SYN:* Zollinger-Ellison syndrome

Reichstein, Tadeus, *1897, joint winner of 1950 Nobel Prize for work related to adrenal cortex hormones.

Reid, Robert W., Scottish anatomist, 1851-1939.

Reid base line – a line drawn from the inferior margin of the orbit to the auricular point and extending backward to the center of the occipital bone.

Reifenstein, Edward C., Jr., U.S. endocrinologist, 1908-1975.

Reifenstein syndrome – a familial form of male pseudohermaphroditism.

NOTES

Reil, Johann C., German physician, neurologist, and histologist, 1759-1813.

circular sulcus of Reil – a semicircular fissure. *SYN:* circular sulcus of insula; limiting sulcus of Reil

island of Reil – an oval region of the cerebral cortex overlying the extreme capsule, lateral to the lenticular nucleus, buried in the depth of the fissura lateralis cerebri (sylvian fissure). *SYN:* insula; insular area; insular cortex

limiting sulcus of Reil – *SYN:* circular sulcus of Reil

Reil ansa – a complex fiber bundle. *SYN:* ansa peduncularis

Reil band – *SYN:* medial lemniscus; septomarginal trabecula

Reil ribbon – *SYN:* medial lemniscus

Reil triangle – *SYN:* lemniscal trigone

Reilly, William A., U.S. pediatrician, *1901.

Alder-Reilly anomaly – *SYN:* Reilly bodies

Reilly bodies – peripheral blood that has basophilic and azurophilic granules in granulocytes that are larger in size than usual. *SYN:* Alder-Reilly anomaly

Reincke, Johann Julius, 19th century German physician.

Mills-Reincke phenomenon – see under Mills, Hiram F.

Reinke, Friedrich B., German anatomist, 1862-1919.

Reinke crystalloids – rod-shaped, crystallike structures with pointed or rounded ends present in the interstitial cells of the testis (Leydig cells) and ovary.

Reinke edema

Reinsch, Adolf, German physician, 1862-1916.

Reinsch test – for arsenic.

Reis, Heinrich Maria Wilhelm, German ophthalmologist, *1872.

Reis-Bücklers corneal dystrophy – an autosomal dominant disorder of Bowman membrane of the cornea.

Reisseisen, Franz D., German anatomist, 1773-1828.

Reisseisen muscles – microscopic smooth muscle fibers in the smallest bronchial tubes.

Reissner, Ernst, German anatomist, 1824-1878.

Reissner fiber – a rodlike, highly refractive fiber running caudally from the subcommissural organ throughout the length of the central canal of the brainstem and spinal cord.

Reissner membrane – separates the cochlear duct from the vestibular canal. *SYN:* vestibular membrane

Reitan, Ralph M., U.S. psychologist, *1922.
Halstead-Reitan battery – see under Halstead

Reiter, Hans Conrad Julius, German bacteriologist and hygienist, 1881-1969.
Fiessinger-Leroy-Reiter syndrome – *SYN:* Reiter syndrome
Reiter disease – *SYN:* Reiter syndrome
Reiter syndrome – association of urethritis, iridocyclitis, mucocutaneous lesions, and arthritis. *SYN:* Fiessinger-Leroy-Reiter syndrome; Reiter disease
Reiter test – a complement-fixation test for syphilis.

Remak, Ernst Julius, German neurologist, 1848-1911.
Remak reflex – plantar flexion of the first three toes with extension of the knee induced by stroking of the upper anterior surface of the thigh.
Remak sign – dissociation of the sensations of touch and of pain in tabes dorsalis.

Remak, Robert, Polish-German anatomist and histologist, 1815-1865.
Remak band
Remak fibers – nerve fibers lacking a myelin sheath but, in common with others, enveloped by a sheath of Schwann cells. *SYN:* unmyelinated fibers
Remak ganglia – (1) groups of nerve cells in the wall of the venous sinus where it joins the right atrium of the heart; (2) autonomic ganglia in nerves of the stomach.
Remak nuclear division – direct division of the nucleus and cell, without the changes in the nucleus that occur in the ordinary process of cell reproduction. *SYN:* amitosis
Remak plexus – a gangliated plexus of unmyelinated nerve fibers, derived chiefly from the superior mesenteric plexus, ramifying in the intestinal submucosa. *SYN:* submucosal plexus

Remondini, D.S.
Osebold-Remondini syndrome – see under Osebold

NOTES

Renaut, Joseph Louis, French physician, 1844-1917.
  Renaut bodies – pale granules found in degenerating nerve fibers in persons with muscular dystrophy.

Rendu, Henri Jules Louis Marie, French physician, 1844-1902.
  Rendu-Osler-Weber syndrome – a disease marked by multiple small telangiectases and dilated venules that develop slowly on the skin and mucous membranes. *SYN:* hereditary hemorrhagic telangiectasia

Renpenning, H., 20th century Canadian physician.
  Renpenning syndrome – X-linked mental retardation with short stature and microcephaly.

Renshaw, Birdsey, 20th century U.S. neurophysiologist.
  Renshaw cells – inhibitory interneurons.

Renwick, T.K., English physician.
  Fisch-Renwick syndrome – see under Fisch
  Renwick-Fisch syndrome – *SYN:* Fisch-Renwick syndrome

Repicci, John A., U.S. dentist and physician.
  Repicci II implant
  Repicci II unicondylar knee

Restorff, Hedwig von, see under von Restorff

Rett, Andreas, Austrian physician, *1924.
  Rett syndrome – a progressive syndrome of autism, dementia, ataxia, and purposeless hand movements.

Retzius, Anders A., Swedish anatomist and anthropologist, 1796-1860.
  cavum retzii – *SYN:* space of Retzius
  Retzius cavity – *SYN:* space of Retzius
  Retzius fibers – stiff fibers in Deiters cells.
  Retzius gyrus – the intralimbic gyrus in the cortical portion of the rhinencephalon.
  Retzius ligament – the deep attachment of the inferior extensor retinaculum in the tarsal sinus. *SYN:* fundiform ligament of foot
  Retzius space – *SYN:* space of Retzius
  Retzius veins – portacaval anastomoses. *SYN:* Ruysch veins
  space of Retzius – the area of loose connective tissue between the bladder with its related fascia and the pubis and anterior abdominal wall. *SYN:* cavum retzii; retropubic space; Retzius cavity; Retzius space

Retzius, Magnus G., Swedish anatomist and anthropologist, 1842-1919.

calcification lines of Retzius – incremental lines of rhythmic deposition of successive layers of enamel matrix during development. *SYN:* lines of Retzius

foramen of Key-Retzius – see under Key, Ernst A.H.

Key-Retzius corpuscles – see under Key, Ernst A.H.

lines of Retzius – *SYN:* calcification lines of Retzius

Retzius foramen – *SYN:* lateral aperture of the fourth ventricle

Retzius striae – dark concentric lines crossing the enamel prisms of the teeth, seen in axial cross sections of the enamel. *SYN:* brown striae; striae parallelae

sheath of Key and Retzius – see under Key, Ernst A.H.

Reuss, August von, Austrian ophthalmologist, 1841-1924.

Reuss color chart – *SYN:* Reuss color table

Reuss color table – obsolete charts that test for deficient color vision. *SYN:* Reuss color chart; Reuss table; Stilling color table

Reuss formula – a means of estimating the percentage of albumin in a fluid.

Reuss table – *SYN:* Reuss color table

Reuss test – for atropine.

Reverdin, Jacques L., Swiss surgeon, 1842-1929.

Reverdin abdominal spatula

Reverdin bunionectomy

Reverdin epidermal free graft

Reverdin graft – small bits of skin of partial or full thickness removed from a healthy area and seeded in a site to be covered. *SYN:* pinch graft

Reverdin holder

Reverdin implant

Reverdin method

Reverdin needle

Reverdin operation

NOTES

Reverdin osteotomy
Reverdin prosthesis
Reverdin skin graft
Reverdin suture needle

Revilliod, Léon, Swiss physician, 1835-1919.
Revilliod sign – in hemiplegia, inability to voluntarily close the eye on the paralyzed side except in conjunction with closure of the other eye. *SYN:* sign of the orbicularis

Rexed, Bror A., Swedish physician, scientist, and public servant, *1914.
lamina of Rexed – a division of the gray matter of the spinal cord into nine laminae and a gray area around the central canal based on cytoarchitectural features.

Reye, Ralph Douglas Kenneth, Australian pediatric pathologist, 1912-1978.
Reye syndrome – an acquired encephalopathy of young children that follows an acute febrile illness, usually influenza or varicella infection.

Reynolds, Osborne, English physicist, 1842-1912.
Reynolds number – a dimensionless number that describes the tendency for a flowing fluid, such as blood, to change from laminar flow to turbulent flow or vice versa.

Reynolds, Telfer B., 20th century U.S. physician.
Reynolds syndrome – coexistence of progressive systemic sclerosis and primary biliary cirrhosis.

Ribbert, Moritz W.H., German pathologist, 1855-1920.
Ribbert theory – that a neoplasm may result when a reduction in tension leads to conditions favorable to uncontrolled growth of cell rests.

Ribbing, Seved, Swedish radiologist, *1902.
Ribbing syndrome – familial osteosclerosis and hyperostosis.

Ribes, François, French physician, 1765-1845.
Ribes ganglion – a small sympathetic ganglion situated on the anterior communicating artery of the brain.

Ribot, T., 19th century French neurologist.
Ribot law – recovery in aphasic multilingual patients comes first in their native language.

Ricci, Vincenzo, Italian physician.
Cacchi-Ricci syndrome – see under Cacchi
Ricci-Cacchi syndrome – *SYN:* Cacchi-Ricci syndrome

Riccò, Annibale, Italian astrophysicist, 1844-1919.
   Riccò law – for small images, light intensity times area equals constant for
      the threshold.

Rich, Arnold R., U.S. pathologist, 1893-1968.
   Hamman-Rich syndrome – *SYN:* usual interstitial pneumonia of Liebow

Richard, Felix Adolphe, Paris surgeon, 1822-1872.
   Richard fringes – *SYN:* fimbriae of uterine tube

Richards, Barry W., 20th century English physician.
   Richards-Rundle syndrome – a nervous system disorder that begins in
      early childhood.

Richards, Dickinson W., joint winner of 1956 Nobel Prize for work related to
circulation and heart catheterization.

Richardson, E.P.
   Rebeitz-Kolodny-Richardson syndrome – see under Rebeitz

Richardson, John Clifford, Canadian neurologist, *1909.
   Richardson rod
   Steele-Richardson-Olszewski disease – *SYN:* Steele-Richardson-
      Olszewski syndrome
   Steele-Richardson-Olszewski syndrome – see under Steele

Riches, Sir Eric William, English urological surgeon.
   Riches bladder syringe
   Riches diathermy forceps

Richet, Charles Robert, 1913 Nobel Prize winner for work related to
anaphylaxis.

Richet, Didier Dominique Alfred, French surgeon, 1816-1891.
   Richet aneurysm
   Richet bandage
   Richet dressing
   Richet operation

NOTES

Richner, Herman, Swiss dermatologist, *1908.
    Richner-Hanhart syndrome – an autosomal disorder with several anomalies and includes mental retardation. *SYN:* type II tyrosinemia

Richter, August G., German surgeon, 1742-1812.
    Monro-Richter line – see under Monro, Alexander, Jr.
    Richter forceps
    Richter hernia – a hernia in which only a portion of the wall of the intestine is engaged. *SYN:* parietal hernia
    Richter-Monro line – *SYN:* Monro-Richter line
    Richter operation
    Richter retractor
    Richter scissors

Richter, Maurice N., U.S. pathologist, *1897.
    Richter syndrome – a high-grade lymphoma developing during the course of chronic lymphocytic leukemia.

Ricketts, Howard T., U.S. pathologist, 1871-1910.
    Rickettsia akari – a species causing human rickettsialpox.
    Rickettsia australis – a species causing a spotted fever.
    Rickettsia conrii – an African species probably causing boutonneuse fever.
    rickettsial – pertaining to or caused by rickettsiae.
    rickettsialpox – an acute disease caused by *Rickettsia akari*; transmitted by the mite.
    Rickettsia prowazekii – a species causing epidemic typhus.
    Rickettsia rickettsii – the agent of Rocky Mountain spotted fever.
    Rickettsia sibirica – the agent of Siberian or North Asian tick typhus.
    Rickettsia tsutsugamushi – a species causing tsutsugamushi disease and scrub typhus.
    Rickettsia typhi – a species causing murine or endemic typhus fever.
    rickettsiosis – infection with rickettsiae.
    rickettsiostatic – an agent inhibitory to the growth of *Rickettsia*.

Rickles, Norman H., U.S. oral pathologist, *1920.
    Rickles test – a colorimetric test for predicting dental caries activity.

Ricord, Phillipe, French physician, 1799-1889.
    Ricord chancre – the first syphilitic chancre.

Riddoch, George, Scottish neurologist, 1889-1947.
    Riddoch mass reflex – leg spasm, involuntary urination, and defecation occurs when there is stimuli to the lower limbs.

Riddoch phenomenon – ability to appreciate a small moving object in an area of the visual field blind to static objects, particularly associated with occipital lobe lesions. *SYN:* Riddoch syndrome

Riddoch syndrome – *SYN:* Riddoch phenomenon

Rideal, Samuel, English chemist and bacteriologist, 1863-1929.

Rideal-Walker coefficient – a figure expressing the disinfecting power of any substance. *SYN:* hygienic laboratory coefficient; phenol coefficient

Rideal-Walker method

Ridgway, Robert, U.S. ornithologist, 1850-1929.

Ridgway color system – method of organizing colors based on the natural color of bird feathers.

Ridley, Humphrey, English anatomist, 1653-1708.

circulus venosus ridleyi – *SYN:* circular sinus

Ridley circle – *SYN:* circular sinus

Ridley sinus – the anterior and posterior anastomoses between the cavernous sinuses. *SYN:* intercavernous sinuses

Riechert, T., 20th century German neurosurgeon.

Riechert-Mundinger apparatus – used in Riechert-Mundinger technique.

Riechert-Mundinger technique – a stereotactic technique that uses the Riechert-Mundinger apparatus to hold the head in place.

Riedel, Bernhard M.C.L., German surgeon, 1846-1916.

Riedel disease – *SYN:* Riedel thyroiditis

Riedel frontal ethmoidectomy

Riedel lobe – tonguelike process extending downward from the right lobe of the liver lateral to the gallbladder. *SYN:* lobus appendicularis; lobus linguiformis

Riedel struma – *SYN:* Riedel thyroiditis

Riedel syndrome – *SYN:* Riedel thyroiditis

Riedel thyroiditis – a rare fibrous induration of the thyroid, with adhesion to adjacent structures, which may cause tracheal compression.

NOTES

SYN: chronic fibrous thyroiditis; ligneous struma; ligneous thyroiditis; Riedel disease; Riedel struma; Riedel syndrome

Rieder, Hermann, German pathologist, 1858-1932.
Rieder cell leukemia – a form of acute granulocytic leukemia.
Rieder cells – abnormal myeloblasts frequently observed in acute leukemia.
Rieder lymphocyte – an abnormal form of lymphocyte with a greatly indented nucleus, usually observed in certain examples of chronic lymphocytic leukemia.

Riegel, Franz, German physician, 1843-1904.
Riegel pulse – a pulse that diminishes in volume during expiration.

Rieger, Herwigh, German ophthalmologist, 1898-1986.
Rieger anomaly – mesodermal dysgenesis of cornea and iris, producing pupillary anomalies, posterior embryotoxon, and secondary glaucoma. *SYN:* iridocorneal mesodermal dysgenesis
Rieger syndrome – Rieger anomaly combined with hypodontia or anodontia and maxillary hypoplasia.

Riehl, Gustav, Austrian dermatologist, 1855-1943.
Riehl melanosis – a brown pigmentary condition of the exposed portions of the skin of the neck and face. *SYN:* Riehl syndrome
Riehl syndrome – *SYN:* Riehl melanosis

Riesman, David, U.S. physician, 1867-1940.
Riesman sign – eyeball softening in comatose diabetic patients.

Rieux, Léon, 19th century French surgeon.
Rieux hernia – a retrocecal hernia.

Rift Valley, section of Kenya where the virus was first discovered in the 1900's.
Rift Valley virus – a virus of the genus *Phlebovirus* that occurs in central and southern Africa in sheep, goats, and cattle; humans may become infected with close contact with infected animals.

Riga, Antonio, Italian physician, 1832-1919.
Fede-Riga disease – *SYN:* Riga-Fede disease
Riga-Fede disease – ulceration of the lingual frenum in teething infants. *SYN:* Fede-Riga disease

Riggs, John Mankey, U.S. dentist, 1810-1885.
Riggs disease – periodontitis.

Riley, Conrad Milton, U.S. pediatrician, *1913.
   Riley-Day syndrome – a congenital syndrome, with specific disturbances
      of the nervous system and aberrations in autonomic nervous system
      function. _SYN:_ familial dysautonomia

Riley, Harris D., Jr., U.S. physician, *1925.
   Smith-Riley syndrome – see under Smith, William R.

Rille, Johann Heinrich, Austrian physician.
   Rille-Comél disease – a form of ichthyosis.

Rindfleisch, Georg E., German physician, 1836-1908.
   Rindfleisch cells – obsolete term for eosinophilic leukocyte.
   Rindfleisch folds – semilunar folds of the serous surface of the
      pericardium, embracing the beginning of the aorta.

Ringer, Sydney, English physiologist, 1835-1910.
   Krebs-Ringer solution – see under Krebs, Sir Hans Adolph
   lactated Ringer injection – used intravenously as a systemic alkalizer
      and a fluid and electrolyte replenisher.
   lactated Ringer solution – a sterile solution of calcium chloride,
      potassium chloride, sodium chloride, and sodium lactate in water.
      SYN: Hartmann solution
   Locke-Ringer solution – see under Locke
   Ringer injection – a sterile solution of sodium chloride, potassium
      chloride, and calcium chloride, used intravenously as a fluid and
      electrolyte replenisher.
   Ringer solution – resembles the blood serum in its salt constituents.

Riniker, P., Swiss pediatrician.
   Glanzmann and Riniker lymphocytophthisis – see under Glanzmann

Rinne, Friedrich Heinrich A., German otologist, 1819-1868.
   Rinne test – a hearing test using a vibrating tuning fork.

NOTES

Riolan, Jean, French anatomist and botanist, 1577-1657.

Riolan anastomosis – the specific portion of the marginal artery of the colon connecting the middle and left colic arteries. *SYN:* Riolan arc (3)

Riolan arc – (1) *SYN:* intestinal arterial arcades; (2) *SYN:* marginal artery of colon; (3) *SYN:* Riolan anastomosis

Riolan arcades – *SYN:* intestinal arterial arcades

Riolan bones – several small sutural bones sometimes present in the petrooccipital suture.

Riolan bouquet – the muscles and ligaments arising from the styloid process.

Riolan muscle – *SYN:* cremaster muscle

Ripault, Louis H.A., French physician, 1807-1856.

Ripault sign – a sign of death consisting of a permanent change in the shape of the pupil produced by unilateral pressure on the eyeball.

Ripstein, Charles, 20th century U.S. surgeon.

Ripstein operation – surgery for rectal prolapse.

Risley, Samuel D., U.S. ophthalmologist, 1845-1920.

Risley pliers

Risley rotary prism – used in examination of ocular muscle imbalance.

Risser, Joseph C., U.S. orthopedic surgeon, 1892-1942.

Risser cast

Risser cast table

Risser frame

Risser grade

Risser jacket – a scoliosis plaster jacket.

Risser localizer scoliosis cast

Risser method

Risser sign

Risser stage

Risser technique

Risser turnbuckle cast

Ritgen, Ferdinand August Marie Franz von, German obstetrician, 1787-1867.

Ritgen maneuver – delivery of a child's head by pressure on the perineum while controlling the speed of delivery by pressure with the other hand on the head.

Ritter, Johann W., German physicist, 1776-1810.

Ritter law – a nerve is stimulated at both the opening and the closing of an electrical current.

Ritter opening tetanus – the contraction that occasionally occurs when a strong current passing through a long stretch of nerve is suddenly interrupted.

Ritter-Rollet phenomenon – on equal electrical stimulation of motor nerve trunks, the flexor and abductor muscle groups react more readily than the extensors and adductors.

Ritter von Rittershain, Gottfried, German physician, 1820-1883.
Ritter disease – *SYN:* Lyell disease
Ritter syndrome – *SYN:* Lyell disease

Rivalta, Fabio, 19th century Italian pathologist.
Rivalta reaction – *SYN:* Moritz test

Rivalta, Sebastiano, Italian veterinarian, 1852-1893.
Rivalta disease – caused in cattle by *Actinomyces bovis*; in humans by *A. israeli.*

Rivero-Carvallo, José Manuel, Mexican cardiologist, *1905.
Carvallo sign – an increase in the intensity of the pansystolic murmur of tricuspid regurgitation during or at the end of inspiration distinguishes tricuspid from mitral involvement.
Rivero-Carvallo effect – inspiratory increase in the systolic murmur of tricuspid insufficiency.

Rivers, William H., English physician, 1864-1922.
Rivers cocktail – an intravenous slow injection used in acute alcoholism. *SYN:* Philadelphia cocktail

Rivière, Lazare (Lazarus), French physician, 1589-1655.
Rivière salt – a deliquescent powder used as a diuretic, diaphoretic, expectorant, systemic, and urinary alkalizer. *SYN:* potassium citrate

Rivinus, August Quirinus, German anatomist, 1652-1723.
Rivinus canals
Rivinus ducts – *SYN:* minor sublingual duct
Rivinus gland – *SYN:* sublingual gland

R

NOTES

Rivinus incisure – *SYN:* tympanic notch
Rivinus ligament– flaccid portion of the tympanic membrane that is
attached to the petrous bone at the notch of Rivinus.
Rivinus membrane – *SYN:* flaccid part of tympanic membrane
Rivinus notch – *SYN:* tympanic notch

Roach, F. Ewing, U.S. prosthodontist, 1868-1960.
Roach clasp – part of a denture or retainer. *SYN:* bar clasp

Roaf, R.
Roaf syndrome – a nonhereditary craniofacial-skeletal disorder
characterized by multiple defects.

Robbins, Frederick Chapman, joint winner of 1954 Nobel Prize for work
related to poliomyelitis virus.

Robert, César Alphonse, French surgeon, 1801-1862.
Robert ligament

Robert, Heinrich L.F., German gynecologist, 1814-1878.
Robert pelvis – obsolete term for a pelvis narrowed transversely in
consequence of the almost entire absence of the alae of the sacrum.

Roberts, John B., U.S. physician, 1852-1924.
Roberts syndrome – autosomal recessive inheritance, with multiple
defects.

Roberts, Maureen, Canadian physician.
Norman-Roberts syndrome – *SYN:* Miller-Dieker syndrome

Roberts, Richard J., joint winner of 1993 Nobel Prize for work related to split
genes.

Roberts, Sir William, English physician, 1830-1899.
Roberts test – for albumin.

Robertshaw, Frank L., 20th century English anesthesiologist.
Robertshaw tube – a variation of Carlen tube.

Robertson, Douglas Moray Cooper Lamb Argyll, Scottish ophthalmologist,
1837-1909.
Argyll Robertson pupil – a form of reflex iridoplegia often present in
tabetic neurosyphilis. *SYN:* Robertson pupil
Robertson pupil – *SYN:* Argyll Robertson pupil

Robertson, William Egbert, U.S. physician, 1869-1956.
Robertson sign – (1) a contraction over the area of the heart of the
pectoralis muscle signaling pending death from cardiac disease;
(2) signals malingering when pupillary dilatation is absent upon placing

pressure on areas identified as painful; (3) demonstrated when the patient has ascites.

Robertson, W.R.B., U.S. geneticist, *1881.

robertsonian translocation – translocation in which the centromeres of two acrocentric chromosomes appear to have fused, forming an abnormal chromosome. *SYN:* centric fusion

Robin, Charles P., French physician, 1821-1885.

Charcot-Robin crystals – *SYN:* Charcot-Leyden crystals

Virchow-Robin space – see under Virchow

Robin, Pierre, French pediatrician, 1867-1950.

Pierre Robin syndrome – micrognathia and abnormal smallness of the tongue, often with cleft palate, severe myopia, congenital glaucoma, and retinal detachment. *SYN:* Robin syndrome

Robin syndrome – *SYN:* Pierre Robin syndrome

Robinow, Meinhard, U.S. physician, *1909.

Robinow dwarfism – *SYN:* Robinow syndrome

Robinow mesomelic dysplasia

Robinow syndrome – dwarfism associated with several facial anomalies. *SYN:* fetal face syndrome; Robinow dwarfism

Robinson, Andrew Ross, U.S. dermatologist, 1845-1924.

Robinson disease – obsolete term for hidrocystoma(s) occurring in the skin of the face, especially in the region of the eyes.

Robinson, Brian F., 20th century English cardiologist.

Robinson index – used to calculate heart work load.

Robinson, E.M.

Robinson syndrome – dysmenorrhea that begins shortly after menarche. *SYN:* dysmenorrhea; unilateral genital atresia

NOTES

Robinson, Frederick Byron, U.S. anatomist, 1857-1910.

Robinson circle – a circle of arteries formed by anastomosing the abdominal aorta, common iliac, hypogastric, uterine, and ovarian arteries.

Robinson, Geoffrey C., Canadian pediatrician, 1878-1940.

Robinson syndrome – sensorineural deafness and other anomalies. *SYN:* familial ectodermal dysplasia

Robinson, Robert A., U.S. orthopedic surgeon, *1914.

Robinson anterior cervical discectomy

Robinson artificial apparatus

Robinson morcellation

Robinson pocket arthrometer

Robinson prosthesis

Robinson spinal arthrodesis

Smith-Robinson anterior approach

Smith-Robinson anterior cervical discectomy

Smith-Robinson anterior fusion

Smith-Robinson cervical fusion

Smith-Robinson interbody arthrodesis

Smith-Robinson interbody fusion

Smith-Robinson operation – see under Smith, G.W.

Smith-Robinson technique

Robison, Robert, English chemist, 1884-1941.

Robison-Embden ester – *SYN:* Robison ester

Robison ester – a key intermediate in glycolysis, glycogenolysis, pentose phosphate shunt, etc. *SYN:* D-glucose 6-phosphate; Robison-Embden ester

Robison ester dehydrogenase – a deficiency of this enzyme can lead to severe hemolytic anemia and favism. *SYN:* glucose 6-phosphate dehydrogenase

Robles, Rudolfo (Valverde), Guatemalan dermatologist, 1878-1939.

Robles disease – onchocerciasis.

Robson, Sir Arthur William Mayo, English surgeon, 1853-1933.

Robson line – imaginary line from the right nipple to the umbilicus.

Robson point – point of greatest tenderness in inflamed gallbladder using Robson line technique.

Robson position – position used in biliary tract surgery.

Rocher, Henri Gaston Louis, French surgeon, *1876.
    Rocher sign – the forward or backward sliding of the tibia indicating laxity
    or tear of the anterior or posterior cruciate ligaments of the knee.
    SYN: drawer sign

Rochon-Duvigneaud, André, French ophthalmologist, 1863-1953.
    Rochon-Duvigneaud syndrome – neurologic disorder resulting from a
    lesion on the floor of the orbit. *SYN:* superior orbital fissure syndrome

Rocky Mountains, mountain range in the United States and Canada.
    Rocky Mountain spotted fever – an acute infectious disease of high
    mortality characterized by frontal and occipital headache; intense
    lumbar pain; malaise; a moderately high continuous fever; and a rash on
    wrists, palms, ankles, and soles from the second to the fifth day, later
    spreading to all parts of the body. *SYN: Rickettsia*

Rodbell, Martin, joint winner of 1994 Nobel Prize for work related to
G-proteins.

Roenheld, L.
    Roenheld syndrome – atypical chest pain and palpitations following a
    meal. *SYN:* postprandial cardiogastritis

Roenne, Henning K.T., Danish ophthalmologist, 1878-1947.
    Roenne nasal step – a visual field defect seen in glaucoma.

Roentgen, Wilhelm K., German physicist and Nobel laureate, 1845-1923.
    roentgen – the international unit of exposure dose for x-rays or gamma
    rays.
    roentgenograph – *SYN:* radiograph
    roentgen ray – *SYN:* x-ray

Roger, Georges Henri, French physiologist, 1860-1946.
    Roger reflex – salivation caused by irritation of the lower end of the
    esophagus. *SYN:* esophagosalivary reflex

Roger, Henri L., French physician, 1809-1891.
    bruit de Roger – *SYN:* Roger murmur

NOTES

maladie de Roger – *SYN:* Roger disease

Roger disease – a congenital cardiac anomaly consisting of a small, isolated, asymptomatic defect of the interventricular septum. *SYN:* maladie de Roger

Roger murmur – a loud pansystolic murmur maximal at the left sternal border, caused by a small ventricular septal defect. *SYN:* bruit de Roger

Rogers, L.E.
Rogers syndrome – *SYN:* thiamine-responsive megaloblastic anemia

Rogers, Oscar H., U.S. physician, 1857-1941.
Rogers sphygmomanometer – a sphygmomanometer with an aneroid barometer gauge.

Röhl, Wilhelm, German physician, 1881-1929.
Röhl marginal corpuscle

Rohr, Karl, Swiss embryologist and gynecologist, *1863.
Rohr stria – layer of fibrinoid in the intervillous spaces of the placenta.

Rokitansky, Karl Freiherr von, Austrian pathologist, 1804-1878.
Mayer-Rokitansky-Küster-Hauser syndrome – see under Mayer, Paul
Rokitansky-Aschoff sinuses – small outpocketings of the mucosa of the gallbladder which extend through the muscular layer.
Rokitansky disease – (1) *SYN:* acute yellow atrophy of the liver; (2) *SYN:* Chiari syndrome
Rokitansky diverticulum
Rokitansky hernia – separation of the muscular fibers of the bowel allowing protrusion of a sac of the mucous membrane.
Rokitansky kidney
Rokitansky-Küster-Hauser syndrome – *SYN:* Mayer-Rokitansky-Küster-Hauser syndrome
Rokitansky pelvis – *SYN:* spondylolisthetic pelvis
Rokitansky tumor

Rolando, Luigi, Italian anatomist, 1773-1831.
fissure of Rolando – a double S-shaped fissure extending obliquely upward and backward on the lateral surface of each cerebral hemisphere at the boundary between frontal and parietal lobes. *SYN:* central sulcus
rolandic epilepsy – a benign autosomal dominant form of epilepsy occurring in children.
Rolando angle – the angle at which the fissure of Rolando meets with the midplane.

Rolando area – the region of the cerebral cortex most immediately influencing movements of the face, neck and trunk, arm, and leg. *SYN:* motor cortex

Rolando cells – the nerve cells in Rolando gelatinous substance of the spinal cord.

Rolando column – a slight ridge on either side of the medulla oblongata related to the descending trigeminal tract and nucleus.

Rolando gelatinous substance – the apical part of the posterior horn of the spinal cord's gray matter, composed largely of very small nerve cells. *SYN:* gelatinous substance

Rolando tubercle – a longitudinal prominence on the dorsolateral surface of the medulla oblongata along the lateral border of the tuberculum cuneatum. *SYN:* tuberculum cinereum

Rolf, Ida, PhD, U.S. biochemist and physical therapist, 1896-1979.
rolfing – deep massage technique.

Roller, Christian F.W., German neurologist and psychiatrist, 1844-1978.
Roller nucleus – lateral nucleus of the accessory nerve.

Rolleston, Sir Humphry D., English physician, 1862-1944.
Rolleston rule – the ideal adult systolic blood pressure is 100 plus half the age, whereas the maximal physiologic pressure is 100 plus the age.

Rollet, Alexander, Austrian physiologist, 1834-1903.
Ritter-Rollet phenomenon – see under Ritter, Johann W.
Rollet stroma – the colorless stroma of the red blood cells.

Rollier, Auguste, Swiss physician, 1874-1954.
Rollier formula – formula used to regulate progressive exposure to natural or artificial ultraviolet radiation.

Romaña, Cecilio, Argentinian physician in Brazil, *1899.
Romaña sign – marked edema of one or both eyelids, thought to be a sensitization response to the bite of a triatomine bug infected with *Trypanosoma cruzi*, and a strong suggestion of acute Charges disease.

R

NOTES

Romano, C., Italian physician, *1923.
   Romano-Ward syndrome – a prolonged Q-T interval in the
      electrocardiogram in children subject to ventricular arrhythmias,
      including ventricular fibrillation. *SYN:* Ward-Romano syndrome
   Ward-Romano syndrome – *SYN:* Romano-Ward syndrome

Romanowsky, Dimitri L., Russian physician, 1861-1921.
   Romanowsky blood stain – prototype of the eosin-methylene blue stains
      for blood smears.

Romberg, E.
   Romberg-Wood syndrome – dyspnea, angina pectoris, shortness of
      breath in otherwise healthy individuals after exertion, cold exposure,
      and/or excitement. *SYN:* primary pulmonary hypertension

Romberg, Mortiz Heinrich von, German physician, 1795-1873.
   facial hemiatrophy of Romberg – *SYN:* Romberg syndrome
   Romberg disease – facial hemiatrophy.
   Romberg-Howship symptom – in cases of incarcerated obturator hernia,
      lancinating pains along the inner side of the thigh to the knee, or down
      the leg to the foot; caused by compression of the obturator nerve.
      SYN: Romberg symptom (2)
   rombergism – *SYN:* Romberg sign
   Romberg sign – a sign of sensory ataxia if a patient standing with heels
      touching cannot maintain balance on closing eyes. *SYN:* rombergism;
      Romberg symptom (1); Romberg test; station test
   Romberg symptom – (1) *SYN:* Romberg sign; (2) *SYN:* Romberg-Howship
      symptom
   Romberg syndrome – atrophy, usually progressive, affecting the tissues
      of one side of the face. *SYN:* facial hemiatrophy of Romberg; Romberg
      trophoneurosis
   Romberg test – *SYN:* Romberg sign
   Romberg trophoneurosis – *SYN:* Romberg syndrome

Römer, Paul H., German bacteriologist, 1876-1916.
   Römer test – for tuberculosis.

Rommelaere, Guillaume, Belgian physician, 1881-1916.
   Rommelaere sign – for sodium chloride and phosphate levels.

Rønne, Henning K.T., Danish ophthalmologist, 1878-1947.
   Rønne nasal step – a nasal visual field defect with one margin
      corresponding to the retinal horizontal medium.

Rood, Margaret S., 20th century U.S. occupational/physical therapist.
Rood method of exercise – therapeutic exercises enhanced by cutaneous stimulation for patients with neuromuscular dysfunction.
Rood technique

Rorschach, Hermann, Swiss psychiatrist, 1884-1922.
Behn-Rorschach test – see under Behn-Eschenburg
Rorschach test – a projective psychological test. *SYN:* inkblot test

Rosai, Juan, U.S. pathologist, *1941.
Rosai-Dorfman disease – *SYN:* sinus histiocytosis with massive lymphadenopathy

Roscoe, Sir Henry E., English chemist, 1833-1915.
Bunsen-Roscoe law – see under Bunsen
Roscoe-Bunsen law – *SYN:* Bunsen-Roscoe law

Rose, Edmund, German physician, 1836-1914.
Rose cephalic tetanus – a type of local tetanus that follows wounds to the face and head. *SYN:* cephalic tetanus

Rose, Frank A., English surgeon, 1873-1935.
Rose position – the patient lies supine with the head falling down over the end of the table, for operations within the mouth or pharynx.

Rose, H.M., U.S. microbiologist, *1906.
Rose-Waaler test – obsolete test for demonstration of rheumatoid arthritis.

Rosenbach, Anton Julius Friedrich, German pathologist, 1842-1923.
erysipeloid of Rosenbach – skin infection.

Rosenbach, Ottomar, German physician, 1851-1907.
Rosenbach disease – (1) *SYN:* Heberden nodes; (2) exostoses on the terminal phalanges of the fingers in osteoarthritis; a specific, usually self-limiting, cellulitis of the hand caused by *Erysipelothrix rhusiopathiae*. *SYN:* erysipeloid
Rosenbach-Gmelin test – *SYN:* Gmelin test

NOTES

Rosenbach law – (1) in affections of the nerve trunks or nerve centers, paralysis of the flexor muscles appears later than that of the extensors; (2) in case of abnormal stimulation of organs with rhythmical functional periodicity.

Rosenbach sign – loss of the abdominal reflex in cases of acute inflammation of the viscera.

Rosenbach test – for bile in the urine.

Rosenberg, Alan L., 20th century U.S. physician.
Rosenberg-Bergstrom syndrome – an autosomal recessive disorder.

Rosenberg, Edward Frank, U.S. physician, *1908.
Hench-Rosenberg syndrome – see under Hench
Rosenberg-Hench syndrome – *SYN:* Hench-Rosenberg syndrome

Rosenberg, L.E.
Rowley-Rosenberg syndrome – see under Rowley

Rosenberg, Roger N., 20th century U.S. physician.
Rosenberg-Chutorian syndrome – characterized by progressive neural hearing loss, optic atrophy, and polyneuropathy that may be accompanied by other neurological disorders.

Rosenmüller, Johann C., German anatomist, 1771-1820.
organ of Rosenmüller – a collection of rudimentary tubules in the mesosalpinx between the ovary and the uterine tube. *SYN:* epoöphoron
Rosenmüller fossa – *SYN:* Rosenmüller recess
Rosenmüller gland – *SYN:* node of Cloquet
Rosenmüller node – *SYN:* node of Cloquet
Rosenmüller recess – a slitlike depression in the membranous pharyngeal wall extending posterior to the opening of the eustachian tube. *SYN:* pharyngeal recess; Rosenmüller fossa
Rosenmüller valve – a fold of mucous membrane guarding the lower opening of the nasolacrimal duct. *SYN:* lacrimal fold

Rosenthal, Curt, neurologist and German psychiatrist, 1892-1937.
Melkersson-Rosenthal syndrome – see under Melkersson
Rosenthal effect – type of self-fulfilling prophecy. *SYN:* Pygmalion effect
Rosenthal syndrome – sleep paralysis that occurs at the moment one falls asleep or awakens.

Rosenthal, Friedrich C., German anatomist, 1780-1829.
basal vein of Rosenthal – a large vein passing along the medial surface of the temporal lobe, from which it receives tributaries. *SYN:* Rosenthal vein; vena basalis

Rosenthal aspiration needle
Rosenthal canal – the winding tube of the bony labyrinth which makes two and a half turns about the modiolus of the cochlea. *SYN:* cochlear canal
Rosenthal vein – *SYN:* basal vein of Rosenthal

Rosenthal, Robert L., U.S. hematologist, *1923.
Rosenthal syndrome – inherited hemorrhagic condition that is caused by coagulation factor XI deficiency.

Roser, Wilhelm, German surgeon, 1817-1888.
Roser-Nélaton line – *SYN:* Nélaton line

Ross, Donald N., U.S. cardiac surgeon, *1922.
Ross procedure – aortic valve replacement using a pulmonic valve autograft.

Ross, Edward Halford, English pathologist, 1875-1928.
Ross bodies – seen in syphilitic blood and tissue fluids.

Ross, Sir George W., Canadian physician, 1841-1931.
Ross-Jones test – for an excess of globulin in the cerebrospinal fluid.

Ross, Sir Ronald, English physician and Nobel laureate, 1857-1932.
Ross cycle – the life cycle of the malaria parasite.

Rossbach, Michael J., German physician, 1842-1894.
Rossbach disease – *SYN:* gastric hyperchlorhydria

Rossolimo, Grigoriy (Grigorij) I., Russian neurologist, 1860-1928.
Rossolimo reflex – a stretch reflex of the toe flexors seen in lesions of the pyramidal tracts. *SYN:* plantar muscle reflex; Rossolimo sign
Rossolimo sign – *SYN:* Rossolimo reflex

Rostan, Léon, French physician, 1790-1866.
Rostan asthma – *SYN:* cardiac asthma

Rotch, Thomas M., U.S. physician, 1848-1914.
Rotch sign – in pericardial effusion, percussion dullness in the fifth intercostal space on the right.

NOTES

Roth, Moritz, Swiss physician and pathologist, 1839-1914.
  Roth spots – a round white retina spot surrounded by hemorrhage in
    bacterial endocarditis and in other retinal hemorrhagic conditions.
  vas aberrans of Roth – an occasional diverticulum of the rete testis or of
    the efferent ductules of the testis.

Roth, Vladimir K., Russian neurologist, 1848-1916.
  Bernhardt-Roth syndrome – *SYN:* Bernhardt disease
  Roth-Bernhardt disease – *SYN:* Bernhardt disease
  Roth disease – *SYN:* Bernhardt disease

Roth, W.
  Roth-Bielschowsky syndrome – complete paralysis of conjugate
    movements of the eyes in one or more directions, except those under
    labyrinthine control. *SYN:* pseudoophthalmoplegia

Rothera, Arthur C.H., English biochemist, 1880-1915.
  Rothera nitroprusside test – for ketone bodies.

Rothmann, Max, German pathologist, 1868-1915.
  Rothmann-Makai syndrome – panniculitis with fat cell necrosis.

Rothmund, August von, German physician, 1830-1906.
  Rothmund syndrome – atrophy, pigmentation, and telangiectasia of the
    skin, usually with juvenile cataract, saddle nose, congenital bone
    defects, disturbance of hair growth, and hypogonadism.
    SYN: poikiloderma atrophicans and cataract; poikiloderma congenitale;
    Rothmund-Thomson syndrome
  Rothmund-Thomson syndrome – *SYN:* Rothmund syndrome

Rothschild, Henri Jacques Nathanial Charles de, French physician,
1872-1923.
  Rothschild sign – (1) loss of eyebrow hair seen in hypothyroidism;
    (2) sternal angle sign seen in tuberculosis.

Rotor, Arturo B., 20th century Philippine internist.
  Rotor syndrome – jaundice appearing in childhood due to impaired biliary
    excretion.

Rouget, Antoine D., 19th century French physiologist.
  Rouget bulb – a venous plexus on the surface of the ovary.

Rouget, Charles M.B., French physiologist, 1824-1904.
  Rouget cell – a cell with several slender processes that embraces the
    capillary wall in amphibia. *SYN:* capillary pericyte
  Rouget muscle – the circular fibers of the ciliary muscle. *SYN:* circular fibers

Rouget-Neumann sheath – the amorphous ground substance between an osteocyte and the lacunar or canalicular wall.

Roughton, Francis J.W., English scientist, 1899-1972.
   Roughton-Scholander apparatus – a syringelike device for analyzing the respiratory gases in a small sample of blood. *SYN:* Roughton-Scholander syringe
   Roughton-Scholander syringe – *SYN:* Roughton-Scholander apparatus

Rougnon de Magny, Nicholas F., French physician, 1727-1799.
   Rougnon-Heberden disease – *SYN:* Heberden angina

Rous, F. Peyton, U.S. pathologist and Nobel laureate, 1879-1970.
   Rous-associated virus – a leukemia virus.
   Rous sarcoma – a fibrosarcoma caused by certain viruses of family Retroviridae. *SYN:* avian sarcoma; Rous tumor
   Rous sarcoma virus – a sarcoma-producing virus of the avian leukosis-sarcoma complex identified by Rous in 1911.
   Rous tumor – *SYN:* Rous sarcoma

Roussy, Gustave, French pathologist, 1874-1948.
   Dejerine-Roussy syndrome – see under Dejerine
   Roussy-Cornil syndrome – occasional lancinating pains, with peripheral weakness, fasciculation, visual disturbance, and ataxia. *SYN:* interstitial hypertrophic neuropathy
   Roussy-Lévy disease – a type of cerebellar ataxia regularly associated with wasting of the calves and intrinsic muscles of the hands, with absent tendon reflexes. *SYN:* Roussy-Lévy syndrome
   Roussy-Lévy syndrome – *SYN:* Roussy-Lévy disease

Rouviere, Henri, French anatomist and embryologist, *1875.
   node of Rouviere – one of the lateral group of retropharyngeal lymph nodes.

NOTES

Roux, César, Swiss surgeon, 1857-1934.
Roux-en-Y anastomosis – a Y-shaped surgical anastomosis involving the small intestine. *SYN:* Roux-en-Y operation
Roux-en-Y gastrectomy
Roux-en-Y gastrojejunostomy
Roux-en-Y hepatic jejunostomy
Roux-en-Y incision
Roux-en-Y loop
Roux-en-Y operation – *SYN:* Roux-en-Y anastomosis
Roux-en-Y pancreatic jejunostomy

Roux, Philibert J., French surgeon, 1780-1854.
Roux method – division of the inferior maxilla in the median line, to facilitate the operation of ablation of the tongue.
Roux sign

Roux, Pierre P.E., French bacteriologist, 1853-1933.
Roux spatula – a very small, nickeled-steel spatula used to transfer bits of infected material to culture tubes.
Roux stain – a double stain for diphtheria bacilli which employs crystal violet or dahlia and methyl green.

Rovighi, Alberto, Italian physician, 1856-1919.
Rovighi sign – fremitus felt on palpation of hepatic hydatid cyst.

Rovsing, Niels Thorkild, Danish surgeon, 1862-1927.
Rovsing operation
Rovsing sign – pain at McBurney point induced in cases of appendicitis by exerting pressure over the descending colon.

Rowland Payne, C.M.E.
Rowland Payne syndrome – pain and weakness in the shoulder; change in voice in women with metastatic breast cancer.

Rowley, P.T.
Rowley-Rosenberg syndrome – growth retardation; reduced muscle and adipose tissue; various degrees of recurrent pulmonary infections; right ventricular hypertrophy.

Rowntree, Leonard G., U.S. physician, 1883-1959.
Rowntree and Geraghty test – *SYN:* phenolsulfonphthalein test

Roy, James Evans, U.S. psychiatrist, *1914.
Friedman-Roy syndrome – see under Friedman, Arnold Phineus

Rozenzweig, Saul, U.S. psychologist, *1907.
Rosenzweig picture-frustration study – a projective test used in psychology.

Rubarth, Sven, Swedish veterinarian, *1905.
Rubarth disease – a disease of dogs caused by canine adenovirus 1.
SYN: infectious canine hepatitis
Rubarth disease virus – causes infectious canine hepatitis in dogs.
SYN: canine adenovirus 1

Rubens, Peter Paul, Flemish painter, 1577-1640.
Rubens flap

Rubin, Edgar J.
Rubin figure – a figure which some see as one goblet; others as two facing profiles. *SYN:* goblet figure

Rubin, Isidor Clinton, U.S. gynecologist, 1883-1958.
Rubin test – an obsolete test of patency of the fallopian tubes.

Rubinstein, Jack Herbert, U.S. child psychiatrist and pediatrician, *1925.
Rubinstein-Taybi syndrome – mental retardation, facial deformities, and cardiac anomaly.

Rubner, Max, German hygienist and biochemist, 1854-1932.
Rubner laws of growth – the rate of growth is proportional to the intensity of the metabolic processes.
Rubner test – for lactose or glucose in the urine.

Rud, Einar, Danish physician, 1892-1933.
Rud syndrome – ichthyosiform erythroderma associated with acanthosis nigricans, dwarfism, hypogonadism, and epilepsy.

Ruffini, Angelo, Italian histologist, 1864-1929.
flower-spray organ of Ruffini – one of the two types of sensory nerve ending (the other being the annulospiral ending) associated with the neuromuscular spindle. *SYN:* flower-spray ending

NOTES

Ruffini corpuscles – sensory end-structures in the subcutaneous connective tissues of the fingers, consisting of an ovoid capsule within which the sensory fiber ends with numerous collateral knobs.

Ruffini papillary endings – papillary endings of the skin's nerve endings.

Rukavinas, J.B.

Rukavinas syndrome – peripheral neuropathy most severely affecting the upper limbs; scleroderma-like changes in the skin of hands and arms; vitreous opacities in the eyes.

Rumpel, Theodor, German physician, 1862-1923.

Leede-Rumpel phenomenon – *SYN:* Rumpel-Leede phenomenon

Rumpel-Leede phenomenon – appearance of petechiae in an area following application of vascular constriction due to capillary fragility or abnormal platelet numbers or function. *SYN:* Leede-Rumpel phenomenon

Rumpel-Leede sign – *SYN:* Rumpel-Leede test

Rumpel-Leede test – a tourniquet test for capillary fragility. *SYN:* bandage sign; Hess test; Rumpel-Leede sign

Rumpf, Heinrich Theodor, German physician, 1851-1923.

Rumpf sign – neurasthenia reaction.

Rundle, A.T., 20th century English physician.

Richards-Rundle syndrome – see under Richards, Barry W.

Rundles, Ralph W., U.S. internist, *1911.

Rundles-Falls syndrome – weakness, tiredness, occasional leg pain, and paresthesias of the feet, associated with pyridoxine deficiency.

Runeberg, Johan W., Finnish physician, 1843-1918.

Runeberg anemia

Runeberg formula – a formula for estimating the percentage of albumin in a serous fluid.

Runyon, Ernest H., 20th century U.S. microbiologist.

Runyon classification – mycobacteria classification. *SYN:* Runyon group

Runyon group – *SYN:* Runyon classification

Rushton, Martin, English pathologist.

Rushton bodies – linear or curved hyaline bodies found within the epithelial lining of odontogenic cysts.

Russell, Albert L., U.S. dentist, *1905.

Russell Periodontal Index – estimates the degree of periodontal disease.

Russell, Alexander, 20th century English pediatrician.

Russell-Silver dwarfism – *SYN:* Silver-Russell syndrome

Russell syndrome – failure of infants and young children to thrive due to suprasellar lesions, commonly astrocytomas of the anterior third ventricle.

Silver-Russell dwarfism – *SYN:* Silver-Russell syndrome

Silver-Russell syndrome – see under Silver

Russell, Gerald F.M., 20th century English physician.

Russell sign – abrasions and scars on the back of the hands of individuals with bulimia, usually due to manual attempts at self-induced vomiting.

Russell, James S. Risien, English physician, 1863-1939.

hooked bundle of Russell – *SYN:* uncinate bundle of Russell

uncinate bundle of Russell – fastigial efferent fibers that terminate in the vestibular nuclei and the reticular formation of the pons and medulla. *SYN:* hooked bundle of Russell; uncinate fasciculus of Russell

uncinate fasciculus of Russell – *SYN:* uncinate bundle of Russell

Russell, Patrick, Irish physician in India, 1727-1805.

Russell viper – characteristically marked, highly venomous snake of southeastern Asia. *SYN:* daboia

Russell viper venom – used as a coagulant in the arrest of hemorrhage from accessible sites in hemophilia.

Russell, R. Hamilton, Australian surgeon, 1860-1933.

Russell-Taylor classification

Russell-Taylor nail

Russell-Taylor rod

Russell traction – an improvement of Buck extension that permits the resultant vector of the applied traction force to be changed, for fractures of the femur.

Russell, William, Scottish physician, 1852-1940.

Russell bodies – small, discrete hyaline bodies that occur frequently in plasma cells in chronic inflammation. *SYN:* fuchsin bodies

NOTES

Russell, William James, English chemist, 1830-1909.
> **Russell effect** – the ability of an agent other than light to make a developable latent image in a photographic film emulsion. *SYN:* photechic effect

Russo, Mario, 19th century Italian physician.
> **Russo reaction** – urine reaction to Russo test in typhoid patients.
> **Russo test**

Rust, Johann N., German surgeon, 1775-1840.
> **Rust disease** – tuberculosis of the two upper cervical vertebrae and their articulations. *SYN:* malum vertebrale suboccipitale; spondylarthrocace; spondylocace
> **Rust phenomenon** – in cancer of the upper cervical vertebrae, the patient supports the head by the hands when changing from the recumbent to the sitting posture or the reverse.
> **Rust sign**

Rutherford, Ernest, English physicist and Nobel laureate, 1871-1937.
> **rutherford** – obsolete term for a unit of radioactivity.

Rutishauser, E., Swiss physician.
> **Martin du Pan-Rutishauser syndrome** – see under Martin du Pan

Ruvalcaba, R.H., U.S. physician, *1934.
> **Ruvalcaba syndrome** – congenital birth defects in male infants.

Ruysch, Frederik, Dutch anatomist, 1638-1731.
> **Ruysch membrane** – the internal layer of the choroidea of the eye, composed of a very close capillary network. *SYN:* choriocapillary layer
> **Ruysch muscle** – the muscular tissue of the fundus of the uterus.
> **Ruysch tube** – a minute tubular cavity opening in the nasal septum.
> **Ruysch veins** – *SYN:* Retzius veins

Ryan, Norbert J., 20th century Australian pathologist.
> **Ryan stain** – a modified trichrome stain for microsporidian spores.

Rye, city in New York where the classification was first identified in 1965.
> **Rye classification** – classification of Hodgkin disease according to lymphocyte predominance, nodular sclerosing, mixed cellularity, and lymphocyte depletion types.

Ryle, John A., English physician, 1889-1950.
> **Ryle tube** – a thin rubber tube used in the giving of a test meal.

Sabin, Albert Bruce, U.S. epidemiologist, 1906-1993.

    Sabin-Feldman dye test – a method for the detection of antitoxoplasma antibody in serum.

    Sabin-Feldman syndrome – chorioretinitis and cerebral calcifications.

    Sabin vaccine – an orally administered vaccine containing live, attenuated strains of poliovirus.

Sabouraud, Raymond Jacques Adrien, French dermatologist, 1864-1938.

    Sabouraud agar – a culture medium for fungi. *SYN:* French proof agar

    Sabouraud-Noiré instrument – an obsolete device for measuring the quantity of x-rays.

    Sabouraud pastils – disks that undergo a color change when exposed to x-rays, previously used to indicate the administered dose.

    Sabouraud syndrome – progressively thinning hair during first 2 months of life; may occur again in adult life. *SYN:* beaded hair

Sacher-Masoch, Leopold von, Austrian attorney and writer, 1836-1895.

    masochism – a form of perversion in which a person experiences pleasure in being abused, humiliated, or mistreated.

    masochist – the passive party in the practice of masochism.

Sachs, Bernard, U.S. neurologist, 1858-1944.

    Tay-Sachs disease – see under Tay

Sachs, Hans, German bacteriologist, 1877-1945.

    Sachs-Georgi test – the first precipitin test for syphilis of diagnostic practicality.

Sachs, M.

    Ghon-Sachs bacillus – *SYN:* Sachs bacillus

    Sachs bacillus – a species found in malignant edema of animals, in human war wounds, and in cases of appendicitis. *SYN: Clostridium septicum*; Ghon-Sachs bacillus

Sachs, Maurice D., U.S. radiologist, *1909.
Hill-Sachs lesion – see under Hill, Harold A.

Sacks, Benjamin, U.S. physician, 1896-1939.
Libman-Sacks endocarditis – see under Libman
Libman-Sacks syndrome – *SYN:* Libman-Sacks endocarditis
Sacks QuickStick catheter
Sacks Single-Step catheter
Sacks-Vine gastrostomy kit
Sacks-Vine PEG system
Sacks-Vine type PEG

Sade, Donatien Alphonse François, Comte de, French soldier, writer, and libertine, 1740-1814.
sadism – a form of perversion in which a person finds pleasure in inflicting abuse and maltreatment.
sadist – one who practices sadism.
sadomasochism – a form of perversion marked by enjoyment of cruelty and/or humiliation in its received or active and/or dispensed and passive form.

Saemisch, Edwin Theodor, German ophthalmologist, 1833-1909.
Saemisch operation
Saemisch section – procedure of transfixing the cornea beneath an ulcer and then cutting from within outward through the base.
Saemisch ulcer – a form of serpiginous keratitis, frequently accompanied by hypopyon.

Saenger, Alfred, German neurologist, 1860-1921.
Saenger pupil
Saenger reflex
Saenger sign – a lost light reflex of the pupil returns after a short time in the dark.

Saenger, Max, Czech obstetrician, 1853-1903.
Saenger macula – a spot of red brighter than the surrounding membrane, at the congested orifice of the duct of Bartholin gland. *SYN:* macula gonorrhoica
Saenger operation – cesarean section followed by careful closure of the uterine wound by three tiers of sutures.
Saenger ovum forceps
Saenger suture
Saenger ulcer

Saethre, Haakon, 20th century Norwegian psychiatrist.
    Saethre-Chotzen syndrome – *SYN:* Chotzen syndrome

Sahli, Hermann, Swiss physician, 1856-1933.
    Sahli method – an original technique for hemoglobin calorimetric measuring.

Saint, Charles F.M., South African radiologist, 1886-1973.
    Saint triad – the concurrence of hiatal hernia, diverticulosis, and cholelithiasis.

Sainton, Raymond, French physician.
    Marie-Sainton syndrome – see under Marie, Pierre

Sakati, Nadia, 20th century Saudi Arabian pediatrician.
    Sakati-Nyhan syndrome – rare syndrome, usually sporadic, featuring craniofacial defects, abnormal limbs, congenital heart defects, patchy alopecia with atrophic skin above the ears, and linear scarlike lesions in the submental areas. *SYN:* Sakati-Nyhan-Tisdale syndrome; Sakati syndrome
    Sakati-Nyhan-Tisdale syndrome – *SYN:* Sakati-Nyhan syndrome
    Sakati syndrome – *SYN:* Sakati-Nyhan syndrome
    Sanjad-Sakati syndrome – see under Sanjad

Sakmann, Bert, joint winner of 1991 Nobel Prize for work related to ion channels in the cell.

Sakurai, Japanese ophthalmologist.
    Sakurai-Lisch nodule – *SYN:* Lisch nodule

Sala, Luigi, Italian zoologist, 1863-1930.
    Sala cells – found in the pericardium.

Salah, M., 20th century Egyptian surgeon.
    Salah sternal puncture needle – a wide-bore needle for obtaining samples of red marrow from the sternum.

S

NOTES

Saldino, Ronald M., U.S. radiologist, *1941.
Langer-Saldino syndrome – see under Langer, Leonard O., Jr.
Saldino-Mainzer syndrome – retinitis pigmentosa, acrodysplasia, nephropathy, and cerebellar ataxia.
Saldino-Noonan syndrome – fatal form of neonatal chondrodystrophy.

Salk, Jonas, U.S. immunologist, 1914-1995.
Salk polio vaccine – *SYN:* Salk vaccine
Salk vaccine – the original poliovirus vaccine. *SYN:* Salk polio vaccine

Salkowski, Ernst Leopold, German physiologic chemist, 1844-1923.
Salkowski test – for carbon monoxide in the blood.

Salmon, Daniel Elmer, U.S. pathologist, 1850-1914.
Salmonella enteritidis – *SYN:* Gärtner bacillus
Salmonella gallinarum – occasionally causes food poisoning or gastroenteritis.
Salmonella hirschfeld – a species causing enteric fever.
Salmonella paratyphi – a species causing enteric fever.
Salmonella schottmulleri – a species causing enteric fever.
SYN: Schottmueller bacillus
Salmonella typhi – *SYN:* Eberth bacillus
Salmonella typhimurium – a species causing food poisoning.

Salmon, Udall J., U.S. obstetrician, *1904.
Meigs-Salmon syndrome – *SYN:* Meigs syndrome

Salter, Robert, 20th century Canadian orthopedist.
Salter fracture (I-VI)
Salter-Harris classification of epiphysial plate injuries – correlates with different prognoses.
Salter innominate osteotomy
Salter operation
Salter osteotomy
Salter technique

Salter, Sir Samuel J.A., English dentist, 1825-1897.
Salter incremental lines – transverse lines sometimes seen in dentin due to improper calcification.

Salus, Robert, Bohemian ophthalmologist, *1877.
Koerber-Salus-Elschnig syndrome – *SYN:* Parinaud I syndrome

Salzmann, Maximilian, German ophthalmologist, 1862-1954.
Salzmann nodular corneal degeneration – prominent nodules of a solid opaque material that stand out from the surface of the cornea.

Sampson, John Albertson, U.S. gynecologist, 1873-1946.
   Sampson cyst – results from local hemorrhage. *SYN:* chocolate cyst

Samuelsson, Bengt I., joint winner of 1982 Nobel Prize for work related to prostaglandins.

Sanarelli, Giuseppe, Italian bacteriologist, 1864-1940.
   Sanarelli phenomenon – *SYN:* generalized Shwartzman phenomenon
   Sanarelli-Shwartzman phenomenon – *SYN:* generalized Shwartzman phenomenon

Sanchez Salorio, Manuel, Spanish ophthalmologist, *1930.
   Sanchez Salorio syndrome – a syndrome characterized by retinal pigmentary dystrophy, cataract, hypotrichosis of the lashes, mental deficiencies, and retarded somatic development.

Sanctis, Carlo De, see under De Sanctis

Sanders, Clarence Elmer, U.S. physician, 1885-1949.
   Sanders oscillating bed – a rocking bed designed to treat patients with peripheral vascular and cardiovascular disease.

Sanders, J., English physician, 1777-1843.
   Sanders sign – constrictive pericarditis with an epigastric pulsation.

Sanders, Murray, U.S. bacteriologist, *1910.
   Sanders disease – *SYN:* keratoconjunctivitis epidemic; Sanders syndrome
   Sanders syndrome – *SYN:* Sanders disease

Sandhoff, K., contemporary German biochemist.
   Sandhoff disease – a lysosomal storage disease. *SYN:* Sandhoff syndrome
   Sandhoff syndrome – *SYN:* Sandhoff disease

Sandifer, Paul, 20th century English radiologist.
   Sandifer syndrome – torticollis in children as a symptom of reflux esophagitis.

S

NOTES

Sandison, J. Calvin, U.S. surgeon, *1899.
   Sandison-Clark chamber – a chamber that can be fitted over a hole punched in a rabbit's ear so that tissue will grow to fill the defect between two transparent plates.

Sandow, Eugene, 1867-1925.
   Sandow apparatus – an elastic extensor apparatus used primarily for upper limb and shoulder girdle exercises.
   Sandow method – method of muscular training. *SYN:* Sandow system
   Sandow system – *SYN:* Sandow method

Sandström, Ivor V., Swedish anatomist, 1852-1889.
   Sandström bodies – *SYN:* parathyroid glands

Sandwith, Fleming Mant, English physician, 1853-1918.
   Sandwith bald tongue – an abnormally clean tongue.

Sanfilippo, Sylvester J., 20th century U.S. pediatrician.
   Sanfilippo syndrome – *SYN:* type III mucopolysaccharidosis

Sanger, Frederick, English biochemist and twice Nobel laureate, *1918.
   Sanger method – sequencing of DNA by employing an enzyme that can polymerase DNA and labeled nucleotides.
   Sanger reagent – *SYN:* fluoro-2,4-dinitrobenzene

Sanger Brown, see under Brown, Sanger

Sanjad, S.A.
   Sanjad-Sakati syndrome – an autosomal recessive disorder characterized by congenital hypoparathyroidism, severe growth failure and dysmorphic features.

San Jose, Hermenia, 20th century Chilean pathologist.
   Maldonado-San Jose stain – see under Maldonado

Sansom, Arthur E., English physician, 1838-1907.
   Sansom sign – in mitral stenosis, apparent duplication of the second heart sound.

Sanson, Louis J., French physician, 1790-1841.
   Purkinje-Sanson images – see under Purkinje
   Sanson images – *SYN:* Purkinje-Sanson images

Santavuori, Pirkko, 20th century Finnish physician.
   Haltia-Santavuori disease – see under Haltia, M.
   Santavuori disease – *SYN:* Haltia-Santavuori disease

Santorini, Giandomenico (Giovanni Domenico), Italian anatomist, 1681-1737.

concha santorini

incisurae santorini – notches in cartilage of external acoustic meatus.

papilla of Santorini – *SYN:* Vater tubercle

Santorini canal – *SYN:* Santorini duct

Santorini cartilage – a conical nodule of elastic cartilage surmounting the apex of each arytenoid cartilage. *SYN:* corniculate cartilage

Santorini concha – a small concha frequently present on the posterosuperior part of the lateral nasal wall. *SYN:* supreme nasal concha

Santorini duct – the excretory duct of the head of the pancreas. *SYN:* accessory pancreatic duct; Santorini canal

Santorini fissures – two vertical fissures in the anterior portion of the cartilage of the external auditory meatus, filled by fibrous tissue. *SYN:* notches in cartilage of external acoustic meatus

Santorini incisures – *SYN:* notches in cartilage of external acoustic meatus

Santorini labyrinth – a venous plexus arising chiefly from the dorsal vein of the penis, situated below the base of the bladder at the sides of the prostate. *SYN:* prostatic venous plexus

Santorini major caruncle – point of opening of the common bile duct and pancreatic duct into the duodenum. *SYN:* major duodenal papilla

Santorini minor caruncle – the site of the opening of the accessory pancreatic duct into the duodenum, located anterior to and slightly superior to the major papilla. *SYN:* minor duodenal papilla

Santorini muscle – draws angle of mouth laterally. *SYN:* risorius muscle

Santorini tubercle – a rounded eminence on the posterior part of the aryepiglottic fold, formed by the underlying corniculate cartilages. *SYN:* corniculate tubercle

Santorini vein – connects the superior sagittal sinus with the tributaries of the superficial temporal vein and other veins of the scalp. *SYN:* parietal emissary vein

S

NOTES

Sappey, Marie P.C., French anatomist, 1810-1896.
Sappey fibers – nonstriated muscular fibers in the check ligaments of the eyeball.
Sappey plexus – a network of lymphatics in the areola of the nipple.
Sappey veins – several small veins arising from cutaneous veins about the umbilicus, running along the round ligament of the liver and terminating as accessory portal veins. *SYN:* paraumbilical veins

Sarason, Seymour Bernard, U.S. psychologist, *1919.
Sarason test anxiety scale – used in psychiatry.

Sartwell, Philip, U.S. epidemiologist, *1908.
Sartwell incubation model – a mathematical model based on empirical observations, showing that incubation periods for communicable diseases have a log-normal distribution.

Satchmo, nickname of Louis Daniel Armstrong, U.S. jazz musician, 1900-1971.
Satchmo syndrome – rupture of orbicularis oris muscle, frequently occurring in musicians who play wind instruments.

Sattler, C. Hubert, Austrian ophthalmologist, 1844-1928.
Sattler elastic layer – the middle layer of the choroid.
Sattler veil – a diffuse edema of the corneal epithelium that may develop after wearing contact lenses.

Saturday, day of the week.
Saturday night palsy syndrome – *SYN:* alcoholic neuropathy
Saturday night paralysis – musculospiral paralysis.

Saundby, Robert, English physician, 1849-1918.
Saundby test – for blood in the stool.

Saunders, Edward W., U.S. physician, 1854-1927.
Saunders disease – acute gastritis in infants due to excessive carbohydrate intake.

Sauvineau, Charles, French ophthalmologist, 1862-1924.
Sauvineau ophthalmoplegia – ocular muscle paralysis caused by a lesion in the medial longitudinal fasciculus.

Savage, Henry, English anatomist and gynecologist, 1810-1900.
Savage perineal body – the fibromuscular mass between the anal canal and the urogenital diaphragm. *SYN:* central tendon of perineum

Savage, Paul Thwaites, English surgeon.
Savage decompressor

Sayre, George P., U.S. ophthalmologist, *1911.
   Kearns-Sayre syndrome – see under Kearns

Sayre, Lewis A., U.S. surgeon, 1820-1900.
   Sayre apparatus
   Sayre bandage
   Sayre elevator
   Sayre jacket – a plaster-of-Paris jacket applied while the patient is
      suspended by the head and axillae.
   Sayre sling – used for head suspension.
   Sayre splint
   Sayre suspension apparatus – obsolete term for Sayre suspension
      traction.
   Sayre suspension traction – spinal traction obtained by vertical
      suspension of the patient by means of a head halter.

Scaglietti, Oscar, Italian orthopedic surgeon, *1906.
   Scaglietti-Dagnini syndrome – *SYN:* Erdheim syndrome

Scanzoni, Friedrich W., German obstetrician, 1821-1891.
   Scanzoni maneuver – forceps rotation and traction in a spiral course, with
      reapplication of forceps for delivery.
   Scanzoni second os – a constriction in the uterus resulting from
      obstructed labor, one of the classic signs of threatened rupture of the
      uterus. *SYN:* pathologic retraction ring

Scardino, Peter L., U.S. urologist, *1915.
   Scardino ureteropelvioplasty
   Scardino vertical flap pyeloplasty – a reconstructive technique for
      correction of uteropelvic obstruction.

Scarff, John E., U.S. neurosurgeon, 1898-1978.
   Stookey-Scarff operation – see under Stookey

NOTES

Scarpa, Antonio, Italian anatomist, orthopedist, and ophthalmologist, 1747-1832.

> **canals of Scarpa** – separate canals for the nasopalatine nerves and vessels.
>
> **fossa scarpae major** – *SYN:* femoral triangle
>
> **Scarpa fascia** – the deeper membranous or lamellar part of the subcutaneous tissue of the lower abdominal wall. *SYN:* membranous layer of superficial fascia
>
> **Scarpa fluid** – the fluid contained within the membranous labyrinth of the inner ear. *SYN:* endolymph
>
> **Scarpa foramina** – two openings in the line of the intermaxillary suture that transmit the nasopalatine nerve.
>
> **Scarpa ganglion** – a collection of bipolar nerve cell bodies forming a swelling on the vestibular part of the eighth nerve in the internal acoustic meatus. *SYN:* vestibular ganglion
>
> **Scarpa habenula** – *SYN:* Haller habenula
>
> **Scarpa hiatus** – a semilunar opening at the apex of the cochlea through which the scala vestibuli and the scala tympani of the cochlea communicate with one another. *SYN:* helicotrema
>
> **Scarpa liquor** – the fluid contained within the membranous labyrinth of the inner ear. *SYN:* endolymph
>
> **Scarpa membrane** – closes the fenestra cochleae or rotunda. *SYN:* secondary tympanic membrane
>
> **Scarpa method** – cure of an aneurysm by ligation of the artery at some distance above the sac.
>
> **Scarpa sheath** – one of the coverings of the spermatic cord, formed of delicate connective tissue and of muscular fibers derived from the internal oblique muscle. *SYN:* cremasteric fascia
>
> **Scarpa staphyloma** – bulging near the posterior pole of the eyeball due to degenerative changes in severe myopia. *SYN:* posterior staphyloma
>
> **Scarpa triangle** – branches of the femoral nerve are distributed within the femoral triangle. *SYN:* femoral triangle; fossa scarpae major

Scatchard, George, U.S. chemist and biochemist, 1892-1973.

> **Scatchard plot** – a graphical representation used in the analysis of binding phenomena.

Schacher, Polycarp G., German physician, 1674-1737.

> **Schacher ganglion** – a small parasympathetic ganglion lying in the orbit between the optic nerve and the lateral rectus muscle. *SYN:* ciliary ganglion

Schachowa, Seraphina, 19th century Russian histologist.
  Schachowa spiral tubes – *SYN:* tubuli renales

Schaeffer, (Schäffer), Max, German neurologist, 1852-1923.
  Schaeffer reflex – great toe dorsiflexion produced by pinching the Achilles tendon.

Schäfer, Erich, German dermatologist, *1897.
  Schäfer syndrome – congenital nail thickening.

Schäfer, Sir Edward A. Sharpey, English physiologist and histologist, 1850-1935.
  Schäfer method – an obsolete method of resuscitation in cases of drowning or asphyxia.

Schäffer, var. of Schaeffer

Schally, Andrew V., joint winner of 1977 Nobel Prize for work related to production of peptide hormone.

Schamberg, Jay Frank, U.S. dermatologist, 1870-1934.
  Schamberg dermatitis – chronic purpura, especially of the legs of men, spreading to form brownish patches. *SYN:* progressive pigmentary dermatosis

Schanz, Alfred, German orthopedic surgeon, 1868-1931.
  Schanz angulation osteotomy
  Schanz brace
  Schanz collar – a tube of material stuffed with cellulose and wound in 3 loops around the neck, forming a collar.
  Schanz collar brace
  Schanz femoral osteotomy
  Schanz operation
  Schanz osteotomy
  Schanz pin
  Schanz screw

NOTES

Schanz syndrome – spinal muscle weakness, pain on pressure over the spinous processes, and a tendency to curvature of the spine.

Schapiro, Heinrich, Russian physician, 1852-1901.
Schapiro sign – in myocardial weakness, no slowing of the pulse occurs when the patient lies down.

Schardinger, Franz, Austrian scientist, 1853-1920.
Schardinger dextrins – the result of action of *Bacillus macerans* on starch.
Schardinger enzyme – a flavoprotein containing molybdenum.
SYN: xanthine oxidase
Schardinger reaction – an example of oxidation in the absence of O_2 with an organic hydrogen acceptor.

Schatzki, Richard, U.S. radiologist, 1901-1992.
Schatzki ring – a contraction ring or incomplete mucosal diaphragm in the lower third of the esophagus, which is occasionally symptomatic.
SYN: Schatzki syndrome
Schatzki syndrome – *SYN:* Schatzki ring

Schaudinn, Fritz R., German bacteriologist, 1871-1906.
Schaudinn fixative – a solution of mercuric chloride, sodium chloride, alcohol, and glacial acetic acid, used on wet smears for cytologic fixation.

Schaumann, Jörgen Nilsen, Swedish physician, 1879-1953.
Besnier-Boeck-Schaumann disease – *SYN:* Besnier-Boeck disease
Besnier-Boeck-Schaumann syndrome – *SYN:* Besnier-Boeck disease
Schaumann bodies – concentrically laminated calcified bodies found in granulomas, particularly in sarcoidosis. *SYN:* conchoidal bodies
Schaumann lymphogranuloma – obsolete term for sarcoidosis.
Schaumann syndrome – *SYN:* Besnier-Boeck disease

Schauta, Friedrich, Austrian gynecologist, 1849-1919.
Schauta-Amreich operation – *SYN:* Schauta operation
Schauta operation – an extensive extirpation of the uterus and the adnexa, using the vaginal approach facilitated by Schuchardt operation.
SYN: Schauta-Amreich operation
Schauta radical vaginal hysterectomy
Schauta-Wertheim operation

Schede, Max, German surgeon, 1844-1902.
Schede clot

Schede method – filling of the defect in bone after removal of a sequestrum or scraping away carious material by allowing the cavity to fill with blood which may become organized.

Schede osteotomy

Scheele, Karl W., Swedish chemist, 1742-1786.

Scheele green – *SYN:* cupric arsenite

Scheffé, Henry, U.S. mathematician, *1907.

Scheffé test – compares the difference between means in the analysis of variance.

Scheibe, A., U.S. physician, *1875.

Scheibe deafness – congenital deafness.

Scheie, Harold Glendon, U.S. ophthalmologist, 1909-1990.

Scheie blade

Scheie cannula

Scheie cataract aspiration

Scheie cautery

Scheie electrocautery

Scheie knife

Scheie needle

Scheie operation

Scheie syndrome – error of mucopolysaccharide related to Hurler syndrome. *SYN:* type IS mucopolysaccharidosis

Scheie trephine

Scheiner, Christoph, German physicist, 1575-1650.

Scheiner experiment – a demonstration of accommodation.

Schellong, Fritz, German physician, 1891-1953.

Schellong-Strisower phenomenon – a reduction of the systolic blood pressure, accompanied sometimes by vertigo, on rising from the horizontal to the erect posture.

Schellong test – for circulatory function.

NOTES

Schenck, Benjamin Robinson, U.S. surgeon, 1873-1920.
    Schenck disease – fungal infection with lymphatic spread to involve musculoskeletal system, gastrointestinal system, and nervous system. *SYN:* Beuermann disease; Beuermann-Gougerot disease; sporotrichosis

Schepelmann, Emil, 20th century German physician.
    Schepelmann sign

Scheuermann, Holger W., Danish surgeon, 1877-1960.
    Scheuermann disease – epiphysial aseptic necrosis of vertebral bodies. *SYN:* adolescent round back; juvenile kyphosis; osteochondritis deformans juvenilis dorsi; Scheuermann syndrome
    Scheuermann juvenile kyphosis
    Scheuermann syndrome – *SYN:* Scheuermann disease

Schick, Bela, Austrian pediatrician in U.S., 1877-1967.
    Schick method – *SYN:* Schick test
    Schick sign
    Schick test – for susceptibility to *Corynebacterium diphtheriae* toxin. *SYN:* Schick method
    Schick test toxin – *SYN:* diagnostic diphtheria toxin

Schiefferdecker, Paul, German anatomist, 1849-1931.
    Schiefferdecker symbiosis theory – theory that there is a symbiosis among the body's tissues.

Schiff, Hugo, German chemist in Florence, 1834-1915.
    Kasten fluorescent Schiff reagents – see under Kasten
    ninhydrin-Schiff stain for proteins
    periodic acid-Schiff stain – a tissue-staining procedure. *SYN:* PAS stain
    Schiff base – condensation products of aldehydes and ketones with primary amine. *SYN:* aldimine
    Schiff reagent – used for aldehydes and in histochemistry to detect polysaccharides, DNA, and proteins.

Schiff, Moritz, German physiologist, 1823-1896.
    Schiff-Sherrington phenomenon – when the spinal cord is transected in the midthoracic region or a little lower, the stretch and other postural reflexes of the upper extremity become exaggerated; if the transection is made in the sacral cord, a similar effect is observed in the lower limbs.

Schiffrin, Arthur, U.S. pathologist, *1904.
    Baehr-Schiffrin disease – *SYN:* Moschcowitz syndrome

Schild, H.O.
    Gaddum and Schild test – see under Gaddum

Schilder, Paul Ferdinand, Austrian neurologist, 1886-1940.
  Addison-Schilder disease – *SYN:* Schilder disease
  Flatau-Schilder disease – *SYN:* Schilder disease
  Schilder disease – encephalitis periaxialis diffusa; progressive demyelinating disorder in adults; early symptom is visual impairment with mental deterioration. *SYN:* Addison-Schilder disease; Flatau-Schilder disease; Schilder syndrome
  Schilder encephalitis
  Schilder syndrome – *SYN:* Schilder disease

Schiller, Walter, Austrian pathologist in U.S., 1887-1960.
  Schiller test – for early carcinoma of the cervix.
  Schiller tumor

Schilling, Robert F., U.S. hematologist, *1919.
  Schilling test – a procedure for determining the amount of B_{12} excreted in the urine. *SYN:* vitamin B_{12} absorption test

Schilling, Victor Theodor Adolf Georg, German hematologist, 1883-1960.
  Schilling band cell – any cell of the granulocytic (leukocytic) series that has a nucleus that could be described as a curved or coiled band. *SYN:* band cell
  Schilling blood count – a method of counting blood. *SYN:* Schilling index
  Schilling index – *SYN:* Schilling blood count
  Schilling type of monocytic leukemia

Schimmelbusch, Curt, German surgeon and pathologist, 1860-1895.
  Schimmelbusch disease – cystic dysplasia of the breast.

Schimmelpenning, G.W., German physician.
  Feuerstein-Mims-Schimmelpenning syndrome – *SYN:* Schimmelpenning-Feuerstein-Mims syndrome
  Schimmelpenning-Feuerstein-Mims syndrome – epidermal nevi. *SYN:* Feuerstein-Mims-Schimmelpenning syndrome; Feuerstein-Mims syndrome

Schiötz, Hjalmar, Norwegian physician, 1850-1927.
Schiötz tonometer – an instrument that measures ocular tension by indicating the ease with which the cornea is indented.

Schirmer, Otto W.A., German ophthalmologist, 1864-1917.
Schirmer test – for tear production, using a strip of filter paper; a measurement of basal and reflex lacrimal gland function.

Schlatter, Carl, Swiss surgeon, 1864-1934.
Osgood-Schlatter disease – see under Osgood
Schlatter disease – *SYN:* Osgood-Schlatter disease
Schlatter-Osgood disease – *SYN:* Osgood-Schlatter disease

Schlemm, Friedrich, German anatomist, 1795-1858.
Schlemm canal – the vascular structure encircling the anterior chamber of the eye and through which the aqueous is returned to the blood circulation. *SYN:* sinus venosus sclerae

Schlesinger, Hermann, Austrian physician, 1868-1934.
Pool-Schlesinger sign – *SYN:* Pool phenomenon
Schlesinger cervical punch
Schlesinger cervical rongeur
Schlesinger clamp
Schlesinger forceps
Schlesinger instrument
Schlesinger punch
Schlesinger rongeur
Schlesinger sign – *SYN:* Pool phenomenon

Schlichter, Jakub G., U.S. internist, *1912.
Schlichter test – for serum bactericidal activity.

Schlösser, Karl, German ophthalmologist, 1857-1925.
Schlösser treatment – for trigeminal neuralgia.

Schmid, Rudi, Swiss-U.S. internist and biochemist, *1922.
McArdle-Schmid-Pearson disease – *SYN:* McArdle syndrome

Schmid, W.
Schmid-Fraccaro syndrome – iris colobomas and anal atresia, associated with an additional acrocentric chromosome. *SYN:* cat's-eye syndrome

Schmidel, Kasimir C., German anatomist, 1718-1792.
Schmidel anastomoses – abnormal channels of communication between the caval and portal venous systems.

Schmidt, Adolph, German physician, 1865-1918.

   Schmidt diet – used to subsequently examine diarrheic stools.

   Schmidt syndrome – one-sided paralysis caused by a lesion of the nucleus ambiguus and the nucleus accessorius. *SYN:* polyglandular autoimmune syndrome

Schmidt, Gerhard, U.S. biochemist, *1900.

   Schmidt-Thannhauser method – a method for fractionation of nucleic acid.

Schmidt, Henry D., U.S. anatomist and pathologist, 1823-1888.

   Schmidt-Lanterman clefts – *SYN:* Schmidt-Lanterman incisures

   Schmidt-Lanterman incisures – funnel-shaped interruptions in the regular structure of the myelin sheath of nerve fibers. *SYN:* Lanterman incisures; Schmidt-Lanterman clefts

Schmidt, Johann F.M., German laryngologist, 1838-1907.

   Schmidt syndrome – unilateral paralysis of a vocal cord, the velum palati, trapezius, and sternocleidomastoid.

Schmidt, Martin Benno, German physician, 1863-1949.

   Schmidt syndrome – the association of primary hypothyroidism, primary adrenocortical insufficiency, and insulin-dependent diabetes mellitus.

Schmincke, Alexander, German pathologist, 1877-1953.

   Schmincke tumor – *SYN:* lymphoepithelioma

Schmitz, Karl Ernst Friedrich, German physician, *1889.

   Schmitz bacillus – *SYN: Shigella dysenteriae* type 2

Schmorl, Christian G., German pathologist, 1861-1932.

   Schmorl bacillus – a bacterial species causing or associated with several necrotic conditions in animals and occasionally in humans. *SYN: Fusobacterium necrophorum*

   Schmorl body

   Schmorl ferric-ferricyanide reduction stain – tests for reducing substances in tissues.

NOTES

Schmorl furrow

Schmorl groove

Schmorl jaundice – kernicterus.

Schmorl nodes

Schmorl nodule – prolapse of the nucleus pulposus through the vertebral body endplate into the spongiosa of the vertebra.

Schmorl picrothionin stain – a stain for compact bone.

Schnabel, Isidor, Austrian ophthalmologist, 1842-1908.

Schnabel atrophy – optic atrophy.

Schnabel cavernous degeneration

Schneeberg, district in Saxony, Germany.

Schneeberg disease – form of pulmonary cancer first discovered in miners who worked in the metal mines of Schneeberg.

Schneider, Conrad Viktor, German anatomist, 1614-1680.

schneiderian membranes – *SYN:* nasal mucosa

Schneider, Franz C., German chemist, 1813-1897.

Schneider carmine – a stain consisting of a 10% solution of carmine in 45% acetic acid, used for fresh chromosome preparations.

Schneider, Richard C., U.S. neurologist.

Schneider catheter

Schneider driver

Schneider extractor

Schneider fixation

Schneider hip arthrodesis

Schneider hip fusion

Schneider intramedullary nail

Schneider medullary nail

Schneider nail driver

Schneider nail shaft reamer

Schneider pelvimeter

Schneider pin

Schneider raspatory

Schneider rod

Schneider self-broaching pin

Schneider-Shiley catheter

Schneider syndrome – cervical spine injury resulting in upper extremity paralysis.

Schnitzler, L., 20th century European physician.
Schnitzler syndrome – tense, generalized chronic urticaria, joint or bone pain, and monoclonal gammopathy of kappa type.

Scholander, Per F., Norwegian physiologist, 1905-1980.
Roughton-Scholander apparatus – see under Roughton
Roughton-Scholander syringe – *SYN:* Roughton-Scholander apparatus
Scholander apparatus – a device used for determining the oxygen and carbon dioxide percentage in 0.5 ml of a respiratory gas.

Scholz, Willibald, German neurologist, 1889-1971.
Scholz disease – obsolete term for the juvenile form of metachromatic leukodystrophy.

Schönbein, Christian F., German chemist, 1799-1868.
Schönbein test – *SYN:* Almén test for blood

Schönlein, Johann Lukas, German physician, 1793-1864.
Henoch-Schönlein purpura – see under Henoch
Henoch-Schönlein syndrome – *SYN:* Henoch-Schönlein purpura
Schönlein disease – *SYN:* Henoch-Schönlein purpura
Schönlein-Henoch syndrome – *SYN:* Henoch-Schönlein purpura
Schönlein purpura – *SYN:* Henoch-Schönlein purpura

Schott, Theodor, German physician, 1850-1921.
Schott treatment – *SYN:* Nauheim treatment

Schottmueller, (Schottmüller), Hugo A.G., German physician, 1867-1936.
Schottmueller bacillus – a species causing enteric fever. *SYN: Salmonella schottmulleri*
Schottmueller disease – an acute infectious disease with symptoms and lesions resembling those of typhoid fever. *SYN:* paratyphoid fever

Schottmüller, var. of Schottmueller

Schrader, Gerhard, German chemist.

schradan – a potent irreversible organophosphate cholinesterase inhibitor used as an insecticide. It was prepared for potential use as a nerve gas. *SYN:* octamethyl pyrophosphoramide

Schreger, Christian H.T., German anatomist and chemist, 1768-1833.

Hunter-Schreger bands – see under Hunter, John
Hunter-Schreger lines – *SYN:* Hunter-Schreger bands
Schreger lines – *SYN:* Hunter-Schreger bands

Schridde, Hermann, German pathologist, *1875.

Schridde cancer hairs – thick lusterless hairs scattered in the beard and the temporal region.

Schroeder, Karl L.E., German gynecologist, 1838-1887.

Schroeder curette
Schroeder operation – excision of diseased endocervical mucosa.
Schroeder scissors
Schroeder tenaculum
Schroeder tenaculum loop
Schroeder uterine sound

Schroeder van der Kolk, see under van der Kolk

Schrön, Otto von, German-born Italian pathologist, 1837-1917.

Schrön granule – structure found in germinal spot of ovum.

Schrötter, Leopold von, Austrian laryngologist, 1837-1908.

Paget-von Schrötter syndrome – see under Paget, Sir James

Schuchardt, Karl A., German surgeon, 1856-1901.

Schuchardt incision
Schuchardt operation – a surgical technique making the upper vagina accessible for fistula closure or radical surgery via the vagina.

Schüffner, Wilhelm, German pathologist in Sumatra, 1867-1949.

Schüffner dots – fine, round, uniform dots characteristically observed in erythrocytes infected with *Plasmodium vivax* and *P. ovale*. *SYN:* Schüffner granules
Schüffner granules – *SYN:* Schüffner dots

Schüller, Artur, Austrian neurologist, 1874-1958.

Hand-Schüller-Christian disease – see under Hand
Schüller disease – *SYN:* Hand-Schüller-Christian disease
Schüller phenomenon – in cases of functional hemiplegia, the patient usually turns to the sound side in walking, but in cases of organic lesion, to the affected side.

Schüller syndrome – *SYN:* Hand-Schüller-Christian disease

Schüller, Karl H.L.A. Max, German surgeon, 1843-1907.
Schüller ducts – inconstant ducts along the side of the female urethra that convey the mucoid secretion of Skene glands to the vestibule. *SYN:* paraurethral ducts

Schulman, Irving, U.S. pediatrician.
Upshaw-Schulman syndrome – see under Upshaw

Schulte, Rudi, German master watchmaker.
Pudenz-Schulte thecoperitoneal shunt

Schultes, var. of Scultetus

Schultz, Arthur R.H., German physician, *1890.
Schultz reaction – *SYN:* Schultz stain
Schultz stain – a stain for cholesterol. *SYN:* Schultz reaction

Schultz, Johann Heinrich, German neurologist and psychiatrist, 1884-1970.
Schultz autogenic training – system of relaxation and awareness of one's body parts and their degree of warmth.
Schultz method

Schultz, Werner, German internist, 1878-1947.
Schultz-Charlton phenomenon – *SYN:* Schultz-Charlton reaction
Schultz-Charlton reaction – the specific blanching of a scarlatina rash at the site of intracutaneous injection of scarlatina antiserum. *SYN:* Schultz-Charlton phenomenon
Schultz-Dale reaction – the contraction of an excised intestinal loop or of an excised strip of virginal uterus from a sensitized animal, which occurs when the tissue is exposed to the specific antigen. *SYN:* Dale reaction

Schultze, Bernhard, German obstetrician, 1827-1919.
Schultze fold – *SYN:* amniotic fold
Schultze knife
Schultze mechanism – expulsion of the placenta with the fetal surface foremost.

NOTES

Schultze phantom – a model of a female pelvis used in demonstrating the mechanism of childbirth and the application of forceps.

Schultze placenta – appears at the vulva with the glistening fetal surface presenting.

Schultze, Friedrich, German physician, 1848-1934.

Schultze-Chvostek sign – *SYN:* Chvostek sign

Schultze sign – *SYN:* Chvostek sign

Schultze, Max Johann, German histologist and zoologist, 1825-1874.

comma bundle of Schultze – a compact bundle composed of descending branches of posterior root fibers located near the border between the fasciculi gracilis and cuneatus of the cervical and thoracic spinal cord. *SYN:* comma tract of Schultze; semilunar fasciculus

comma tract of Schultze – *SYN:* comma bundle of Schultze

Schultze cells – *SYN:* olfactory receptor cells

Schultze membrane – the specialized olfactory receptive area. *SYN:* region of olfactory mucosa

Schultze sign – in latent tetany, tapping the tongue causes its depression with a concave dorsum. *SYN:* tongue phenomenon

Schumm, Otto, early 20th century German chemist.

Schumm test – used to detect methemalbumin.

Schütz, Erich, German biochemist, *1902.

Schütz law – *SYN:* Schütz rule

Schütz rule – the rate of an enzyme reaction is proportional to the square root of the enzyme concentration. *SYN:* Schütz law

Schütz, Hugo, early 20th century German neurologist anatomist.

Schütz bundle – thin, poorly myelinated nerve fibers reciprocally connecting the periventricular zone of the hypothalamus with ventral parts of the central gray substance of the midbrain. *SYN:* dorsal longitudinal fasciculus

Schwabach, Dagobert, German otologist, 1846-1920.

Schwabach test – a hearing test using a series of five tuning forks of different tones.

Schwalbe, Gustav A., German anatomist, 1844-1916.

Schwalbe corpuscle – *SYN:* taste bud

Schwalbe fissure

Schwalbe foramen

Schwalbe membrane

Schwalbe nucleus

Schwalbe ring – the periphery of the cornea. *SYN:* anterior limiting ring
Schwalbe sheath
Schwalbe spaces – the spaces within the internal sheath of the optic
nerve filled with cerebrospinal fluid and continuous with the
subarachnoid space. *SYN:* intervaginal space of optic nerve

Schwann, Theodor, German histologist and physiologist, 1810-1882.
Schwann cells – cells of ectodermal (neural crest) origin that compose a
continuous envelope around each nerve fiber of peripheral nerves.
SYN: neurilemma cells
Schwann cell unit – a single Schwann cell and all of the axons lying in
troughs indenting its surface.
schwannoma – *SYN:* neurilemoma; neuroschwannoma
Schwann tumor
Schwann white substance – the lipid material present in the myelin
sheath of nerve fibers; the medulla of bones and other organs.
sheath of Schwann – a cell that enfolds one or more axons of the
peripheral nervous system. *SYN:* neurilemma

Schwartz, Henry, U.S. neurosurgeon, *1909.
Schwartz tractotomy – a medullary spinothalamic tractotomy.

Schwartz, Oscar, U.S. pediatrician, *1919.
Schwartz-Jampel-Aberfeld syndrome – *SYN:* Schwartz-Jampel syndrome
Schwartz-Jampel syndrome – myotonic chondrodystrophy.
SYN: Schwartz-Jampel-Aberfeld syndrome
Schwartz syndrome – multiple congenital disorders.

Schwartz, R. Plato, orthopedic surgeon, 1892-1965.
Schwartz method – system of locomotor exercises for children with
cerebral palsy.

Schwartz, Samuel, U.S. physician, *1916.
Watson-Schwartz test – see under Watson, Cecil J.

NOTES

Schwartz, William, U.S. physician, *1922.
Schwartz-Bartter syndrome – complication of oat cell bronchogenic carcinoma that results in a dilutional hyponatremia, caused by inappropriate antidiuretic hormone secretion.

Schwartze, Hermann Hugo Rudolf, German otologist, 1837-1910.
Schwartze sign – erythema and hypervascularity in otosclerosis due to the formation of new stapes.

Schweigger-Seidel, Franz, German physiologist, 1834-1871.
sheath of Schweigger-Seidel – (1) a spherical or spindle-shaped condensation of phagocytic macrophages in a reticular stroma investing the wall of the splenic arterial capillaries; (2) the outer end of the inner segment of the retinal rods and cones. *SYN:* ellipsoid

Schweninger, Ernst, German dermatologist, 1850-1924.
Schweninger-Buzzi anetoderma – sudden appearance of bluish-white, balloonlike lesions, soft and readily indented.
Schweninger method – a method suggested to reduce obesity by restricting intake of fluid.

Scopoli, G.A., Italian naturalist, 1723-1788.
scopolia – the dried rhizome and roots of *Scopolia carniolica*, an herb of Austria and neighboring European countries; resembles belladonna in pharmacologic action.

Scott, Bruce A., U.S. orthotist at Craig Rehabilitation Hospital, Englewood, CO.
Scott-Craig orthosis – a hip stabilizing knee-ankle-foot orthosis.

Scott, Charles I., Jr., U.S. pediatrician, *1934.
Aarskog-Scott syndrome – see under Aarskog

Scott, H. William, U.S. surgeon, *1916.
Scott operation – a jejunoileal bypass for morbid obesity.

Scottish Rite, Hospitals for Children, located throughout the U.S., owned by a division of the Masonic system.
Scottish Rite brace
Scottish Rite hip orthosis
Scottish Rite splint

Scott-Wilson, H., English scientist.
Scott-Wilson reagent – an alkaline solution of mercuric cyanide and silver nitrate used in the detection of acetone.

Scribner, Belding H., U.S. nephrologist, *1921.
    Quinton-Scribner shunt – see under Quinton
    Scribner shunt – connection of an artery to the cephalic vein via a short extracorporeal catheter.

Scultetus, (originally Schultes), Johann, German surgeon, 1595-1645.
    Scultetus bandage – applied to the thorax or abdomen. *SYN:* many-tailed bandage
    Scultetus binder
    Scultetus position – supine position on an inclined plane, with head low.

Seashore, Carl Emil, U.S. psychologist, 1866-1949.
    Seashore measures of musical talent tests – given to determine the components of musical aptitude.
    Seashore test – a test in which the individual must discriminate between two sounds.

Sebileau, Pierre, French anatomist, 1860-1953.
    Sebileau hollow – depression between the inferior aspect of the tongue and the sublingual glands.
    Sebileau muscle – deep fibers of the dartos tunic that pass into the scrotal septum.

Seckel, Helmut Paul George, German physician, 1900-1960.
    Seckel dwarfism – *SYN:* Seckel syndrome
    Seckel syndrome – an autosomal recessive disorder. *SYN:* Seckel dwarfism

Secrétan, H., Swiss surgeon, 1856-1916.
    Secrétan syndrome – traumatic, recurrent edema or hemorrhage of the dorsum of the hand.

Seeligmüller, Otto L.G.A., German neurologist, 1837-1912.
    Seeligmüller sign – contraction of the pupil on the affected side in facial neuralgia.

S

NOTES

Seessel, Albert, U.S. embryologist, 1850-1910.
   Seessel pocket – the part of the embryonic foregut extending cephalad to the level of the oral plate and caudal to the pituitary diverticulum.
   SYN: preoral gut
   Seessel pouch

Séguin, Edouard, French-U.S. psychiatrist, 1812-1880.
   Séguin formboard – a board with cutouts into which corresponding-shaped blocks of geometric forms are placed.

Seidel, Erich, German ophthalmologist, 1882-1946.
   Seidel scotoma – a form of Bjerrum scotoma.
   Seidel sign – a sickle-shaped scotoma appearing as an upward or downward extension of the blind spot.

Seignette, Pierre, French apothecary, 1660-1719.
   Seignette salt – a mild saline cathartic, used as an ingredient in compound effervescent powders. _SYN:_ potassium sodium tartrate

Seiler, Carl, Swiss laryngologist and anatomist in U.S., 1849-1905.
   Seiler cartilage – a small rod of cartilage attached to the vocal process of the arytenoid cartilage.
   Seiler knife
   Seiler tonsillar knife

Seip, Martin Fredrik, Norwegian pediatrician.
   Lawrence-Seip syndrome – see under Lawrence

Seitelberger, Franz, Austrian neuropathologist, *1916.
   Seitelberger disease – demyelination of the pyramidal tracts.
   SYN: neuroaxonal degeneration; Seitelberger syndrome
   Seitelberger syndrome – _SYN:_ Seitelberger disease

Seitz, Ernest, German bacteriologist, *1885.
   Seitz filter – an asbestos filter used for removing bacteria.

Seldinger, Sven Ivar, Swedish radiologist, *1921.
   Seldinger cardiac catheterization
   Seldinger catheter
   Seldinger intubation technique
   Seldinger method
   Seldinger needle
   Seldinger retrograde wire
   Seldinger technique – a method of percutaneous insertion of a catheter into an artery or vein.
   Seldinger wire

Selivanoff, (Seliwanow), Feodor, Russian chemist, *1859.
　Selivanoff test – for fructosuria. *SYN:* resorcinol test

Seliwanow, var. of Selivanoff

Sellick, Brian A., 20th century English anesthetist.
　Sellick maneuver – pressure applied to the cricoid cartilage to prevent
　　regurgitation during tracheal intubation in the anesthetized patient.

Selter, Paul, German pediatrician, 1866-1941.
　Selter disease – *SYN:* acrodynia

Selye, Hans, Austrian endocrinologist in Canada, 1907-1982.
　adaptation syndrome of Selye – general nonspecific adaptation of the
　　organism in response to specific stimuli, which trigger physiological
　　changes in the endocrine and other organ systems due to prolonged
　　and intense stress. *SYN:* Selye syndrome
　Selye syndrome – *SYN:* adaptation syndrome of Selye

Semelaigne, Georges, French physician, *1892.
　Debré-Semelaigne syndrome – *SYN:* Kocher-Debré-Semelaigne
　　syndrome
　Kocher-Debré-Semelaigne syndrome – see under Kocher

Semliki Forest, forest in Uganda where the virus is transmitted by
mosquitos.
　Semliki Forest virus – an alphavirus in the family *Togaviridae* rarely
　　associated with human disease.

Semon, Richard W., German biologist, 1859-1908.
　Semon-Hering theory – the theory that stimuli leave definite traces on the
　　protoplasm of the animal or plant that persist after the stimuli cease.
　　SYN: mnemic hypothesis

Semon, Sir Felix, German laryngologist in England, 1849-1921.
　Gerhardt-Semon law – see under Gerhardt, Carl
　Semon law – an obsolete law regarding injury to the recurrent laryngeal
　　nerve.

NOTES

Semple, Sir David, English physician, 1856-1937.
  Semple vaccine – a modification of the original rabies vaccine.

Senear, Francis E., U.S. dermatologist, 1889-1958.
  Senear-Usher disease – *SYN:* Senear-Usher syndrome
  Senear-Usher syndrome – an eruption involving sun-exposed skin, especially the face. *SYN:* pemphigus erythematosus; Senear-Usher disease

Sengstaken, Robert W., U.S. neurosurgeon, *1923.
  Sengstaken-Blakemore tube – a tube with three lumens used for emergency treatment of bleeding esophageal varices.

Senior, Boris, South African pediatrician.
  Senior-Løken syndrome – congenital nephronophthisis with retinitis pigmentosa.

Seoul, city in Korea where the virus was first isolated.
  Seoul virus – a species of Hantavirus causing hemorrhagic fever with renal syndrome.

Sergent, Emile, French physician, 1867-1943.
  Bernard-Sergent syndrome – *SYN:* acute adrenocortical insufficiency
  Sergent white line – a pale streak appearing within 30 to 60 seconds after stroking the skin with a fingernail and lasting for several minutes, a sign of diminished arterial tension. *SYN:* white line

Serrati, Serafino, 18th century Italian physicist.
  Serratia – a genus of anaerobic bacteria that contain gram-negative rods.
  Serratia marcescens – a species found in water, soil, milk, foods, and insects; significant cause of hospital-acquired infection.

Serres, Antoine E.R.A., French anatomist, 1786-1868.
  rests of Serres – remnants of dental lamina epithelium entrapped within the gingiva.
  Serres angle – the angle between the pterygoid processes and the base of the skull. *SYN:* metafacial angle
  Serres glands – epithelial cell rests found in the subepithelial connective tissue in the palate of the newborn, similar to those found in the gingivae.

Sertoli, Enrico, Italian histologist, 1842-1910.
  Sertoli-cell-only syndrome – the absence from the seminiferous tubules of the testes of germinal epithelium, Sertoli cells alone being present. *SYN:* Del Castillo syndrome

Sertoli cells – elongated cells in the seminiferous tubules to which spermatids are attached during spermiogenesis. *SYN:* nurse cells

Sertoli cell tumor – a testicular tumor. *SYN:* androblastoma

Sertoli columns

Servetus, Miguel, Spanish anatomist and theologian, 1511-1553.

Servetus circulation – obsolete term for pulmonary circulation.

Settegast, H., 20th century German radiologist.

Settegast position – radiographic technique using axial projection to image vertical fractures of patella and articular surfaces of femoropatellar articulation.

Sever, James Warren, U.S. surgeon, 1878-1964.

Sever disease – calcaneoapophysitis.

Sever modification of Fairbank technique

Sever operation

Severinghaus, John W., U.S. physiologist and anesthesiologist, *1922.

Severinghaus electrode – commonly used to analyze arterial blood samples. *SYN:* carbon dioxide electrode

Sézary, Albert, French dermatologist, 1880-1956.

Sézary-Bouvrain syndrome – *SYN:* Sézary syndrome

Sézary cell – an atypical T lymphocyte seen in the peripheral blood in Sézary syndrome.

Sézary erythroderma – *SYN:* Sézary syndrome

Sézary syndrome – a variant of mycosis fungoides. *SYN:* Sézary-Bouvrain syndrome; Sézary erythroderma

Shaffer, A., U.S. biochemist, 1881-1960.

Shaffer-Hartmann method – an obsolete method for the quantitative determination of glucose in biological fluids.

Sharp, Phillip A., *1943, joint winner of 1993 Nobel Prize for work related to split genes.

NOTES

Sharpey, William, Scottish physiologist and histologist, 1802-1880.
Sharpey fibers – bundles of collagenous fibers that pass into the outer circumferential lamellae of bone or the cementum of teeth.
SYN: perforating fibers

Shaver, Cecil Gordon, Canadian physician, *1901.
Shaver disease – a pulmonary condition due to the occupational inhalation of bauxite fumes. *SYN:* bauxite pneumoconiosis

Sheehan, Harold Leaming, English pathologist, 1900-1988.
Sheehan syndrome – hypopituitarism arising from a severe circulatory collapse postpartum, with resultant pituitary necrosis. *SYN:* postpartum pituitary necrosis syndrome; thyrohypophysial syndrome

Sheldon, Joseph H., English pediatrician, 1920-1964.
Freeman-Sheldon syndrome – *SYN:* craniocarpotarsal dystrophy

Sheldon, William H., U.S. psychologist, 1898-1970.
Sheldon constitutional theory of personality – theory used in psychology/psychiatry.

Shemin, David, U.S. biochemist, *1911.
Shemin cycle – *SYN:* glycine-succinate cycle

Shenton, Edward Warren Hine, English radiologist, 1872-1955.
Shenton line – a curved line formed by the top of the obturator foramen and the inner side of the neck of the femur, seen on an anteroposterior frontal x-ray of a normal hip joint.

Shepherd, Francis John, Canadian surgeon, 1851-1929.
Shepherd fracture – a fracture of the posterior process of the talus, sometimes mistaken for a displacement of the os trigonum.

Shepardson, H.C.
Escamilla-Lisser-Shepardson syndrome

Sherman, Harry Mitchell O'Neill, U.S. surgeon, 1854-1921.
Sherman block test
Sherman bone plate
Sherman bone screw
Sherman knife
Sherman plate
Sherman plates and screws
Sherman screw
Sherman screwdriver
Sherman suction tube

Sherman, Henry C., U.S. biochemist, 1875-1955.

Sherman-Bourquin unit of vitamin B$_2$ – equivalent to 0.001 to 0.007 mg of riboflavin.

Sherman-Munsell unit – a rat growth unit.

Sherman unit – unit of vitamin C, minimum protective dose.

Sherren, James, English surgeon, 1872-1946.

Ochsner-Sherren regime – see under Ochsner, Albert John

Sherren triangle – an area of skin hyperesthesia found in acute appendicitis.

Sherrington, Sir Charles Scott, English physiologist and Nobel laureate, 1857-1952.

Liddell-Sherrington reflex – see under Liddell

Schiff-Sherrington phenomenon – see under Schiff, Moritz

Sherrington law – every dorsal spinal nerve root supplies a particular area of the skin.

Sherrington phenomenon – after the muscles of the leg have been deprived of their motor innervation, stimulation of the sciatic nerve causes slow contraction of the muscles.

Shiga, Kiyoshi, Japanese bacteriologist, 1870-1957.

Shiga bacillus – *SYN: Shigella dysenteriae*

Shiga-Kruse bacillus – *SYN: Shigella dysenteriae*

Shigella – a genus of nonmotile, aerobic to facultatively anaerobic bacteria (family Enterobacteriaceae), all of whose species produce dysentery.

Shigella boydii – a species found in feces of symptomatic individuals.

Shigella dysenteriae – a species causing dysentery in humans and in monkeys. *SYN:* Shiga bacillus; Shiga-Kruse bacillus

Shigella flexneri – a species found in the feces of symptomatic individuals and of convalescents or carriers; the most common cause of dysentery epidemics and sometimes of infantile gastroenteritis. *SYN:* Flexner bacillus; paradysentery bacillus

NOTES

Shigella sonnei – a species causing mild dysentery and also summer diarrhea in children. *SYN:* Sonne bacillus

shigellosis – bacillary dysentery caused by bacteria of the genus *Shigella*.

Shiley, D.B., 20th century U.S. engineer.
Schneider-Shiley catheter
Shiley cardioplegia system
Shiley catheter
Shiley catheter distention system
Shiley cuffless fenestrated tube
Shiley cuffless tracheostomy tube
Shiley decannulation plug
Shiley distention kit
Shiley endotracheal tube
Shiley guiding catheter
Shiley heart valve
Shiley Infusaid pump
Shiley JL-4 guiding catheter
Shiley JR-4 guiding catheter
Shiley laryngectomy tube
Shiley low-pressure cuffed tracheostomy tube
Shiley MultiPro catheter
Shiley neonatal tracheostomy tube
Shiley oxygenator
Shiley pediatric tracheostomy tube
Shiley pressure-relief adapter
Shiley sump tube
Shiley tracheostomy tube
Shiley valve

Shipley, Walter C., U.S. psychiatrist, *1903.
Shipley-Hartford scale – a test of intellectual and conceptual aptitude.

Shirodkar, N.V., Indian obstetrician and gynecologist, 1900-1971.
Shirodkar needle
Shirodkar operation – a cerclage procedure done by pursestring suturing of an incompetent cervical os with a nonabsorbent suture material.
Shirodkar probe
Shirodkar suture

Shokeir, M.K.H.
Pena-Shokeir II syndrome – see under Pena

Shone, John D., 20th century English cardiologist.

Shone anomaly – coarctation of the aorta, subaortic stenosis, and stenosing ring of the left atrium found in association with a parachute mitral valve.

Shone complex – an obstructive lesion of the mitral valve complex, with left ventricular outflow obstruction and coarctation of the aorta.

Shone syndrome – the association of obstructive lesions of the mitral valve complex, with left ventricular outflow obstruction and coarctation of the aorta.

Shope, Richard E., U.S. pathologist, 1902-1966.

Shope fibroma – a connective tissue tumor of cottontail rabbits caused by a poxvirus of the genus *Leporipoxvirus.* *SYN:* rabbit fibroma

Shope fibroma virus – a poxvirus of the genus *Leporipoxvirus*, closely related to vaccinia and myxoma viruses, that causes Shope fibroma. *SYN:* rabbit fibroma virus

Shope papilloma – a papillomatous growth found in wild cottontail rabbits.

Shope papilloma virus – a papillomavirus infecting wild cottontail rabbits.

Short, D.S.

Short syndrome – alternating bradycardia tachycardia.

Shouldice, Edward Earl, Canadian surgeon, 1890-1965.

Shouldice repair – surgical repair of inguinal hernias using 4-layered imbricated repair of inguinal canal. *SYN:* Canadian repair

Shprintzen, Robert J., 20th century U.S. geneticist.

Shprintzen syndrome – *SYN:* velocardiofacial syndrome

Shrapnell, Henry J., English anatomist, 1761-1841.

Shrapnell membrane – triangular part of tympanic membrane between the malleolar folds. *SYN:* flaccid part of tympanic membrane

S

NOTES

Shulman, Lawrence Edward, U.S. rheumatologist, *1919.
  Shulman syndrome – induration and edema of the connective tissues of the extremities, usually appearing following exertion. _SYN:_ eosinophilic fasciitis

Shwachman, Harry, U.S. pediatrician, 1910-1986.
  Shwachman-Diamond syndrome – _SYN:_ Shwachman syndrome
  Shwachman syndrome – an autosomal recessive disorder characterized by sinusitis, bronchiectasis, pancreatic insufficiency, neutropenia, short stature, and skeletal changes, with radiographic findings of metaphyseal flaring of the long bones. _SYN:_ Shwachman-Diamond syndrome

Shwartzman, Gregory, Russian bacteriologist in U.S., 1896-1965.
  generalized Shwartzman phenomenon – death occurs in an animal that has been injected with a primary injection of endotoxin-containing filtrate and secondary injection given intravenously 24 hours apart.
    SYN: Sanarelli phenomenon; Sanarelli-Shwartzman phenomenon
  Sanarelli-Shwartzman phenomenon – _SYN:_ generalized Shwartzman phenomenon
  Shwartzman phenomenon – a rabbit injected intradermally with a small quantity of endotoxin followed by a second intravenous injection 24 hours later will develop a hemorrhagic and necrotic lesion at the site of the first injection. _SYN:_ Shwartzman reaction
  Shwartzman reaction – _SYN:_ Shwartzman phenomenon

Shy, George Milton, U.S. neurologist, 1919-1967.
  Shy-Drager syndrome – a progressive disorder involving the autonomic system, characterized by hypotension, external ophthalmoplegia, iris atrophy, incontinence, anhidrosis, impotence, tremor, and muscle wasting.
  Shy-Magee syndrome – progressive muscle disease that begins in the first year of life.

Sia, R.H.P., U.S. physician, 1895-1970.
  Sia test – for macroglobulins.

Siamese twins, named for Eng and Chang (1811-1874) who were born in Siam (now Thailand).

Sibson, Francis, English anatomist, 1814-1876.
  Sibson aortic vestibule – the anterosuperior portion of the left ventricle of the heart immediately below the aortic orifice. _SYN:_ aortic vestibule
  Sibson aponeurosis – _SYN:_ suprapleural membrane
  Sibson fascia – _SYN:_ suprapleural membrane

Sibson groove – a groove occasionally seen on the outer side of the thorax, formed by the prominent lower border of the pectoralis major muscle.

Sibson muscle – an occasional independent muscular fasciculus between the scalenus anterior and medius and having the same action and innervation. *SYN:* scalenus minimus muscle

Sicard, Jean Anasthase, French physician, 1872-1929.
Collet-Sicard syndrome – see under Collet

Sidbury, James B., U.S. pediatrician, *1922.
Sidbury syndrome – enzyme deficiency that causes decreased oxidation of butyric and *n*-hexanoic acids.

Siegert, Ferdinand, German pediatrician, 1865-1946.
Siegert sign – shortness and inward curvature of the terminal phalanges of the fifth fingers in Down syndrome.

Siegle, Emil, German otologist, 1833-1900.
Siegle otoscope – an ear speculum.

Siekert, Robert George, U.S. neurologist, *1924.
Millikan-Siekert syndrome – see under Millikan

Siemens, Hermann Werner, German dermatologist, 1891-1969.
Christ-Siemens-Touraine syndrome – see under Christ
Hallopeau-Siemens syndrome

Siemens, Sir William, English engineer, 1823-1883.
siemens (S) – the SI unit of electrical conductance.

Siemerling, Ernst, German physician, 1857-1931.
Siemerling nucleus – a subdivision of the oculomotor nucleus complex.

Sigault, Jean René, French obstetrician, *1740.
Sigault operation – enlarging the pelvic outlet by division of the symphysis pubis to facilitate childbirth. *SYN:* symphysiotomy

NOTES

Siggaard-Andersen, Ole, Danish clinical biochemist, *1932.
Siggaard-Andersen nomogram – used to predict acid-base composition of blood.

Signorelli, Angelo, Italian physician, 1876-1952.
Signorelli sign – tenderness on pressure in the glenoid fossa in front of the mastoid process in meningitis.

Silber, Robert H., U.S. biochemist, *1915.
Porter-Silber chromogens – see under Porter, Curt C.
Porter-Silber chromogens test – see under Porter, Curt C.
Porter-Silber reaction – see under Porter, Curt C.

Silfverskiöld, Nils G., Swedish orthopedist, 1888-1957.
Silfverskiöld syndrome – osteochondrodystrophy, with only slight vertebral changes but with shortened and curved long bones of the extremities.

Siltzbach, Louis, U.S. physician, 1906-1980.
Kveim-Siltzbach antigen – *SYN:* Kveim antigen

Silver, Henry K., U.S. pediatrician, *1918.
Russell-Silver dwarfism – *SYN:* Silver-Russell syndrome
Silver-Russell dwarfism – *SYN:* Silver-Russell syndrome
Silver-Russell syndrome – a disorder characterized by low birth weight, late closure of the anterior fontanel, bilateral bodily asymmetry, clinodactyly of the fifth fingers, triangular facies, and carp mouth. *SYN:* Russell-Silver dwarfism; Silver-Russell dwarfism

Silverman, Frederic Noah, U.S. pediatrician, *1914.
Silverman syndrome – *SYN:* Currarino-Silverman syndrome
Currarino-Silverman syndrome – see under Currarino

Silverman, Irving, U.S. surgeon, *1904.
Silverman needle – long, thin needle with central trocar and outer, hollow sheath used to obtain percutaneous liver biopsy specimens.

Silverman, Leslie, U.S. engineer, 1914-1966.
Silverman-Lilly pneumotachograph – measures flow in terms of the proportional pressure drop across a resistance consisting of a very fine mesh screen.

Silverman, William A., 20th century U.S. pediatrician.
Caffey-Silverman syndrome – *SYN:* Caffey syndrome
Silverman score

Silvester, Henry Robert, English physician, 1829-1908.
Silvester method – an artificial respiration technique.

Simmonds, Franklin Adin, English orthopedic surgeon.
Simmonds test – tests the Achilles tendon.

Simmonds, Morris, German physician, 1855-1925.
Simmonds disease – anterior pituitary insufficiency due to trauma, vascular lesions, or tumors. *SYN:* hypophysial cachexia; pituitary cachexia; Simmonds syndrome
Simmonds syndrome – *SYN:* Simmonds disease

Simmons, James S., U.S. bacteriologist, 1890-1954.
Simmons citrate medium – a diagnostic medium used in the differentiation of species of Enterobacteriaceae, based on their ability to utilize sodium citrate as the sole source of carbon.

Simon, Charles E., U.S. physician, 1866-1927.
Simon sign – the movements of the diaphragm that are dissociated from those of the thorax in incipient meningitis in children.

Simon, George, English radiologist.
Simon foci – calcified caseous nodules found at the apices of children with pulmonary tuberculosis.

Simon, Gustav, German surgeon, 1824-1876.
Simon incision
Simon perineorrhaphy
Simon position – for vaginal examination.
Simon speculum

Simon, Richard, 20th century U.S. oncologist.
Norton-Simon hypothesis – see under Norton, Larry

Simon, Théodore, French physician, 1873-1961.
Binet-Simon scale – see under Binet

S

NOTES

Simonart, Pierre J.C., Belgian obstetrician, 1817-1847.
   Simonart bands – weblike band of tissue partially filling the gap between the medial and lateral portions of a cleft lip.
   Simonart ligaments – *SYN:* Simonart threads
   Simonart threads – strands of amniotic tissue adherent to the embryo or fetus. *SYN:* amniotic bands; Simonart ligaments

Simons, Arthur, German physician, *1877.
   Barraquer-Simons disease – *SYN:* Barraquer disease
   Simons disease – *SYN:* Barraquer disease

Simpson, J.L., U.S. physician.
   Simpson syndrome – X-linked dysmorphia syndrome. *SYN:* bulldog syndrome

Simpson, Sir James Y., Scottish obstetrician, 1811-1870.
   Simpson forceps – obstetrical forceps.
   Simpson uterine sound – a slender flexible metal rod.

Sims, J. Marion, U.S. gynecologist, 1813-1883.
   Sims anoscope
   Sims cannula
   Sims curette
   Sims dilator
   Sims double-ended retractor
   Sims double-ended speculum
   Sims knife
   Sims needle
   Sims plug
   Sims position – facilitates vaginal examination. *SYN:* English position; lateral recumbent position; semiprone position
   Sims probe
   Sims proctoscope
   Sims retractor
   Sims scissors
   Sims sound
   Sims speculum
   Sims suction tip
   Sims suture
   Sims tenaculum
   Sims uterine sound – a slender flexible sound.
   Sims vaginal decompressor
   Sims vaginal speculum

Sindbis, village in Egypt where the fever was first observed in the 1950's.
   Sindbis fever – a febrile illness of humans in Africa, Australia, and other countries, caused by the Sindbis virus, and characterized by arthralgia, rash, and malaise.
   Sindbis virus – the type species of the genus Alphavirus, in the family *Togaviridae*.

Sinding-Larsen, Christian Magnus Falsen, Norwegian physician, 1866-1930.
   Sinding-Larsen-Johansson syndrome – apophysitis of the distal pole of the patella.

Singer, H.D., U.S. physician.
   Moschcowitz-Singer-Symmers syndrome – *SYN:* Moschcowitz syndrome

Singleton, Edward B., U.S. radiologist.
   Singleton-Merten syndrome – calcification of the aortic arch, with enlargement of the heart.

Sipple, John H., U.S. physician, *1930.
   Sipple syndrome – pheochromocytoma, medullary carcinoma of the thyroid, and neural tumors. *SYN:* multiple endocrine neoplasia, type 2

Sippy, Bertram W., U.S. physician, 1866-1924.
   Sippy diet – formerly used in the initial stages of treatment of peptic ulcer.

Siris, Evelyn, U.S. radiologist, 1914-1987.
   Coffin-Siris syndrome – see under Coffin

Sister Mary Joseph Dempsey, superintendent at Saint Mary's Hospital, Mayo Clinic, and surgical assistant to Dr. William Mayo, c. 1928, 1856-1929.
   Sister Joseph nodule – malignant intraabdominal neoplasm metastatic to the umbilicus. *SYN:* Sister Mary Joseph nodule
   Sister Mary Joseph nodule – *SYN:* Sister Joseph nodule

Sisto, Genaro, Argentinian pediatrician.
   Sisto sign – constant crying by infants with congenital syphilis.

NOTES

Sistrunk, Walter Ellis, U.S. surgeon, 1880-1933.
Sistrunk band retractor
Sistrunk dissecting scissors
Sistrunk double-ended retractor
Sistrunk operation – excision of the thyroglossal cyst and duct, including the midportion of the hyoid bone through or near which the duct traverses.
Sistrunk procedure
Sistrunk retractor
Sistrunk scissors

Siwe, Sture August, Swedish pediatrician, 1897-1966.
Abt-Letterer-Siwe syndrome – *SYN:* Letterer-Siwe disease
Letterer-Siwe disease – see under Letterer
Letterer-Siwe syndrome – *SYN:* Letterer-Siwe disease

Sjögren, Henrik Samuel Conrad, Swedish ophthalmologist, 1899-1986.
Gougerot-Sjögren disease – *SYN:* Sjögren syndrome
Sjögren disease – *SYN:* Sjögren syndrome
Sjögren syndrome – keratoconjunctivitis sicca, dryness of mucous membranes, telangiectasias or purpuric spots on the face, and bilateral parotid enlargement, seen in menopausal women. *SYN:* Gougerot-Sjögren disease; sicca syndrome; Sjögren disease

Sjögren, Karl Gustaf Torsten, Swedish physician, 1859-1939.
Marinesco-Sjögren-Garland syndrome – see under Marinesco
Marinesco-Sjögren syndrome – see under Marinesco
Sjögren-Larsson syndrome – congenital ichthyosis in association with oligophrenia and spastic paraplegia.
Sjögren syndrome – *SYN:* Marinesco-Sjögren syndrome
Torsten Sjögren syndrome – *SYN:* Marinesco-Sjögren-Garland syndrome
Torsten syndrome – *SYN:* Marinesco-Sjögren syndrome

Sjöqvist, O., Swedish neurosurgeon, 1901-1954.
Sjöqvist tractotomy – division of the descending fibers of the trigeminal tract in the medulla. *SYN:* trigeminal tractotomy

Skene, Alexander J.C., U.S. gynecologist, 1838-1900.
ducts of Skene glands – inconstant ducts along the side of the female urethra that convey the mucoid secretion of Skene glands to the vestibule. *SYN:* paraurethral ducts
Skene glands – numerous mucous glands in the wall of the female urethra. *SYN:* glands of the female urethra

Skene tubules – the embryonic urethral glands that are the female homologue of the prostate.

Skillern, Penn Gaskell, U.S. surgeon, *1882.
Skillern cannula
Skillern forceps
Skillern fracture – fracture of distal radius with greenstick fracture of neighboring portion of ulna.
Skillern phimosis forceps
Skillern probe
Skillern punch
Skillern sinus curette
Skillern sphenoid cannula
Skillern sphenoid probe

Skinner, Burrhus Frederic, U.S. psychologist, 1904-1990.
Skinner box – an experimental apparatus in which an animal presses a lever to obtain a reward or receive punishment.
skinnerian conditioning – an experimenter waits for the target response to be conditioned to occur spontaneously, immediately after which the organism is given a reinforcer reward. *SYN:* operant conditioning

Sklowsky, E.L., 20th century German physician.
Sklowsky symptom – the rupture of a varicella vesicle on very slight pressure with the finger.

Skoda, Joseph, Bohemian clinician in Vienna, 1805-1881.
Skoda crackles – bronchial sounds heard in pneumonia.
skodaic resonance – a peculiar, high-pitched sound, less musical than that obtained over a cavity, elicited by percussion just above the level of a pleuritic effusion. *SYN:* Skoda sign; Skoda tympany
Skoda rale – a rale in a bronchus, heard through an area of consolidated tissue in pneumonia.
Skoda sign – *SYN:* skodaic resonance
Skoda tympany – *SYN:* skodaic resonance

NOTES

Slater, Robert James, Canadian-U.S. pediatrician, *1923.
   Bearn-Kunkel-Slater syndrome – *SYN:* Bearn-Kunkel syndrome

Slocumb, Charles Henry, U.S. physician, *1905.
   Slocumb syndrome – *SYN:* Perkoff syndrome

Sluder, Greenfield, U.S. laryngologist, 1865-1928.
   Sluder guillotine tonsillectomy

Sluder, Greenfield.
   Sluder neuralgia – *SYN:* sphenopalatine neuralgia

Sly, William S., U.S. pediatrician, *1932.
   Sly syndrome – beta-glucuronidase deficiency that causes short stature
      with hepatosplenomegaly and frequent pulmonary infections; may also
      cause slow development, coarse facies, and clouded corneas. *SYN:* type
      VII mucopolysaccharidosis

Slyke, Donald D. Van, see under Van Slyke

Smellie, William, English obstetrician, 1697-1763.
   Smellie scissors – obsolete term for lance-pointed shears with external
      cutting edges, used for fetal craniotomy.

Smith, (origin unknown).
   Smith-Boyde operation – see under Boyce, William H.

Smith, Allan J., 20th century English physician.
   Smith-Strang disease – autosomal recessive disease with onset of loss of
      response to stimuli, mental deterioration, edema, and white hair shortly
      after birth. *SYN:* methionine malabsorption syndrome; oasthouse urine
      disease

Smith, Ann C.M., 20th century U.S. genetics counselor.
   Smith-Magenis syndrome – a rare form of mental retardation.

Smith, David W., U.S. pediatrician, 1926-1981.
   Marshall-Smith syndrome – *SYN:* Marshall syndrome
   Mulvihill-Smith syndrome – see under Mulvihill
   Smith-Lemli-Opitz syndrome – mental retardation, small stature,
      anteverted nostrils, ptosis, male genital anomalies, and syndactyly of the
      second and third toes.

Smith, Eustace, English physician, 1835-1914.
   Eustace Smith sign – *SYN:* Smith sign
   Smith sign – indicates presence of enlarged bronchial glands if murmur
      can be auscultated over manubrium when patient's neck is in full
      extension. *SYN:* Eustace Smith sign

Smith, G.W., U.S. neurosurgeon, 1917-1964.
  Smith aneurysmal clip
  Smith-Robinson anterior approach
  Smith-Robinson anterior cervical discectomy
  Smith-Robinson anterior fusion
  Smith-Robinson cervical fusion
  Smith-Robinson interbody arthrodesis
  Smith-Robinson interbody fusion
  Smith-Robinson operation – interbody spinal fusion through an anterior
    cervical approach.
  Smith-Robinson technique

Smith, Hamilton Othanel, joint winner of 1978 Nobel Prize for work related to
restriction enzymes.

Smith, Henry, Irish-born English military surgeon in India, 1862-1948.
  Smith cataract extraction
  Smith cataract knife
  Smith eye speculum
  Smith hook
  Smith-Indian operation – a surgical technique for removal of cataract
    within the capsule. *SYN:* Smith operation
  Smith intraocular implant lens
  Smith-Leiske cross-action intraocular lens forceps
  Smith lens
  Smith lens expressor
  Smith lid expressor
  Smith lid retracting hook
  Smith operation – *SYN:* Smith-Indian operation
  Smith orbital floor implant

Smith, John Ferguson, see under Ferguson Smith, John

Smith, Lucian A.
  Achor-Smith syndrome – see under Achor

Smith, M.J.V., 20th century U.S. urologist.
  Smith pessary

Smith, Robert William, Irish surgeon, 1807-1873.
  Smith fracture – fracture of the radius near its lower articular surface, with displacement of the fragment toward the volar aspect.

Smith, Sir Thomas, English orthopedic surgeon, 1833-1909.
  Tom Smith arthritis – septic arthritic condition that occurs in infancy.

Smith, Theobald, U.S. pathologist, 1859-1934.
  Theobald Smith phenomenon – guinea pigs that had survived use for diphtheria antitoxin standardization were highly susceptible to subsequent inoculation of horse serum.

Smith, William R., 20th century U.S. physician.
  Smith-Riley syndrome – multiple hemangiomas, macrocephaly, and blurred optic disks.

Smith-Petersen, Marius N., U.S. surgeon, 1886-1953.
  Smith ankle prosthesis
  Smith bone clamp
  Smith clamp
  Smith dislocation
  Smith drill
  Smith flexor pollicis longus abductor plasty
  Smith fracture
  Smith-Petersen acromioplasty
  Smith-Petersen approach
  Smith-Petersen cannulated nail
  Smith-Petersen capsule retractor
  Smith-Petersen cervical fusion
  Smith-Petersen chisel
  Smith-Petersen cup
  Smith-Petersen cup arthroplasty
  Smith-Petersen curved gouge
  Smith-Petersen curved osteotome
  Smith-Petersen fracture pin
  Smith-Petersen hammer
  Smith-Petersen hemiarthroplasty
  Smith-Petersen hip cup prosthesis
  Smith-Petersen incision
  Smith-Petersen laminectomy rongeur
  Smith-Petersen mallet

Smith-Petersen nail – a flanged nail for pinning a fracture of the neck of the femur.

Smith-Petersen nail with Lloyd adapter

Smith-Petersen osteotome

Smith-Petersen osteotomy

Smith-Petersen pin

Smith-Petersen plate

Smith-Petersen prosthesis

Smith-Petersen reamer

Smith-Petersen rongeur

Smith-Petersen sacroiliac joint fusion

Smith-Petersen spatula

Smith-Petersen straight gouge

Smith-Petersen straight osteotome

Smith-Petersen synovectomy

Smith-Petersen technique

Smith-Petersen transarticular nail

Smith-Petersen tucker

Smith physical capacities evaluation

Smith prosthesis

Smith scissors

Smith STA-peg

Smith technique

Sneddon, Ian Bruce, English dermatologist, 1923-1987.

Sneddon syndrome – a cerebral arteriopathy of unknown etiology, characterized by noninflammatory intimal hyperplasia of medium-size vessels.

Sneddon-Wilkinson disease – a chronic pruritic anular eruption of sterile vesicles and pustules beneath the stratum corneum. *SYN:* subcorneal pustular dermatosis

Snell, George Davis, 1903-1996, joint winner of 1980 Nobel Prize for work related to cell structures and regulation of immunological reactions.

Snell, Simeon, English ophthalmologist, 1851-1909.

> **Snell law** – for two given media, the sine of the angle of incidence bears a constant relation to the sine of the angle of refraction. *SYN:* law of refraction

Snellen, Hermann, Dutch ophthalmologist, 1834-1908.

> **Snellen chart** – used to test visual acuity.
> **Snellen conventional reform implant**
> **Snellen entropion forceps**
> **Snellen eye implant**
> **Snellen letters**
> **Snellen operation**
> **Snellen reform eye**
> **Snellen sign** – bruit heard on auscultation over the eye in a patient with Graves disease.
> **Snellen soft contact lens**
> **Snellen suture**
> **Snellen test types** – square black symbols employed in testing the acuity of distant vision.
> **Snellen vectis**

Snodgrass, Warren, late 20th century U.S. physician.

> **Snodgrass procedure** – tubularization of the incised urethral plate.

Snyder, Marshall L., U.S. microbiologist, 1907-1969.

> **Snyder test** – a colorimetric test for determining dental caries activity or susceptibility. *SYN:* colorimetric caries susceptibility test

Soave, F., 20th century Italian pediatric surgeon.

> **Soave operation** – endorectal pull-through for treatment of congenital megacolon.

Soderbergh, G., Swedish physician, *1878.

> **Soderbergh pressure reflex** – seen in pyramidal tract lesions that is brought on by firm downward stroking of the ulna.

Soemmerring, Samuel Thomas von, German anatomist, 1755-1830.

> **ring of Soemmerring** – a mass of lenticular fibers enclosed between the anterior and posterior portion of the lenticular capsule, leaving the pupillary area relatively free.

Soemmerring ganglion – a large cell mass extending forward over the dorsal surface of the crus cerebri from the rostral border of the pons into the subthalamic region. *SYN:* substantia nigra

Soemmerring ligament – small fibers attaching the lacrimal gland to the periorbita.

Soemmerring muscle – a fasciculus occasionally passing from the thyrohyoid muscle to the isthmus of the thyroid gland. *SYN:* levator muscle of thyroid gland

Soemmerring spot – an oval area of the sensory retina at the center of which is the central fovea, which contains only retinal cones. *SYN:* macula retinae

Soffer, Louis J., U.S. internist, *1904.
   Sohval-Soffer syndrome – see under Sohval

Sohval, Arthur R., U.S. internist, 1904-1985.
   Sohval-Soffer syndrome – hypogonadism, gynecomastia, skeletal anomalies, and mental retardation, without chromosomal abnormality.

Solente, G., 20th century French physician.
   Touraine-Solente-Golé syndrome – see under Touraine

Somogyi, Michael, U.S. biochemist, 1883-1971.
   Somogyi effect – in diabetes, a rebound phenomenon of reactive hyperglycemia in response to a preceding period of relative hypoglycemia.
   Somogyi method
   Somogyi unit – a measure of the level of activity of amylase in blood serum.

Sondermann, R., 20th century German ophthalmologist.
   Sondermann canal – a blind outpouching of Schlemm canal, extending toward the anterior chamber of the eye.

Sonne, Carl, Danish bacteriologist, 1882-1948.
   Sonne bacillus – *SYN: Shigella sonnei*

NOTES

Sonne dysentery – dysentery due to infection by *Shigella sonnei.*

Sörensen, Sören P.L., Danish chemist, 1868-1939.
    Sörensen scale – the negative logarithm of the hydrogen ion concentration, used as a scale for expressing acidity and alkalinity. *SYN:* pH scale

Soret, Charles, French radiologist, 1854-1931.
    Soret band – the absorption band of all porphyrins at about 400 nm.
    Soret phenomenon – in a solution kept in a long, upright tube at room temperature, the upper part being the warmer, is also the more concentrated.

Sorsby, Arnold, English ophthalmologist, 1900-1980.
    Sorsby macular degeneration – hereditary macular degeneration that occurs during the fifth decade of life. *SYN:* familial pseudoinflammatory macular degeneration
    Sorsby syndrome – congenital macular coloboma and apical dystrophy of the extremities.

Sotos, Juan F., U.S. pediatrician, *1927.
    Sotos syndrome – cerebral gigantism and generalized large muscles in childhood, with mental retardation and defective coordination.

Sottas, Jules, French neurologist, 1866-1943.
    Dejerine-Sottas disease – see under Dejerine
    Dejerine-Sottas neuropathy – *SYN:* Dejerine-Sottas disease

Soulier, Jean Pierre, French hematologist, 1915-1985.
    Bernard-Soulier syndrome – see under Bernard, Jean

Souques, Alexandre Achille, French neurologist, 1860-1944.
    Souques phenomenon – *SYN:* Souques sign
    Souques sign – lack of leg extension when patient sitting in chair is quickly pushed over backward; seen in advanced striatal dysfunction. *SYN:* Souques phenomenon

Southern, M.E., 20th century English biologist.
    Southern blot analysis – a procedure to separate and identify DNA sequences.

Southey, Reginald, English physician, 1835-1899.
    Southey tubes – obsolete cannulas of small caliber thrust by a trocar into the subcutaneous tissues to drain the fluid of anasarca.

Souttar, Sir Henry Sessions, English surgeon, 1875-1964.
    Souttar tube

Souttar valvotomy – pioneer procedure in heart surgery.

Spalding, Alfred Baker, U.S. obstetrician and gynecologist, 1874-1942.
  Spalding sign – indication of fetal death in utero if bones of skull are seen to be overriding each other on radiography.

Spallanzani, Lazaro, Italian priest and scientist, 1729-1799.
  Spallanzani law – the younger the individual, the greater is the regenerative power of its cells.

Spatz, Hugo, German neurologist and psychiatrist, 1888-1969.
  Hallervorden-Spatz disease – *SYN:* Hallervorden-Spatz syndrome
  Hallervorden-Spatz syndrome – see under Hallervorden

Spearman, Charles Edward, English psychologist, 1863-1945.
  Spearman correlation coefficient – statistical measure used to assess significance of differences between groups.

Spee, Ferdinand Graf von, German embryologist, 1855-1937.
  curve of Spee – the anatomic curvature of the mandibular occlusal plane. *SYN:* von Spee curve
  Spee embryo
  von Spee curve – *SYN:* curve of Spee

Spencer Wells, Sir Thomas, English surgeon, 1818-1897.
  Spencer Wells forceps

Spengler, Carl, Swiss physician, 1861-1937.
  Spengler fragments – tuberculous sputum that contains small discoid bodies.

Spens, Thomas, Scottish physician, 1764-1842.
  Spens syndrome – *SYN:* Adams-Stokes syndrome

Sperry, Roger Wolcott, U.S. researcher, 1913-1994, winner of 1981 Nobel Prize for medicine and physiology.

S

Spiegelberg, Otto, German gynecologist, 1830-1881.
  Spiegelberg criteria – for differentiating ovarian from other ectopic pregnancies.

Spieghel, var. of Spigelius

Spiegler, Eduard, Austrian dermatologist, 1860-1908.
  Ancell-Spiegler cylindroma – *SYN:* Brooke disease (1)
  Ancell-Spiegler syndrome – *SYN:* Brooke disease (1)
  Spiegler-Fendt pseudolymphoma – a soft red to violaceous skin nodule often involving the head, caused by dense infiltration of the dermis by lymphocytes and histiocytes. *SYN:* benign lymphocytoma cutis; Spiegler-Fendt sarcoid
  Spiegler-Fendt sarcoid – *SYN:* Spiegler-Fendt pseudolymphoma

Spielmeyer, Walter, German neurologist, 1879-1935.
  Spielmeyer acute swelling – a form of degeneration of nerve cells in which the cell body and its processes swell and stain palely and diffusely.
  Spielmeyer-Stock disease – *SYN:* Batten disease
  Spielmeyer-Vogt disease – *SYN:* Batten disease
  Vogt-Spielmeyer disease – *SYN:* Batten disease

Spigelius, Adrian (van der Spieghel), Flemish anatomist in Padua, 1578-1625.
  spigelian hernia – abdominal hernia through the semilunar line.
    SYN: lateral ventral hernia
  Spigelius line – the slight groove in the external abdominal wall parallel to the lateral edge of the rectus sheath. *SYN:* linea semilunaris
  Spigelius lobe – a small lobe of the liver situated posteriorly between the sulcus for the vena cava and the fissure for the ligamentum venosum. *SYN:* lobus caudatus

Spiller, William G., U.S. neurologist, 1864-1940.
  Frazier-Spiller operation – see under Frazier

Spinelli, Pier G., Italian gynecologist, 1862-1929.
  Spinelli operation – an operation splitting the anterior wall of the prolapsed uterus and reversing the organ preliminary to reduction.

Spitz, Sophie, U.S. pathologist, 1910-1956.
  Spitz nevus – a benign, slightly pigmented or red superficial small skin tumor. *SYN:* epithelioid cell nevus; spindle cell nevus

Spitzer, Alexander, Austrian anatomist, 1868-1943.
   Spitzer theory – an interpretation of the partitioning of the heart of
      mammalian embryos, primarily on the basis of recapitulations of the
      adult structural pattern of lower forms.

Spitzka, Edward C., U.S. neurologist, 1852-1914.
   column of Spitzka-Lissauer – *SYN:* Spitzka marginal tract
   Spitzka marginal tract – a longitudinal bundle of thin, unmyelinated and
      poorly myelinated fibers capping the apex of the posterior horn of the
      spinal gray matter. *SYN:* column of Spitzka-Lissauer; dorsolateral
      fasciculus; Spitzka marginal zone
   Spitzka marginal zone – *SYN:* Spitzka marginal tract
   Spitzka nucleus – *SYN:* Perlia nucleus

Spitzy, Hans, Austrian orthopedic surgeon, 1872-1956.
   Spitzy button – a device used in correction of postural defect. *SYN:* Spitzy
      spike
   Spitzy spike – *SYN:* Spitzy button

Spix, Johann B., German anatomist, 1781-1826.
   Spix spine – a pointed tongue of bone overlapping the mandibular
      foramen, giving attachment to the sphenomandibular ligament.
      SYN: lingula of mandible

Splendore, Alfonso, Brazilian physician, 1871-1953.
   Lutz-Splendore-Almeida disease – see under Lutz
   Splendore-Hoeppli phenomenon – radiating or anular eosinophilic
      deposits of host-derived materials and possibly of parasite antigens,
      which form around fungi, helminths, or bacterial colonies in tissue.

Spooner, William A., clergyman in Church of England, 1844-1930.
   spoonerism – misuse or inappropriate word usage, or transposition of
      syllables.

Spranger, Jurgen W., German physician.
   Maroteaux-Spranger-Wiedemann syndrome – see under Maroteaux

NOTES

Sprengel, Otto G.K., German surgeon, 1852-1915.
Sprengel anomaly
Sprengel deformity – *SYN:* Sprengel shoulder
Sprengel shoulder – congenital elevation of the scapula. *SYN:* Sprengel deformity; Sprengel syndrome
Sprengel syndrome – *SYN:* Sprengel shoulder

Sprinz, Helmuth, German-born U.S. pathologist, *1911.
Sprinz-Dubin syndrome – *SYN:* Dubin-Johnson syndrome
Sprinz-Nelson syndrome – *SYN:* Dubin-Johnson syndrome

Spurway, John, 19th century English physician.
Spurway syndrome – osteogenesis imperfecta.

Squire, Truman Hoffman, U.S. surgeon, 1823-1899.
Squire catheter
Squire sign

Ssabanejew, Ivan, 19th century Russian surgeon.
Ssabanejew-Frank operation – a method of performing gastrostomy.

Stader, Otto, U.S. veterinary surgeon, *1894.
Stader pin
Stader pin guide
Stader splint – a splint used primarily in veterinary medicine.

Staderini, Rutilio, 19th century Italian neuroanatomist.
Staderini nucleus – a small collection of nerve cells in the medulla oblongata lying lateral to the hypoglossal nucleus. *SYN:* intercalated nucleus

Stafne, Edward C., U.S. oral pathologist, 1894-1981.
Stafne bone cyst – an indentation on the lingual surface of the mandible within which lies a portion of the submandibular gland. *SYN:* lingual salivary gland depression

St. Agatha, patron saint of those with breast disease, torture victims, nurses, and jewelers.
St. Agatha disease – disease of the female breast.

Stahl, Friedrich K., German physician, 1811-1873.
Stahl ear – a deformed external ear regarded as a stigma of degenerate constitution.

Stähli, Jean, Swiss ophthalmologist, *1890.
Hudson-Stähli line – see under Hudson

Stahr, Hermann, German anatomist and pathologist, 1868-1947.
   Stahr gland – lymph node located next to facial artery.

Stainton, C.W., U.S. dentist.
   Stainton-Capdepont syndrome – *SYN:* Capdepont syndrome

Stamey, Thomas A., U.S. surgeon.
   Stamey test – test used to detect unilateral renal disease.

Stamey, Thomas Alexander, U.S. urologist, *1928.
   Stamey needle
   Stamey procedure – retropubic urethropexy using needle suspension in
      stress incontinence.
   Stamey test – measure of unilateral urine volume and *para*-
      aminohippurate concentration when assessing kidney.

Stanford, American University where the test was revised for use in the U.S.
   Stanford-Binet intelligence scale – a standardized test for the
      measurement of intelligence. *SYN:* Binet test

Stanger, J., German tanner.
   Stanger bath – a hydrogalvanic bath.

Stanley, Edward, English surgeon, 1793-1862.
   Stanley cervical ligaments – fibers of the capsule of the hip joint reflected
      onto the neck of the femur.

Stanley Way, see under Way, Stanley

Stannius, Herman F., German biologist, 1808-1883.
   Stannius ligature

St. Anthony the Abbot, patron saint of domestic animals, gravediggers,
and hermits.
   St. Anthony fire – any of several inflammations or gangrenous skin
      conditions. *SYN:* ergotism; Milian sign

Stargardt, Karl Bruno, German ophthalmologist, 1875-1927.

NOTES

Stargardt disease – juvenile macular degeneration. *SYN:* Stargardt syndrome

Stargardt syndrome – *SYN:* Stargardt disease

Starling, Ernest Henry, English physiologist, 1866-1927.

Frank-Starling curve – *SYN:* Starling curve

Starling curve – a graph in which cardiac output or stroke volume is plotted against mean atrial or ventricular end-diastolic pressure. *SYN:* Frank-Starling curve

Starling equilibrium

Starling hypothesis

Starling law of the heart – the energy liberated by the heart when it contracts is a function of the length of its muscle fibers at the end of diastole. *SYN:* law of the heart

Starling law of the intestine – food causes a band of constriction proximally and relaxation distally, resulting in a peristaltic wave.

Starling reflex – tapping the volar surfaces of the fingers causes flexion.

Starr, Albert, U.S. physician, *1926.

Starr ball heart prosthesis

Starr ball heart valve

Starr-Edwards aortic valve prosthesis

Starr-Edwards ball valve prosthesis

Starr-Edwards ball-cage valve

Starr-Edwards disk valve prosthesis

Starr-Edwards heart valve

Starr-Edwards mitral prosthesis

Starr-Edwards pacemaker

Starr-Edwards prosthesis

Starr-Edwards prosthetic aortic valve

Starr-Edwards prosthetic mitral valve

Starr-Edwards Silastic valve

Starr-Edwards silicone rubber ball valve

Starr-Edwards valve – a cage and ball artificial cardiac valve with high reliability and durability, first used to replace the mitral valve. *SYN:* Starr valve

Starr fixation forceps

Starr forceps

Starr valve – *SYN:* Starr-Edwards valve

Stas, Jean-Servais, Belgian chemist, 1813-1891.
  Stas-Otto method – used for extraction of alkaloids from plants and animal bodies.

Staub, Hans, Swiss internist, 1890-1967.
  Staub-Traugott effect – in normal persons, a drop in blood glucose which follows a second oral dose of glucose given 30 minutes or so after the first. *SYN:* Staub-Traugott phenomenon
  Staub-Traugott phenomenon – *SYN:* Staub-Traugott effect

Stauffer, Maurice H., 20th century U.S. gastroenterologist.
  Stauffer syndrome – elevation of liver function tests, in the absence of metastatic disease, due to cholestasis in renal cell cancer patients. *SYN:* Grawitz tumor

St. Clair of Assisi, patron saint of eyes, television, telegraph, and telephone.
  St. Clair forceps

Stearns, A. Warren, U.S. physician, 1885-1959.
  Stearns alcoholic amentia – a temporary alcoholic mental disorder resembling delirium tremens but lasting for a longer time and showing a greater degree of amnesia and other mental defects.

Stearns, Genevieve, U.S. physician.
  Boyd-Stearns syndrome – see under Boyd

Steele, John C., Canadian neurologist, d. 1968.
  Steele-Richardson-Olszewski disease – *SYN:* Steele-Richardson-Olszewski syndrome
  Steele-Richardson-Olszewski syndrome – a progressive neurologic disorder characterized by a supranuclear paralysis of vertical gaze, retraction of eyelids, exophoria under cover, dysarthria, and dementia. *SYN:* progressive supranuclear palsy; Steele-Richardson-Olszewski disease

S

Steell, Graham, English physician, 1851-1942.
  Graham Steell murmur – an early diastolic murmur of pulmonic insufficiency secondary to pulmonary hypertension. *SYN:* Steell murmur
  Steell murmur – *SYN:* Graham Steell murmur

Steenbock, Harry, U.S. physiologist and chemist, 1886-1967.
  Steenbock unit – a unit of vitamin D.

Steidele, Raphael J., 18th century Austrian physician.
  Steidele complex – *SYN:* Steidele syndrome
  Steidele syndrome – absence of the aortic arch. *SYN:* Steidele complex

Stein, Irving Freiler, Sr., U.S. gynecologist, *1887.
  Stein-Leventhal syndrome – a condition commonly characterized by hirsutism, obesity, menstrual abnormalities, infertility, and enlarged ovaries. *SYN:* polycystic ovary syndrome

Stein, Stanislav A.F. von, Russian otologist, *1855.
  Stein test – in cases of labyrinthine disease the patient is unable to stand or to hop on one foot with his/her eyes shut.

Steinberg, I.
  Steinberg thumb sign – in Marfan syndrome, when the thumb is held across the palm of the same hand it projects well beyond the ulnar surface of the hand.

Steinbrinck, W., 20th century German physician.
  Chédiak-Steinbrinck-Higashi anomaly – *SYN:* Chédiak-Steinbrinck-Higashi syndrome
  Chédiak-Steinbrinck-Higashi syndrome – see under Chédiak

Steindler, Arthur, U.S. orthopedic surgeon, 1878-1959.
  Steindler arthrodesis
  Steindler effect
  Steindler elbow arthrodesis
  Steindler flexorplasty
  Steindler matrixectomy
  Steindler operation
  Steindler procedure
  Steindler release
  Steindler stripping
  Steindler technique
  Steindler wrist fusion

Steiner, L., German physician.
  Steiner tumor – *SYN:* auricular tumor

Steinert, (Steinhert), Hans, German physician, *1875.
    Curschmann-Batten-Steinert syndrome – see under Curschmann
    Steinert disease – a chronic, slowly progressing disease marked by atrophy of the muscles, failing vision, lenticular opacities, ptosis, slurred speech, and general muscular weakness. *SYN:* myotonic dystrophy
    Steinert myotonic dystrophy
    Steinert syndrome

Steinhert, var. of Steinert

Steinmann, Fritz, Swiss surgeon, 1872-1932.
    Steinmann calibrated pin
    Steinmann extension
    Steinmann fixation pin
    Steinmann holder
    Steinmann nail
    Steinmann pin – used to transfix bone for traction or fixation.
    Steinmann pin chuck
    Steinmann pin fixation
    Steinmann pin with ball bearing
    Steinmann pin with Crowe pilot point
    Steinmann pin with pin chuck
    Steinmann test
    Steinmann traction
    Steinmann tractor

Stellwag, Carl von Carion, Austrian ophthalmologist, 1823-1904.
    Stellwag sign – infrequent and incomplete blinking in Graves disease.

Stender, Wilhelm P., 19th century German manufacturer of scientific apparatus.
    Stender dish – a flat shallow vessel used in staining sections.

Stensen, Niels, Danish anatomist, 1638-1686.
    Stensen canal
    Stensen duct – *SYN:* parotid duct

NOTES

Stensen experiment – an experiment on an animal in which the blood supply is cut off from the lumbar region of the spine.
Stensen foramen – *SYN:* incisive foramen
Stensen plexus – the parotid duct's venous structure.
Stensen veins – *SYN:* vortex veins

Stent, Charles R, English dentist, 1845-1901.
Stent graft – an inlay skin graft, or a skin graft held in place by a tie-over dressing.

Stern, Heinrich, U.S. physician, 1868-1918.
Stern posture – supine position, with the head extended and lowered over the end of the table.

Sternberg, George M., U.S. bacteriologist, 1838-1915.
Reed-Sternberg cells – see under Reed, Dorothy
Sternberg cells – *SYN:* Reed-Sternberg cells
Sternberg-Reed cells – *SYN:* Reed-Sternberg cells

Sternberg, Karl, Austrian pathologist, 1872-1935.
Sternberg lymphoma – mediastinal mass that resembles acute lymphatic leukosarcoma. *SYN:* Sternberg syndrome
Sternberg syndrome – *SYN:* Sternberg lymphoma

Stevens, Albert Mason, U.S. pediatrician, 1884-1945.
Stevens-Johnson syndrome – a bullous form of erythema multiforme. *SYN:* Baader dermatostomatitis; ectodermosis erosiva pluriorificialis; erythema multiforme bullosum; erythema multiforme exudativum; erythema multiforme major

Stevens, Stanley Smith, U.S. psychophysicist, 1906-1973.
Stevens power law – a logarithm used in psychology/psychiatry.

Stewart, Fred Waldorf, U.S. physician, 1894-1991.
Stewart-Treves syndrome – angiosarcoma arising in arms, affected by postmastectomy lymphedema.

Stewart, George N., Canadian-U.S. scientist, 1860-1930.
Hamilton-Stewart formula – *SYN:* Stewart-Hamilton method
Hamilton-Stewart method – *SYN:* Stewart-Hamilton method
Stewart test – estimation of the amount of collateral circulation in case of an aneurysm of the main artery of a limb.
Stewart-Hamilton method – a method for measuring cardiac output. *SYN:* Hamilton-Stewart formula; Hamilton-Stewart method; indicator dilution method

Stewart, R.M., 20th century English neurologist.
    Stewart-Morel syndrome – *SYN:* Morgagni syndrome

Stewart, Sir James Purves, English physician, 1869-1949.
    Stewart granuloma – *SYN:* Wegener granulomatosis

Stewart, Thomas Grainger, English neurologist, 1877-1957.
    Stewart-Holmes sign – in cerebellar disease, the inability to check a
        movement when passive resistance is suddenly released. *SYN:* rebound
        phenomenon

St. Giles, patron saint of lepers, physically challenged people, paupers, and
blacksmiths.
    St. Giles disease – *SYN:* leprosy

St. Helenia's Island, site where first cases were observed.
    St. Helenia cellulitis syndrome – intense burning in legs, headache and
        rigor accompany.

Sticker, Georg, German physician, 1860-1960.
    Sticker disease – a mild infectious exanthema of childhood caused by
        Parvovirus B19. *SYN:* erythema infectiosum

Stickler, Gunnar B., U.S. pediatrician, *1925.
    Stickler syndrome – *SYN:* hereditary progressive arthroophthalmopathy

Stieda, Alfred, German surgeon, 1869-1945.
    Pellegrini-Stieda disease – *SYN:* Pellegrini disease
    Stieda disease
    Stieda fracture

Stieda, Ludwig, German anatomist, 1837-1918.
    Stieda process – a projection of the talus bearing medial and lateral
        tubercles. *SYN:* posterior process of talus

Stierlin, Eduard, German surgeon, 1878-1919.
    Stierlin sign – repeated emptying of the cecum seen radiographically.

NOTES

Stiles, Walter S., English physicist, 1901-1985.

Stiles-Crawford effect – light that enters through the center of the pupil produces a greater visual effect than light that enters obliquely.

Still, Sir George F., English physician, 1868-1941.

Still-Chauffard syndrome – *SYN:* Chauffard syndrome

Still disease – a form of juvenile chronic arthritis.

Still murmur – an innocent musical murmur.

Stiller, Berthod, Hungarian physician, 1837-1922.

Stiller rib – *SYN:* Stiller sign

Stiller sign – floating tenth rib. *SYN:* costal stigma; Stiller rib

Stilling, Benedict, German anatomist, 1810-1879.

Stilling canal – a minute canal running through the vitreous from the discus nervi optici to the lens. *SYN:* hyaloid canal

Stilling column – *SYN:* Stilling nucleus

Stilling gelatinous substance – the central gray matter of the spinal cord surrounding the central canal. *SYN:* central and lateral intermediate substance

Stilling nucleus – a column of large neurons located in the base of the posterior gray column of the spinal cord, extending from the first thoracic through the second lumbar segment. *SYN:* Stilling column; thoracic nucleus

Stilling raphe – the transverse interdigitations of fiber bundles across the anterior median fissure of the medulla oblongata at the decussation of the pyramidal tracts.

Stilling, Jakob, German ophthalmologist, 1842-1915.

Stilling color table – *SYN:* Reuss color table

Stilling test – used in ophthalmology.

Stimson, Lewis A., U.S. surgeon, 1844-1917.

Stimson technique – method to reduce anterior dislocation of humerus at shoulder.

Stirling, William, English histologist and physiologist, 1851-1932.

Stirling modification of Gram stain – a stable aniline-crystal violet stain.

St. Jude, patron saint of desperate situations and hospitals.

St. Jude bileaflet prosthetic valve

St. Jude composite valve graft

St. Jude mitral valve prosthesis

St. Jude valve

St. Louis, city in Missouri, where the disease was first observed in 1933.
  St. Louis encephalitis – *SYN:* St. Louis syndrome
  St. Louis syndrome – encephalitis. *SYN:* St. Louis encephalitis

St. Luke, patron saint of physicians, surgeons, artists, sculptors, painters, notaries, glass workers, butchers, and brewers.
  St. Luke retractor
  St. Luke rongeuer

St. Mark, patron saint of notaries, Egypt, and Venice, Italy.
  St. Mark clamp
  St. Mark excision
  St. Mark incision

Stock, Wolfgang, German ophthalmologist, 1874-1956.
  Spielmeyer-Stock disease – see under Spielmeyer
  Stock eye trephine
  Stock operation

Stocker, Frederick William, U.S. ophthalmologist, 1893-1974.
  Stocker cyclodiathermy needle
  Stocker line – a fine line of pigment in the corneal epithelium near the head of a pterygium.
  Stocker operation

Stockholm, city in Sweden where the syndrome was first reported in 1973.
  Stockholm syndrome – emotional involvement that occurs between hostage and perpetrator.

Stoerk, Karl, Austrian laryngologist, 1832-1899.
  Stoerk blennorrhea – chronic catarrh of the upper air passages with hypertrophy of the mucous membrane and submucosa.

Stoffel, Adolf, German orthopedic surgeon, 1880-1937.
  Stoffel operation – division of certain motor nerves for the relief of spastic paralysis.

S

NOTES

Stokes, Sir George Gabriel, English physicist and mathematician, 1819-1903.

 stoke – unit of kinematic viscosity.

 Stokes law – relationship of the rate of fall of a small sphere in a viscous fluid.

 Stokes lens – used to diagnose astigmatism.

Stokes, Sir William, Irish surgeon, 1839-1900.

 Gritti-Stokes amputation – see under Gritti

 Stokes amputation – modification of the Gritti-Stokes amputation so that the line of section of the femur is slightly higher.

Stokes, William, Irish physician, 1804-1878.

 Adams-Stokes disease – *SYN:* Adams-Stokes syndrome

 Adams-Stokes syncope – see under Adams, Robert

 Adams-Stokes syndrome – see under Adams, Robert

 Cheyne-Stokes breathing – *SYN:* Cheyne-Stokes respiration

 Cheyne-Stokes psychosis – see under Cheyne

 Cheyne-Stokes respiration – see under Cheyne

 Morgagni-Adams-Stokes syndrome – *SYN:* Adams-Stokes syndrome

 Stokes-Adams disease – *SYN:* Adams-Stokes syndrome

 Stokes-Adams syndrome – *SYN:* Adams-Stokes syndrome

 Stokes law – a muscle lying above an inflamed mucous or serous membrane is frequently the seat of paralysis.

Stokvis, Barend J.E., Dutch physician and physiologist, 1834-1902.

 Stokvis disease – *SYN:* enterogenous cyanosis

Stookey, Byron, U.S. neurosurgeon, 1887-1966.

 Queckenstedt-Stookey test – see under Queckenstedt

 Stookey cranial rongeur

 Stookey reflex

 Stookey retractor

 Stookey-Scarff operation – establishes an opening from the third ventricle to the prechiasmal and interpeduncular cisterns. *SYN:* third ventriculostomy

Storm van Leeuwen, William, Dutch pharmacologist, 1882-1933.

 Storm van Leeuwen chamber – a room that is free of airborne antigens, used to treat patients with allergies.

Strachan, William H.W., English physician, 1857-1921.

 Strachan syndrome – polyneuritis caused by dietary deprivation.

Strandberg, James Victor, Swedish dermatologist, 1883-1942.
Grönblad-Strandberg syndrome – see under Grönblad

Strang, Leonard Birnie, English physician, *1925.
Smith-Strang disease – see under Smith, Allan J.

Strassburg, Gustav A., German physiologist, *1848.
Strassburg test – for bile in the urine.

Strassman, Paul F., German gynecologist, 1866-1938.
Strassman phenomenon – obsolete term for failure of placental detachment in the third stage of labor.

Stratton, George Malcolm, U.S. psychologist, 1865-1957.
Stratton experiment – visual and tactual motor study technique.

Straus, Isidore, French physician, 1845-1896.
Straus reaction – a diagnostic test for glanders.
Straus sign – in facial paralysis, if an injection of pilocarpine is followed by sweating on the affected side later than on the other, the lesion is peripheral.

Strauss, Alfred A., psychologist.
Strauss syndrome – behavioral characteristics of brain-injured children.

Strauss, Hermann, German physician, 1868-1944.
Strauss phenomenon – fat in chylous ascites is the result of eating fatty foods.

Strauss, Lotte, U.S. pathologist, 1913-1985.
Churg-Strauss syndrome – see under Churg
Strauss-Churg-Zak syndrome – *SYN:* Churg-Strauss syndrome

Sträussler, E., Austrian physician.
Gerstmann-Sträussler-Scheinker syndrome
Gerstmann-Sträussler syndrome – see under Gerstmann

NOTES

Streeter, George L., U.S. embryologist, 1873-1948.
    Streeter bands – strands of amniotic tissue adherent to the embryo or fetus. *SYN:* amniotic bands
    Streeter developmental horizon(s) – a term borrowed from geology and archeology by Streeter to define 23 developmental stages in young human embryos, from fertilization through the first 2 months.
    Streeter dysplasia

Streiff, Enrico Bernard, Swiss ophthalmologist, 1908-1988.
    Hallermann-Streiff-François syndrome – *SYN:* Hallermann-Streiff syndrome
    Hallermann-Streiff syndrome – see under Hallermann

Stroganoff, Vasili V., Russian obstetrician, 1857-1938.
    Stroganoff method – obsolete term for treatment of eclampsia.

Stromeyer, Georg Friedrich Ludwig, German surgeon, 1804-1876.
    Stromeyer cephalohematocele – subperiosteal tissue mass with communication to venous sinuses.
    Stromeyer hook – device used for elevation of zygomatic arch fractures.

Strong, Edward K., Jr., U.S. psychologist, *1884.
    Strong vocational interest test – matches an individual's specific likes, dislikes, and interests to those characteristic of persons working in each of a number of vocations.

Strontian, a town in Scotland for which the element is named.
    strontium (Sr) – a metallic element, atomic no. 38.

Stroop, J.R., psychologist.
    Stroop test – used in psychology/psychiatry.

Stroud, Bert B., 19th century U.S. physiologist, anatomist, and zoologist.
    Stroud pectinated area – obsolete term for the area of the anal canal lying just below the rectal columns.

Strümpell, Ernst Adolf von, German physician, 1853-1925.
    Fleischer-Strümpell ring – *SYN:* Kayser-Fleischer ring
    Marie-Strümpell disease – *SYN:* Strümpell-Marie disease
    Strümpell disease – arthritis and osteitis deformans involving the spinal column. *SYN:* acute epidemic leukoencephalitis; spondylitis deformans
    Strümpell-Marie disease – arthritis of the spine, resembling rheumatoid arthritis, that may progress to bony ankylosis. *SYN:* ankylosing spondylitis; Marie-Strümpell disease

Strümpell phenomenon – dorsal flexion of the great toe in a paralyzed limb when the limb is drawn up against the body, flexing knee and hip. *SYN:* tibial phenomenon

Strümpell reflex – stroking the abdomen or thigh causes flexion of the leg and adduction of the foot.

Strümpell-Westphal disease – *SYN:* Wilson disease

Westphal-Strümpell pseudosclerosis – *SYN:* Wilson disease

Struthers, Sir John, Scottish anatomist, 1823-1899.

ligament of Struthers – a fibrous band located on the medial aspect of the distal humerus.

Stryker, Garold V., U.S. pathologist, *1896.

Stryker-Halbeisen syndrome – reddish, scaling, macular eruption on the head and upper trunk due to vitamin B complex deficiency.

Stryker, Homer H., U.S. orthopedic surgeon, 1894-1980.

mini-Stryker power drill

Stryker bed – *SYN:* Stryker frame

Stryker cast cutter

Stryker CircOlectric bed

Stryker drill

Stryker fracture frame

Stryker fracture table

Stryker frame – holds the patient and permits turning in various planes without individual motion of parts. *SYN:* Stryker bed

Stryker leg exerciser

Stryker power instrumentation

Stryker saw – a rapidly oscillating saw used for cutting bone or plaster casts.

Stryker screw

Stuart, surname of the patient in which factor was first discovered.

Stuart factor – *SYN:* Stuart-Prower factor

Stuart-Prower factor – factor X. *SYN:* Stuart factor

Student, pseudonym for William Sealy Gossett, English research chemist and statistician.

> **Student t test** – assesses the difference between, or the equality of, two or more population means.

Sturge, William Allen, English physician, 1850-1919.

> **Sturge-Kalischer-Weber syndrome** – *SYN:* Sturge-Weber syndrome
> **Sturge syndrome**
> **Sturge-Weber disease** – *SYN:* Sturge-Weber syndrome
> **Sturge-Weber syndrome** – a triad of (1) congenital flame nevus in the distribution of the trigeminal nerve, usually unilateral; (2) homolateral meningeal angioma with intracranial calcification and neurologic signs; and (3) angioma of the choroid, often with secondary glaucoma. *SYN:* cephalotrigeminal angiomatosis; encephalotrigeminal angiomatosis; Sturge-Kalischer-Weber syndrome; Sturge-Weber disease

Sturm, Johann C., German physician and mathematician, 1635-1703.

> **Sturm conoid** – in optics, the pattern of rays formed after passage through a spherocylindrical combination.
> **Sturm interval** – the distance between the anterior and posterior focal lines in a spherocylindrical lens combination.

Sturmdorf, Arnold, U.S. gynecologist, 1861-1934.

> **Sturmdorf amputation of the cervix**
> **Sturmdorf colporrhaphy**
> **Sturmdorf needle**
> **Sturmdorf operation** – conical removal of the endocervix.
> **Sturmdorf reamer**
> **Sturmdorf suture**

St. Vincent, patron saint of charitable organizations.

> **St. Vincent forceps**
> **St. Vincent tube clamp**

St. Vitus, patron saint against oversleeping, danger from animals, and of actors.

> **St. Vitus dance** – chorea and dancing mania.

Sucquet, J.P., French anatomist, 1840-1870.

> **Sucquet anastomoses** – *SYN:* Sucquet-Hoyer canals
> **Sucquet canals** – *SYN:* Sucquet-Hoyer canals
> **Sucquet-Hoyer anastomoses** – *SYN:* Sucquet-Hoyer canals
> **Sucquet-Hoyer canals** – arteriovenous anastomoses controlling blood flow in the glomus bodies in the digits. *SYN:* Hoyer anastomoses; Hoyer

canals; Sucquet anastomoses; Sucquet canals; Sucquet-Hoyer anastomoses

Sudeck, Paul Hermann Martin, German surgeon, 1866-1938.

Sudeck atrophy – atrophy of bones, commonly of the carpal or tarsal bones, following a slight injury such as a sprain. *SYN:* acute reflex bone atrophy; posttraumatic osteoporosis; Sudeck syndrome

Sudeck critical point – region in the colon between the supply of the sigmoid arteries and that of the superior rectal artery.

Sudeck disease

Sudeck syndrome – *SYN:* Sudeck atrophy

Sugiura, M., 20th century Japanese surgeon.

Sugiura procedure – esophageal transection with paraesophageal devascularization for esophageal varices.

Suker, George Franklin, 20th century U.S. ophthalmologist.

Suker cyclodialysis spatula

Suker iris forceps

Suker knife

Suker sign – seen in Graves disease.

Sulkowitch, Hirsh W., U.S. physician, *1906.

Sulkowitch reagent – for the detection of calcium in the urine. *SYN:* Sulkowitch test

Sulkowitch test – *SYN:* Sulkowitch reagent

Sulston, John E., English scientist, *1942, joint winner of 2002 Nobel Prize for work related to genetic regulation of organ development and cell death.

Sulzberger, Marion Baldur, U.S. dermatologist, 1895-1983.

Bloch-Sulzberger disease – see under Bloch, Bruno

Bloch-Sulzberger syndrome – *SYN:* Bloch-Sulzberger disease

Sulzberger-Garbe disease – resembles an exudative form of eczema described in Jewish males with oval lesions on the penis, trunk, and face. *SYN:* Sulzberger-Garbe syndrome

NOTES

Sulzberger-Garbe syndrome – *SYN:* Sulzberger-Garbe disease

Sumner, Franklin W., 20th century English surgeon.
   Sumner sign – slight increase in tonus of the abdominal muscles, an early indication of inflammation of the appendix, stone in the kidney or ureter, or a twisted pedicle of an ovarian cyst.

Sutherland, Earl W., Jr., 1915-1974, winner of 1971 Nobel Prize in medicine or physiology for work related to hormones.

Sutton, Richard Lightburn, Jr., U.S. dermatologist, 1908-1990.
   Sutton disease – *SYN:* Sutton nevus
   Sutton nevus – a benign melanocytic nevus in which involution occurs with a central brown mole surrounded by a uniformly depigmented zone or halo. *SYN:* halo nevus; Sutton disease
   Sutton ulcer – a solitary, deep, painful ulcer of the buccal or genital mucous membrane.

Sutton, Willy, U.S. bank robber.
   Sutton law – principle of going to the most likely diagnosis.

Suzanne, Jean G., French physician, *1859.
   Suzanne gland – a small mucous gland in the floor of the mouth.

Svedberg, Theodor, Swedish chemist and Nobel laureate, 1884-1971.
   Svedberg equation
   Svedberg unit – a sedimentation constant.

Swan, Harold James C., U.S. cardiologist, *1922.
   Swan discission knife
   Swan-Ganz balloon flotation catheter
   Swan-Ganz bipolar pacing catheter
   Swan-Ganz catheter – a thin (5-Fr), flexible, flow-directed catheter using a balloon to carry it through the heart to a pulmonary artery.
   Swan-Ganz flow-directed catheter
   Swan-Ganz pacing TD catheter
   Swan lancet
   Swan needle

Sweat, Faye, 20th century pathologist.
   Puchtler-Sweat stain – see under Puchtler

Swediaur, Francois X., Austrian physician, 1748-1824.
   Swediaur disease – *SYN:* Albert disease

Swedish, named for the country of its origin, Sweden.
   Swedish massage – traditional massage.

Sweeney, Anne, U.S. scientist.
   Nance-Sweeney syndrome – see under Nance

Sweet, Robert Douglas, 20th century English dermatologist.
   Sweet disease – *SYN:* acute febrile neutrophilic dermatosis; Sweet syndrome
   Sweet syndrome – *SYN:* Sweet disease

Swenson, Orvar, U.S. surgeon, *1909.
   Swenson operation – definitive surgical correction of Hirschsprung disease.

Swift, Harry, Australian pediatrician, 1858-1937.
   Swift disease – *SYN:* Feer disease

Swindle, Percy Ford, U.S. physiologist, 1889-1916.
   Swindle ghost – prolonged afterimage.

Swyer, Paul R., U.S. pediatrician, *1921.
   Swyer-James-Macleod syndrome – *SYN:* Swyer-James syndrome (2)
   Swyer-James syndrome – (1) radiographic evidence that density of one lung is markedly less than the other because of the presence of air trapped during expiration. *SYN:* Macleod syndrome; (2) hyperlucency of one lung from obliterating bronchiolitis. *SYN:* Swyer-James-Macleod syndrome

Sydenham, Thomas, English physician, 1624-1689.
   Sydenham chorea – a postinfectious chorea appearing several months after a streptococcal infection, with subsequent rheumatic fever. *SYN:* Sydenham disease; Sydenham syndrome
   Sydenham cough
   Sydenham disease – *SYN:* Sydenham chorea
   Sydenham syndrome – *SYN:* Sydenham chorea

Sylvest, Ejnar, Norwegian physician, 1880-1931.
   Sylvest disease – an acute infectious disease usually occurring in epidemic form. *SYN:* epidemic pleurodynia

Sylvius, Franciscus, Dutch physician, 1614-1672.
   aqueduct of Sylvius

S

NOTES

fossa of Sylvius
sylvian angle
sylvian fissure – *SYN:* lateral cerebral sulcus
sylvian line
sylvian point
sylvian valve – *SYN:* valve of inferior vena cava
sylvian ventricle – *SYN:* cavity of septum pellucidum
vallecula sylvii

Syme, James, Scottish surgeon, 1799-1870.
Syme amputation – amputation of the foot at the ankle joint. *SYN:* Syme operation
Syme amputation prosthesis
Syme ankle disarticulation amputation
Syme foot prosthesis
Syme operation – *SYN:* Syme amputation
Syme procedure
Syme prosthesis
Syme prosthetic foot
terminal Syme procedure
two-stage Syme amputation

Symington, Johnson, Scottish anatomist, 1851-1924.
Symington anococcygeal body – a musculofibrous band that passes between the anus and the coccyx. *SYN:* anococcygeal ligament

Symmers, Douglas, U.S. pathologist, 1879-1952.
Brill-Symmers disease – see under Brill
Moschcowitz-Singer-Symmers syndrome – *SYN:* Moschcowitz syndrome

Symmers, William St. Claire, English pathologist, 1863-1937.
Symmers clay pipestem fibrosis – a characteristic pipe-shaped fibrosis formed around hepatic portal veins. *SYN:* pipestem fibrosis

Symonds, Percival Mallon, U.S. psychologist, 1893-1960.
Symonds picture-study test – projective test for adolescents, used in psychology/psychiatry.

Syms, Parker, U.S. surgeon, 1860-1933.
Syms traction
Syms tractor – a collapsible rubber bag and tube used to draw an enlarged prostate into an operative wound.

Szabo, Diorys, Hungarian physician, 1856-1918.
Szabo sign – sciatic sensory loss along the lateral aspect of the foot.

Taenzer, Paul Rudolf, German dermatologist, 1858-1919.

    Taenzer stain – an orcein solution used for staining elastic tissue.
        SYN: Unna-Taenzer stain

    Unna-Taenzer stain – *SYN:* Taenzer stain

Tagliacozzi, Gaspare, Italian surgeon, 1546-1599.

    tagliacotian operation – method of rhinoplasty utilizing a flap from the arm.

Tait, Robert L., English gynecologist, 1845-1899.

    Tait law – an obsolete dictum that an exploratory laparotomy should be performed in every case of obscure pelvic or abdominal disease that threatens health or life.

Takahara, Shigeo, 20th century Japanese otolaryngologist.

    Takahara disease – *SYN:* Takahara syndrome

    Takahara syndrome – chronic severe mouth infection. *SYN:* Takahara disease; acatalasia

Takamine, Jokichi, Japanese-born U.S. chemist, 1860-1938.

    Taka-diastase – an amylase that has been used clinically as a digestive aid. *SYN:* α-amylase

Takata, Maki, Japanese pathologist, *1892.

    Takata-Ara test – for globulin in cerebrospinal fluid.

Takayama, Masao, Japanese physician, *1872.

    Takayama stain – used for identification of blood stains.

Takayasu, Michishige, Japanese ophthalmologist, 1860-1938.

    Takayasu disease – *SYN:* Takayasu pulseless disease

    Takayasu pulseless disease – obliterative arteritis, primarily of the carotid and subclavian arteries. *SYN:* Takayasu disease; Takayasu syndrome

    Takayasu syndrome – *SYN:* Takayasu pulseless disease

NOTES

Takeuchi, K., Japanese physician.
   Nishimoto-Takeuchi syndrome – *SYN:* Nishimoto disease

Takos, Greek physician.
   Petzetakis-Takos syndrome – see under Petzetakis

Talbot, William Henry Fox, English scientist, 1800-1877.
   Plateau-Talbot law – see under Plateau

Tamm, Igor, U.S. virologist, 1922-1971.
   Tamm-Horsfall mucoprotein – the matrix of urinary casts derived from
      the secretion of renal tubular cells.
   Tamm-Horsfall protein

Tangier Island, an island in the Chesapeake Bay where the first patient was
diagnosed.
   Tangier disease – *SYN:* analphalipoproteinemia

Tanner, James, English pediatrician.
   Tanner developmental scale – *SYN:* Tanner growth chart
   Tanner growth chart – a series of charts showing distribution of
      parameters of physical development for children by sex, age, and stages
      of puberty. *SYN:* Tanner developmental scale
   Tanner stage – stage of puberty on the Tanner growth chart.

Tanner, Norman Cecil, English surgeon.
   Tanner incision
   Tanner slide

Tapia, Antonio, Spanish otolaryngologist, 1875-1950.
   Tapia syndrome – unilateral paralysis of the larynx, velum palati, and
      tongue, with atrophy of the latter.
   Tapia vagohypoglossal palsy

Tar, Aloys, Hungarian physician, *1886.
   Tar symptom – the low lung borders lie as deeply with moderate
      exhalation as in the upright position of the lungs with deep inhalation.

Tardieu, Auguste Abroise, French physician, 1818-1879.
   Tardieu ecchymoses – subpleural and subpericardial petechiae or
      ecchymoses (or both), as observed in the tissues of persons who have
      been asphyxiated. *SYN:* Tardieu petechiae; Tardieu spots
   Tardieu petechiae – *SYN:* Tardieu ecchymoses
   Tardieu spots – *SYN:* Tardieu ecchymoses
   Tardieu test

Tarin, Pierre, French anatomist, 1725-1761.

> **Tarin space** – a dilation of the subarachnoid space in front of the pons. *SYN:* interpeduncular cistern

> **Tarin tenia** – a slender, compact fiber bundle that connects the amygdala with the hypothalamus and other basal forebrain regions. *SYN:* terminal stria

> **Tarin valve** – a thin sheet of white matter hidden by the cerebellar tonsil and attached along the peduncle of the flocculus and to the nodulus of the vermis. *SYN:* inferior medullary velum

Tarlov, Isadore Max, U.S. surgeon, 1905-1977.

> **Tarlov cyst** – a perineural cyst found in the proximal radicles of the lower spinal cord.

> **Tarlov nerve elevator**

Tarnier, Étienne Stephane, French obstetrician, 1828-1897.

> **Tarnier forceps** – a type of axis-traction forceps.

Tarui, Seiichiro, Japanese physician, *1927.

> **Tarui disease** – marked by exercise intolerance in childhood, hemolysis, and hyperuricemia. *SYN:* glycogen storage disease VII

Tatum, Edward Lawrie, 1909-1975, joint winner of 1958 Nobel Prize for work related to genetics.

Taussig, Helen B., U.S. pediatrician, 1898-1986.

> **Blalock-Taussig operation** – see under Blalock

> **Blalock-Taussig shunt** – see under Blalock

> **Taussig-Bing disease** – *SYN:* Taussig-Bing syndrome

> **Taussig-Bing syndrome** – complete transposition of the aorta with a left-sided pulmonary artery overriding the left ventricle and ventricular septal defect, right ventricular hypertrophy, anteriorly situated aorta, and posteriorly situated pulmonary artery. *SYN:* Taussig-Bing disease

Tawara, K. Sunao, Japanese pathologist, 1873-1952.

> **His-Tawara system** – see under His, Wilhelm, Jr.

NOTES

node of Aschoff and Tawara – see under Aschoff

Tawara node – *SYN:* node of Aschoff and Tawara

Tay, Warren, English physician, 1843-1927.

Tay cherry-red spot – the ophthalmoscopic appearance of the normal choroid beneath the fovea centralis. *SYN:* cherry-red spot

Tay-Sachs disease – cerebral sphingolipidosis, infantile type. *SYN:* infantile G_{M2} gangliosidosis

Taybi, Hooshang, U.S. pediatrician and radiologist, *1919.

Rubinstein-Taybi syndrome – see under Rubinstein

Taybi syndrome

Taylor, Charles Fayette, U.S. orthopedic surgeon, 1827-1899.

Taylor apparatus – *SYN:* Taylor back brace

Taylor back brace – a steel spinal support. *SYN:* Taylor apparatus; Taylor splint

Taylor clavicle support

Taylor-Knight brace

Taylor procedure

Taylor retractor

Taylor spinal frame

Taylor spine brace

Taylor splint – *SYN:* Taylor back brace

Taylor technique

Taylor thoracolumbosacral orthosis

Taylor, H.C., Jr.

Taylor syndrome – various areas of congestive dysfunction, possibly psychogenic in origin.

Taylor, Robert W., U.S. dermatologist, 1842-1908.

Taylor disease – diffuse idiopathic cutaneous atrophy.

Teale, Thomas P., English surgeon, 1801-1868.

Teale amputation – amputation of the forearm, thigh, or leg.

Teichmann, Ludwig, German histologist, 1823-1895.

Teichmann crystals – used in microscopic detection of blood. *SYN:* chlorohemin crystals

Teichmann test – used to detect blood.

TeLinde, Richard W., U.S. gynecologist, *1894.

TeLinde operation – *SYN:* modified radical hysterectomy

Temin, Howard Martin, joint winner of 1975 Nobel Prize for work related to tumor viruses and cell material.

Tenckhoff, H., 20th century U.S. nephrologist.
   Tenckhoff catheter – thin, hollow, Silastic tube usually placed into peritoneal cavity for peritoneal dialysis.

ten Horn, C., 20th century Dutch surgeon.
   ten Horn sign – pain caused by gentle traction on the right spermatic cord, indicative of appendicitis.

Tenon, Jacques R., French pathologist and oculist, 1724-1816.
   Tenon capsule – *SYN:* fascial sheath of eyeball
   Tenon space – the space between the fascial sheath of the eyeball and the sclera. *SYN:* episcleral space

Terman, Lewis Madison, U.S. psychologist, 1877-1956.
   Terman-McNemar test of mental ability – a group intelligence scale.

Terrey, Mary, 20th century U.S. physician.
   Lowe-Terrey-MacLachlan syndrome – *SYN:* Lowe syndrome

Terrien, Felix, French ophthalmologist, 1872-1940.
   Terrien marginal degeneration – a form of marginal corneal degeneration.
   Terrien-Viel syndrome – recurrent glaucoma, unilateral.

Terrier, Louis-Félix, French surgeon, 1837-1908.
   Courvoisier-Terrier syndrome – obsolete syndrome.
   rier valve – a valvelike fold between the gallbladder and the cystic duct.

Terry, Theodore L., U.S. ophthalmologist, 1899-1946.
   Terry syndrome – *SYN:* retinopathy of prematurity

Terson, Albert, French ophthalmologist, 1867-1935.
   Terson forceps
   Terson glands – *SYN:* conjunctival glands
   Terson speculum

NOTES

Terson syndrome – hemorrhage into the vitreous of the eye.

Teschen, district in Czechoslovakia where the disease was first described in 1929.

    Teschen disease virus – a picornavirus causing Teschen disease of pigs. *SYN:* infectious porcine encephalomyelitis virus

Tesla, Nikola, Serbian-U.S. electrical engineer, 1856-1943.

    tesla – in the SI system, the unit of magnetic flux density.

    Tesla current – *SYN:* high-frequency current

    Tesla magnet

    Tesla measurement

Tessier, Paul, 20th century French physician.

    Tessier bone bender

    Tessier craniofacial instruments

    Tessier craniofacial operation

    Tessier elevator

    Tessier facial dysostosis operation

    Tessier osteotomy

Teutleben, F.E.K. von, German anatomist, *1842.

    Teutleben ligament – *SYN:* pulmonary ligament

Thal, Alan P., U.S. surgeon, *1925.

    Thal procedure – correction of a benign stricture of the lower esophagus.

Thane, Sir George D., English anatomist, 1850-1930.

    Thane method – for indicating the position of the central sulcus of the brain.

Thannhauser, Siegfried Josef, German-U.S. internist, 1885-1962.

    Hauptmann-Thannhauser syndrome – see under Hauptmann

Thayer, James D.

    Thayer-Martin agar – used for transport and primary isolation of *Neisseria gonorrhoeae* and *Neisseria meningitides*. *SYN:* Thayer-Martin medium

    Thayer-Martin medium – *SYN:* Thayer-Martin agar

Thaysen, Thornwald Einar Hess, Danish physician, 1883-1936.

    Gee-Thaysen disease – see under Gee

    Thaysen syndrome – *SYN:* Maclennan syndrome

Thebesius, Adam C., German physician, 1686-1732.

    thebesian foramina – a number of fossae in the wall of the right atrium containing the openings of minute intramural veins. *SYN:* foramina of the venae minimae

thebesian valve – a delicate fold of endocardium at the opening of the coronary sinus into the right atrium. *SYN:* valve of coronary sinus

thebesian veins – numerous small valveless venous channels that open directly into the chambers of the heart from the capillary bed in the cardiac wall, enabling a form of collateral circulation unique to the heart. *SYN:* venae cordis minimae

Theden, Johann C.A., German surgeon, 1714-1797.
Theden method – treatment of aneurysms or of large sanguineous effusions by compression of the entire limb with a roller bandage.

Theile, Friedrich W., German anatomist, 1801-1879.
Theile canal – a passage in the pericardial sac between the origins of the great vessels, formed as a result of the flexure of the heart tube. *SYN:* transverse pericardial sinus

Theile glands – small, mucous, tubuloalveolar glands in the mucosa of the larger bile ducts and especially in the neck of the gallbladder. *SYN:* glands of biliary mucosa

Theile muscle – *SYN:* superficial transverse perineal muscle

Theiler, Max, South African microbiologist in the U.S. and Nobel laureate, 1899-1972.
Theiler disease – (1) *SYN:* mouse encephalomyelitis; (2) *SYN:* equine serum hepatitis

Theiler mouse encephalomyelitis virus – a virus in the family Picornaviridae. *SYN:* Theiler virus

Theiler virus – *SYN:* Theiler mouse encephalomyelitis virus

Theobald Smith, see under Smith, Theobald

Theorell, Axel Hugo Theodor, 1903-1982, winner of 1955 Nobel Prize for work related to oxidation enzymes.

Thévenard, André, French physician, 1898-1952.
Thévenard syndrome

NOTES

Thibierge, Georges, French physician, 1856-1926.
Thibierge-Weissenbach syndrome – calcinosis, Raynaud phenomenon, esophageal motility disorders, sclerodactyly, and telangiectasia. *SYN:* CREST syndrome

Thiemann, H., early 20th century German physician.
Thiemann disease – *SYN:* Thiemann syndrome
Thiemann syndrome – avascular necrosis of the epiphyses of phalanges of fingers or toes. *SYN:* familial arthropathy of the fingers or toes; Thiemann disease

Thier, Carl Jörg, German physician.
Weyers-Thier syndrome – see under Weyers

Thiers, Joseph, French physician, *1885.
Achard-Thiers syndrome – see under Achard

Thiersch, Karl, German surgeon, 1822-1895.
Ollier-Thiersch graft – *SYN:* Ollier graft
Thiersch canaliculi – minute channels in newly formed reparative tissue.
Thiersch graft – *SYN:* Ollier graft
Thiersch graft operation – *SYN:* Thiersch operation
Thiersch implant
Thiersch knife
Thiersch medium split free graft
Thiersch method
Thiersch operation – the application of a partial thickness skin graft. *SYN:* Thiersch graft operation
Thiersch prosthesis
Thiersch suture
Thiersch thin split free graft
Thiersch wire

Thiry, Ludwig, Austrian physiologist, 1817-1897.
Thiry fistula – *SYN:* Thiry-Vella fistula
Thiry-Vella fistula – experimental isolation of a segment of intestine in a dog or other animal. *SYN:* Thiry fistula; Vella fistula

Thoma, Richard, German histologist, 1847-1923.
Thoma ampulla – a dilation of the arterial capillary beyond the sheathed artery of the spleen.
Thoma fixative – nitric acid in 95% alcohol, used for decalcifying bone in the preparation of histologic specimens.
Thoma law – the development of blood vessels is governed by dynamic forces acting on their walls.

Thoma-Zeiss apparatus – *SYN:* Abbé-Zeiss apparatus

Thomas, André Antoine Henri, French neurologist, 1867-1963.
  André Thomas sign – pinching trapezius muscle causes piloerection cephalad to spinal cord lesion.

Thomas, Edward Donnall, *1920, joint winner of 1990 Nobel Prize for work related to cell and organ transplantation.

Thomas, Hugh Owen, English surgeon, 1834-1891.
  Thomas Allis forceps
  Thomas brace
  Thomas cervical collar brace
  Thomas classification
  Thomas collar
  Thomas collar cervical orthosis
  Thomas extrapolated bar graft
  Thomas fracture frame
  Thomas full-ring splint
  Thomas heel
  Thomas hinged splint
  Thomas hyperextension frame
  Thomas Kapsule instruments
  Thomas knee splint
  Thomas Kodel sling
  Thomas posterior splint
  Thomas procedure
  Thomas ring
  Thomas sign
  Thomas splint – a long leg splint extending from a ring at the hip to beyond the foot.
  Thomas splint with Pearson attachment
  Thomas suspension splint
  Thomas test

Thomas test of function
Thomas walking brace
Thomas wrench

Thomas, M., French physician.
Bureau-Barrière-Thomas syndrome – see under Bureau

Thomas, Terry, 20th century English comedic film actor.
Terry Thomas sign – *SYN:* David Letterman sign

Thompson, Frederick R., U.S. orthopedic surgeon, 1907-1983.
Thompson anterolateral approach
Thompson anteromedial approach
Thompson approach
Thompson arthroplasty
Thompson excision
Thompson femoral head prosthesis
Thompson femoral neck prosthesis
Thompson fracture frame
Thompson frame
Thompson hemiarthroplasty hip prosthesis
Thompson hip endoprosthesis system
Thompson hip prosthesis
Thompson hip prosthesis forceps
Thompson modification of Denis Browne splint
Thompson posterior radial approach
Thompson prosthesis
Thompson quadriceps plasty
Thompson resection
Thompson sign
Thompson splint
Thompson squeeze test of Achilles tendon
Thompson telescoping V osteotomy
Thompson test

Thompson, Sir Henry, English surgeon, 1820-1904.
bandaletta of Thompson – thickened inferior margin of the transversalis fascia. *SYN:* iliopubic tract
Thompson test – for extent of gonorrhea infection. *SYN:* two-glass test

Thomsen, Asmus J., Danish physician, 1815-1896.
Thomsen disease – a hereditary disease marked by tonic spasms that occur when voluntary movement is attempted. *SYN:* Thomsen myotonia congenita

Thomsen myotonia congenita – *SYN:* Thomsen disease

Thomson, Frederick H., English physician, 1867-1938.
Thomson sign – *SYN:* Pastia sign

Thomson, Matthew Sidney, English dermatologist, 1894-1969.
Rothmund-Thomson syndrome – *SYN:* Rothmund syndrome

Thorel, Christen, German physician, 1880-1935.
Thorel bundle – a cardiac muscle bundle.

Thormählen, Johann, 19th century German physician.
Thormählen test – for melanin.

Thorn, George W., U.S. physician, *1906.
Thorn syndrome – a rare disorder resulting from renal tubular damage.
SYN: salt-losing nephritis
Thorn test – putative test of adrenal cortical function.

Thorndike, Edward Lee, U.S. psychologist and lexicographer, 1874-1949.
Thorndike handwriting scale – a series of handwriting samples that compares an individual's handwriting.
Thorndike trial and error learning – a theory used in psychology.

Thornwaldt, var. of Tornwaldt

Thost, Arthur, German physician, *1854.
Unna-Thost syndrome – see under Unna, Paul Gerson

Throckmorton, Thomas Bentley, U.S. neurologist, 1885-1961.
Throckmorton reflex – causes extension of the great toe and flexion of the other toes by stroking the dorsum of the foot.
Throckmorton sign – corticospinal tract response characterized by dorsiflexion of toes.

Thudichum, John Lewis William, German-born English physician, 1829-1901.
Thudichum test – used to detect creatine.

NOTES

Thure Brandt, see under Brandt, Thure

Thygeson, Phillips, U.S. ophthalmologist, *1903.
Thygeson disease – epithelial punctate keratitis associated with viral conjunctivitis. *SYN:* superficial punctate keratitis

Tièche, Max, Swiss dermatologist, 1878-1938.
Jadassohn-Tièche nevus – see under Jadassohn

Tiedemann, Friedrich, German anatomist, 1781-1861.
Tiedemann gland – one of two mucoid-secreting tubuloalveolar glands on either side of the lower part of the vagina. *SYN:* greater vestibular gland
Tiedemann nerve – a sympathetic nerve accompanying the central artery of the retina in the optic nerve.
Tiedemann rongeur

Tietze, Alexander, German surgeon, 1864-1927.
Tietze disease – *SYN:* Tietze syndrome
Tietze syndrome – inflammation and painful nonsuppurative swelling of a costochondral junction. *SYN:* peristernal perichondritis; Tietze disease

Tillaux, Paul Jules, French surgeon, 1834-1904.
spiral of Tillaux – an imaginary line connecting the insertions of the recti muscles of the eye.
Tillaux disease
Tillaux fracture

Tinbergen, Nikolaas, 1907-1988, joint winner of 1973 Nobel Prize for work related to social behavior.

Tinel, Jules, French neurologist, 1879-1952.
Tinel sign – a sensation of tingling felt in the distal extremity of a limb with percussion over the site of an injured nerve, indicating a partial lesion or early regeneration in the nerve. *SYN:* Tinel test
Tinel suture
Tinel test – *SYN:* Tinel sign

Tisdale, W.K., U.S. physician.
Sakati-Nyhan-Tisdale syndrome – *SYN:* Sakati-Nyhan syndrome

Tiselius, Arne, Swedish biochemist and Nobel laureate, 1902-1971.
Tiselius apparatus – used to separate proteins in solution by electrophoresis.
Tiselius electrophoresis cell – the special container in a Tiselius apparatus containing the solution to be analyzed by electrophoresis.

Tissot, Jules, early 20th century French physiologist.
   Tissot spirometer – a large water-sealed spirometer designed for accumulating expired gas over a long period of time.

Tizzoni, Guido, Italian physician, 1853-1932.
   Tizzoni stain – used as a test for iron in tissue.

Tobey, George L., Jr., U.S. otolaryngologist, 1881-1947.
   Ayer-Tobey test
   Tobey-Ayer test

Tod, David, English surgeon, 1794-1856.
   Tod muscle – *SYN:* oblique auricular muscle

Todaro, Francesco, Italian anatomist, 1839-1918.
   Todaro tendon – an inconstant tendinous structure that extends from the right fibrous trigone of the heart toward the valve of the inferior vena cava.

Todd, John Launcelot, Canadian physician, 1876-1949.
   Todd body – eosinophilic cytoplasmic inclusions found in amphibian erythrocytes.

Todd, Robert B., English physician, 1809-1860.
   Todd paralysis – paralysis of temporary duration that occurs in the limb(s) involved in jacksonian epilepsy after the seizure. *SYN:* Todd postepileptic paralysis
   Todd postepileptic paralysis – *SYN:* Todd paralysis

Toison, J., French histologist, 1858-1950.
   Toison stain – a blood diluent and leukocyte stain also used for erythrocyte counts.

Toker, Cyril, U.S. pathologist, *1930.
   Toker cell – an epithelial cell with clear cytoplasm found in 10% of normal nipples.

NOTES

Toldt, Karl, Austrian anatomist, 1840-1920.
Toldt fascia – continuation of Treitz fascia behind the body of the pancreas.
Toldt membrane – the anterior layer of the renal fascia.
white line of Toldt – junction of parietal peritoneum with Denonvilliers fascia.

Tolman, Edward Chase, U.S. psychologist, 1886-1959.
Tolman purposive behaviorism – combination of Gestalt concepts.

Tolosa, Eduardo S., 20th century Spanish neurosurgeon.
Tolosa-Hunt syndrome – cavernous sinus syndrome produced by an idiopathic granuloma.

Tom Smith, see under Smith, Sir Thomas

Tomes, Sir Charles S., English dentist, 1846-1928.
Tomes processes – processes of the enamel cells.

Tomes, Sir John, English dentist and anatomist, 1815-1895.
Tomes fibers – the processes of the pulpal cells which are contained within the dentinal tubules. *SYN:* dentinal fibers
Tomes granular layer – a thin layer of dentin adjacent to the cementum.

Tomkins, Silvan S., U.S. psychologist, *1911.
Tomkins-Horn picture arrangement test – test in which an individual arranges three sketches in a sensible sequence.

Tommaselli, Salvatore, Italian physician, 1834-1906.
Tommaselli disease – hemoglobinuria and pyrexia due to quinine intoxication.

Tonegawa, Susumu, *1939, winner of 1987 Nobel Prize for work related to antibodies.

Tooth, Howard H., English physician, 1856-1925.
Charcot-Marie-Tooth disease – see under Charcot
Tooth disease – *SYN:* Charcot-Marie-Tooth disease

Töpfer, Alfred E., German physician, *1858.
Töpfer test – an obsolete test for free hydrochloric acid in the gastric contents.

Topinard, Paul, French anthropologist, 1830-1912.
Topinard facial angle – ophryospinal facial angle.
Topinard line – runs between the glabella and the mental point.

Topolanski, Alfred, Austrian ophthalmologist, 1861-1960.
　Topolanski sign – congestion of the pericorneal region of the eye in
　　Graves disease.

Torek, Franz J.A., U.S. surgeon, 1861-1938.
　Keetley-Torek operation – *SYN:* Torek operation
　Torek operation – a two-stage operation for bringing down an
　　undescended testicle. *SYN:* Keetley-Torek operation

Torkildsen, Arne, Norwegian neurosurgeon, *1899.
　Torkildsen operation
　Torkildsen shunt – a ventriculocisternal shunt.
　Torkildsen shunt procedure
　Torkildsen ventriculocisternostomy

Tornwaldt, (Thornwaldt), Gustavus Ludwig, German physician, 1843-1910.
　Tornwaldt abscess – chronic infection of the pharyngeal bursa.
　Tornwaldt cyst – a cystic notochordal remnant found inconstantly in the
　　posterior wall of the nasopharynx at the lower end of the pharyngeal
　　tonsil. *SYN:* pharyngeal bursa
　Tornwaldt disease – inflammation or obstruction of the pharyngeal bursa
　　or an adenoid cleft with the formation of a cyst containing pus.
　Tornwaldt syndrome – nasopharyngeal discharge, occipital headache,
　　and stiffness of posterior cervical muscles, with halitosis due to chronic
　　infection of the pharyngeal bursa.

Torrance, Ellis Paul, U.S. psychologist, *1915.
　Torrance tests of creative thinking – batteries of test items that use
　　creative thinking with words, pictures, and sounds.

Torre, Douglas P., U.S. dermatologist, *1919.
　Muir-Torre syndrome – *SYN:* Torre syndrome
　Torre syndrome – multiple sebaceous gland neoplasms associated with
　　multiple visceral malignancies. *SYN:* Muir-Torre syndrome

T

NOTES

Torricelli, Evangelista, Italian scientist, 1608-1647.
torr – a unit of pressure.
torricellian vacuum – a vacuum above the mercury in a barometer tube.

Torsten Sjögren, see under Sjögren, Karl Gustaf Torsten

Toti, Addeo, early 20th century Italian ophthalmologist.
Toti operation – corrects stenosis of the lacrimal duct.

Toulouse-Lautrec, Henri de, French painter and lithographer, 1864-1901.
Toulouse-Lautrec disease – an autosomal recessive disease of bone.

Toupet, A., French surgeon.
Toupet fundoplication – a partial posterior fundoplication in which the stomach edge is secured to the esophagus.

Touraine, Albert, French dermatologist, 1883-1961.
Christ-Siemens-Touraine syndrome – see under Christ
Touraine-Solente-Golé syndrome – primary form of osteoarthropathy marked by clubbing of fingers, new bone formation, and synovial effusions.

Tourette, see under Gilles de la Tourette

Tournay, Auguste, French ophthalmologist, 1878-1969.
Tournay phenomenon – dilation of the pupil in the abducting eye on extreme lateral gaze. *SYN:* Gianelli sign; Tournay sign
Tournay sign – *SYN:* Tournay phenomenon

Tourtual, Kaspar, Prussian anatomist, 1802-1865.
Tourtual membrane – the elastic fibra membrane that extends from the ventricular fold of the larynx upward to the aryepiglottic fold. *SYN:* quadrangular membrane
Tourtual sinus – the interval between the palatoglossal and palatopharyngeal arches above the tonsil, most obvious after the tonsil has regressed in the adult. *SYN:* supratonsillar fossa

Touton, Karl, German dermatologist, 1858-1934.
Touton giant cell – a xanthoma cell in which the multiple nuclei are grouped around a small island of nonfoamy cytoplasm.

Tovell, Ralph M., U.S. anesthesiologist, 1901-1967.
Tovell tube – a tracheal tube.

Towne, Edward B., U.S. otolaryngologist, 1883-1957.
Towne projection – anteroposterior radiographic projection devised to demonstrate the occipital bone, foramen magnum, and dorsum sellae,

as well as the petrous ridges. *SYN:* half-axial projection; half-axial view; Towne view

Towne view – *SYN:* Towne projection

Toynbee, Joseph, English otologist, 1815-1866.

Toynbee corpuscles – connective tissue cells found between the laminae of fibrous tissue in the cornea. *SYN:* corneal corpuscles

Toynbee maneuver – swallowing or blowing while the nose is pinched closed and the mouth is shut opens the ears.

Toynbee muscle – draws the handle of the malleus medialward, tensing the tympanic membrane to protect it from excessive vibration by loud sounds. *SYN:* tensor tympani muscle

Toynbee tube – a tube by which an otologist can listen to the sounds in a patient's ear during politzerization.

Trager, Milton, U.S. physician.

Trager work – a form of massage therapy.

Trantas, Alexios, Greek ophthalmologist, 1867-1960.

Horner-Trantas dots – see under Horner, Johann Friedrich

Trantas dots – pale, grayish red, uneven nodules of gelatinous aspect at the limbal conjunctiva in vernal conjunctivitis.

Trapp, Julius, Russian pharmacist, 1815-1908.

Trapp formula – *SYN:* Häser formula

Trapp-Häser formula – *SYN:* Häser formula

Traube, Ludwig, German physician and pathologist, 1818-1876.

Traube bruit – a triple cadence to the heart sounds at rates of 100 beats per minute or more, usually indicative of serious disease. *SYN:* gallop

Traube corpuscle – a hypochromic, crescent-shaped erythrocyte, probably resulting from artifactual rupture of a red cell with loss of hemoglobin. *SYN:* achromocyte

Traube double tone – a double sound heard on auscultation over the femoral vessels in cases of aortic and tricuspid insufficiency.

T

NOTES

Traube dyspnea – obsolete term for inspiratory dyspnea with maximal expansion of the chest and a slow respiratory rhythm.

Traube-Hering curves – rhythmical variations in blood pressure. *SYN:* Traube-Hering waves

Traube-Hering waves – *SYN:* Traube-Hering curves

Traube plugs – *SYN:* Dittrich plugs

Traube semilunar space – a crescentic space about 12 cm wide, just above the costal margin.

Traube sign – a double sound or murmur heard in auscultation over arteries in significant aortic regurgitation.

Traugott, Carl, German internist, *1885.

Staub-Traugott effect – see under Staub

Staub-Traugott phenomenon – *SYN:* Staub-Traugott effect

Trautmann, Moritz F., German otologist, 1832-1902.

Trautmann triangular space – the area of the temporal bone bounded by the sigmoid sinus, the superior petrosal sinus, and a tangent to the posterior semicircular canal. *SYN:* triangle of Trautmann

triangle of Trautmann – *SYN:* Trautmann triangular space

Treacher Collins, see under Collins

Treitz, Wenzel, Bohemian pathologist, 1819-1872.

Treitz arch – a sickle-shaped fold of peritoneum that forms the anterior boundary of the paraduodenal recess. *SYN:* paraduodenal fold

Treitz fascia – fascia behind the head of the pancreas.

Treitz fossa – an inconstant depression in the peritoneum extending posterior to the cecum. *SYN:* subcecal fossa

Treitz hernia – hernia in the subperitoneal tissues. *SYN:* duodenojejunal hernia

Treitz ligament – *SYN:* suspensory muscle of duodenum

Treitz muscle – *SYN:* suspensory muscle of duodenum

Trélat, Ulysse, French surgeon, 1828-1890.

Leser-Trélat sign – see under Leser

Trélat stools – stools streaked with blood, occurring in proctitis.

Trenaunay, Paul, French physician, *1875.

Klippel-Trenaunay-Weber syndrome – see under Klippel

Trendelenburg, Friedrich, German surgeon, 1844-1924.

Brodie-Trendelenburg test – see under Brodie, Sir Benjamin C.

reverse Trendelenburg position – supine position, without flexing or extending, in which the head is higher than the feet.

steep Trendelenburg position

Trendelenburg cannula

Trendelenburg gait

Trendelenburg limp

Trendelenburg lurch

Trendelenburg operation – pulmonary embolectomy.

Trendelenburg position – a supine position on the operating table, used during and after operations in the pelvis or for shock.

Trendelenburg sign – in congenital dislocation of the hip or in hip abductor weakness, the pelvis will sag on the side opposite to the dislocation when the hip and knee of the normal side is flexed.

Trendelenburg symptom – a waddling gait in paresis of the gluteal muscles, as in progressive muscular dystrophy. *SYN:* Trendelenburg waddle

Trendelenburg tampon

Trendelenburg test – a test of the valves of the leg veins.

Trendelenburg vein ligation

Trendelenburg waddle – *SYN:* Trendelenburg symptom

Tresilian, Frederick J., English physician, 1862-1926.

Tresilian sign – a reddish prominence at the orifice of Stensen duct, noted in mumps.

Trethowan, W.H., English orthopedic surgeon, 1882-1934.

Trethowan line – along the upper border of the femoral neck on hip x-ray, failure to enter the head indicates slipped upper femoral epiphysis.

Trethowan metatarsal osteotomy

Treves, Norman, U.S. surgeon, 1894-1964.

Stewart-Treves syndrome – see under Stewart, Fred Waldorf

Treves, Sir Frederick, English surgeon, 1853-1923.

bloodless field of Treves

Treves fold – a fold of peritoneum bounding the ileocecal or ileoappendicular fossa. *SYN:* ileocecal fold

NOTES

Treves intestinal clamp

Trevor, David, English orthopedic surgeon, 1906-1988.
  Trevor disease – epiphysealis hemimelica, affects ankles and knees leading to limitation of motion. *SYN:* tarsoepiphyseal aclasis

Tripier, Léon, French surgeon, 1842-1891.
  Tripier amputation – a modification of Chopart amputation, in that a part of the calcaneus is also removed.

Troisier, Charles-Emile, French physician, 1844-1919.
  Troisier ganglion – lymph node immediately above the clavicle, palpably enlarged as the result of a metastasis from a malignant neoplasm. *SYN:* Troisier node
  Troisier-Hanot-Chauffard syndrome – hypertrophic cirrhosis of the liver associated with diabetes mellitus; excess melanin or iron pigment deposition in tissues causes dark brown pigmentation of skin.
  Troisier node – *SYN:* Troisier ganglion
  Troisier sign – Troisier ganglion enlargement.

Troland, L.T., U.S. physicist, 1889-1932.
  troland – a unit of visual stimulation at the retina equal to the illumination per square millimeter of pupil received from a surface of 1 lux brightness.

Trolard, Paulin, French anatomist, 1842-1910.
  Trolard vein – a large communicating vein between the superficial middle cerebral vein and the superior sagittal sinus. *SYN:* superior anastomotic vein
  vein of Trolard

Tröltsch, Anton F. von, German otologist, 1829-1890.
  Tröltsch corpuscles – minute spaces resembling corpuscles between the radial fibers of the drum membrane of the ear.
  Tröltsch fold – one of two ligamentous bands that mark the boundary between the tense and the flaccid portions of the tympanic membrane. *SYN:* mallear fold
  Tröltsch pockets – *SYN:* Tröltsch recesses
  Tröltsch recesses – slitlike spaces on the tympanic wall between the anterior and posterior malleolar folds and the tympanic membrane. *SYN:* anterior recess of tympanic membrane; posterior recess of tympanic membrane; Tröltsch pockets

Trömner, Ernest L.O., German neurologist, 1868-1949.
    Trömner reflex – a modified Rossolimo reflex, seen in pyramidal tract lesions, with moderate spasticity.

Trotter, W.
    Trotter syndrome – nasopharyngeal tumor.

Trousseau, Armand, French physician, 1801-1867.
    Trousseau-Lallemand bodies – *SYN:* Lallemand bodies (2)
    Trousseau point – painful neuralgia at the spinous process of the vertebra below which arises the offending nerve.
    Trousseau sign – in latent tetany, the occurrence of carpopedal spasm accompanied by paresthesia, elicited when the upper arm is compressed.
    Trousseau spot – a line of redness resulting from drawing a point across the skin, especially notable in cases of meningitis. *SYN:* meningitic streak
    Trousseau syndrome – thrombophlebitis migrans associated with visceral cancer. *SYN:* Nygaard-Brown syndrome

Trueta, Joseph, Spanish surgeon, *1897.
    Trueta shunt

Trunecek, Karel, Czech physician, *1865.
    Trunecek sign – palpable impulse of the subclavian artery near the point of origin of the sternomastoid muscle in cases of aortic sclerosis.

Tubbs, Oswald Sydney, English surgeon.
    Tubbs dilator

Tübingen, a town in Germany.
    Tübingen perimeter – a bowl perimeter in which a static stimulus was increased in intensity until detected.

Tucker, Ervin Alden, U.S. obstetrician, 1862-1902.
    Tucker-McLean forceps – a type of axis-traction forceps.

Tuffier, Marin Théodore, French surgeon, 1857-1929.
    Tuffier test – *SYN:* Hallion test

NOTES

Tulare, county in California where the disease was first discovered.

    tularemia – a disease that is transmitted to humans from rodents through the bite of a deer fly or other bloodsucking insects, or through the handling of an infected animal carcass. *SYN:* deer-fly disease; deer-fly fever; Pahvant Valley fever; Pahvant Valley plague; rabbit fever

Tullio, Pietro, 20th century Italian physician.

    Tullio phenomenon – momentary vertigo caused by any loud sound, notably occurring in cases of active labyrinthine fistula.

Tulp, Nicholas (Nicolaus Tulpius), Dutch anatomist, 1593-1674.

    Tulp valve – the bilabial prominence of the terminal ileum into the large intestine at the cecocolic junction as seen in cadavers. *SYN:* ileocecal valve

Tulpius, var. of Tulp

Tuohy, Edward B., 20th century U.S. anesthesiologist.

    Tuohy aortography needle

    Tuohy-Borst adapter

    Tuohy-Borst introducer

    Tuohy needle – used to place catheters into the subarachnoid or epidural space.

Türck, Ludwig, Austrian neurologist, 1810-1868.

    Türck bundle – uncrossed fibers forming a small bundle in the pyramidal tract. *SYN:* Türck column; Türck tract

    Türck column – *SYN:* Türck bundle

    Türck degeneration – degeneration of a nerve fiber and its sheath distal to the point of injury or section of the axon.

    Türck tract – *SYN:* Türck bundle

Turcot, Jacques, Canadian surgeon, *1914.

    Turcot syndrome – a rare and distinctive form of multiple intestinal polyposis associated with brain tumors.

Türk, Siegmund, 20th century Swiss ophthalmologist.

    Ehrlich-Türk line – see under Ehrlich

Türk, Wilhelm, Austrian hematologist, 1871-1916.

    Türk cell – a relatively large immature cell found in circulating blood only in pathologic conditions. *SYN:* irritation cell; Türk leukocyte

    Türk leukocyte – *SYN:* Türk cell

Turner, George Grey, English surgeon, 1877-1951.
    Grey Turner sign – local areas of discoloration about the umbilicus and in the region of the loins, in acute hemorrhagic pancreatitis and other causes of retroperitoneal hemorrhage.

Turner, Henry H., U.S. endocrinologist, 1892-1970.
    Turner syndrome – a syndrome with chromosome count 45 and only one X chromosome. *SYN:* XO syndrome

Turner, Joseph G., English dentist, d. 1955.
    Turner tooth – enamel hypoplasia involving a solitary permanent tooth.

Turner, Sir William, English anatomist, 1832-1916.
    intraparietal sulcus of Turner – *SYN:* Turner sulcus
    Turner sulcus – a horizontal sulcus that divides the parietal lobe into superior and inferior parietal lobules. *SYN:* intraparietal sulcus of Turner

Turner, U.C., U.S. surgeon.
    Hefke-Turner sign – see under Hefke
    Turner-Hefke sign – *SYN:* Hefke-Turner sign
    Turner pin
    Turner prosthesis

Turyn, Felix, Polish physician, *1899.
    Turyn sign – pain in buttocks on dorsal bending of 1st toe, indicative of sciatica.

Tuttle, James P., U.S. surgeon, 1857-1913.
    Tuttle proctoscope – a tubular rectal speculum illuminated at its distal extremity.

Tweed, Charles H., U.S. orthodontist, 1895-1970.
    Tweed edgewise treatment
    Tweed triangle – defined by facial and dental landmarks.

Twort, Frederick W., English bacteriologist, 1877-1950.
    Twort-d'Herelle phenomenon – the lysis of bacteria by bacteriophage. *SYN:* bacteriophagia; d'Herelle phenomenon; Twort phenomenon

NOTES

Twort phenomenon – *SYN:* Twort-d'Herelle phenomenon

Tyndall, John, English physicist, 1820-1893.

Tyndall effect – *SYN:* Tyndall phenomenon

tyndallization – exposure to a temperature of 100°C (flowing steam) for a definite period, usually an hour, on each of several days. *SYN:* fractional sterilization

Tyndall light – light that is reflected by gas- or liquid-suspended particles.

Tyndall phenomenon – the visibility of floating particles in gases or liquids when illuminated by a ray of sunlight and viewed at right angles to the illuminating ray. *SYN:* Tyndall effect

Tyrode, Maurice V., U.S. pharmacologist, 1878-1930.

Tyrode solution – a modified Locke solution used to irrigate the peritoneal cavity.

Tyrrell, Frederick, English anatomist and surgeon, 1797-1843.

Tyrrell fascia – a fascial layer that extends superiorly from the central tendon of the perineum to the peritoneum between the prostate and rectum. *SYN:* rectovesical septum

Tyson, Edward, English anatomist, 1649-1708.

Tyson glands – sebaceous glands of the corona glandis and inner surface of the prepuce, which produce smegma. *SYN:* preputial glands

Tzanck, Arnault, Russian dermatologist, 1886-1954.

Tzanck cells – acantholytic epithelial cells seen in the Tzanck test.

Tzanck test – the examination of fluid from a bullous lesion for Tzanck cells.

Uehlinger, E., Swiss pathologist, *1899.
    Meyenburg-Altherr-Uehlinger syndrome – *SYN:* Meyenburg disease

Uffelmann, Jules, German physician, 1837-1894.
    Uffelmann reagent – a 2% solution of phenol in water and aqueous ferric chloride.
    Uffelmann test – determines amount of lactic acid in gastric fluid.

Uhl, Henry S.M., U.S. internist, *1921.
    Uhl anomaly – *SYN:* Uhl syndrome
    Uhl syndrome – congenital malformation of the heart. *SYN:* Uhl anomaly

Uhtoff, Wilhelm, German ophthalmologist, 1853-1927.
    Uhtoff sign – *SYN:* Uhtoff symptom
    Uhtoff symptom – a damaged nerve that often has a lowered shut-down temperature. *SYN:* Uhtoff sign

Ullmann, Emerich, Hungarian surgeon, 1861-1937.
    Ullmann line – the line of displacement in spondylolisthesis.
    Ullmann syndrome – a systemic angiomatosis due to multiple arteriovenous malformations.

Ullrich, Otto, German physician, 1894-1957.
    Bonnevie-Ullrich syndrome – see under Bonnevie
    Morquio-Ullrich disease – *SYN:* Morquio syndrome
    Ullrich drill guard
    Ullrich forceps
    Ullrich laminectomy retractor
    Ullrich self-retaining retractor
    Ullrich tubing clamp

Ultzmann, Robert, German urologist, 1842-1889.
    Ultzmann test – for bile pigments.

NOTES

Ulysses, Greek mythological character.
 Ulysses syndrome – the ill effects of extensive diagnostic investigations performed because of a false-positive result in the course of routine laboratory screening.

Umber, Friedrich, German physician, 1871-1946.
 Umber test – to determine scarlet fever.

Underwood, Michael, English pediatrician, 1737-1820.
 Underwood disease – *SYN:* Underwood syndrome
 Underwood syndrome – neonatal sclerema. *SYN:* Underwood disease

Unna, Marie, German physician.
 Marie Unna syndrome – childhood hair loss. *SYN:* Unna syndrome
 Unna syndrome – *SYN:* Marie Unna syndrome

Unna, Paul Gerson, German dermatologist and staining expert, 1850-1929.
 Unna disease – *SYN:* seborrheic dermatitis
 Unna mark – a pale vascular birthmark found on the nape of the neck in 25% to 50% of normal persons. *SYN:* nape nevus
 Unna-Pappenheim stain – a contrast stain used to detect RNA and DNA in tissue sections; used to demonstrate plasma cells during chronic inflammation.
 Unna stain – an alkaline methylene blue stain for plasma cells.
 Unna syndrome – *SYN:* seborrheic dermatitis
 Unna-Taenzer stain – *SYN:* Taenzer stain
 Unna-Thost syndrome – uniform keratoderma of the palms and soles, usually presenting in the first six months of life.

Unschuld, Paul, German internist, 1835-1905.
 Unschuld sign – a tendency toward cramps in the calves of the legs.

Unverricht, Heinrich, German physician, 1853-1912.
 Unverricht disease – a progressive myoclonic epilepsy. *SYN:* Unverricht syndrome
 Unverricht syndrome – *SYN:* Unverricht disease

Upshaw, Jefferson D., U.S. hematologist.
 Upshaw-Schulman syndrome – congenital microangiopathic hemolytic anemia and thrombocytopenia.

Urbach, Erich, Austrian-U.S. allergist and dermatologist, 1893-1946.
 Oppenheim-Urbach disease – see under Oppenheim, Moriz
 Urbach-Oppenheim disease – *SYN:* Oppenheim-Urbach disease
 Urbach-Wiethe disease – autosomal recessive disorder characterized by disturbance of lipid metabolism. *SYN:* lipoid proteinosis

Urban, Jerome A., surgeon, *1914.
>   **Urban operation** – extended radical mastectomy, including en bloc resection of internal mammary lymph nodes, part of the sternum, and costal cartilages.
>   **Urban retractor**

Usher, Barney, Canadian dermatologist, 1899-1978.
>   **Senear-Usher disease** – *SYN:* Senear-Usher syndrome
>   **Senear-Usher syndrome** – see under Senear

Usher, Charles Howard, English ophthalmologist, 1865-1942.
>   **Usher syndrome** – sensorineural hearing loss and retinitis pigmentosa.

Vaduz, city in Liechtenstein.

    Vaduz hand – below-the-elbow prosthesis with a myoelectric hand.
    SYN: French electric hand

Valentin, Gabriel Gustav, German-Swiss physiologist, 1810-1883.

    Valentin corpuscles – small bodies, probably amyloid, found occasionally in nerve tissue.

    Valentin ganglion – a ganglion on the superior alveolar nerve.

    Valentin nerve – connects the pterygopalatine ganglion with the abducens nerve.

Valentine, Ferdinand C., U.S. surgeon, 1851-1909.

    Valentine irrigation tube

    Valentine irrigator

    Valentine position – a supine position on a table used to facilitate urethral irrigation.

    Valentine test – the bladder is emptied by passing urine into a series of 3-ounce test tubes, and the contents of the first and the last are examined. *SYN:* three-glass test

    Valentine tube

Valleix, François L.I., French physician, 1807-1855.

    Valleix points – various points in the course of a nerve, pressure upon which is painful in cases of neuralgia.

Valsalva, Antonio M., Italian anatomist, 1666-1723.

    aneurysm of sinus of Valsalva – a congenital thin-walled tubular out-pouching usually in the right or noncoronary sinus with an entirely intracardiac course.

    teniae of Valsalva – the three bands in which the longitudinal muscular fibers of the large intestine, except the rectum, are collected. *SYN:* teniae coli

Valsalva antrum – a cavity in the petrous portion of the temporal bone. *SYN:* mastoid antrum

Valsalva ligaments – the three ligaments that attach the auricle to the side of the head. *SYN:* auricular ligaments

Valsalva maneuver – any forced expiratory effort against a closed airway.

Valsalva muscle – a band of vertical muscular fibers on the outer surface of the tragus of the ear. *SYN:* tragicus muscle

Valsalva sinus – the space between the superior aspect of each cusp of the aortic valve and the dilated portion of the wall of the ascending aorta. *SYN:* aortic sinus

Valsalva test – when the heart is monitored during the Valsalva maneuver, there is a characteristic complex sequence of cardiocirculatory events, departure from which indicates disease or malfunction.

van Bogaert, Ludo, Belgian neurologist, *1897.
  Canavan-van Bogaert-Bertrand disease – *SYN:* Canavan disease
  Divry-van Bogaert disease – see under Divry
  Nyssen-van Bogaert-Meyer syndrome – see under Nyssen
  van Bogaert disease
  van Bogaert encephalitis – a rare chronic, progressive encephalitis that affects primarily children and young adults, caused by the measles virus. *SYN:* subacute sclerosing panencephalitis

van Buchem, Francis Steven Peter, Dutch internist, 1897-1979.
  van Buchem syndrome – an inherited skeletal dysplasia. *SYN:* generalized cortical hyperostosis

van Buren, William H., U.S. surgeon, 1819-1883.
  van Buren disease – *SYN:* Peyronie disease
  van Buren sound – a standard sound used for urethral calibration or dilation.

van Creveld, Simon, Dutch pediatrician, 1894-1971.
  Ellis-van Creveld syndrome – see under Ellis, Richard White Bernard

van Deen, Izaak A., Dutch physiologist, 1804-1869.
  van Deen test – *SYN:* Almén test for blood

van de Graaf, Robert Jemison, U.S. engineer and physicist, 1901-1967.
  van de Graaf generator – high voltage electrostatic generator.

van den Bergh, A.A. Hymans, Dutch physician, 1869-1943.
  van den Bergh reaction – *SYN:* van den Bergh test
  van den Bergh test – for bilirubin. *SYN:* van den Bergh reaction

van der Hoeve, Jan, Dutch ophthalmologist, 1878-1952.
   van der Hoeve syndrome – conduction hearing loss caused by temporal bone changes.

van der Kolk, Jacobus Ludwig Conrad Schroeder, Dutch physician, 1797-1862.
   van der Kolk law – in a mixed nerve, the sensory fibers are distributed to the parts moved by the muscles controlled by the motor fibers.

van der Spieghel, see under Spigelius

van der Velden, Reinhardt, German physician, 1851-1903.
   van der Velden test – for free hydrochloric acid.

van der Waals, Johannes D., Dutch physicist and Nobel laureate, 1837-1923.
   van der Waals forces – explains deviations from ideal gas behavior seen in real gases. *SYN:* London forces

Vane, Sir John R., joint winner of 1982 Nobel Prize for work related to prostaglandins.

van Ekenstein, W.A., 19th century scientist.
   Lobry de Bruyn-van Ekenstein transformation – see under Lobry de Bruyn

van Ermengen, Emile P., Belgian bacteriologist, 1851-1932.
   van Ermengen stain – a method for staining flagella.

van Gieson, Ira, U.S. histologist and bacteriologist, 1865-1913.
   van Gieson stain – a mixture of acid fuchsin in saturated picric acid solution, used in collagen staining.

van Gogh, Vincent, Dutch artist, 1853-1890.
   van Gogh syndrome – *SYN:* Münchausen syndrome

van Helmont, Jean B., Flemish physician and chemist, 1577-1644.
   van Helmont mirror – obsolete term for central tendon of diaphragm.

V

van Horne, Jan (Johannes), Dutch anatomist, 1621-1670.
  van Horne canal – the largest lymph vessel in the body, beginning at the cisterna chyli at about the level of the second lumbar vertebra. *SYN:* thoracic duct

Van Neck, M., Belgian physician.
  Van Neck disease – ischiopubic osteochondritis in children and adolescents. *SYN:* Odelberg disease; Van Neck-Odelberg disease; Van Neck-Odelberg syndrome
  Van Neck-Odelberg disease – *SYN:* Van Neck disease
  Van Neck-Odelberg syndrome – *SYN:* Van Neck disease

Van Slyke, Donald D., U.S. biochemist, 1883-1971.
  slyke – a unit of buffer value, the slope of the acid-base titration curve of a solution.
  Van Slyke apparatus – determines the amount of respiratory gases in the blood.
  Van Slyke formula – the value obtained when the square root of the urine flow is multiplied by the urine urea concentration and divided by the whole blood urea concentration. *SYN:* standard urea clearance

van't Hoff, Jacobus H., Dutch chemist and Nobel laureate, 1852-1911.
  Le Bel-van't Hoff rule – see under Le Bel
  van't Hoff equation – equation for osmotic pressure of dilute solutions for any reaction.
  van't Hoff law – in stereochemistry, all optically active substances have one or more multivalent atoms united to four different atoms or radicals so as to form in space an unsymmetrical arrangement.
  van't Hoff theory – that substances in dilute solution obey the gas laws.

Vaquez, Louis H., French physician, 1860-1936.
  Vaquez disease – a chronic form of polycythemia characterized by bone marrow hyperplasia. *SYN:* polycythemia vera

Varmus, Harold E., joint winner of 1989 Nobel Prize for work related to oncogenes.

Varolius, Constantius (Costanzio), Italian anatomist and physician, 1543-1575.
  pons varolii – in neuroanatomy, that part of the brainstem between the medulla oblongata caudally and the mesencephalon rostrally. *SYN:* pons
  valve of Varolius – the bilabial prominence of the terminal ileum into the large intestine at the cecocolic junction as seen in cadavers. *SYN:* ileocecal valve

Vater, Abraham, German anatomist and botanist, 1684-1751.

duct of Vater – *SYN:* Bochdalek duct

Vater ampulla – the dilation within the major duodenal papilla that normally receives both the common bile duct and the main pancreatic duct. *SYN:* hepatopancreatic ampulla

Vater corpuscles – small oval bodies in the skin of the fingers, in the mesentery, tendons, and elsewhere sensitive to pressure. *SYN:* lamellated corpuscles; pacinian corpuscles; Vater-Pacini corpuscles

Vater fold – a fold of mucous membrane in the duodenum just above the greater duodenal papilla.

Vater-Pacini corpuscles – *SYN:* Vater corpuscles

Vater tubercle – duodenal papilla. *SYN:* papilla of Santorini

Vedder, Edward B., U.S. physician, 1878-1952.

Vedder sign – loss of sensation in the anterior lower leg, pain on calf pressure, loss of knee jerk, and difficulty rising from a squatting position caused by beriberi.

Veillon, Adrien, French bacteriologist, 1864-1931.

Veillonella – a genus of nonmotile, non–spore-forming, anaerobic bacteria.

Veillonella alcalescens **subsp.** *alcalescens* – a bacterial subspecies found primarily in the mouths of humans but occasionally in the buccal cavity of rabbits and rats.

Veillonella alcalescens **subsp.** *dispar* – a subspecies found in the mouths and respiratory tracts of humans.

Veillonella atypica – *SYN:* *Veillonella parvula* subsp. *atypica*

Veillonellaceae – a family of nonmotile, non–spore-forming, anaerobic bacteria containing gram-negative cocci.

Veillonella parvula – a bacterial species found normally as a harmless parasite in the natural cavities, especially the mouths and digestive tracts of humans and other animals.

Veillonella parvula **subsp.** *atypia* – a bacterial subspecies found in the buccal cavity of rats and humans. *SYN:* *Veillonella atypica*

Veillonella parvula subsp. *parvula* – a bacterial subspecies found in the mouth, or intestinal or respiratory tract of humans.

Veillonella parvula subsp. *rodentium* – a bacterial subspecies found in the buccal cavity and intestinal tract of hamsters, rats, and rabbits. *SYN: Veillonella rodentium*

Veillonella rodentium – *SYN: Veillonella parvula* subsp. *rodentium*

Vella, Luigi, Italian physiologist, 1825-1886.
Thiry-Vella fistula – see under Thiry
Vella fistula – *SYN:* Thiry-Vella fistula

Velpeau, Alfred A.L.M., French surgeon, 1795-1867.
Velpeau axillary lateral view
Velpeau axillary radiograph
Velpeau bandage – serves to immobilize arm to chest wall, with the forearm positioned obliquely across and upward on front of chest.
Velpeau canal – passage through the layers of the lower abdominal wall that transmits the spermatic cord in the male and the round ligament in the female. *SYN:* inguinal canal
Velpeau cast
Velpeau deformity
Velpeau dressing
Velpeau fossa – a wedge-shaped space with its base toward the perineum. *SYN:* ischiorectal fossa
Velpeau hernia – femoral hernia in which the intestine is in front of the blood vessels.
Velpeau shoulder immobilizer
Velpeau sling
Velpeau stockinette
Velpeau tendon transfer
Velpeau wrap

Venable, Charles Scott, U.S. surgeon.
Venable plates and screws
Venable screw
Venable-Stuck fracture pin
Venable-Stuck nail

Venn, John, English logician and philosopher, 1834-1923.
Venn diagram – pictorial representation of the extent to which two or more quantities or concepts are mutually inclusive and exclusive.

Venturi, Giovanni B., Italian physicist, 1746-1822.
Venturi apparatus

Venturi aspiration vitrectomy device
Venturi bobbin myringotomy tube
Venturi collar button myringotomy tube
Venturi effect – term applied to the operation of a Venturi tube and similar systems.
Venturi grommet myringotomy tube
Venturi insufflator
Venturi mask
Venturi meter – a device for measuring flow of a fluid.
Venturi pediatric myringotomy tube
Venturi spirometer
Venturi tube – a tube with a specially streamlined constriction.
Venturi ventilator

Verbrugge, Jean, Belgian orthopedic surgeon, 1896-1964.
Verbrugge bone-holding clamp
Verbrugge clamp
Verbrugge forceps
Verbrugge needle
Verbrugge retractor

Verga, Andrea, Italian neurologist, 1811-1895.
cavum vergae – *SYN:* Verga ventricle
Verga ventricle – an inconstant, horizontal, slitlike space between the posterior one-third of the corpus callosum and the underlying commissura fornicis resulting from failure of these two commissural plates to fuse completely during fetal development. *SYN:* cavum psalterii; cavum vergae; sixth ventricle

Verheyen, Philippe, Flemish anatomist, 1648-1710.
stellulae verheyenii – *SYN:* venulae stellatae
Verheyen stars – the star-shaped groups of venules in the renal cortex. *SYN:* venulae stellatae

NOTES

Verhoeff, Frederick H., U.S. ophthalmologist, 1874-1968.
    Verhoeff advancement
    Verhoeff capsule forceps
    Verhoeff cataract forceps
    Verhoeff dissecting scissors
    Verhoeff elastic tissue stain
    Verhoeff expressor
    Verhoeff operation
    Verhoeff scissors
    Verhoeff sclerotomy
    Verhoeff suture

Verner, John, U.S. internist, *1927.
    Verner-Morrison syndrome – watery diarrhea, hypokalemia, and achlorhydria associated with secretion of vasoactive intestinal polypeptide by a pancreatic islet-cell tumor in the absence of gastric hypersecretion. *SYN:* watery diarrhea, hypokalemia, and achlorhydria (WDHA) syndrome

Vernet, Maurice, French neurologist, 1887-1974.
    Vernet syndrome – paralysis of the motor components of the glossopharyngeal, vagus, and accessory cranial nerves, most commonly the result of head injury.

Verneuil, Aristide A., French surgeon, 1823-1895.
    hidradenitis axillaris of Verneuil – an axillary abscess.
    Verneuil neuroma – a nodular enlargement of the cutaneous nerves.

Vernier, Pierre, French mathematician, 1580-1637.
    Vernier acuity – detection of displacement of a portion of a line.

Verocay, José, Czech pathologist, 1876-1927.
    Verocay bodies – hyalinized acellular areas seen microscopically in neurilemomas.

Vesalius, Andreas (Andre), Flemish anatomist, 1514-1564.
    Vesalius bone – the tuberosity of the fifth metatarsal bone sometimes existing as a separate bone. *SYN:* os vesalianum
    Vesalius foramen – a minute inconstant foramen in the greater wing of the sphenoid bone. *SYN:* foramen venosum
    Vesalius vein – the emissary vein passing through the foramen venosum.

Vicat, L.J., French engineer, 1786-1861.
    Vicat needle – a device for obtaining the setting time of plaster and other materials.

Vicq d'Azyr, Félix, French anatomist, 1748-1794.

    Vicq d'Azyr bundle – a compact, thick bundle of nerve fibers that passes from the mamillary body to terminate in the anterior nucleus of the thalamus. *SYN:* mamillothalamic fasciculus

    Vicq d'Azyr centrum semiovale – the great mass of white matter composing the interior of the cerebral hemisphere. *SYN:* centrum semiovale

    Vicq d'Azyr foramen – a small triangular depression at the lower boundary of the pons that marks the upper limit of the median fissure of the medulla oblongata. *SYN:* foramen cecum medullae oblongatae

Victor, (origin unknown).

    Victor-Michaelis-Menten equation – *SYN:* Michaelis-Menten equation

Victoria, Queen of England from 1837-1901.

    Victoria blue – any of several blue diphenyl naphthylmethane derivatives used as a stain in histology.

Vidal, Jean Baptiste Emile, French dermatologist, 1825-1893.

    Vidal disease – obsolete term for lichen simplex chronicus.

Vidius, Guidi (Guido), Italian anatomist and physician, 1500-1569.

    vidian artery – *SYN:* artery of pterygoid canal

    vidian canal – an opening through the base of the medial pterygoid process of the sphenoid bone through which pass the artery, vein, and nerve of the pterygoid canal. *SYN:* pterygoid canal

    vidian nerve – the nerve constituting the parasympathetic and sympathetic root of the pterygopalatine ganglion. *SYN:* nerve of pterygoid canal

    vidian vein – a vein accompanying the nerve and artery through the pterygoid canal and emptying into the pharyngeal venous plexus. *SYN:* vein of pterygoid canal

Viel, P.

    Terrien-Viel syndrome – see under Terrien

NOTES

Vierordt, Karl, German physiologist, 1818-1884.

Vierordt law – principle used to determine two-point threshold for a stimulus.

Vierra, J.P., 20th century Brazilian dermatologist.

Vierra sign – yellowing and canalization of the nail.

Vieussens, Raymond de, French anatomist, 1641-1715.

valve of Vieussens – a prominent valve in the great cardiac vein where it turns around the obtuse margin to become the coronary sinus.

Vieussens annulus – *SYN:* Vieussens ring

Vieussens ansa – *SYN:* Vieussens loop

Vieussens centrum – the great mass of white matter composing the interior of the cerebral hemisphere. *SYN:* centrum semiovale

Vieussens foramina – a number of fossae in the wall of the right atrium, containing the openings of minute intramural veins. *SYN:* foramina of the venae minimae

Vieussens ganglia – the largest and highest group of prevertebral sympathetic ganglia, located on the superior part of the abdominal aorta, on either side of the origin of the celiac artery. *SYN:* celiac ganglia

Vieussens isthmus – *SYN:* Vieussens ring

Vieussens limbus – *SYN:* Vieussens ring

Vieussens loop – a nerve cord connecting the middle cervical and stellate sympathetic ganglia, forming a loop around the subclavian artery. *SYN:* ansa subclavia; Vieussens ansa

Vieussens ring – a muscular ring surrounding the fossa ovalis in the wall of the right atrium of the heart. *SYN:* limbus fossae ovalis; Vieussens annulus; Vieussens isthmus; Vieussens limbus

Vieussens valve – the thin layer of white matter stretching between the two superior cerebellar peduncles forming the roof of the superior recess of the fourth ventricle. *SYN:* superior medullary velum

Vieussens veins – the small superficial veins of the heart. *SYN:* innominate cardiac veins

Vieussens ventricle – a slitlike, fluid-filled space of variable width between the left and right transparent septum. *SYN:* cavity of septum pellucidum

Vigotsky, Lev Semionovich, Russian psychologist, 1896-1934.

Vigotsky test – used to study thinking and concept formation process; also used to detect ability to think in abstract and to detect thought disturbance.

Vilanova, Xavier, Spanish physician.

Vilanova-Pinol Aguadé syndrome – small, painless, subcutaneous nodules on the anterolateral aspect of the leg, usual onset one to 20 days following tonsillitis or pharyngitis.

Villaret, Maurice, French neurologist, 1877-1946.

Villaret syndrome – retropharyngeal or retroparotid space lesion that causes unilateral paralysis of cervical sympathetic nerves 9-12.

Vincent, Henri, French physician, 1862-1950.

Vincent angina – an ulcerative infection of the oral soft tissues, including the tonsils and pharynx, caused by fusiform and spirochetal organisms.

Vincent bacillus

Vincent disease – *SYN:* necrotizing ulcerative gingivitis

Vincent spirillum – the spirillum or spirochete found in association with Vincent bacillus.

Vincent tonsillitis – angina limited chiefly to the tonsils, caused by Vincent organisms (bacillus and spirillum).

Vincent white mycetoma – mycetoma caused by *Actinomadura madurae* and occurring in North Africa, India, Argentina, and Cuba.

Vineberg, Arthur M., Canadian thoracic surgeon, *1903.

Vineberg procedure – implantation of the internal mammary artery into the myocardium to improve blood flow to the heart.

Vinson, Porter P., U.S. surgeon, 1890-1959.

Plummer-Vinson syndrome – see under Plummer

Vipond, French physician.

Vipond sign – generalized adenopathy occurring during the period of incubation of various exanthemas of childhood.

Virchow, Rudolf, German pathologist and politician, 1821-1902.

Virchow angle – an angle formed by the meeting of a line drawn from the middle of the nasofrontal suture to the base of the anterior nasal spine, with a line drawn from this last point to the center of the external auditory meatus. *SYN:* Virchow-Holder angle

Virchow cells – (1) the lacunae in osseous tissue containing the bone cells; also the bone cells themselves; (2) connective tissue cells between the laminae of fibrous tissue in the cornea. *SYN:* corneal corpuscles; Virchow corpuscles

Virchow corpuscles – *SYN:* Virchow cells (2)

Virchow crystals – yellow-brown, amber, or burnt orange crystals of hematoidin, frequently observed in extravasated blood in tissues.

Virchow disease – acute congenital encephalitis, a condition in which the head is abnormally large. *SYN:* megacephaly

Virchow-Hassall bodies – *SYN:* Hassall bodies

Virchow-Holder angle – *SYN:* Virchow angle

Virchow law – there is no special or distinctive neoplastic cell inasmuch as the component cells of neoplasms originate from preexisting forms.

Virchow node – a firm, palpable supraclavicular lymph node that may be the first recognized presumptive evidence of a malignant neoplasm in one of the viscera. *SYN:* signal node

Virchow psammoma – a firm, cellular neoplasm derived from fibrous tissue of the meninges, choroid plexus, and certain other brain structures. *SYN:* psammomatous meningioma

Virchow-Robin space – a tunnel-like extension of the subarachnoid space surrounding blood vessels that pass into the brain or spinal cord from the subarachnoid space. *SYN:* His perivascular space

Virchow triad – factors predisposing vascular thrombosis.

Vladimiroff, Vladimir D., Russian surgeon, 1837-1903.
Mikulicz-Vladimiroff amputation – see under Mikulicz
Vladimiroff-Mikulicz amputation – *SYN:* Mikulicz-Vladimiroff amputation

Voges, Daniel Wilhelm Otto, German physician, *1867.
Voges-Proskauer reaction – a chemical reaction used in testing for the production of acetyl methyl carbinol by various bacteria.

Vogt, Alfred, Swiss ophthalmologist, 1879-1943.
limbal girdle of Vogt – corneal opacity that occurs in an arc concentric pattern.
Vogt-Koyanagi-Harada syndrome – systemic inflammatory eye condition. *SYN:* VKH syndrome
Vogt-Koyanagi syndrome – bilateral uveitis with iritis and glaucoma, premature graying of the hair, alopecia, vitiligo, and dysacusia. *SYN:* oculocutaneous syndrome; uveocutaneous syndrome

Vogt, Cécile, 1875-1962 and Oskar, 1870-1959, German neurologists.
  Vogt syndrome – a type of cerebral palsy. *SYN:* double athetosis

Vogt, Heinrich, German neurologist, *1875.
  Spielmeyer-Vogt disease – *SYN:* Batten disease
  Vogt-Spielmeyer disease – *SYN:* Batten disease

Vogt, Karl, German physiologist, 1817-1895.
  Vogt angle – a craniometric angle formed by the nasobasilar and
    alveolonasal lines.

Vohwinkel, H.H., 20th century German dermatologist.
  Vohwinkel syndrome – *SYN:* mutilating keratoderma

Voigt, Christian A., Austrian anatomist, 1809-1890.
  Voigt line – *SYN:* Futcher line

Volhard, Franz, German physician, 1872-1950.
  Volhard test – for renal function.

Volkmann, Alfred W., German physiologist, 1800-1877.
  Volkmann canals – vascular canals in compact bone that are not
    surrounded by concentric lamellae of bone.
  Volkmann membrane

Volkmann, Richard, German surgeon, 1830-1889.
  Volkmann bone curette
  Volkmann bone hook
  Volkmann cheilitis – an acquired disorder, of unknown etiology of the
    lower lip, characterized by swelling, ulceration, crusting, mucous gland
    hyperplasia, abscesses, and sinus tracts. *SYN:* cheilitis glandularis
  Volkmann claw hand deformity
  Volkmann contracture – ischemic contracture resulting from irreversible
    necrosis of muscle tissue, produced by a compartment syndrome.
  Volkmann fracture
  Volkmann ischemia
  Volkmann ischemic contracture

NOTES

Volkmann ischemic paralysis
Volkmann rake retractor
Volkmann splint
Volkmann spoon – a sharp spoon for scraping away carious bone or other diseased tissue.
Volkmann subluxation

Vollmer, Herman, U.S. pediatrician, 1896-1959.
Vollmer test – a tuberculin patch test.

Volpe, Anthony R., U.S. dentist, *1932.
Volpe-Manhold Index – an index for comparing the amount of dental calculus in individuals.

Volta, Alessandro, Italian physicist, 1745-1827.
volt (V, v) – the unit of electromotive force.

Voltolini, Friedrich E.R., German laryngologist, 1819-1889.
Voltolini disease – disease of the labyrinth leading to deaf-mutism in young children.

von Behring, see under Behring, Emil A. von

von Békésy, see under Békésy, Georg von

von Bergmann, see under Bergmann, Gustav von

von Brunn, see under Brunn, Albert von

von Bruns, see under Bruns, Ludwig von

von Ebner, Victor, Austrian histologist, 1842-1925.
Ebner glands – serous glands of the tongue opening in the bottom of the trough surrounding the circumvallate papillae.
Ebner reticulum – a network of nucleated cells in the seminiferous tubules.
imbrication lines of von Ebner – incremental lines in the dentin of the tooth that reflect variations in mineralization during dentin formation. *SYN:* incremental lines of von Ebner
incremental lines of von Ebner – *SYN:* imbrication lines of von Ebner

von Economo, Constantin, Austrian neurologist, 1876-1931.
Economo disease – *SYN:* von Economo disease
von Economo disease – the basis for postencephalitic parkinsonism, suspected to be of viral origin. *SYN:* Economo disease; encephalitis lethargica; polioencephalitis infectiva; sleeping sickness

von Gierke, see under Gierke, Edgar von

von Graefe, see under Graefe, Albrecht von

von Hansemann, D.P., German pathologist, 1858-1920.
Hansemann macrophages – large cells associated with a granulomatous condition primarily affecting the urinary tract.

von Heine, Jacob, German orthopedist, 1800-1879.
Heine-Medin disease – poliomyelitis or infantile paralysis.

von Hippel, Eugen, German ophthalmologist, 1867-1939.
Hippel keratoplasty
Hippel trephine
von Hippel disease – retinal hemangiomatosis.
von Hippel-Lindau syndrome – a type of phacomatosis, consisting of hemangiomas of the retina associated with hemangiomas or hemangioblastomas primarily of the cerebellum and walls of the fourth ventricle, occasionally involving the spinal cord. *SYN:* cerebroretinal angiomatosis; Lindau disease

von Jaksch, Rudolf, Czech physician, 1855-1947.
von Jaksch anemia – childhood acute hemolytic anemia.

von Kossa, Julius, 19th century Austrian-Hungarian pathologist.
Kossa stain – *SYN:* von Kossa stain
von Kossa stain – for calcium in mineralized tissue. *SYN:* Kossa stain

von Linné, see under Linné, Carl von

von Mayer, Julius Robert, German physician, 1814-1878.
mayer – heat capacity unit.

von Meyenburg, see under Meyenburg, H. von

von Ostertag, Robert, German veterinarian, 1864-1940.
Ostertagia – genus of stomach worms that are found primarily in cattle.
ostertagiasis – infection caused by *Ostertagia. SYN:* ostertagiosis

von Pirquet, Clemens P., Austrian physician, 1874-1929.
von Pirquet test – an early test for tuberculosis.

V

NOTES

von Recklinghausen, see under Recklinghausen, Friedrich Daniel von

von Restorff, Hedwig, German psychologist.
   von Restorff effect – memory process theory.

von Rittershain, see under Ritter von Rittershain, Gottfried

von Sacher-Masoch, see under Sacher-Masoch, Leopold von

von Schrötter, see under Schrötter, Leopold von

von Spee, see under Spee, Ferdinand Graf von

von Willebrand, Erik Adolph, Finnish physician, 1870-1949.
   von Willebrand disease – a hemorrhagic diathesis characterized by the tendency to bleed primarily from mucous membranes.

Voorhees, James D., U.S. obstetrician, 1869-1929.
   Voorhees bag – once used for manipulation of the uterus.

Voorhoeve, N., Dutch radiologist, 1879-1927.
   Voorhoeve disease – linear striations seen radiographically in the metaphyses of long and flat bones. *SYN:* osteopathia striata

Voss, D.E.
   Knott-Voss method of exercise – *SYN:* Kabat method of exercise

Vossius, Adolf, German pathologist, 1855-1925.
   Vossius lenticular ring – a ring-shaped opacity found on the anterior lens capsule after contusion of the eye.

Vulpian, Edme Felix Albert, French physician, 1826-1887.
   Vulpian atrophy – progressive spinal muscular atrophy beginning in the shoulder. *SYN:* scapulohumeral atrophy

Vvdenskii, var. of Wedensky

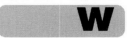

Waage, P., Norwegian chemist, 1833-1900.
Guldberg-Waage law – see under Guldberg

Waaler, Erik, Norwegian biologist *1903.
Rose-Waaler test – see under Rose, H.M.

Waardenburg, Petrus Johannes, Dutch ophthalmologist, 1886-1979.
Waardenburg syndrome – *SYN:* Mende syndrome

Wachendorf, Eberhard J., German botanist and anatomist, 1702-1758.
Wachendorf membrane – the protoplasmic boundary of all cells that
controls permeability and may serve other functions through surface
specializations. *SYN:* cell membrane; pupillary membrane

Wachstein, Max, U.S. histologist and pathologist, 1905-1965.
Wachstein-Meissel stain for calcium-magnesium-ATPase – enzyme
activity is generally demonstrated at cell membranes.

Wächter, Herman J.G., German pathologist, *1878.
Bracht-Wächter bodies – see under Bracht
Bracht-Wächter lesion – see under Bracht

Wada, John A., Japanese-Canadian neurosurgeon, *1924.
Wada test – unilateral internal carotid injection of amobarbital to determine
the laterality of speech.

Waddington, Conrad, English embryologist and geneticist, 1905-1975.
waddingtonian homeostasis – *SYN:* homeorrhesis

Wadsworth, Guy W., Jr., U.S. psychologist, *1901.
Humm-Wadsworth Temperament Scale – personality inventory.

Wagner, Hans, Swiss ophthalmologist, *1905.
Wagner disease – progressive liquefaction and destruction of the vitreous
humor with grayish-white preretinal membranes, myopia, cataract,

retinal detachment, and hyperpigmentation and hypopigmentation. *SYN:* hyaloideoretinal degeneration; Wagner syndrome

Wagner syndrome – *SYN:* Wagner disease

Wagner-Jauregg, Julius, winner of 1927 Nobel Prize for work related to malaria inoculation for treating dementia paralytica.

Wagstaffe, William, English surgeon, 1843-1910.
Wagstaffe fracture – fracture with displacement of the medial malleolus.

Waksman, Selman Abraham, winner of 1952 Nobel Prize for discovery of streptomycin.

Walcher, Gustav A., German obstetrician, 1856-1935.
Walcher position – obsolete term for a supine position of the parturient woman, with the lower extremities falling over the edge of the table.

Wald, George, joint winner of 1967 Nobel Prize for work related to the eye.

Waldenström, Jan G., Swedish physician, *1906.
Waldenström macroglobulinemia – *SYN:* hyperglobulinemic purpura; Waldenström purpura; Waldenström syndrome
Waldenström purpura – *SYN:* Waldenström macroglobulinemia
Waldenström syndrome – *SYN:* Waldenström macroglobulinemia
Waldenström test – a test for porphyrin in the urine.

Waldenström, Johann Henning, Swedish surgeon, *1877.
Waldenström disease – juvenile osteochondritis.

Waldeyer, Heinrich G. von, German anatomist and pathologist, 1836-1921.
Waldeyer fascia – rectal fascia.
Waldeyer fluid
Waldeyer forceps
Waldeyer fossae
Waldeyer glands – glands near the margins of the eyelids.
Waldeyer sheath – *SYN:* Waldeyer space
Waldeyer space – the tubular space between the bladder wall and the intramural portion of the ureter. *SYN:* Waldeyer sheath
Waldeyer sulcus
Waldeyer throat ring – the broken ring of lymphoid tissue, formed of the lingual, faucial, and pharyngeal tonsils. *SYN:* lymphoid ring
Waldeyer tract – *SYN:* Waldeyer zonal layer
Waldeyer zonal layer – a longitudinal bundle of thin, unmyelinated and poorly myelinated fibers capping the apex of the posterior horn of the spinal gray matter. *SYN:* dorsolateral fasciculus; Waldeyer tract

Walker, Arthur Earl, U.S. neurologist, *1907.
Dandy-Walker syndrome – see under Dandy
Walker tractotomy – a mesencephalic spinothalamic tractotomy.
Walker-Warburg syndrome – a congenital disorder, usually fatal before age one.

Walker, James, English gynecologist, *1916.
Walker chart – a system of plotting the relative fetal and placental sizes.

Walker, J.T. Ainslie, English chemist, 1868-1930.
Rideal-Walker coefficient – see under Rideal
Rideal-Walker method

Walker, William A., U.S. pediatrician, *1937.
Marden-Walker syndrome – see under Marden

Wallace, Alexander Burns, Scottish plastic surgeon, *1903.
Wallace rule of nines – a guide to assist estimating proportion of body surface affected by burns.

Wallenberg, Adolf, German physician, 1862-1949.
Wallenberg syndrome – a syndrome usually due to thrombosis.
    SYN: posterior inferior cerebellar artery syndrome

Waller, Augustus V., English physiologist, 1816-1870.
wallerian degeneration – degenerative changes in the distal segment of a peripheral nerve fiber when its continuity with its cell body is interrupted by a focal lesion. *SYN:* orthograde degeneration; secondary degeneration

Walsh, Patrick Craig, U.S. urologist, *1938.
neurovascular bundle of Walsh – the anatomic structure composed of capsular arteries and veins to the prostate and cavernous nerves that provides the macroscopic landmark used during nerve-sparing radical pelvic surgery.
Walsh procedure – nerve-sparing radical retropubic prostatectomy.

Walshe, J.J., U.S. physician.
Magoss-Walshe syndrome – see under Magoss

Walthard, Max, Swiss gynecologist, 1867-1933.

Walthard cell rest – a nest of epithelial cells occurring in the peritoneum of the uterine tubes or ovary.

Walther, August F., German anatomist, 1688-1746.

Walther canals – from 8 to 20 small ducts of the sublingual salivary gland that open into the mouth on the surface of the sublingual fold. *SYN:* minor sublingual ducts; Walther ducts

Walther ducts – *SYN:* Walther canals

Walther ganglion – the most inferior, unpaired ganglion of the sympathetic trunk. *SYN:* ganglion impar

Walther plexus – the portion of the internal carotid plexus in the cavernous sinus. *SYN:* intracavernous plexus

Walther, Augustine Friedrich, German surgeon and gynecologist, 1688-1746.

Walther catheter

Walther clamp

Walther dilator

Walther forceps

Walther sound

Walther tissue forceps

Walther trocar

Wang, Chung Yik, Chinese pathologist, 1889-1931.

Wang test – a quantitative test for indican.

Wangensteen, Owen H., U.S. surgeon, 1898-1981.

Wangensteen apparatus

Wangensteen awl

Wangensteen carrier

Wangensteen clamp

Wangensteen colostomy

Wangensteen dissector

Wangensteen drain

Wangensteen drainage – continuous drainage by suction through an indwelling gastric or duodenal tube.

Wangensteen dressing

Wangensteen duodenal tube

Wangensteen forceps

Wangensteen herniorrhaphy

Wangensteen needle

Wangensteen needle holder

Wangensteen suction – a modified siphon that maintains constant negative pressure, used with a duodenal tube for the relief of gastric and intestinal distention. *SYN:* Wangensteen tube

Wangensteen tissue inverter

Wangensteen trocar

Wangensteen tube – *SYN:* Wangensteen suction

Warburg, Mette, 20th century Danish ophthalmologist.

Norrie-Warburg syndrome – *SYN:* Norrie disease

Walker-Warburg syndrome – see under Walker, Arthur Earl

Warburg, Otto, German biochemist and Nobel laureate, 1883-1970.

Barcroft-Warburg apparatus – *SYN:* Warburg apparatus

Barcroft-Warburg technique – *SYN:* Warburg apparatus

Warburg apparatus – measures the oxygen consumption of incubated tissue slices by manometric measurement of changes in gas pressure produced by oxygen absorption in an enclosed flask. *SYN:* Barcroft-Warburg apparatus; Barcroft-Warburg technique

Warburg-Lipmann-Dickens-Horecker shunt – *SYN:* Dickens shunt

Warburg old yellow enzyme – a flavoprotein oxidizing NADPH to $NADP^+$. *SYN:* NADPH dehydrogenase

Warburg respiratory enzyme – a system of cytochromes and their oxidases that participate in respiratory processes. *SYN:* Atmungsferment

Warburg theory – that the development of cancer is due to irreversible damage to the respiratory mechanism of cells, leading to the selective multiplication of cells with increased glycolytic metabolism, both aerobic and anaerobic.

Ward, Frederick O., English osteologist, 1818-1877.

Ward triangle – an area of diminished density in the trabecular pattern of the neck of the femur.

Ward, Owen C., 20th century Irish pediatrician.

Romano-Ward syndrome – see under Romano

Ward-Romano syndrome – *SYN:* Romano-Ward syndrome

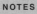

Wardrop, James, English surgeon, 1782-1869.
  Wardrop disease – acute onychia occurring spontaneously in debilitated
    patients, or in response to slight trauma. *SYN:* onychia maligna
  Wardrop method – for treatment of aneurysm.

Warfarin, Wisconsin Alumni Research Foundation (WARF).
  Warfarin – oral anticoagulant, named for the foundation.

Warm Springs, named for the Warm Springs Foundation in Georgia, where
the crutch was made.
  Warm Springs crutch – *SYN:* Everett crutch

Warren, W. Dean, U.S. surgeon, 1924-1989.
  Warren flap
  Warren incision
  Warren-Mack rotating drill
  Warren shunt – anastomosis of the splenic end of the divided splenic vein
    to the left renal vein. *SYN:* distal splenorenal shunt

Wartenberg, Robert, German neurologist, 1887-1956.
  Wartenberg sign
  Wartenberg symptom – intense pruritus of the tip of the nose and nostrils
    in cases of cerebral tumor.

Warthin, Aldred S., U.S. pathologist, 1866-1931.
  Warthin area
  Warthin-Finkeldey cells – giant cells with multiple overlapping nuclei,
    found in lymphoid tissue in measles, especially during the prodromal
    stage. *SYN:* Finkeldey cells
  Warthin-Starry silver stain – a stain for spirochetes in which preparations
    are incubated in 1% silver nitrate solution followed by a developer.
  Warthin-Starry staining method
  Warthin tumor – a benign glandular tumor, usually arising in the parotid
    gland. *SYN:* adenolymphoma

Wasmann, Adolphus, 19th century German anatomist.
  Wasmann glands – branched tubular glands lying in the mucosa of the
    fundus and body of the stomach. *SYN:* gastric glands

Wassermann, August P. von, German bacteriologist, 1866-1925.
  provocative Wassermann test – an obsolete test of historical interest
    only.
  Wassermann antibody – evoked during syphilitic infection.
  Wassermann reaction – *SYN:* Wassermann test

Wassermann test – a complement-fixation test used in the diagnosis of syphilis. *SYN:* Wassermann reaction

Waterhouse, Rupert, English physician, 1873-1958.
Friderichsen-Waterhouse syndrome – *SYN:* Waterhouse-Friderichsen syndrome
Waterhouse-Friderichsen syndrome – a condition characterized by vomiting, diarrhea, extensive purpura, cyanosis, tonic-clonic convulsions, and circulatory collapse. *SYN:* acute fulminating meningococcal septicemia; Friderichsen syndrome; Friderichsen-Waterhouse syndrome

Waters, Charles Alexander, U.S. radiologist, 1888-1961.
Waters view radiograph – *SYN:* maxillary sinus radiograph

Waters, Edward G., U.S. obstetrician and gynecologist, *1898.
Waters operation – an extraperitoneal cesarean section with a supravesical approach.
Waters position

Waterston, David J., English thoracic and pediatric surgeon, *1910.
Waterston operation – a surgically created anastomosis between the pulmonary artery and the ascending aorta to palliate adult tetralogy of Fallot.
Waterston shunt – creation of a narrow opening between the ascending aorta and the subjacent right pulmonary artery.

Watson, Cecil J., U.S. physician, 1901-1983.
Watson-Schwartz test – urine test using Ehrlich reagent for acute intermittent porphyria.

Watson, James Dewey, U.S. geneticist and Nobel laureate, *1928.
Watson-Crick helix – the helical structure assumed by two strands of deoxyribonucleic acid. *SYN:* DNA helix; double helix; twin helix

Watson-Jones, Sir Reginald, English orthopedic surgeon, 1902-1972.
Watson-Jones anterior approach

Watson-Jones approach
Watson-Jones arthrodesis
Watson-Jones bone gouge
Watson-Jones bone lever
Watson-Jones classification of tibial tubercle avulsion fracture
Watson-Jones dressing
Watson-Jones elevator
Watson-Jones fracture repair
Watson-Jones frame
Watson-Jones gouge
Watson-Jones guide pin
Watson-Jones incision
Watson-Jones lateral approach
Watson-Jones ligament reconstruction
Watson-Jones nail
Watson-Jones operation
Watson-Jones procedure
Watson-Jones reconstruction
Watson-Jones repair
Watson-Jones tibial fracture classification
Watson-Jones traction
Watson-Jones tractor

Watt, James, Scottish engineer, 1736-1819.
    watt (W) – the SI unit of electrical power.

Way, Stanley, English obstetrician-gynecologist.
    Stanley Way procedure – a radical vulvectomy.
    Way operation

Weber, Ernst Heinrich, German physiologist and anatomist, 1795-1878.
    Fechner-Weber law – *SYN:* Weber-Fechner law
    Weber experiment – if the peripheral end of the divided vagus nerve is stimulated, the heart is arrested in diastole.
    Weber-Fechner law – the intensity of a sensation varies by a series of equal increments as the strength of the stimulus is increased geometrically. *SYN:* Fechner-Weber law; Weber law
    Weber law – *SYN:* Weber-Fechner law
    Weber paradox – if a muscle is loaded beyond its power to contract, it may elongate.

Weber, Frederick Parkes, English physician, 1863-1962.
    Klippel-Trenaunay-Weber syndrome – see under Klippel

Rendu-Osler-Weber syndrome – see under Rendu
Sturge-Kalischer-Weber syndrome – *SYN:* Sturge-Weber syndrome
Sturge-Weber disease – *SYN:* Sturge-Weber syndrome
Sturge-Weber syndrome – see under Sturge
Weber-Christian disease – a group of conditions with recurrent subcutaneous nodules, with or without fever or suppuration, followed by depression of the overlying skin. *SYN:* Christian disease (2); nodular nonsuppurative panniculitis
Weber-Cockayne syndrome – epidermolysis bullosa of the hands and feet.

Weber, Friedrich Eugen, German otologist, 1823-1891.
Weber test – determines unilateral hearing loss by using a vibrating tuning fork.

Weber, Helga, German physician.
Mietens-Weber syndrome – see under Mietens

Weber, Moritz Ignaz, German anatomist, 1795-1875.
Weber glands – muciparous glands at the border of the tongue on either side posteriorly.
Weber organ – a minute pouch in the prostate opening on the summit of the seminal colliculus. *SYN:* prostatic utricle

Weber, Rainer, 20th century U.S. pathologist.
Weber stain – a modified trichrome stain for microsporidian spores.

Weber, Sir Hermann David, English physician, 1823-1918.
Weber sign – *SYN:* Weber syndrome
Weber syndrome – midbrain tegmentum lesion characterized by ipsilateral oculomotor nerve paresis and contralateral paralysis of the extremities, face, and tongue. *SYN:* Weber sign

Weber, Wilhelm E., German physicist, 1804-1891.
Weber point – a point situated 1 cm below the promontory of the sacrum, believed by Weber to represent the center of gravity of the body.

NOTES

Weber triangle – an area on the sole of the foot.

Webster, John, English chemist, 1878-1927.
Webster test – for trinitrotoluene in the urine.

Webster, John C., U.S. gynecologist, 1863-1950.
Webster operation – *SYN:* Baldy operation

Wechsler, David, U.S. psychologist, *1896.
Wechsler Adult Intelligence Scale – modification of the Wechsler-Bellevue scale.
Wechsler-Bellevue scale – a measure of general intelligence superseded by the Wechsler Adult Intelligence Scale and its subsequent revision.
Wechsler Intelligence Scale for Children – intelligence test for children between the ages of 5 years to 15 years, 11 months.
Wechsler Intelligence Scale for Children-Revised
Wechsler intelligence scales – scales for the measurement of general intelligence in children and adults.
Wechsler Memory Scale
Wechsler Preschool and Primary Scale of Intelligence – intelligence test for children between the ages 4 years to 6 years, 6 months.

Wecker, Louis H. de, see under de Wecker

Wedensky, (Vvdenskii), Nikolai I., Russian neurophysiologist, 1852-1922.
Wedensky effect – a relatively long enhancing effect following application of a maximal shock or stimulus to a neuromuscular preparation.
Wedensky facilitation – the additive effect of a series of electric shocks.
Wedensky inhibition – inhibition of muscle response as a result of a series of rapidly repeated stimuli to the motor nerve.

Weeks, John E., U.S. ophthalmologist, 1853-1949.
Koch-Weeks bacillus – see under Koch, Robert
Weeks bacillus – *SYN:* Koch-Weeks bacillus

Wegener, Friedrich, German pathologist, 1907-1990.
Wegener granulomatosis – characterized by necrotizing granulomas and ulceration of the upper respiratory tract, with purulent rhinorrhea, nasal obstruction, and sometimes with otorrhea, hemoptysis, pulmonary infiltration and cavitation, and fever.

Wegner, Friedrich R.G., German pathologist, 1843-1917.
Wegner disease – inflammation of the epiphyseal line associated with congenital syphilis. *SYN:* syphilitic osteochondritis
Wegner line – a narrow whitish line at the junction of the epiphysis and diaphysis of a long bone, related to syphilitic epiphysitis.

Weibel, Ewald R., Swiss physician, *1929.
Weibel-Palade bodies – rod-shaped bundles of microtubules seen by electron microscopy in vascular endothelial cells.

Weichselbaum, Anthony, Austrian pathologist, 1845-1920.
Fraenkel-Weichselbaum pneumococcus – *SYN:* Fraenkel pneumococcus
Weichselbaum coccus – a species found in the human nasopharynx, the causative agent of meningococcal meningitis. *SYN: Neisseria meningitidis*

Weidel, Hugo, Austrian chemist, 1849-1899.
Weidel reaction – a reaction showing the presence of xanthine.

Weigert, Carl, German pathologist, 1845-1904.
Weigert-Gram stain – a stain for bacteria in tissues in which sections are stained in alum-hematoxylin, then in eosin, aniline methyl violet, and Lugol solution.
Weigert iodine solution – an iodine-potassium iodide mixture used as a reagent to alter crystal and methyl violet so that they are retained by certain bacteria and fungi.
Weigert iron hematoxylin stain
Weigert law – the loss or destruction of a part or element in the organic world is likely to result in compensatory replacement and overproduction of tissue during the process of regeneration or repair.
   SYN: overproduction theory
Weigert stain – dye used in the study of myelinated axons.
Weigert stain for actinomyces
Weigert stain for elastin
Weigert stain for fibrin
Weigert stain for myelin
Weigert stain for neuroglia

Weigl, Egon, Romanian-born psychologist.
Weigl-Goldstein-Scheerer test – a concept formation test.

Weil, Adolf, German physician, 1848-1916.
Larrey-Weil disease – *SYN:* Weil disease

Weil disease – leptospirosis. *SYN:* infectious icterus; infectious jaundice; Larrey-Weil disease

Weil, Edmund, Austrian physician, 1880-1922.
Weil-Felix reaction – *SYN:* Weil-Felix test
Weil-Felix test – for the presence and type of rickettsial disease. *SYN:* Weil-Felix reaction

Weil, Ludwig A., German dentist, 1849-1895.
Weil basal layer – the layer beneath the odontoblasts of the tooth. *SYN:* Weil basal zone
Weil basal zone – *SYN:* Weil basal layer

Weill, Georges, French ophthalmologist, 1866-1952.
Weill-Marchesani syndrome – *SYN:* Marchesani syndrome
Weill syndrome – *SYN:* Adie syndrome

Weill, Jean A., French physician, *1903.
Leri-Weill disease – *SYN:* dyschondrosteosis
Leri-Weill syndrome – *SYN:* dyschondrosteosis

Weinberg, Michel, French pathologist, 1868-1940.
Weinberg reaction – a complement fixation test of the presence of hydatid disease.

Weinberg, Wilhelm, German physician, 1862-1937.
Hardy-Weinberg equilibrium – see under Hardy, Godfrey H.
Hardy-Weinberg law – see under Hardy, Godfrey H.

Weingarten, R.J., German physician.
Weingarten syndrome – tropical pulmonary eosinophilia.

Weir, Robert F., U.S. surgeon, 1838-1927.
Weir operation – obsolete term for appendicostomy.

Weir Mitchell, see under Mitchell, Silas Weir

Weisbach, Albin, Austrian anthropologist, 1837-1914.
Weisbach angle – a craniometric angle formed by the junction at the alveolar point of lines passing from the basion and from the middle of the frontonasal suture.

Weismann, August Friedrich Leopold, German biologist, 1834-1914.
weismannism – theory of the noninheritance of acquired characteristics.

Weiss, Nathan, Austrian physician, 1851-1883.
Weiss gold dilator
Weiss sign – *SYN:* Chvostek sign

Weiss, Soma, U.S. physician, 1898-1942.
   Charcot-Weiss-Baker syndrome – see under Charcot
   Mallory-Weiss lesion – see under Mallory, George Kenneth
   Mallory-Weiss syndrome – see under Mallory, George Kenneth
   Mallory-Weiss tear – *SYN:* Mallory-Weiss lesion

Weissenbach, Raymond Joseph Emil, French physician, 1885-1963.
   Thibierge-Weissenbach syndrome – see under Thibierge

Weissenbacher, G., Austrian physician.
   Weissenbacher-Zweymüller syndrome – multiple congenital anomalies.
     SYN: otospondylomegaepiphyseal dysplasia

Weitbrecht, Josias, German-Russian anatomist, 1702-1747.
   Weitbrecht cartilage – the articular disk of fibrocartilage usually found
     between the acromial end of the clavicle and the medial border of the
     acromion. *SYN:* articular disk of acromioclavicular joint
   Weitbrecht cord – *SYN:* Weitbrecht ligament
   Weitbrecht fibers – one of several longitudinal folds of the articular
     capsule of the hip joint. *SYN:* retinaculum capsulae articularis coxae
   Weitbrecht foramen – an opening in the articular capsule of the shoulder
     joint, communicating with the subtendinous bursa of the subscapularis
     muscle.
   Weitbrecht ligament – a slender band extending from the lateral part of
     the coronoid process of the ulna distad and laterad to the radius
     immediately distal to the bicipital tuberosity. *SYN:* oblique ligament of
     elbow joint; Weitbrecht cord

Welander, Lisa, Swedish neurologist, *1909.
   Kugelberg-Welander disease – see under Kugelberg
   Welander myopathy
   Wohlfart-Kugelberg-Welander disease – *SYN:* Kugelberg-Welander
     disease

Welch, William H., U.S. pathologist, 1850-1934.
   Clostridium welchii – *SYN:* Welch bacillus

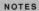
NOTES

Welch bacillus – the chief causative agent of gas gangrene, also one of the most common causes of food poisoning in the U.S. *SYN: Clostridium perfringens*; *Clostridium welchii*

Welcker, Hermann, German anthropologist and anatomist, 1822-1898.
Welcker angle – the anterior inferior angle of the parietal bone.
SYN: sphenoidal angle of parietal bone

Weller, Thomas Huckle, joint winner of 1954 Nobel Prize for work related to the poliomyelitis virus.

Wells, G.C., 20th century English dermatologist.
Wells syndrome – recurrent cellulitis followed by brawny edematous skin lesions. *SYN:* eosinophilic cellulitis

Wells, Michael Vernon, 20th century English physician.
Muckle-Wells syndrome – see under Muckle

Wenckebach, Karel F., Dutch internist, 1864-1940.
Wenckebach block – *SYN:* Wenckebach phenomenon
Wenckebach period – a sequence of cardiac cycles in the electrocardiogram ending in a dropped beat due to A-V block.
Wenckebach phenomenon – progressive lengthening of conduction time in cardiac tissue, with ultimate dropping of a beat. *SYN:* Wenckebach block

Wenzel, Joseph, German anatomist and physiologist, 1768-1808.
Wenzel ventricle – a slitlike, fluid-filled space of variable width between the left and right transparent septum. *SYN:* cavity of septum pellucidum

Wepfer, Johann J., 1620-1695.
Wepfer glands – small, branched, coiled tubular glands in the duodenum that secrete an alkaline mucoid substance that serves to neutralize gastric juice. *SYN:* duodenal glands

Werdnig, Guido, Austrian neurologist, 1862-1919.
Werdnig-Hoffmann disease – *SYN:* Werdnig-Hoffmann muscular atrophy
Werdnig-Hoffmann muscular atrophy – progressive dysfunction of the anterior horn cells in the spinal cord and brainstem cranial nerves, with profound weakness and bulbar dysfunction. *SYN:* infantile spinal muscular atrophy; Werdnig-Hoffmann disease

Werlhof, Paul G., German physician, 1699-1767.
Werlhof disease – obsolete term for idiopathic thrombocytopenic purpura.

Wermer, Paul, U.S. internist, 1898-1975.
  Wermer syndrome – Zollinger-Ellison syndrome with additional endocrine and glandular disorders.

Wernekinck, Friedrich C.G., German anatomist and physician, 1798-1835.
  Wernekinck commissure – the decussation of the brachia conjunctiva before their entrance into the red nucleus of the tegmentum.
  Wernekinck decussation – the decussation of the left and right superior cerebellar peduncles in the tegmentum of the caudal mesencephalon. *SYN:* decussation of superior cerebellar peduncles

Werner, F.F., early 20th century German chemist.
  Werner test – *SYN:* thyroid suppression test

Werner, Otto, German physician, 1879-1936.
  Werner disease – hereditary disorder characterized by premature aging. *SYN:* progeria adultorum; Werner syndrome
  Werner syndrome – *SYN:* Werner disease

Wernicke, Karl, German neurologist, 1848-1905.
  Gayet-Wernicke syndrome – *SYN:* Wernicke syndrome
  Wernicke aphasia – impairment in the comprehension of spoken and written words. *SYN:* Bastian aphasia; sensory aphasia
  Wernicke area – *SYN:* Wernicke center
  Wernicke center – the region of the cerebral cortex thought to be essential for understanding and formulating coherent, propositional speech. *SYN:* sensory speech center; Wernicke area; Wernicke field; Wernicke region; Wernicke zone
  Wernicke cramp – psychogenic muscle cramp. *SYN:* cramp neurosis
  Wernicke disease – *SYN:* Wernicke syndrome
  Wernicke encephalopathy – *SYN:* Wernicke syndrome
  Wernicke field – *SYN:* Wernicke center
  Wernicke-Korsakoff encephalopathy
  Wernicke-Korsakoff syndrome – the coexistence of Wernicke and Korsakoff syndromes.

NOTES

Wernicke-Mann hemiplegia – extremity hemiplegia that is partial.
  SYN: Wernicke-Mann paralysis
Wernicke-Mann paralysis – *SYN:* Wernicke-Mann hemiplegia
Wernicke radiation – the massive, fanlike fiber system passing from the
  lateral geniculate body of the thalamus to the visual cortex. *SYN:* optic
  radiation
Wernicke reaction – in hemianopia, a reaction due to damage of the optic
  tract, consisting in loss of pupillary constriction when the light is directed
  to the blind side of the retina. *SYN:* Wernicke sign
Wernicke region – *SYN:* Wernicke center
Wernicke sign – *SYN:* Wernicke reaction
Wernicke syndrome – a condition encountered in chronic alcoholics,
  characterized by disturbances in ocular motility, pupillary alterations,
  nystagmus, and ataxia with tremors. *SYN:* Gayet disease; Gayet-Wernicke
  syndrome; superior hemorrhagic polioencephalitis; Wernicke disease;
  Wernicke encephalopathy;
Wernicke zone – *SYN:* Wernicke center

Wertheim, Ernst, Austrian gynecologist, 1864-1920.
  Schauta-Wertheim operation
  Wertheim clamp
  Wertheim deep surgery scissors
  Wertheim forceps
  Wertheim hysterectomy
  Wertheim needle holder
  Wertheim operation – a radical surgery for carcinoma of the uterus.
  Wertheim vaginal forceps

Werther, J., 20th century German physician.
  Werther disease – recurrent eruption of vesicles, papules, and
  papulonecrotic lesions on the buttocks and extensor surfaces of the
  extremities, accompanied by fever, sore throat, diarrhea, and
  eosinophilia. *SYN:* dermatitis nodularis necrotica

Wesselsbron, a town in South Africa where the causative agent for the fever
was first isolated.
  Wesselsbron disease – *SYN:* Wesselsbron fever
  Wesselsbron fever – a mosquito-borne disease of sheep and humans
  caused by the Wesselsbron disease virus. *SYN:* Wesselsbron disease;
  Wesselsbron virus
  Wesselsbron virus – *SYN:* Wesselsbron fever

West, Charles, English physician, 1816-1898.

  West syndrome – an encephalopathy in infancy characterized by infantile spasms, arrest of psychomotor development, and hypsarhythmia.

Westberg, Friedrich, 19th century German physician.

  Westberg space – the space surrounding the origin of the aorta which is invested with the pericardium.

Westergren, Alf, Swedish physician, *1891.

  Westergren method – a procedure for estimating the sedimentation rate of red blood cells in fluid blood.

  Westergren sedimentation rate

West Nile, a province in Uganda where the virus was first discovered in 1937.

  West Nile encephalitis virus – a Flavivirus in the family Flaviviridae.
    SYN: West Nile virus

  West Nile fever – a febrile illness caused by West Nile virus, a member of the family Flaviviridae, and characterized by headache, fever, maculopapular rash, myalgia, lymphadenopathy, and leukopenia; spread by *Culex* mosquitoes.

  West Nile virus – *SYN:* West Nile encephalitis virus

Westphal, Karl Friederich Otto, German neuroanatomist and psychiatrist, 1833-1890.

  Edinger-Westphal nucleus – see under Edinger

  Erb-Westphal sign – see under Erb

  Strümpell-Westphal disease – *SYN:* Wilson disease

  Westphal ataxia – *SYN:* Westphal-Leyden syndrome

  Westphal disease – *SYN:* Wilson disease

  Westphal-Erb sign – *SYN:* Erb-Westphal sign

  Westphal-Leyden syndrome – absence of knee jerk reflex characteristic of neurosyphilitic disease. *SYN:* Leyden ataxia; Westphal ataxia

  Westphal phenomenon – *SYN:* Erb-Westphal sign

  Westphal-Piltz phenomenon – *SYN:* Piltz sign

W

NOTES

Westphal pseudosclerosis – *SYN:* Wilson disease
Westphal pupillary reflex – *SYN:* Piltz sign
Westphal sign – *SYN:* Erb-Westphal sign
Westphal-Strümpell pseudosclerosis – *SYN:* Wilson disease

Wetzel, Norman C., U.S. pediatrician, 1897-1984.
Wetzel grid – chart of growth, plotting height, weight, physical fitness and related aspects of young and adolescent children.

Wever, Ernest Glen, U.S. psychologist, *1902.
Wever-Bray effect – *SYN:* Wever-Bray phenomenon
Wever-Bray phenomenon – action potentials in the acoustic nerve that correspond to auditory stimuli reaching the cochlea. *SYN:* Wever-Bray effect

Weyers, Helmut, 20th century German pediatrician.
Weyers-Thier syndrome – microphthalmia, colobomas, or anophthalmia with small orbit, twisted face due to unilateral dysplasia of maxilla, macrostomia with malformed teeth and malocclusion, vertebral malformations, and branched and hypoplastic ribs. *SYN:* oculovertebral dysplasia

Wharton, Thomas, English anatomist and physician, 1614-1673.
Wharton duct – of the salivary gland. *SYN:* submandibular duct
Wharton jelly – the mucous connective tissue of the umbilical cord.

Wheatstone, Charles, English physicist, 1802-1875.
Wheatstone bridge – an apparatus for measuring electrical resistance.

Wheeler, Henry Lord, U.S. chemist, 1867-1914.
Wheeler-Johnson test – cystosine or uracil when treated with bromine yields dialuric acid which gives a green color with excess of barium hydroxide.

Wheeler, John M., U.S. ophthalmologist, 1879-1938.
Wheeler cyclodialysis system
Wheeler cystotome
Wheeler discission knife
Wheeler eye implant
Wheeler eye sphere implant
Wheeler graft material
Wheeler halving procedure
Wheeler incision
Wheeler knife
Wheeler malleable-shape knife

Wheeler method – a surgical procedure for correction of cicatricial ectropion.
Wheeler prosthesis
Wheeler spatula
Wheeler vessel forceps

Wheelhouse, Claudius G., English surgeon, 1826-1909.
Wheelhouse operation – obsolete term for external urethrotomy via an external opening in the perineum or penile skin. *SYN:* external urethrotomy

Wheelock, Frank Cawthore, Jr., U.S. physician, *1918.
McKittrick-Wheelock syndrome – *SYN:* McKittrick syndrome

Whipple, Allen Oldfather, U.S. surgeon, 1881-1963.
Whipple incision
Whipple operation – excision of all or part of the pancreas together with the duodenum. *SYN:* pancreatoduodenectomy
Whipple pancreatectomy
Whipple triad – diagnostic of pancreatic insulinoma.

Whipple, George Hayt, U.S. pathologist and Nobel laureate, 1878-1976.
Whipple disease – a rare disease characterized by steatorrhea, frequently generalized lymphadenopathy, arthritis, fever, and cough.

Whitaker, Robert, English surgeon, *1939.
Whitaker test – a pressure-perfusion test in the upper urinary tract to demonstrate impediment of flow.

White, Cleveland, U.S. physician.
Marshall-White syndrome – see under Marshall, Wallace

White, Harry H., U.S. physician.
May-White syndrome – see under May, Duane L.

White, Paul Dudley, U.S. cardiologist, 1886-1973.
Bland-White-Garland syndrome – see under Bland
Lee-White method – see under Lee, Roger I.

NOTES

McGinn-White sign – see under McGinn, Louis
Wolff-Parkinson-White syndrome – see under Wolff, Louis

Whitehead, Walter, English surgeon, 1840-1913.
Whitehead deformity – circumferential mucosal ectropion at the anus following Whitehead operation.
Whitehead operation – excision of hemorrhoids by two circular incisions above and below involved veins, allowing normal mucosa to be pulled down and sutured to anal skin.

Whitfield, Arthur, English dermatologist, 1867-1947.
Whitfield ointment – a combination of salicylic and benzoic acids used to treat superficial dermatophyte infection of the skin.

Whitman, Royal, U.S. surgeon, 1857-1946.
Whitman arch support
Whitman arthroplasty
Whitman femoral neck reconstruction
Whitman fracture appliance
Whitman fracture frame
Whitman frame – similar to the Bradford frame but with curved sides.
Whitman operation
Whitman osteotomy
Whitman paralysis
Whitman plate
Whitman talectomy procedure
Whitman technique

Whitmore, Alfred, English surgeon, 1876-1946.
Whitmore bacillus – a species found in cases of melioidosis in humans and other animals and in soil and water in tropical regions.
SYN: Pseudomonas pseudomallei
Whitmore disease – an infectious disease of rodents in India and Southeast Asia that is caused by *Pseudomonas pseudomallei* and is communicable to humans. *SYN:* melioidosis

Whitnall, Samuel E., English anatomist, 1876-1952.
Whitnall tubercle – *SYN:* orbital tubercle of zygomatic bone

Whitney, Donald Ransom, U.S. statistician, *1915.
Mann-Whitney test – see under Mann, Henry Berthold

Wiberg, Gunnar, Swedish orthopedic surgeon, 1902-1988.
angle of Wiberg – frontal radiographic view of the pelvis measuring the relationship between the femoral head and the acetabulum.

Wickham, Louis-Frédéric, French dermatologist, 1861-1913.
   Wickham striae – fine whitish lines having a network arrangement on the surface of lichen planus papules.

Widal, Georges Fernand Isidor, French physician, 1862-1929.
   Gruber-Widal reaction – *SYN:* Widal reaction
   Hayem-Widal syndrome – see under Hayem
   Widal and Abrami test – for paroxysmal hemoglobinuria.
   Widal reaction – agglutination reaction as applied to the diagnosis of typhoid. *SYN:* Gruber reaction; Gruber-Widal reaction
   Widal syndrome – *SYN:* Hayem-Widal syndrome

Wiedemann, Hans Rudolf, German pediatrician, *1915.
   Beckwith-Wiedemann syndrome – see under Beckwith
   Maroteaux-Spranger-Wiedemann syndrome – see under Maroteaux
   Wiedemann syndrome – deformities in neonates caused by thalidomide ingestion during pregnancy.

Wiener, H.
   tract of Münzer and Wiener – see under Münzer

Wieschaus, Eric F., joint winner of 1995 Nobel Prize for work related to genetics and early development of embryo.

Wiesel, Torsten N., joint winner of 1981 Nobel Prize for work related to vision.

Wiethe, Camillo, Austrian otologist, 1888-1949.
   Urbach-Wiethe disease – see under Urbach

Wigand, J. Heinrich, German obstetrician and gynecologist, 1766-1817.
   Wigand maneuver – assisted breech delivery with pressure above the symphysis while the fetus lies astraddle the operator's other arm.
   Wigand version

Wilbrand, H. German neuroophthalmologist, 1851-1935.
   Charcot-Wilbrand syndrome – see under Charcot

NOTES

Wilcoxon, Frank, U.S. chemist and statistician, 1892-1962.
    Wilcoxon test – nonparametric test.

Wilde, Sir William R.W., Irish oculist and otologist, 1815-1876.
    Wilde cords – transverse markings on the corpus callosum.
    Wilde triangle – area at the anterior inferior part of the tympanic
       membrane. *SYN:* pyramid of light

Wilder, Helenor C., 20th century U.S. scientist.
    Wilder stain for reticulum – a silver impregnation technique in which
       reticulum appears as black, well-defined fibers without beading and with
       a relatively clear background.

Wilder, Joseph, U.S. neuropsychiatrist, *1895.
    Wilder law of initial value – the direction of response of a body function to
       any agent depends to a large degree on the initial level of that function.
       SYN: law of initial value

Wilder, William H., U.S. ophthalmologist, 1860-1935.
    Wilder band spreader
    Wilder dilating forceps
    Wilder dilator
    Wilder lens hook
    Wilder lens loop
    Wilder lens scoop
    Wilder loupe
    Wilder retractor
    Wilder scleral depressor
    Wilder scleral self-retaining retractor
    Wilder sign – a slight twitch of the eyeball when changing its movement
       from abduction to adduction or the reverse, noted in Graves disease.
    Wilder trephine

Wildermuth, Hermann A., German psychiatrist, 1852-1907.
    Wildermuth ear – an ear in which the helix is turned backward and the
       anthelix is prominent.

Wildervanck, L.S., 20th century Dutch geneticist.
    Wildervanck syndrome – a congenital short neck on girls associated with
       paralysis of the external ocular muscles and with perceptive deafness.
       SYN: cervicooculoacoustic syndrome

Wildi, Erwin, Swiss physician.
    Morel-Wildi syndrome – see under Morel, Ferdinand

Wilhelmy, Ludwig F., German scientist, 1812-1864.
  Wilhelmy balance – a device for measuring surface tension used in a Langmuir trough to study pulmonary surfactant.

Wilke, F., German ophthalmologist.
  Meesmann-Wilke disease – *SYN:* Meesmann dystrophy
  Meesmann-Wilke syndrome – *SYN:* Meesmann dystrophy

Wilkie, David P.D., Scottish surgeon, 1882-1938.
  Wilkie artery – the right colic artery when it occasionally crosses the duodenum.
  Wilkie disease – partial or complete block of the superior mesenteric artery. *SYN:* superior mesenteric artery syndrome
  Wilkie syndrome

Wilkins, Lawson, U.S. physician, 1894-1963.
  Wilkins disease – congenital hyperplasia of the adrenals.

Wilkinson, Daryl Sheldon, 20th century English dermatologist.
  Sneddon-Wilkinson disease – see under Sneddon

Wilkinson, Robert H., English physician, *1926.
  Moncrieff-Wilkinson syndrome – *SYN:* Moncrieff syndrome

Wilkinson, Scott J., U.S. physician.
  Wilkinson syndrome – cyanosis in infants who are otherwise apparently healthy.

Wilks, Sir Samuel, English physician, 1824-1911.
  Wilks syndrome – *SYN:* myasthenia gravis

Willebrand, Erik A. von, see under von Willebrand

Willett, J. Abernethy, English obstetrician, 1872-1932.
  Willett clamp
  Willett forceps – obsolete term for a traction forceps used to treat placenta previa.

W

Willi, Heinrich, Swiss pediatrician, 1900-1971.
　Prader-Willi syndrome – see under Prader

Williams, Anna, U.S. bacteriologist, 1863-1955.
　Park-Williams bacillus – see under Park, William H.
　Park-Williams fixative – see under Park, William H.
　Williams stain – a stain for Negri bodies.

Williams, J.C.P., 20th century New Zealand cardiologist.
　Williams syndrome – multiple congenital disorders.

Williams, Paul C., U.S. orthopedic surgeon, 1900-1978.
　Williams back brace – a thoracolumbosacral brace.
　Williams brace
　Williams discectomy
　Williams discography
　Williams flexion exercise
　Williams interlocking Y nail
　Williams orthosis
　Williams procedure
　Williams rod
　Williams screwdriver
　Williams self-retaining retractor

Williamson, Carl S., U.S. surgeon, 1896-1952.
　Mann-Williamson operation – see under Mann, Frank C.
　Mann-Williamson ulcer – see under Mann, Frank C.

Williamson, Oliver K., English physician, 1866-1941.
　Williamson sign – blood pressure is lower in the leg than it is in the arm
　　on the same side of the body where there is pneumothorax or large
　　pleural effusion. *SYN:* Williamson test
　Williamson test – *SYN:* Williamson sign

Willis, Thomas, English physician, 1621-1675.
　accessorius willisii – nerve that arises by two sets of roots: cranial,
　　emerging from the side of the medulla, and spinal, emerging from the
　　ventrolateral part of the first five cervical segments of the spinal cord.
　　SYN: accessory nerve
　chordae willisii – *SYN:* Willis cords
　circle of Willis – an anastomotic circle of arteries at the base of the brain.
　　SYN: arterial circle of cerebrum
　Willis centrum nervosum – the largest and highest group of prevertebral
　　sympathetic ganglia, located on the superior part of the abdominal
　　aorta. *SYN:* celiac ganglia

Willis cords – several fibrous cords crossing the superior sagittal sinus. *SYN:* chordae willisii

Willis pancreas – a portion of the head of the pancreas formed by the superior mesenteric artery and abdominal aorta. *SYN:* uncinate process of pancreas

Willis paracusis – the apparent increase in auditory acuity of a deaf person to conversation in noisy surroundings due to a companion's unconscious voice raising. *SYN:* false paracusis

Willis pouch – obsolete term for lesser omentum.

Williston, Samuel Wendell, U.S. paleontologist, 1852-1918.
Williston law – as the vertebrate scale is ascended, the number of bones in the skull is reduced.

Wilms, Max, German surgeon, 1867-1918.
Wilms syndrome – *SYN:* Wilms tumor
Wilms tumor – a malignant renal tumor of young children. *SYN:* adenomyosarcoma; embryoma of the kidney; nephroblastoma; Wilms syndrome

Wilson, Clifford, English physician, *1906.
Kimmelstiel-Wilson disease – *SYN:* Kimmelstiel-Wilson syndrome
Kimmelstiel-Wilson syndrome – see under Kimmelstiel

Wilson, Frank Norman, U.S. cardiologist, 1890-1952.
Wilson block – the most common form of right bundle-branch block.

Wilson, James, English anatomist, physiologist, and surgeon, 1765-1821.
Wilson muscle – (1) certain fibers of the levator ani; (2) *SYN:* sphincter urethrae

Wilson, Miriam G., U.S. pediatrician, *1922.
Wilson-Mikity syndrome – a respiratory disorder occurring in small, premature infants. *SYN:* pulmonary dysmaturity syndrome

Wilson, Samuel Alexander Kinnier, U.S.-born English neurologist, 1878-1937.
Kinnier Wilson disease – *SYN:* Wilson disease (1)

NOTES

Wilson disease – (1) disorder characterized by cirrhosis, degeneration in the basal ganglia of the brain, and deposition of green pigment in the periphery of the cornea. *SYN:* Kinnier Wilson disease; Strümpell-Westphal disease; Westphal disease; Westphal pseudosclerosis; Westphal-Strümpell pseudosclerosis; Wilson syndrome; (2) generalized exfoliation with scaling of the skin and usually with erythema. *SYN:* exfoliative dermatitis

Wilson syndrome – *SYN:* Wilson disease

Wilson, Sir William J.E., English dermatologist, 1809-1884.
 Wilson lichen – eruption of flat-topped, shiny, violaceous papules on flexor surfaces, male genitalia, and buccal mucosa of unknown cause. *SYN:* lichen planus

Wimshurst, James, English engineer, 1822-1903.
 Wimshurst machine – generates static electricity.

Winckel, Franz K.L.W. von, German physician, 1837-1911.
 Winckel disease – hemoglobinuria of the newborn.

Windigo, (Wittigo), legendary human-like monster that lives in the forests of Quebec, Canada.
 Windigo psychosis – severe anxiety neurosis with special reference to food, manifested in melancholia, violence, and obsessive cannibalism, occurring among Canadian Indians.

Winiwarter, Felix von, German surgeon, 1852-1931.
 Winiwarter-Buerger disease – *SYN:* Buerger disease

Winkler, Max, Swiss physician, 1875-1952.
 Winkler disease – a benign, chronic, small, painful nodule on the helix of the ear in elderly white males. *SYN:* chondrodermatitis nodularis chronica helicis; Winkler syndrome
 Winkler syndrome – *SYN:* Winkler disease

Winslow, Jacob Benignus, Danish anatomist, physicist, and surgeon in Paris, 1669-1760.
 stellulae winslowii – capillary whorls in the lamina choroidocapillaris from which arise the venae vorticosae. *SYN:* Winslow stars
 Winslow foramen – the passage below and behind the portal hepatis connecting the two sacs of the peritoneum. *SYN:* epiploic foramen
 Winslow ligament – the cordlike ligament that passes from the lateral epicondyle of the femur to the head of the fibula. *SYN:* fibular collateral ligament

Winslow pancreas – a portion of the head of the pancreas formed by the superior mesenteric artery and abdominal aorta. *SYN:* uncinate process of pancreas

Winslow stars – *SYN:* stellulae winslowii

Winterbottom, Thomas Masterman, English physician, 1765-1859.
    Winterbottom sign – swelling of the posterior cervical lymph nodes, characteristic of early stages of African trypanosomiasis.

Winternitz, Wilhelm, Austrian physician, 1835-1917.
    Winternitz sound – a double-current catheter in which water at any desired temperature circulates.

Wintersteiner, Hugo, Austrian ophthalmologist, 1865-1918.
    Wintersteiner rosettes – found only in retinal embryonic tumors.

Wintrobe, Maxwell M., U.S. hematologist, *1901.
    Wintrobe hematocrit – using one tube, hematocrit and erythrocyte sedimentation rate is measured.

Wirsung, Johann G., German anatomist in Padua, 1600-1643.
    Wirsung canal – *SYN:* Wirsung duct
    Wirsung duct – the excretory duct of the pancreas. *SYN:* pancreatic duct; Wirsung canal

Wiskott, Alfred, 20th century German pediatrician.
    Wiskott-Aldrich syndrome – a fatal X-linked immunodeficiency disorder occurring in male children. *SYN:* Aldrich syndrome

Wissler, Hans, Swiss pediatrician, *1906.
    Wissler-Fanconi syndrome – toxic allergic hypersensitivity.
    Wissler syndrome – high intermittent fever and rash in children and adolescents.

Wistar, Caspar, U.S. biologist, 1760-1818, after whom the Wistar Institute is named.
    Wistar rats – an inbred strain of rats used for research.

NOTES

Wittigo, var. of Windigo

Witzel, Friedrich O., German surgeon, 1865-1925.
Witzel jejunostomy

Wohlfahrt, Peter, German medical writer, d. 1726.
Wohlfahrtia – a genus of larviparous dipterous flesh flies of which some species' larvae breed in ulcerated surfaces and flesh wounds of humans and animals.
Wohlfahrtia magnifica – widely distributed obligatory flesh fly whose tissue-destroying maggots invade wounds or head cavities of humans and domestic animals.
Wohlfahrtia nuba – a facultative flesh fly of Old World distribution, found in head wounds or cavities but not in dermal sores.
Wohlfahrtia opaca – *SYN: Wohlfahrtia vigil*
Wohlfahrtia vigil – produces cutaneous myiasis in human infants in the northern U.S. and southern Canada by larvae that penetrate the skin and cause boillike lesions. *SYN: Wohlfahrtia opaca*
wohlfahrtiosis – infection of humans and animals with larvae of flies of the genus *Wohlfahrtia.*

Wohlfart, Gunnar, Swedish neurologist, 1910-1961.
Gamstorp-Wohlfart syndrome – see under Gamstorp
Wohlfart-Kugelberg-Welander disease – *SYN:* Kugelberg-Welander disease

Wolf, A., 20th century U.S. pathologist.
Wolf-Orton bodies – intranuclear inclusion bodies seen in cells of malignant neoplasms, especially those of glial cell origin.

Wolfe, John R., Scottish ophthalmologist, 1824-1904.
Krause-Wolfe graft – *SYN:* Krause graft
Wolfe eye forceps
Wolfe graft – a full-thickness skin graft without any subcutaneous fat. *SYN:* Wolfe-Krause graft
Wolfe-Krause graft – *SYN:* Wolfe graft
Wolfe method
Wolfe prosthesis
Wolfe ptosis operation

Wolff, Julius, German anatomist, 1836-1902.
Wolff law – changes in bone function are followed by changes in internal architecture.
Wolff vasogenic theory

Wolff, Kaspar F., German embryologist in Russia, 1733-1794.

wolffian body – one of three excretory organs appearing in the evolution of vertebrates. *SYN:* canal of Oken; corpus of Oken; mesonephros

wolffian cyst – a cyst lying in the broad ligaments of the uterus and arising from any mesonephric structures.

wolffian duct – a duct in the embryo draining the mesonephric tubules. *SYN:* mesonephric duct

wolffian rest – remnants of the wolffian duct in the female genital tract that give rise to cysts. *SYN:* mesonephric rest

wolffian ridge – one of the paired longitudinal ridges developing in the dorsal body wall of the embryo. *SYN:* urogenital ridge

wolffian tubules – *SYN:* Kobelt tubules

Wolff, Louis, U.S. cardiologist, 1898-1972.

Wolff-Chaikoff block – blocking of the organic binding of iodine and its incorporation into hormone caused by large doses of iodine. *SYN:* Wolff-Chaikoff effect

Wolff-Chaikoff effect – *SYN:* Wolff-Chaikoff block

Wolff-Parkinson-White syndrome – an electrocardiographic pattern sometimes associated with paroxysmal tachycardia. *SYN:* preexcitation syndrome

Wölfler, Anton, Bohemian surgeon, 1850-1917.

Wölfler gland – *SYN:* accessory thyroid gland

Wolfram, Donald J., U.S. physician, *1910.

Wolfram syndrome – autosomal recessive disorder characterized by juvenile diabetes mellitus and optic atrophy. The acronym DIDMOAD is used to describe the syndrome (diabetes insipidus, diabetes mellitus, optic atrophy and deafness).

Wolfring, Emilj F. von, Polish ophthalmologist, 1832-1906.

Wolfring glands – accessory lacrimal ducts that lie above the tarsal plate.

Wollaston, William H., English physician and physicist, 1766-1828.

Wollaston doublet – a combination of two planoconvex lenses in the eyepiece of a microscope designed to correct the chromatic aberration.

Wollaston theory – a theory that the semidecussation of the optic nerves at the chiasm is proved by the homonymous hemianopia seen in brain lesions.

Wolman, Moske, Israeli neuropathologist, *1914.

Wolman disease – lipidosis caused by deficiency of liposomal acid lipase activity. *SYN:* cholesterol ester storage disease

Wolman xanthomatosis

Woltman, Henry William, U.S. neurologist, 1889-1964.

Kernohan-Woltman syndrome – see under Kernohan

Moersch-Woltman syndrome – see under Moersch

Woltman-Kernohan syndrome – *SYN:* Kernohan-Woltman syndrome

Wood, (origin unknown).

Romberg-Wood syndrome – see under Romberg, E.

Wood, Paul.

Wood units – a simplified measurement of pulmonary vascular resistance that uses pressures instead of more complicated units.

Wood, Robert, U.S. physicist, 1868-1955.

Wood glass – a glass containing nickel oxide, used in Wood lamp.

Wood lamp – an ultraviolet lamp used to detect by fluorescence hairs infected with species of *Microsporum*.

Wood light – ultraviolet light produced by Wood lamp.

Woodworth, Robert Sessions, U.S. psychologist, 1869-1962.

Woodworth-Mathews personal data sheet – a personality inventory.

Woolf, B., 20th century English biochemist.

Woolf-Lineweaver-Burk plot – *SYN:* Lineweaver-Burk plot

Woolner, Thomas, English sculptor, 1826-1892.

Woolner tip – a point projecting upward and posteriorly from the free outcurved margin of the helix a little posterior to its upper end. *SYN:* tip of auricle

Woringer, Frédéric, French dermatologist, 1903-1964.

Woringer-Kolopp disease – a benign localized form of lymphoma. *SYN:* pagetoid reticulosis

Worm, Ole, Danish anatomist, 1588-1654.
   wormian bones – small irregular bones found along the sutures of the cranium, particularly related to the parietal bone. *SYN:* sutural bones

Wormley, Theodore G., U.S. chemist, 1826-1897.
   Wormley test – for alkaloids.

Worth, Claud, English ophthalmologist, 1869-1936.
   Worth amblyoscope – the original amblyoscope.
   Worth strabismus forceps

Woulfe, Peter, English chemist, 1727-1803.
   Woulfe bottle – a bottle with two or three necks, used in a series, connected with tubes, for working with gases.

Wright, Basil Martin, 20th century English physician.
   Wright peak flow meter
   Wright respirometer – an inferential meter used to measure tidal and minute volume.

Wright, Irving S., U.S. physician, *1901.
   Wright syndrome – numbness, paresthesias, and erythema with weakness and pain of the arm and hand. *SYN:* subcoracoid-pectoralis minor tendon syndrome.

Wright, James Homer, U.S. pathologist, 1871-1928.
   Wright stain – a mixture of eosinates of polychromed methylene blue used in staining of blood smears.

Wright, Marmaduke Burr, U.S. obstetrician, 1803-1879.
   Wright version – a cephalic version employed in cases of shoulder presentation.

Wrisberg, Heinrich A., German anatomist and gynecologist, 1739-1808.
   nerve of Wrisberg
   Wrisberg cartilage – a small, nonarticulating rod of elastic cartilage. *SYN:* cuneiform cartilage

Wrisberg ganglia – parasympathetic ganglia of the cardiac plexus. *SYN:* cardiac ganglia

Wrisberg lesion

Wrisberg ligament – the band that passes posterior to the posterior cruciate ligament. *SYN:* posterior meniscofemoral ligament

Wrisberg nerve – *SYN:* medial brachial cutaneous nerve; nervus intermedius

Wrisberg tubercle – a rounded eminence on the posterior part of the aryepiglottic fold. *SYN:* cuneiform tubercle

Wucherer, Otto, German physician, 1820-1873.
Wuchereria – genus of filarial nematodes.
Wuchereria bancrofti – the bancroftian filaria.
wuchereriasis – infection with worms of the genus *Wuchereria*.

Wunderlich, Carl R.A., German physician, 1815-1877.
Wunderlich syndrome – traumatic perirenal hematoma.

Wundt, Wilhelm Max, German psychologist/physiologist, 1932-1920.
Wundt curve – an illusion in which straight lines appear to be curved.

Wurster, Casimir, German chemist, 1856-1913.
Wurster reagent – filter paper impregnated with tetramethyl-p-phenylenediamine, which turns blue in the presence of ozone or hydrogen peroxide.
Wurster test – for tyrosine.

Wyatt, W.
Brushfield-Wyatt disease – see under Brushfield

Wyburn-Mason, Roger, 20th century English physician.
Wyburn-Mason syndrome – arteriovenous malformation on the cerebral cortex, retinal arteriovenous angioma and facial nevus.

Wyman, Jeffries, U.S. biochemist, *1901.
Monod-Wyman-Changeux model – see under Monod

Yerkes, Robert Mearns, U.S. psychobiologist, 1876-1956.
   Yerkes discrimination box – used to study visual discrimination in
      animals.
   Yerkes-Dodson law – rule regarding task performance.

Yersin, Alexandre Émil Jean, Swiss bacteriologist and surgeon, 1863-1943.
   Yersinia enterocolitica – a species causing yersiniosis.
   Yersinia pestis – a species causing plague. *SYN:* Kitasato bacillus
   Yersinia pseudotuberculosis – a species causing pseudotuberculosis in
      birds and rodents; rarely in humans. *SYN: Pasteurella pestis*
   yersiniosis – infectious disease caused by *Yersinia enterocolitica*.

Young, Hugh H., U.S. urologist, 1870-1945.
   Young approach
   Young clamp
   Young cystoscope
   Young dilator
   Young dissector
   Young epispadias repair – *SYN:* Young operation (2)
   Young operation – (1) perineal prostatectomy. *SYN:* Young perineal
      prostatectomy; (2) epispadias repair. *SYN:* Young epispadias repair
   Young perineal prostatectomy – *SYN:* Young operation (1)
   Young prostatic tractor
   Young vastectomy

Young, J.
   Young-Paxson syndrome – traumatic uteroplacental damage.

Young, Thomas, English physician and physicist, 1773-1829.
   Young-Helmholtz theory of color vision – a theory that there are three
      color-perceiving elements in the retina: red, green, and blue.
      SYN: Helmholtz theory of color vision
   Young modulus – a type of modulus of elasticity.

NOTES

Young rule – an obsolete rule to determine a child's medication dose.

Young, W.G., U.S. endocrinologist and anatomist, 1899-1965.
  Young syndrome – obstructive azoospermia manifested by infertility and sinopulmonary infection.

Young, William John, 20th century Australian biochemist.
  Harden-Young ester – see under Harden

Ytterby, village in Sweden.
  ytterbium (Yb) – a metallic element of the lanthanide group, atomic no. 70.
  yttrium (Y) – a metallic element, atomic no. 39.
  yttrium-90 – an artificial radioactive isotope with a physical half-life of 2.67 days.

Yvon, Paul, French physician and chemist, 1848-1913.
  Yvon test – for alkaloids.

Zaffaroni, Alejandro, Uruguayan-U.S. chemist and biochemist, *1923.
   Zaffaroni system – a chromatographic system for the separation of steroids.

Zaglas, John, 19th century anatomist's assistant in Edinburgh, Scotland.
   Zaglas ligament – a short, thick, fibrous band extending from the posterior superior spine of the ilium to the second transverse tubercle of the sacrum.

Zahn, Friedrich W., German pathologist, 1845-1904.
   lines of Zahn – riblike markings seen by the naked eye on the surface of antemortem thrombi. *SYN:* striae of Zahn
   striae of Zahn – *SYN:* lines of Zahn
   Zahn infarct – a pseudoinfarct of the liver due to obstruction of a branch of the portal vein.

Zahorsky, John, U.S. physician, 1871-1963.
   Zahorsky disease – a skin disorder.

Zak, Frederick G., U.S. physician.
   Strauss-Churg-Zak syndrome – *SYN:* Churg-Strauss syndrome

Zambusch, Leo von, 20th century German physician.
   generalized pustular psoriasis of Zambusch – an extensive exacerbation of psoriasis. *SYN:* pustular psoriasis

Zander, Jonas Gustav Wilhelm, Swedish physician, 1835-1920.
   Zander apparatus – equipment used for exercise therapy.
   Zander exercise – passive, active, or resistive exercise.

Zang, Christoph Bonifacius, Austrian surgeon, 1772-1835.
   Zang metatarsal cap
   Zang metatarsal cap implant
   Zang space – supraclavicular fossa.

Zange, Johannes, German otorhinolaryngologist, 1880-1969.
Kindler-Zange syndrome – *SYN:* Zange-Kindler syndrome
Zange-Kindler syndrome – neurological disorder resulting from blockage of cerebrospinal fluid in the cisterna magna. *SYN:* Kindler-Zange syndrome

Zappert, Julius, Austrian physician, 1867-1942.
Zappert counting chamber – a special standardized glass slide used for counting cells and other particulate material in a measured volume of fluid.

Zaufal, Emanuel, Czech physician, 1833-1910.
Zaufal bone rongeur
Zaufal sign – saddle-nose defect.

Zavanelli, William, 20th century U.S. obstetrician.
Zavanelli maneuver – *SYN:* cephalic replacement

Zeeman, Pieter, Dutch physicist and Nobel laureate, 1865-1943.
Zeeman effect – the splitting of spectral lines into three or more symmetrically placed lines when the light source is subjected to a magnetic field.

Zeis, Eduard, Dresden ophthalmologist, 1807-1868.
Zeis glands – sebaceous glands opening into the follicles of the eyelashes.
zeisian sty – inflammation of one of the Zeis glands.

Zeiss, Carl, German optician, 1816-1888.
Abbé-Zeiss apparatus – see under Abbé, Ernst Karl
Thoma-Zeiss apparatus – *SYN:* Abbé-Zeiss apparatus

Zellweger, Hans U., U.S. pediatrician, 1909-1990.
Fanconi-Albertini-Zellweger syndrome – see under Fanconi
Zellweger syndrome – *SYN:* cerebrohepatorenal syndrome

Zenker, Friedrich Albert von, German pathologist, 1825-1898.
formol-Zenker fixative – Zenker fixative in which glacial acetic acid has been replaced by formalin.
Zenker degeneration – a form of severe hyaline degeneration or necrosis in skeletal muscle, occurring in severe infections. *SYN:* waxy degeneration; Zenker necrosis
Zenker diverticulum – common diverticulum of the esophagus, arises between the inferior pharyngeal constrictor and the cricopharyngeus muscle. *SYN:* pharyngoesophageal diverticulum
Zenker fixative – a rapid fixative.

Zenker necrosis – *SYN:* Zenker degeneration

Zenker paralysis – paresthesia and paralysis in the area of the external popliteal nerve.

Ziegler, Samuel Louis, U.S. ophthalmologist, 1861-1925.
Ziegler blade
Ziegler cautery
Ziegler cilia forceps
Ziegler dilator
Ziegler ectropion repair
Ziegler eye speculum
Ziegler forceps
Ziegler iridectomy
Ziegler iris knife
Ziegler lacrimal probe
Ziegler needle
Ziegler operation
Ziegler probe
Ziegler puncture
Ziegler wash bottle

Ziehen, Georg T., German psychiatrist, 1862-1950.
Ziehen-Oppenheim disease – a disorder beginning in childhood or adolescence marked by muscular contractions that distort the spine and hips. *SYN:* dystonia musculorum deformans

Ziehl, Franz, German bacteriologist, 1857-1926.
Ziehl-Neelsen stain – a method for staining acid-fast bacteria.
Ziehl stain – a carbol-fuchsin solution of phenol and basic fuchsin used to demonstrate bacteria and cell nuclei.

Zielke, K., 20th century German orthopedic surgeon.
Zielke bifid hook
Zielke derotator bar
Zielke gouge

NOTES

Z

Zielke instrumentation
Zielke instrumentation for scoliosis spinal fusion
Zielke pedicular instrumentation
Zielke rod
Zielke screw
Zielke technique

Ziemann, Hans R.P., German pathologist, 1865-1939.
Ziemann dots – fine dots seen in erythrocytes in malariae malaria.
SYN: Ziemann stippling
Ziemann stippling – *SYN:* Ziemann dots

Ziemssen, Hugo Wilhelm von, German physician, 1829-1902.
Ziemssen motor point

Zieve, Leslie, U.S. physician, *1915.
Zieve syndrome – transient jaundice, hemolytic anemia, and hyperlipemia associated with acute alcoholism in patients with cirrhosis or a fatty liver.

Zimmerlin, Franz, Swiss physician, 1858-1932.
Zimmerlin atrophy – hereditary progressive muscular atrophy in which the atrophy begins in the upper half of the body.

Zimmermann, Karl W., German histologist, 1861-1935.
polkissen of Zimmermann – mesangial cells that fill the triangular space between the macula densa and the afferent and efferent arterioles of the juxtaglomerular apparatus. *SYN:* extraglomerular mesangium
Zimmermann corpuscle – *SYN:* Zimmermann elementary particle
Zimmermann elementary particle – a disklike cytoplasmic fragment found in the peripheral blood where it functions in clotting. *SYN:* platelet; Zimmermann corpuscle; Zimmermann granule
Zimmermann granule – *SYN:* Zimmermann elementary particle

Zimmermann, Wilhelm, German physician, *1910.
Zimmermann reaction – a chemical reaction between methylene ketones and aromatic polynitro compounds in alkaline solutions.
SYN: Zimmermann test
Zimmermann test – *SYN:* Zimmermann reaction

Zinkernagel, Rolf M., joint winner of 1996 Nobel Prize for work related to immunity.

Zinn, Johann Gottfried, German anatomist, 1727-1759.
Zinn artery – *SYN:* central artery of retina
Zinn corona – *SYN:* Zinn vascular circle
Zinn ligament – *SYN:* Zinn ring

Zinn membrane – the anterior layer of the iris.

Zinn ring – a fibrous ring that surrounds the optic canal and the medial part of the superior orbital fissure. *SYN:* common tendinous ring; Zinn ligament; Zinn tendon

Zinn tendon – *SYN:* Zinn ring

Zinn vascular circle – a network of branches of the short ciliary arteries on the sclera around the point of entrance of the optic nerve. *SYN:* vascular circle of optic nerve; Zinn corona

Zinn zonule – a series of delicate meridional fibers arising from the inner surface of the orbiculus ciliaris and that run in bundles between and in a very thin layer over the ciliary processes. *SYN:* ciliary zonule

Zinsser, Hans, U.S. bacteriologist and immunologist, 1878-1940.
   Brill-Zinsser disease – see under Brill

Ziprkowski, L., Israeli physician.
   Ziprkowski-Margolis syndrome – recessive sex-linked gene disorder characterized by partial albinism and deaf mutism.

Zivert, A.K., physician from the Ukraine.
   Zivert syndrome – *SYN:* Kartagener syndrome

Zollinger, Robert M., U.S. surgeon, 1903-1992.
   Zollinger-Ellison syndrome – peptic ulceration with gastric hypersecretion and non–beta cell tumor of the pancreatic islets, sometimes associated with familial polyendocrine adenomatosis. *SYN:* Reichmann disease

   Zollinger-Ellison tumor – a non–beta cell tumor of pancreatic islets causing the Zollinger-Ellison syndrome.

   Zollinger leg holder
   Zollinger multipurpose tissue forceps
   Zollinger splint

Zöllner, Johann F., German physicist, 1834-1882.
   Zöllner lines – figures devised to show the possibility of optical illusions.

NOTES

Z

Zondek, Bernhardt, German obstetrician and gynecologist, 1891-1966.
   Aschheim-Zondek test – see under Aschheim
   Zondek-Aschheim test – *SYN:* Aschheim-Zondek test

Zoon, Johannes Jacobus, Dutch dermatologist, *1902.
   balanitis of Zoon – benign circumscribed balanitis characterized
      microscopically by subepithelial plasma cell infiltration and clinically by
      small erythematous papular lesions. *SYN:* plasma cell balanitis; Zoon
      erythroplasia
   Zoon erythroplasia – *SYN:* balanitis of Zoon

Zsigmondy, Richard, Austrian-German chemist and Nobel laureate,
1865-1929.
   brownian-Zsigmondy movement – *SYN:* brownian movement
   Zsigmondy test – *SYN:* Lange test

Zuckerkandl, Emil, Austrian anatomist, 1849-1910.
   organs of Zuckerkandl – *SYN:* Zuckerkandl bodies
   Zuckerkandl bodies – small masses of chromaffin tissue found near the
      sympathetic ganglia along the aorta. *SYN:* organs of Zuckerkandl;
      paraaortic bodies
   Zuckerkandl convolution – *SYN:* subcallosal gyrus
   Zuckerkandl fascia – the posterior layer of the renal fascia.

Zuelzer, Wolf W., U.S. hematologist, *1909.
   Zuelzer-Ogden syndrome – hematologic disorder in infants.
      SYN: megaloblastic anemia in infants
   Zuelzer syndrome – autosomal recessive trait characterized by the
      association of eosinophilia, leukocytosis, and hypergammaglobulinemia
      in infants and young children. *SYN:* familial eosinophilia

Zumbusch, Leo von, German dermatologist, 1874-1940.
   Zumbusch psoriasis – pustular psoriasis.

Zweymüller, E., Austrian physician.
   Weissenbacher-Zweymüller syndrome – see under Weissenbacher

device
Charnley d., 134
Venturi aspiration vitrectomy d.,
725

dextrins
Schardinger d., 632

diabetes
Lancereaux d., 404
Mosler d., 500

diagonal
Broca d. band, 102

diagram
Venn d., 724

dialysis
LeVeen d. shunt, 421

diameter
Baudelocque d., 53

diaphragm
Åkerlund d., 9
Bucky d., 110

diarrhea
Brainerd d., 96

diathermy
Riches d. forceps, 597

diathesis
Dupuytren d., 201

diazo
Ehrlich d. reagent, 210

diet
Atkins d., 32
Banting d., 45
Bristol d. therapy, 101
Feingold d., 228
Jenny Craig d., 160
Kempner rice d., 376
Minot-Murphy d., 486
Ornish reversal d., 533
Pritikin d., 572
Schmidt d., 637
Sippy d., 659

dilating
Mixter d. probe, 487
Wilder d. forceps, 756

dilation
Anel lacrimal duct d., 22

dilator
Amplatz fascial d., 18
Bonney cervical d., 88
Bowman lacrimal d., 93
Bozeman d., 94
Braasch ureteral d., 95
Cooley coronary d., 152
Cooley d., 152
Cooley pediatric d., 152
Cooley valve d., 152
DeBakey vascular d., 178
Gerbode d., 268
Gerbode mitral d., 268
Gerbode mitral valvulotomy d.,
268
Gerbode valve d., 268
Goodell d., 283
Gouley d., 286
Guyon d., 298
Hanks d., 306
Heath d., 315
Hegar d., 317
Jackson triangular brass d.,
356
Kelly uterine d., 375
Kollmann d., 390
Laborde tracheal d., 401
Le Fort d., 415
Mixter d., 487
Murphy d., 506
Nettleship d., 514
Phillips d., 558
Plummer d., 563
Potts d., 569
Potts expansile d., 569
Pratt d., 570
Puestow d., 574
Ramstedt d., 583
Sims d., 658
Tubbs d., 711
Walther d., 738
Weiss gold d., 746
Wilder d., 756
Young d., 767
Ziegler d., 771

diogenis
poculum d., 188

diplobacillus
Morax-Axenfeld d., 34, 495

diplococcus
Neisser d., 512

direct Coombs test, 153

director
Leksell d., 417
Pratt d., 570
Putti-Platt d., 562, 576

disarticulation
Syme ankle d. amputation, 690

discectomy
Robinson anterior cervical d.,
606
Smith-Robinson anterior
cervical d., 606, 663
Williams d., 758

discission
Castroviejo d. knife, 127
Moncrieff d., 491
Parker d. knife, 543
Parker serrated d. knife, 543
Swan d. knife, 688
Wheeler d. knife, 752

discography
Williams d., 758

discrimination
Yerkes d. box, 767

disease
Acosta d., 5
Adams-Stokes d., 5, 682
Addison-Biermer d., 6
Addison d., 6
Addison-Schilder d., 6, 634
Aguecheek d., 8
Akureyri d., 9
Albers-Schönberg d., 10
Albert d., 10
Albright d., 11
Aleutian d., 12
Alexander d., 13
Alibert d. I, 13
Alibert d. II, 13
Alibert d. III, 13
Almeida d., 15
Alpers d., 15
Alzheimer d., 16
Anders d., 19
Andersen d., 20
Anderson-Fabry d., 20, 223

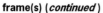

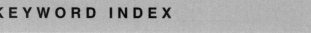

newborn
Parrot atrophy of the n., 544

newton, 516

niche
Haudek n., 312

night
Saturday n. palsy syndrome, 628
Saturday n. paralysis, 628

nines
Wallace rule of n., 737

ninhydrin
n.-Schiff stain for proteins, 634

nipple
Kock n., 388
Kock n. valve, 388
Paget disease of the n., 538

nitroprusside
Rothera n. test, 614

nobelium (No), 520

***Nocardia*, 520**
N. brasiliensis, 520
N. dacryoliths, 520

Nocardiaceae, 520

Nocardiasis bovine farcy, 520

nocardiosis, 520

node(s)
Babès n., 37
Bouchard n., 91
Calot n., 120
Dürck n., 202
Féréol n., 229
Flack n., 235
Ghon n., 271
Haygarth n., 314
Hensen n., 324
Keith and Flack n., 375
Keith n., 375
Koch n., 388
Meynet n., 480
n. of Aschoff and Tawara, 30
n. of Cloquet, 144
n. of Ranvier, 584
n. of Rouviere, 615
Osler n., 534
Parrot n., 544

Patey axillary n. dissection, 547
Rosenmüller n., 612
Schmorl n., 637
Tawara n., 694
Troisier n., 710
Virchow n., 730

nodosities
Haygarth n., 314
Heberden n., 316

nodular
Salzmann n. corneal
degeneration, 624

nodule(s)
Albini n., 11
Arantius n., 25
Aschoff n., 30
Babès n., 37
Bianchi n., 71
Bohn n., 86
Busacca n., 115
Caplan n., 122
Cruveilhier n., 164
Dalen-Fuchs n., 170
Heberden n., 316
Hoboken n., 334
Jeanselme n., 361
Lisch n., 428
malpighian n., 451
Morgagni n., 497
Peyer n., 556
Sakurai-Lisch n., 428, 623
Schmorl n., 638
Sister Joseph n., 659
Sister Mary Joseph n., 659

***Noguchia*, 520**
N. granulosis, 520

noise
Bárány n. apparatus, 45
Bárány n. apparatus whistle, 45

nomenclature
linnaean system of n., 427

nomogram
d'Ocagne n., 189
Radford n., 581
Siggaard-Andersen n., 656

non-Hodgkin
n.-H. lymphoma, 334

notch
Hutchinson crescentic n., 347
Kernohan n., 377
Rivinus n., 604

nuclear
Pelger-Huët n. anomaly, 550
Remak n. division, 593

nucleoid
Lavdovsky n., 413

nucleus, nuclei
basal n. of Ganser, 261
Bekhterev n., 60
Blumenau n., 83
Burdach n., 113
Clarke n., 142
convergence n. of Perlia, 553
Deiters n., 180
Edinger-Westphal n., 208
Gudden tegmental n., 294
interstitial n. of Cajal, 118
Klein-Gumprecht shadow n., 383
Monakow n., 490
n. basalis of Ganser, 261
n. of Darkschewitsch, 172
n. of Goll, 282
n. of Luys, 440
Onuf n., 531
Perlia n., 553
Roller n., 608
Schwalbe n., 642
Siemerling n., 655
Spitzka n., 671
Staderini n., 672
Stilling n., 680

number
Avogadro n., 34
Brinell hardness n., 100
Hehner n., 317
Hounsfield n., 341
Kestenbaum n., 378
Koettstorfer n., 389
Loschmidt n., 434
Mach n., 443
Mohs hardness n., 489
Reichert-Meissl n., 591
Reynolds n., 596

nystagmus
Bruns n., 108
Cheyne n., 136

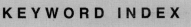

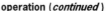

otoplasty
Alexander o., 12

otoscope
Politzer o., 565
Siegle o., 655

outrigger
Bunnell o. splint, 112

oval area of Flechsig, 236

ovarian
Billroth o. retractor, 75
Emmet o. trocar, 215

ovum
Peters o., 554
Saenger o. forceps, 622

oxidation
Meyerhof o. quotient, 480

oxygenator
Lillehei-DeWall o., 426
Shiley o., 652

Oxyspirura mansoni, 453

pascal, 545

passer
Bunnell tendon p., 112
Gallie tendon p., 259
Ober tendon p., 525

passing
Codman wire-p. drill, 146

paste
Lassar p., 411

Pasteurella, **546**
P. aerogenes, 546
P. multocida, 546
P. pestis, 546
P. "SP", 546
P. tularensis, 546

pasteurellosis, 546

pasteurization, 546

pasteurizer, 546

pastils
Sabouraud p., 621

patch(es)
Bitot p., 78
Carrel p., 125
Hutchinson p., 348
MacCallum p., 443
Peyer p., 556

patellar
Chandler p. advancement, 131

patent
Cooley p. ductus clamp, 152
Cooley p. ductus forceps, 152
DeBakey p. ductus clamp, 178

pathway
Embden-Meyerhof p., 215
Embden-Meyerhof-Parnas p.,
215, 479, 544
Mishima dual p. theory, 486

peak
Cupid bow p., 165
Wright p. flow meter, 765

pearls
Elschnig p., 214

Epstein p., 216
Laënnec p., 402

pecqueti
receptaculum p., 550

pectinated
Stroud p. area, 684

pediatric
Allis Micro-Line p. forceps, p15
Cooley p. clamp, 152
Cooley p. dilator, 152
Cooley tangential p. forceps,
152
Shiley p. tracheostomy tube,
652
Venturi p. myringotomy tube,
725

pedicle
Filatov-Gillies tubed p., 232

peel
Jessner chemical p., 363
Monheit combination p., 492

PEG
Moss G-tube P. kit, 500
Moss P. kit, 500

pelvimeter
DeLee p., 181
Schneider p., 638
McDonald p., 468

pelvis
Deventer p., 184
Nägele p., 509
Otto p., 535
Robert p., 604
Rokitansky p., 608

penis
Paget disease of the p., 538

pentalogy of Fallot, 224

perception
Frostig Developmental Test of
Visual P., 254

percussion
Lerch p., 419
Murphy p., 506

perforated
Casser p. muscle, 126

perforating
Chandler spinal p. forceps, 131

perforator
Cushing p., 166
Cushing p. drill, 166
hunterian p., 345
Joseph p., 367
Politzer ear p., 564

performance
Arthur Point Scale of P., 29
Leishman International P. Scale,
417
Pintner-Paterson scale of p.
tests, 561

perfusor
Belsey p., 61

pericardial
Carpentier-Edwards p. valve,
125, 208

perimeter
Goldmann p., 281
Tübingen p., 711

perineal
Carcassonne p. ligament, 123
Savage p. body, 628
Young p. prostatectomy, 767

perineorrhaphy
Simon p., 657

period
Oedipus p., 527
Wenckebach p., 748

periodic acid-Schiff stain, 634

periodontal
Kirkland p. pack, 381
Russell P. Index, 618

periosteal
Brophy p. elevator, 104
Cobb p. elevator, 144
Cushing p. elevator, 166
Davidson p. elevator, 173
Dean p. elevator, 177
Hibbs p. elevator, 329

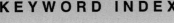

W